DRUG DELIVERY SYSTEMS

Second Edition

Pharmacology and Toxicology: Basic and Clinical Aspects

Mannfred A. Hollinger, Series Editor
University of California, Davis

Published Titles

Cell-Penetrating Peptides, 2002, Ülo Langel
PARP as a Therapeutic Target, 2002, Jie Zhang
Immune Interferon: Properties and Clinical Applications, 2002, Roumen Tsanev
   and Ivan Ivanov
Molecular Bases of Anesthesia, 2001, Eric Moody and Phil Skolnick
Biomedical Applications of Computer Modeling, 2001, Arthur Christopoulos
Cell Death: The Role of PARP, 2000, Csaba Szabó
Manual of Immunological Methods, 1999, Pauline Brousseau, Yves Payette,
   Helen Tryphonas, Barry Blakley, Herman Boermans, Denis Flipo, Michel Fournier
CNS Injuries: Cellular Responses and Pharmacological Strategies, 1999, Martin Berry
   and Ann Logan
*Infectious Diseases in Immunocompromised Hosts,*1998, Vassil St. Georgiev
Pharmacology of Antimuscarinic Agents, 1998, Laszlo Gyermek
Basis of Toxicity Testing, Second Edition, 1997, Donald J. Ecobichon
Anabolic Treatments for Osteoporosis, 1997, James F. Whitfield and Paul Morley
Antibody Therapeutics, 1997, William J. Harris and John R. Adair
Muscarinic Receptor Subtypes in Smooth Muscle, 1997, Richard M. Eglen
Antisense Oligodeonucleotides as Novel Pharmacological Therapeutic Agents, 1997,
   Benjamin Weiss
Airway Wall Remodelling in Asthma, 1996, A.G. Stewart
Drug Delivery Systems, 1996, Vasant V. Ranade and Mannfred A. Hollinger
Brain Mechanisms and Psychotropic Drugs, 1996, Andrius Baskys and Gary Remington
Receptor Dynamics in Neural Development, 1996, Christopher A. Shaw
Ryanodine Receptors, 1996, Vincenzo Sorrentino
Therapeutic Modulation of Cytokines, 1996, M.W. Bodmer and Brian Henderson
Pharmacology in Exercise and Sport, 1996, Satu M. Somani
Placental Pharmacology, 1996, B. V. Rama Sastry
Pharmacological Effects of Ethanol on the Nervous System, 1996, Richard A. Deitrich
Immunopharmaceuticals, 1996, Edward S. Kimball
Chemoattractant Ligands and Their Receptors, 1996, Richard Horuk
Pharmacological Regulation of Gene Expression in the CNS, 1996, Kalpana Merchant
Experimental Models of Mucosal Inflammation, 1995, Timothy S. Gaginella
Human Growth Hormone Pharmacology: Basic and Clinical Aspects, 1995,
   Kathleen T. Shiverick and Arlan Rosenbloom
Placental Toxicology, 1995, B. V. Rama Sastry
Stealth Liposomes, 1995, Danilo Lasic and Frank Martin
TAXOL®: Science and Applications, 1995, Matthew Suffness
Endothelin Receptors: From the Gene to the Human, 1995, Robert R. Ruffolo, Jr.
*Alternative Methodologies for the Safety Evaluation of Chemicals in the
   Cosmetic Industry,*1995, Nicola Loprieno
Phospholipase A$_2$ in Clinical Inflammation: Molecular Approaches to Pathophysiology,
   1995, Keith B. Glaser and Peter Vadas
Serotonin and Gastrointestinal Function, 1995, Timothy S. Gaginella and
   James J. Galligan

Pharmacology and Toxicology: Basic and Clinical Aspects

Published Titles (*Continued*)

DRUG DELIVERY SYSTEMS

Second Edition

Vasant V. Ranade
Mannfred A. Hollinger

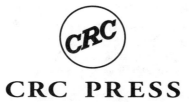

CRC PRESS

Boca Raton   London   New York   Washington, D.C.

Library of Congress Cataloging-in-Publication Data

Ranade, Vasant V.
Drug delivery systems / Vasant V. Ranade, Mannfred A. Hollinger.—2nd ed.
p. ; cm. — (Pharmacology and toxicology)
Includes bibliographical references and index.
ISBN 0-8493-1433-X (alk. paper)
1. Drug delivery systems. I. Hollinger, Mannfred A. II. Title. III. Pharmacology &
toxicology (Boca Raton, Fla.)
[DNLM: 1. Drug Delivery Systems. WB 340 R185d 2003]
RS199.5.D77 2003
615.5′8—dc202003048997

Visit the CRC Press Web site at www.crcpress.com

© 2004 by CRC Press LLC
Lewis Publishers is an imprint of CRC Press LLC

No claim to original U.S. Government works
International Standard Book Number 0-8493-1433-X
Library of Congress Card Number 2003048997
Printed in the United States of America 1 2 3 4 5 6 7 8 9 0
Printed on acid-free paper

Preface to the First Edition

The introduction of the first successful drug delivery system brought about tremendous interest in the usage of delivery systems for entry of drugs into the systemic circulation of the body. Several drug delivery products followed into the marketplace and many are now in different stages of product development. Lately, a plethora of drug delivery departments and companies have emerged partly as a result of surging interest in generic drug development and continued technological advances are occurring in this area of pharmaceutical research.

The main goal of this book has been to collect current information in one volume to further research in drug delivery and to serve as an introduction to the various systems. The aim has also been simply to identify areas of potential and real improvement in the drug treatment of disease as well as to review the different approaches and methods of assessment of novel drug delivery.

This book contains introductory and state-of-the-art information on liposomes, monoclonal antibodies, use of polymers, implants, oral, transdermal, miscellaneous, intranasal, and ocular forms of drug delivery. Finally, a literature review on the regulatory and global aspects of drug delivery systems is presented. Obviously, in this rapidly expanding field, several important omissions must have occurred despite our efforts to include significant advances known by early 1994, when most of the literature was collected. We hope this effort will prove to be of value to scientists, clinicians, and product development personnel seeking information in this area and this compilation of the introductory data should serve as a useful resource tool.

The research ideas and concepts described in this book are not our own and neither do we make any claims indicating such a notion nor do we seek any credit. We are indebted to scientists and authors for their permission to use or include their research work. Particularly, we express our appreciation to the following: Drs. G. Gregoriadis, U. Persson, F.H. Roerdink, R.L. Juliano and D. Mufson for liposomes, Drs. E. Tomlinson, J. Schlom, W. Lebherz, G.F. Rowland and T. Suzuta for monoclonal antibodies, Drs. F.G. Hutchinson and J.B. Lloyd for use of polymers, Drs. F. Theeuwes and M. Sefton for implants, Drs. D. Ganderton and S.S. Davis for oral drug delivery, Dr. B.W. Barry for transdermal drug delivery, Drs. Y.W. Chien, K.S.E. Su and D. Proctor for intranasal and ocular drug delivery, Capsugel Americas and SoloHill Engineering Company for miscellaneous forms of drug delivery and Dr. R. Tetzlaff for regulatory and global aspects for drug delivery systems. Also, our special thanks are to the management of *Journal of Clinical Pharmacology*, Pharmaceutical Technology, Controlled Release Society, Noyes Data Corporation, and Ellis Horwood Ltd. for allowing us to include information from the abstracts and articles published in their journals.

Because of the exhaustive nature of the topics discussed in this book, it may be apparent that omissions of expression of our thanks to researchers might have occurred, but it is certainly not intentional; we apologize for that. We also would like to thank Drs. J. Somberg, A. Laddu, R. Gokhale, R. Chorvat, J. Plattner, Mr. B. Shah and Ms. S. Fradin for their support, interest and cooperation and we are grateful to CRC Press Inc for all the enthusiasm to complete this undertaking. Finally, we would like to express our deep sense of gratitude to our wives, Usha and Georgia, for their efforts in assisting us whenever their help was called for throughout this endeavor.

Preface

Inclusion of the material on drug delivery systems is organized based mainly on the uniqueness, originality, and potential application of the basic research toward commmercialization and ultimate product introduction into the market. Every researched example in a particular delivery system is not included — although it merits inclusion — because such an effort would result in a voluminous book on each subject. This is beyond the intention or scope of this book, which is meant to serve simply as an introduction of a particular area to a researcher who is not an expert but would like to "get to know" an area of interest. The reader is requested to understand the background of the production of this book before he or she attempts to form an opinion on the subject matter presented.

In this second edition, every attempt is made to include material published between 1995 and 2002. The content has been expanded to provide integrated coverage of the topics in the first edition and to introduce the reader to new topics of general scientific interest.

The authors thank all their associates for their continued support during the preparation of this book.

Authors

Vinayak (Vasant) V. Ranade, Ph.D., is director of chemical sciences for Academic Pharmaceuticals, Inc. in Lake Bluff, Illinois. He also holds a faculty position in the Department of Pharmacology at Rush-Presbyterian-St. Luke's Medical Center in Chicago.

Dr. Ranade earned his Ph.D. degree in organic chemistry from the University of Bombay in 1965 and received his postdoctoral training in the College of Pharmacy at the University of Michigan, Ann Arbor. He has worked as a research chemist for Abbott Laboratories, Mallinckrodt Inc., and DuPont Critical Care.

Dr. Ranade is a member of the American Chemical Society, APhA Academy of Pharmaceutical Sciences and the honorary society, Sigma Xi. He was awarded the Council of Scientific and Industrial Research Fellowship, and was elected fellow of the American Institute of Chemists. He was the co-recipient of the Genia Czerniak Prize for Nuclear Medicine and Radiopharmacology.

Dr. Ranade has been a reviewer for a number of scientific jounals, and his biography is listed in *Who's Who* and *American Men and Women of Science and Technology*. He has presented research work at the American Chemical Society, the APhA Academy of Pharmaceutical Sciences, and the American College of Cardiology and Pharmacology meetings. He has published more than 90 papers including original and review articles, book chapters, and abstracts. He is the recipient of several U.S. patents, and his research work has also been included in Canadian and European patents. He co-authored the first edition of this book titled *Drug Delivery Systems* published by CRC Press in 1995.

Dr. Ranade's significant contributions to pharmaceutical research and development include synthesis of tumor imaging agents, formulations of cardiovascular and diuretic drugs, and chiral chromatographic separations of a variety of drugs. Dr. Ranade is also a consultant in the areas of chemical and pharamaceutical technology for some industrial organizations, securities market analysis companies, and research institutes in the U.S.

Mannfred A. Hollinger, Ph.D., is currently a professor emeritus in the Department of Medical Pharmacology and Toxicology, School of Medicine, University of California, Davis. Dr. Hollinger is the former editor of *Current*

Topics in Pulmonary Pharmacology and Toxicology, Focus on Pulmonary Pharmacology and Toxicology, and *Yearbook of Pharmacology,* and assistant editor of *The Journal of Pharmacology and Experimental Therapeutics.* Dr. Hollinger serves on the editorial advisory board of *The Journal of Pharmacology and Experimental Therapeutics, Research Communications in Chemical Pathology and Pharmacology,* and *The Journal of the American College of Toxicology.* Dr. Hollinger is, at present, the series editor of *Pharmacology and Toxicology: Basic and Clinical Aspects* published by CRC Press. He is a member of the American Society of Pharmacology and Experimental Therapeutics and the Society of Toxicology.

Born in Chicago, he earned his B.S. degree from North Park College in 1961 and his M.S. (1965) and Ph.D. (1967) degrees from Loyola University. He was employed by Baxter Laboratories from 1961 to 1963. From 1967 to 1969, Dr. Hollinger was a postdoctoral research fellow in the Department of Pharmacology, Stanford University Medical School. Since coming to Davis in 1969, Dr. Hollinger has participated in several team-taught courses to undergraduate, graduate, and medical students.

While at Davis, Dr. Hollinger has published numerous research papers as well as a monograph on respiratory pharmacology and toxicology. He continues to serve as a referee for many of the principal pharmacology and toxicology journals. Dr. Hollinger was the recipient of a Burroughs-Wellcome Visiting Scientist Fellowship to Southampton, England in 1986 as well as a National Institutes of Health Fogarty Senior International Fellowship to Heidelberg, Germany in 1988. Dr. Hollinger currently resides in Oro Valley, Arizona.

Contents

Section five: Regulatory considerations and global outlook

section one

Site-specific drug delivery

chapter one

Site-specific drug delivery using liposomes as carriers*

Contents

I.   Introduction

Over the past three decades, significant advances have been made in drug delivery technology. This effort, pioneered by Alza Laboratories of Palo Alto, California,[1,2] among others, has been accelerated in recent years due to the substantial decline in the development of new drug entities.

Drug delivery has now become a multidisciplinary science consisting of biopharmaceutics and pharmacokinetics. Great strides have also been made

* Adapted from Ranade, V.V., Drug delivery systems. 1. Site specific drug delivery using liposomes as carriers, *J. Clin. Pharmacol.*, 29, 685, 1989. With permission of the *J. Clin. Pharmacol.*, and J.B. Lippincott Publishing Company, Philadelphia, PA.

by physical biochemists, pharmacists, and other pharmaceutical research scientists working in university and industrial laboratories.[3-6]

The underlying principle that drug delivery technology, per se, can bring both therapeutic and commercial value to health care products has been widely accepted. Recently, large pharmaceutical companies have been losing their market share to generic competitors with increasing rapidity after their patents expire. This has created an intense need for presenting "old" drugs in new forms and utilizing novel forms of delivery. As a result, companies developing new drug delivery systems seem to enjoy a good return on their investment in the form of increased revenues and market share.[7]

In the U.S., the Drug Price Competition and Patent Term Restoration Act (also known as ANDA-Exclusivity Provisions Act) was passed in 1984. This provided new incentives to manufacturers who can distinguish their products from the competition, with features such as longer dosage schedules, improved safety profiles, new indications for existing drugs, and new combinations.[8]

The following chapters, which focus on the area of research and development in the drug delivery field, have been divided into five sections:

1. Site-specific drug delivery
2. Polymers and implantable drug delivery systems
3. Oral drug delivery
4. Transdermal, intranasal, ocular, and miscellaneous drug delivery systems
5. Regulatory considerations and global outlook

Drug delivery, which takes into consideration the carrier, the route, and the target, has evolved into a strategy of processes or devices designed to enhance the efficacy of therapeutic agents through controlled release. This may involve enhanced bioavailability, improved therapeutic index, or improved patient acceptance or compliance. Drug delivery, or controlled release, has been defined by Flynn as "the use of whatever means possible, be it chemical, physiochemical, or mechanical, to regulate a drug's access rate to the body's central compartment, or in some cases, directly to the involved tissues."[9]

Tomlinson[10] has emphasized features such as exclusive delivery to specific components, access to primarily inaccessible sites, protection of body from unwanted deposition, controlled rate and modality of delivery to pharmacological receptors, and reduction in the amount of active principal employed. Tomlinson[10,11] has also described the properties that are needed for site-specific carriers, as well as properties that are biological, drug-related, and carrier-related.

II. Liposomes in drug delivery

A. Regional drug delivery

Most efforts to make drug therapy more efficient by direct delivery of drugs to affected tissues have focused on local or regional injection techniques, such as intra-arterial or infusions into body cavities, such as the peritoneum. The benefits of regional therapy include reducing systemic toxicity and achieving peak drug levels directly at the target site. However, these methods of administration have met with limited success. For example, although intra-arterial injections effectively concentrate drugs at certain tumor sites, in others the drug is cleared from the system so rapidly that the benefits are not realized. Currently, pharmaceutical researchers are trying to design drug delivery systems that will localize drugs and affect only the afflicted tissues. A carrier system that has received considerable attention in this regard is liposomes.[12–17]

B.   Chemical characteristics of liposomes

Liposomal affinity for various tissues can be modified by synthesizing liposomes containing phospholipids with various fatty-acid chain configurations. These microparticles may be either solid or liquid at defined temperatures.[18,19] Altering the charge on the liposome vesicle can greatly influence its distribution in the body. Negatively charged vesicles, for example, enter the cell by fusion. This allows the drug to be discharged into the cell cytoplasm. Neutral vesicles, on the other hand, are incorporated into the cell by phagocytosis. This exposes the drug to the lysosomal hydrolytic system of the cells. Positive- and neutral-liposomal vesicles are cleared more slowly than those negatively charged.

What is a liposome made of and how does it look? The liposome is a microparticulate, ranging in size from 0.03 μm to 10 μm, consisting of a bilayer of phospholipid encapsulating an aqueous space. A variety of amphipathic lipid molecules can be used to form the bilayer.[20] The lipid molecules arrange themselves by exposing their polar head groups towards the water phase. Hydrophobic hydrocarbon moieties adhere together in the bilayer, thus forming close, concentric, bimolecular lipid leaflets separating aqueous compartments.

Drug molecules can either be encapsulated in the aqueous space or intercalated into the bilayer (see Figure 1.1 and Figure 1.2). The exact location of the drug in the liposome depends upon the physiochemical characteristics of the drug and the composition of the constituent lipids.[21] Stable liposomes from phospholipids are formed only at temperatures above the "gel to liquid-crystalline" phase transition temperature (Tc). This represents the melting point of the acyl chains. All phospholipids have a characteristic Tc, which is contingent upon the nature of the polar head group and on the length and degree of unsaturation of the acyl chains.[21,22] Above the transition temperature, phospholipids form a liquid-crystalline phase that constitutes increased mobility of the acyl chains. A reduction in temperature below the Tc creates a transition to a more rigid gel state. This results in restrained mobility of the tightly packed acyl chains. When the liquid molecules arrange themselves to form closed bilayer structures containing water and solutes, drugs are trapped between the adjacent planes of the polar head

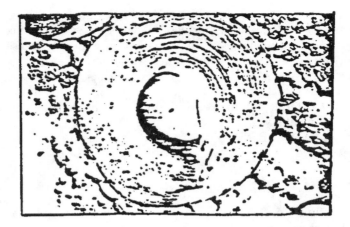

Figure 1.1 Schematic of a bilayer vesicle or liposome. (From *Pharmaceutical Technology*, Conf. Proc., The Latest Developments in Drug Delivery Systems, Oct. 1985. With permission.)

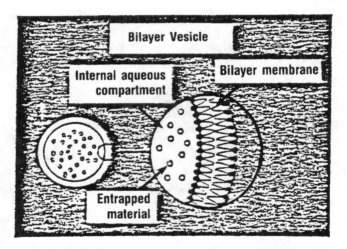

Figure 1.2 A micrograph view of a liposome. (Reprinted by permission of The Liposome Company, Inc., Princeton, NJ.)

groups. This compartmentalization has been discussed in detail by Roerdink et al.[14]

C.   Phospholipids

A variety of phospholipids can be used to prepare liposomes. The lipid most widely used is phosphatidylcholine,[23,24] which has been used individually or in combination with cholesterol. Cholesterol is known to condense the packing of phospholipids in bilayers above the Tc. Cholesterol also reduces the permeability of the bilayers to encapsulated compounds.

Negatively charged lipids, such as stearylamine, are usually used in order to provide a surface charge to the liposomes. For drug molecules encapsulated in the aqueous space, the bilayer serves as a diffusion barrier, permitting the liposomes to serve as a rate-controlling input device. Papahadjopoulos and co-workers have done pioneering research in trying to establish and develop the liposomal delivery system from experimental therapeutics to clinical applications.[25-29] The introduction of this delivery system directly to the target site (such as the eye, lung, or bladder) is a well-established approach for treating local diseases, and liposomes have been shown to play a beneficial role when applied in this way.

III. The liposome-drug concept

A. Liposome size

Liposomes have been used via a variety of administration routes, including intravenous, intramuscular, intraperitoneal, and oral.[30-32] However, IV injection is the most widely utilized route. The half-life of liposomes in the vascular system can range from a few minutes to many hours, depending on the size and lipid composition of the vesicles.

Following IV administration, small liposomes (0.1 to 1.0 μm) are taken up preferentially by cells of the reticuloendothelial system (RES), located principally in the liver and spleen,[33] whereas liposomes larger than 3.0 μm are deposited in the lungs.[34] This preferential uptake of smaller-size liposomes by cells of the RES system has been utilized to deliver chemotherapeutic agents to macrophages and tumors of the liver.[14]

Alternative physical approaches based upon the ability to destabilize the liposome bilayer have led to the design of heat-sensitive, light-sensitive, and pH-sensitive liposomes.[35-37]

B. Targeting ligands

The chemical approach to achieving site-specific delivery requires that the liposome has a targeting ligand bound to its surface, thereby enabling it to attach preferentially to the target site. A variety of targeting ligands have been proposed for this purpose, including antitumor monoclonal antibodies (MAb), carbohydrates, vitamins, and transport proteins.[38] Only carbohydrate and MAb-modified liposomes have thus far shown promise in achieving targeting specificity.

Successful targeting of liposomes to cells other than those belonging to the RES is fairly restricted, but appears to include hepatocytes and circulating red blood cells.[39] A high degree of specific liposome-cell association has been obtained *in vitro* by coating the vesicles with cell-specific ligands, such as MAbs or F(ab¹)₂ fragments (see Figure 1.3).[40-42]

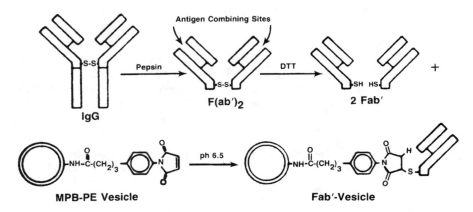

Figure 1.3 Illustration of the chemical-coupling methodology for antibody/liposomes. (From *Pharmaceutical Technology*, Conf. Proc., The Latest Developments in Drug Delivery Systems, Oct. 1985. With permission.)

C.   Problems

In vivo, the obstacles to successful targeting that have to be overcome are substantial. First, the liposomes have to escape nonspecific clearance by the RES cells. Second, the vesicles have to cross the capillary endothelium and the basement membrane. Third, many cell types, including most tumor cells, display a low endocytotic capacity. Since it has been found that endocytosis is the dominant mechanism of liposome-cell interaction, this is a serious limitation to the successful application of liposomes as a drug delivery system.[14]

Small-size liposomes may serve as drug carriers to liver parenchymal cells by virtue of their capacity to penetrate the liver's fenestrated endothelium. Once taken up by the cells, liposomes may be degraded in the lysosomal compartment. Liposome-encapsulated drugs, when resistant to the intralysosomal environment, may slowly leak out of the lysosomes into the cytosol and may become available to exert their therapeutic action. Drugs may also be released from liposomes phagocytized by macrophages.

Another important aspect of the liposome-drug relationship involves reducing toxicity of the liposome-encapsulated agent. This is particularly important for antineoplastic agents with low therapeutic indices, such as adriamycin or antimicrobial drugs like amphotericin B.[43–45]

D.   Manufacturing issues

Liposomes are phospholipid vesicles composed of one or more phospholipid bilayer membranes and they carry aqueous or lipid drugs. The lipids are both hydrophobic and lipophilic in aqueous media, and their hydrophobic regions sequestrate into spherical bilayers. These layers are referred to as lamellae. Liposomes vary in charge and their size, depending on the method of preparation and the lipids used.

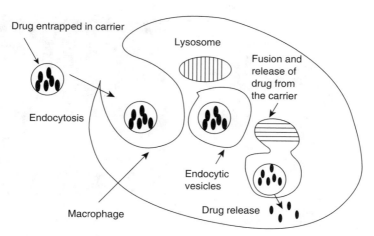

Figure 1.4 Schematic of phagocytosis of particulate carriers by macrophages. Macrophages take up the carriers by the process of endocytosis. Drugs are released from the carriers following intralysosomal degradation of the carriers. (With permission, Elsevier, *J. Control. Rel.*, 79, 29–40, 2002.)

Two major methods are usually used to make liposomal systems for drug incorporation. The first method deals with hydration of a lipid followed by high-intensity agitation using sonication or a high-shear propeller. Liposomes are subsequently sized by filtration or extrusion. In the second method, a phospholipid is first dissolved in an organic solvent and then added to an aqueous medium by vigorous agitation. The organic solvent is removed under vacuum, and the resulting liposomal dispersion or emulsion is sized by filtration or extrusion. Generally, the first method yields multiple lamellae (see Figure 1.4).

Liposomes produced by the high-encapsulation injection process are found to exhibit a broad size distribution in the range of 0.2 to 1.5 µm; downsizing such liposomes results in a loss of encapsulated materials. An alternative method involves the extrusion of a heterogeneous population of fairly large liposomes through polycarbonate membranes under moderate pressures. This technique can reduce a heterogeneous population to a suspension of vesicles that exhibit a mean particle size near that of the pores through which they are extruded (see Figure 1.5).

Incorporation of drugs into liposomes is achieved by using one of the three primary mechanisms: encapsulation, partitioning, and reverse loading. Encapsulation is useful for water-soluble drugs, and it involves hydration of a lipid with an aqueous solution of a drug. The dissolved drug remains in the intralamellar spaces. In the process of partitioning, the drug is dissolved along with the phospholipids in a suitable organic solvent. It is then dried first or added directly to the aqueous phase. The residual solvent is removed in a vacuum. The reverse-loading process is used for weak acidic drugs that exist in both charged and uncharged forms, depending on the

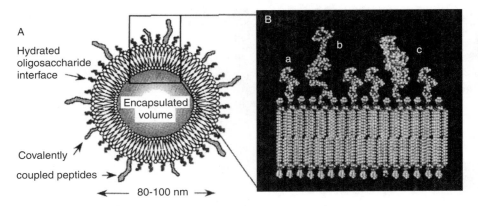

Figure 1.5 Molecular schematic of a surface-modified liposomal drug delivery vehicle for intravascular targeting. (A) The liposome surface consists of a glycocalyx-like oligosaccharide layer to minimize nonspecific interactions and peptide ligands to mediate selective receptive targeting. (B) Composite molecular model showing glycolipids hydrating the surface of the phospholipid bilayer (a), an RGD peptide coupled to the liposome through a poly(ethylene oxide) spacer (b), and a hypothetical coagulation factor VII peptide for targeting endothelial TF (c). (With permission, Elsevier, *J. Control. Rel.*, 78, 235–247, 2002.)

pH of the environment. Such drug molecules are added to an aqueous phase in the uncharged state to permeate into liposomes. The pH is then adjusted to create a charge on the drug molecule. The charged drug molecule is not lipophilic enough to pass through the lipid bilayer and return to the external medium (see Figure 1.6).

Concentrations of the drug and lipids in the vesicles, measurements of captured volume, size distribution, and lamellarity characterize lipid vesicles. The size of liposomes is an important aspect in measuring liposome-complement interactions. The complement system is not known to discriminate according to the liposomal size. Mean vesicle size and size distribution are important parameters for the physical properties and biological fate of liposomes and their entrapped substances *in vivo*. One of the most commonly used methods to determine size and size distribution is light-scattering analysis. Newer methods use laser light scattering. If the liposomes are monodisperse, light-scattering analysis is used. For heterogeneous liposomes, accurate estimate of their size–frequency distribution is necessary. Other systems, such as dispersion, emulsions, and suspensions, are used frequently (see Figure 1.7).

By utilizing a dehydration–rehydration process, a number of molecules can be quantitatively entrapped into the aqueous phase of liposomes. Small, unilamellar vesicles are mixed with a solution of the drug and used for entrapment. The mixture is dehydrated by freeze drying, and the powder thus obtained is rehydrated under controlled conditions. Microfluidization of the drug containing dehydration–rehydration vesicles in the presence of

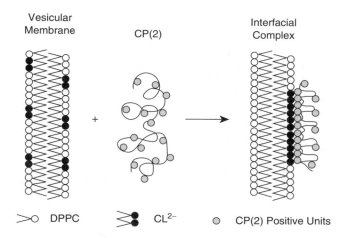

Figure 1.6 Adsorption of CP(2) on the membrane of liquid mixed-negative vesicles (schematic presentation). (With permission, Elsevier, *J. Control. Rel.*, 78, 267–271, 2002.)

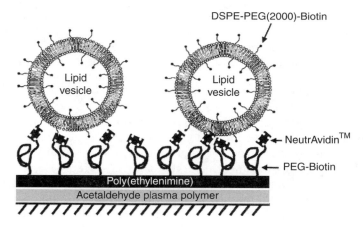

Figure 1.7 Schematic drawing (not to scale) of the multilayer construct used for immobilizing PEG-biotinylated liposomes onto solid polymeric carrier materials via NeutrAvidin™ binding. (With permission, Elsevier, *J. Control. Rel.*, 80, 179–195, 2002.)

nonentrapped solute generates smaller vesicles. In gene delivery, cationic liposomes that interact with negatively charged nucleic acid polymers are used. Relatively homogenous and physically stable suspensions can be obtained by carefully controlling the complex conditions.

Liposome stability is determined by using controlled systems, which are stabilized electrostatically, sterically, or electrosterically. Besides normal colloids, self-assembling colloids can undergo fusion or phase change after aggregation. Liposome dispersions exhibit both physical and chemical stability. Physically stable formulations preserve both liposomal size distribution and the quantity of the material entrapped. Stability depends on the

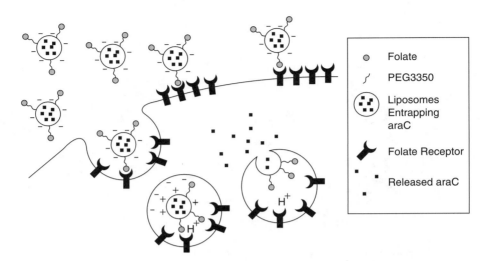

Figure 1.8 Possible mechanism of intracellular araC delivery by FR-targeted, cationic, lipid-based, pH-sensitive liposomes. At first, the folate-derivatized liposomes are taken into the cell by binding to the FRs on the plasma membrane and FR-mediated endocytosis. This is followed by acidification of the endosome, which results in protonation of the anionic lipid component and generation of a net positive surface charge on the liposomes. Finally, the electrostatic interactions between the liposomal and endosomal membranes result in bilayer fusion and the cytosolic delivery of the encapsulated araC. (With permission, Elsevier, *J. Control. Rel.*, 80, 309–319, 2002.)

mechanical properties of the liposomal membranes, their thermodynamics, and colloidal properties of the system. Often, stability tests stress a system to limits beyond those to which the product will ever be subjected.

High-temperature testing (greater than 25°C; see Figure 1.8) is frequently used for heterogeneous products. Phase-transition temperatures for a liposomal system are critical, but the changes, should this occur, are reversible. On the other hand, under frozen conditions, ice crystals are formed. Certain polymers are known to retard or suppress ice crystal growth. Aging studies involving determinations of zeta potential and dielectric constants are usually performed. These analyses determine the status of structural alterations in liposomal vesicles. In summary, in liposomal preparations, each test condition indicating stability of the vesicles should express conditions for microscopic observation (e.g., flocculation), particle-size profiles, rheological profiles, extent of leakage, and chemical and physical stability.

IV. Liposomes as carriers of therapeutic agents

A. Application

Since 1972, when Gregoriadis proposed the use of liposomes as carriers of enzymes in the treatment of lysosomal storage diseases, the application of liposomes has been extended to a variety of drugs, such as antineoplastic agents,[16,46,47] antimicrobial compounds,[42,48] and immunomodulators.[49-52] In addition to utilizing liposomes as drug carriers in the treatment of intracellular infections,[53] liposomes have also been used as carriers of amphotericin B in the treatment of mycotic infections, such as histoplasmosis,[54] cryptococcosis, and candidiasis.[54] Lopez-Berestein et al.[55] reported that liposomal amphotericin B is effective in the treatment of candida and aspergillus infections in leukemia patients who have not responded to the nonencapsulated drug. The increase in amphotericin's efficacy by encapsulation in liposomes is associated with reduced toxicity.[56]

Incorporation of lipophilic amphotericin within liposomes might result in a facilitated transfer of the drug to fungal cells. In turn, this selective transfer of amphotericin from liposomes to fungal cells may form the molecular basis of the reduced toxicity. Other factors, such as altered kinetics or tissue distribution, may also play an important role.[57]

Antibacterial activity with liposome encapsulation has been reported by Sunamoto and co-workers (in experimental Legionnaires' disease).[58] They showed that uptake of IV-injected liposomes by circulating monocytes and alveolar macrophages can be increased by coating the vesicles with a palmitoyl derivative of amylopectin. After IV injection, the amylopectin-modified liposomes were found to preferentially distribute in the lungs.

Macrophages have an affinity for liposomes, and this property has been utilized in the use of these vesicles as carriers of immunomodulators to create macrophages cytotoxic to metastatic tumor cells. As a result, macrophages serve as an important barrier against the proliferation and metastatic spread of tumor cells. Activation of macrophages to induce tumor cytotoxicity occurs as a result of exposure to a variety of immunomodulating substances, such as lymphokines,[59] γ-interferon, and muramyl dipeptide (MDP).[60-63]

Liposomes are known to increase the adjuvant activity of MDP. Adjuvants are nonspecific immune stimulants that boost immunoresponses to weak antigenic molecules. MDP micelles, for example, are highly potent adjuvants in tests for vaccination against bovine viral diarrhea. Although it is unknown how this process occurs, activated macrophages can selectively kill tumor cells. Activated macrophages have been considered in the management of metastatic cancer, which is often seriously hampered by the biological heterogeneity of tumor cells with respect to growth rate and sensitivity to various cytotoxic drugs.

Although preliminary results with liposome-encapsulated immunomodulators are encouraging, successful application in the treatment of patients with liver metastasis may be hampered by unfavorable macrophage-to-tumor cell ratios in many metastatic tumors.[64] Therefore, it would appear that therapeutic regimens designed to stimulate macrophage-mediated tumor cytotoxicity will have to be used in combination with other treatment modalities.[65-67]

Successful targeting of liposomes, at least to solid tumors located outside the main circulatory system, faces numerous challenges. As described by

Roerdink et al.,[14] selective introduction of antineoplastic drugs into tumor cells *in vivo* by means of liposomes is currently a difficult task. However, application of liposomes as a drug delivery system for antitumor drugs may be of great benefit in diminishing toxicity of encapsulated compounds by altering their pharmacokinetics or tissue distribution. In addition, liposomes can serve as a sustained- or controlled-release system for cytostatic drugs, such as cytosine arabinoside. The therapeutic effect of this cell-cycle-specific drug is enhanced by liposomal encapsulation, possibly by maintaining therapeutically favorable drug levels for a prolonged period of time following leakage from the liposomes, or, alternatively, from macrophages that have phagocytosed the drug-loaded liposomes.

A promising example of a liposomal delivery system for an antitumor drug has been the use of doxorubicin in liposome-encapsulated form.[14] Doxorubicin, an anthracycline antibiotic, is useful in the treatment of a variety of solid neoplasms, lymphomas, and leukemias. Its clinical use, however, is limited by its cardiotoxicity. Several investigators have shown that entrapment of doxorubicin within liposomes greatly reduces its cardiotoxicity without loss of antitumor activity.[68–71] The mechanism responsible for doxorubicin's increased therapeutic index is not fully understood, but may involve low uptake of the liposomal drug by the myocardium[14] or prolonged release of the drug from macrophage depots.[72]

While in the bloodstream, liposomes may be susceptible to destabilizing effects of serum proteins, resulting in the escape of encapsulated water-soluble compounds. In addition, high-density lipoproteins (HDL) have been found to penetrate liposomal bilayers. This process is accompanied by loss of phosphatidylcholine from the liposomes to the HDL.[73,74]

High susceptibility to phosphapidylcholine loss was found at the gel-to-liquid phase-transition temperatures of the liposomal lipids, while both above and below those temperatures the liposomes were relatively stable.[75] Net loss of phospholipid can be prevented by incorporation of cholesterol into the liposomal membranes, thereby causing obstruction to penetration of serum lipoproteins. This may result in an increased stability of liposomes.[76]

B.   Manufacturers

Table 1.1 presents a list of liposome technology-based research and development firms, their products, and indications for their usage.[77]

In addition to those presented in the table, the following industrial establishments are also involved in liposome delivery research and development: American Bioproducts, American Lecithin Co., Applied Genetics, Argus Pharmaceuticals, Becton Dickinson & Co., Bristol-Myers Squibb, Brocades Pharma ESCA Agenetics Corp., Fountain Pharmaceuticals, Genzyme Corp., IGI, Inc., Nichiyu Liposome Co., Pharmos Ltd., RibiImmunochem Research, Inc., Schering AG, Schering-Plough Corp., Somatogen, Inc., Structure Probe, and Vical, Inc. According to FIND/SVP's report on the total

Table 1.1 Summary of activity in liposome usage

Corporation	Product	Indications
Fujisawa	Vestar's liposomal formulation of amphotericin B (AmBisome)	Systemic fungal infections
Vestar	MiKasome — aminoglycoside antibiotic, amikacin	Drug-resistant tuberculosis
	Hemoglobin	Blood substitute
	Cyclosporine	Multidrug resistance to cancer chemotherapy
	Liposomes linked to specific proteins	Affinity for sites on diseased cells
	Liposomes coated with a specific viral receptor protein	AIDS and other viral diseases
	Boron isotope of mass 10	Cancer therapy
	Vescan	MRI enhancer in animal tumors
Teijin-Taisho	Epoprostanol derivatives	Myocardial infarction
	Isocarbacyclin	Cerebrovascular orders, chronic arterial obstruction in rats
ImmunoTherapeutics	Glucosamyl muramyl analog	Delivery to the monocyte/macrophage system in cancer chemotherapy
Ciba-Geigy	Muramyl tripeptide	Cancer therapy Metastatic melanoma
Genset	Development of liposomes	For antisense delivery
Liposome Technology Activators	Amphosil (amphotericin B)	aspergillosis infections
	Plasminogen streptokinase reversed	In canines, encapsulated local ischemia
	Amphotericin B cholesterol sulfate-based delivery system (known as ABCD), amphotericin B colloidal dispersion	Leishmaniasis
	(5,12-naphthacenedione) doxorubicin (Lip-Dox)	Advanced cancer patients
	Stealth liposomes (Doxil)	Kaposi's sarcoma
	Metered dose technology Liposome inhalation products	Respiratory and systemic diseases
	Albuterol, Salbutamol (inhaled liposomal formulations)	Beta 2 adrenoreceptor agonist (asthma)

Table 1.1 Summary of activity in liposome usage (Continued)

Corporation	Product	Indications
Technology Unlimited	Development of liposomes	Delivery of water and lipid-soluble material to skin, oral cavity, lungs, digestive tract, vagina, urinary, bladder, liver solid tumors, and HIV-infected cells
The Liposome Co.	Defensins, potent antifungal and antiviral peptides isolated from human neutrophils	Cryptococcal infections in AIDS patients
	Gentamicin — (aminoglycoside antibiotic) TLC G-65	*Mycobacterium avium intracellulare* (MAI) infections in AIDS patients
	Amphotericin B (AB lipid complex) ABLC	Fungal infections in AIDS and cancer patients
The Liposome Co.	TLC I-16, nonionic, iodinated contrast agent	Liver imaging in CT scans, potential in the detection of liver metastases in patients with advanced breast, colon, and lung cancer
Univax & Micro Vesicular Systems	Novasome liposome technology for vaccines	Bacterial and viral vaccines (e.g., for pseudomonas, HIV)
	Liposomal adjuvant system using TLC A-60	Human influenza vaccine
	TLC C-53 (prostaglandin E)	Acute inflammatory and veso-occlusive conditions

market for liposomal pharmaceuticals and diagnostics for 1995, anti-infectives will occupy 75.2% of the market, followed by anticancers (18.8%), diagnostics (5.0%), and respiratory (1.0%). The total market for pharmaceutical and diagnostic liposomes reached an estimated $18 million in 1991, and this is expected to grow dramatically as new products gain regulatory approval. The overall market for drug delivery systems is observed to reach $399 million in 1995.

In Table 1.2, liposomal and conventional formulations of amphotericin B are compared in transplant recipients with systemic fungal infections.[78]

V. Recent advances

Recent studies and examples of liposomal formulations containing various entrapped ingredients are as follows:[79–81]

Table 1.2 Formulation

Parameter	Liposomal	Conventional
Number of Patients	29	29
Graft losses[a]	6/11 (55%)	14/16 (88%)
Mean duration of antifungal treatment	21.3 days	21 days
Adverse reaction reports	3 in 3 patients	
Deaths	9	17
Survival rates		
Liver transplant	71.4% (n = 7)	20.0% (n = 5)
Kidney transplant	72.7% (n = 11)	62.5% (n = 16)
Bone marrow transplant	63.6% (n = 11)	12.5% (n = 8)

[a] Kidney or pancreas transplant only.

L-NDDP (cis-bis-neodecanoato-*trans*-R,4–1, 2-Daminocyclohexane plati-num), vincristine (in stealth liposome), cytochalasin B, vaginal antifungal agents, such as miconazole, steroidal liposomes from sterols, such as choles-terol, vitamin D, steroid hormones and fluorinated steroids, benzylpenicillin, topical and in-aerosol devices for anti-inflammatories, beclomethasone dipropionate, dexamethasone palmitate, bronchodilators, such as metapro-terenol (Metasome) and terbutaline, indomethacin, daunorubicin (Cerbu-dine), radiopharmaceutical VS-101, cisplatin (Platinol), minoxidil, calcitonin, camptothecin,[111] indium, cephalothin, nystatin, α-tocopherol, α-tocopherol nicotinate, vitamins A and E, tin mesoporphyrin, cyclosporin A (aerosol formulation), apolipoprotein B,5-fluoro-2′-deoxyuridine and its pro-drug, 3–5′-*O*-dipalmitoyl derivative, (dpFUdR) corticosteroids, 14-*O*-palmi-toyl-hydroxyrubicin, plasmid DNA, glutathione, idarubicin, dideoxyinosine triphosphate, bovine somatotropin, antimonial drug meglumine antimonate for leishmaniasis, hamycin, Novasome vaccines, 2–133-Interleukin 2, imida-zolidines, and dyphylline.[77]

A.   Highlights of current research

- Liposome products to deliver medication to the eye (e.g., dry eye syndrome)[82,83] or gastrointestinal tract have been described.[77]
- Animal studies have been carried out using liposomes and heat application to deliver anticancer drugs. Anticancer drug-contain-ing liposomes are injected into the bloodstream. At temperatures a few degrees above normal, the liposomes melt, allowing drugs to leak out.[85]
- Primaquin (an antimalarial agent) has been coupled to a liver cell-tar-geting peptide to form a complex that can be encapsulated.[86,87]
- A new liposomal product known as pro-liposome has been devel-oped that has a significantly stronger membrane.[82]
- Multivesicular liposomes for the administration of anticancer agents have been developed. These liposomes are composed of multiple,

nonconcentric, aqueous chambers, allowing more efficient drug entrapment and improved incorporation of drugs, including cytarabine and bleomycin.[14]

- Battelle has developed a process to dehydrate drug-encapsulated liposomes, allowing storage as a stable powder that can be reconstituted when required for drug delivery.[77]
- Macromolecular carriers and liposomes have been covalently coupled to monoclonal antibodies targeted against cardiac myosin heavy chain. Deferoxamine-modified polymers were bound tightly with ^{67}Ga and ^{68}Ga radioisotopes.[88]
- The penetration behavior of liposomes (prepared from NAT 106) incorporated with proteins has been investigated *in vivo* utilizing MAbs. Within 20 minutes of topical application to young pig skin, an even distribution through all skin layers was demonstrated.[89]
- Dioleoyl-N-(monoethoxy polyethyleneglycol succinyl)-phosphatidylethanolamine (PGE-PE) (mol wt of PEG = 5000), an amphipathic polymer, can be incorporated into the liposome membrane and significantly prolong the blood circulation time of the liposome.[90]
- Two rat MAbs, 34A and 201B, that specifically bind to a surface glycoprotein (gp112) of the pulmonary endothelial cell surface, have been coupled to unilamellar liposomes (immunoliposomes) of approximately 0.25 μm in diameter. Time-course studies reveal that 34A liposomes bind to lung antigens within 1 min after injection, indicating that binding takes place during the first few passages through the lung capillary bed.[91]
- The MAb DAL K29 against a human renal cell carcinoma associated cell surface antigen has been covalently linked to small unilamellar lipid vesicles (SUV) containing the antifolate methotrexate, with full retention of antibody activity.[92]
- Two T lymphocyte cell surface molecules, CD4 and CD7, have been studied as targets for the specific delivery of drugs from antibody-directed liposomes. The efficiency of uptake by peripheral lymphocytes, thymocytes, and two CEM sublines (CEM.MRS and CEM-T4) of anti-CD4 and anti-CD7 liposomes containing methotrexate have been evaluated by methotrexate-mediated inhibition of the incorporation of d-[3H]Urd into DNA. This was compared with similar liposomes targeted to MHC-encoded HLA class I molecules, which are known to be taken up efficiently by T cells.[93]
- Generation of cytotoxic T lymphocytes (CTL) *in vitro* and tumor-rejection responses by sensitization of semisyngenic mice with tumor antigen reconstituted liposomes has been investigated. Liposomes were prepared from a crude butanol extract of BALBRVD leukemia cells and egg phosphatidylcholine (PC): 1,2-Dimyristoylamido-1,2-Deoxyphosphatidylcholine (DDPC) (3:2), or dimyristoylphosphatidylcholine (DMPC):DDPC (1:4).[94]

- A new method for the elimination of mononuclear phagocytic cells from cell suspensions has been described. By making use of liposome-encapsulated dichloromethylene diphosphonate, macrophages were effectively removed from spleen cell suspensions. This effect was not observed when using the free-drug or control liposomes.[95]
- Comparative studies of the preparation of immunoliposomes with the use of two bifunctional coupling agents and investigation of *in vitro* immunoliposome target cell binding by cytofluorometry and electron microscopy have been carried out. The specificity of the binding of B8–24.3-liposomes to EL4 target cells was visualized by scanning electron microscopy. Antibody-mediated endocytic uptake of immunoliposomes was demonstrated.[96]
- The potential of small unilamellar liposomes coupled to antitumor MAbs to accumulate in solid tumor tissue has been tested in two systems: a human malignant melanoma xenografted into nude mice and a syngeneic murine lymphoma ESb.Mp exhibiting spontaneous metastasis to the liver. Both MAbs tested were partly released from immunoliposomes within a few hours and produced a constant level of circulating antibody.[97]
- A differentiation inducer, sodium butyrate (SB), encapsulated in liposomes conjugated covalently to an MAb directed to CD19 antigen has been successfully targeted to human lymphoma cell lines SKLY-18 and Ramos grown *in vitro* and *in vivo* in nude mice. Various control liposomes (lacking SB or antibody, or coupled to an irrelevant antibody) are not effective targeters. In view of the limited number of tumor-specific antigens, targeting of differentiation inducers rather than cytotoxic drugs to tumor cells may provide a useful approach for conversion of highly malignant to less malignant tumors.[98]
- A technique for loading certain types of drug molecules into preformed liposomes has been described. The drug must be amphiphatic and exist in a charged, protonated form. Liposome suspensions are formed with a higher concentration of ammonium ions within the liposome than in the external aqueous phase, thus establishing a pH gradient across the liposome boundary. The amphiphatic drug molecule is added to the suspension and, because of the pH gradient, is preferentially loaded in the core of the liposome.[99]
- Liposomes targeted to the liver have been prepared with a high content of a nonionic surfactant. This formulation was prepared by mixing soybean phosphatidylcholine, α-tocopherol, and ethoxylated hydrogenated castor oil (HCO-60) in methanol, concentrating the mixture under vacuum, and then shaking it with water. Transport to rat liver after IV administration was claimed to be approximately twice as high for liposomes containing castor oil ethoxylate as for controls without surfactant.[100]
- The extent to which liposomes promote the permeability of insulin through the nasal mucosa with or without pretreatment with sodium

glycocholate (an enhancer of nasal absorption) has been studied. Results indicate that sodium glycocholate remaining in the nasal mucosa causes the lysis of liposomes that come to the surface of the nasal mucosa and the subsequent release of insulin from the liposome. The relatively high level of insulin in the mucosal surface caused permeation of insulin through the mucosa.[101]

- The release of 5(6)-carboxyfluorescein (CF) from liposomes and phospholipid peroxidation against time in the presence of different concentrations of collagen, albumin, and γ-globulin has been studied. Results indicate that collagen decreases liposome permeability by an antioxidant effect and also by a specific interaction with phospholipids. Collagen provides nonspecific protection against the detergent-induced release of CF from liposomes. Thus, a liposome-collagen complex may provide an improved drug delivery system.[102]

- Removal of intravenously injected liposomes from the circulation has been achieved by cells of the mononuclear phagocyte system (i.e., RES). On exposure to blood, liposomes become coated with plasma proteins. Some of these proteins (opsonins) are thought to become determinants for subsequent recognition by mononuclear phagocytes. The review by Patel provides a critical discussion of factors that control opsonization of liposomes and their phagocytosis *in vivo* and *in vitro*.[103]

- The distribution of 2-imidazolines in neutral dimyristoylphoaphatidylcholine (DMPC) liposomes in negatively charged liposomes containing dicetylphosphate (DCP) or phosphatidylserine (PS) and in positively charged liposomes containing stearylamine (STA) has been investigated. Electrophoretic mobilities of multilamellar liposomes were measured as a function of drug concentration. The results indicate the relative importance of the membrane surface characteristics on partitioning behavior and the membrane transport behavior of the 2-imidazoline drugs.[104]

- The effect of P_o (a cell-adhesion molecule from avian peripheral nerve myelin) on the rate of interaction of liposomes with human M21 melanoma cells has been studied. Liposome uptake by the cells was quantitated using radioactive lipids and liposome entrapped drugs under various conditions. The results suggest that the attachment of liposomes to the cell surface can increase their drug delivery potential. This may be the result of triggering binding endocytic processes or a temporary permeability increase of liposome and cellular membrane, thereby leading to enhanced uptake.[105]

- Liposomes have been prepared containing two lipophilic drugs, dl-α-tocopherol nicotinate (TN) and the anti-inflammatory substance, L440. In the case of TN liposomes, oleoyl-hydrolyzed animal protein (OHAP) was added in order to control the vesicle size. The skin penetration ability of both drugs from liposomal gels into human stratum corneum was determined *in vivo* by a stripping method and compared with conventional galenical formulations. The anti-inflammatory effect of the released L440 was examined in the ear edema model in mice. The penetration tests showed significantly higher absorption rates for both drugs after application of the liposomal preparations in comparison to other topical formulations. However, only a slight relationship between drug permeation into the stratum corneum and liposome diameter was observed.[106]

- The pulmonary delivery of liposomes has recently been reviewed. The technological aspects of delivering liposomes to the lungs are discussed, including the characterization of liposome-containing aerosols and the potential advantages and disadvantages of the various methods that have been employed for their generation. Studies indicate that liposomes can be effectively deposited in the human respiratory tract, wherein they may remain for prolonged periods. Prolonged retention in the airways may markedly alter the pharmacokinetics of liposome-associated materials, thereby increasing local concentrations while decreasing levels at sites distant from the lung. The future potential for such systems, including the possibilities for selective drug delivery to specific cell populations within the lung, has yet to be determined.[107]

- Treatment of pulmonary diseases using the immunosuppressive drug cyclosporin A (CsA) is limited, in part, by poor penetration into the lungs following oral or intravenous administration and by the development of limiting renal, hepatic, and other toxicity following prolonged administration. CsA aerosol delivery may provide an alternate route of local administration that could improve treatment and reduce systemic toxicity. The total CsA dosage administered via aerosol is expected to be less than the conventional oral or intravenous dosage routes. Lipophilic CsA prepared with different phosphatidylcholine liposome formulations has been studied in this regard.[108]

- Liposomes composed of dioleolylphoaphatidylethanolamine, 1,2-Dipalmitoylsuccinylglycerol with polyethylene glycol are pH-sensitive, plasma-stable and have a long circulation time in the blood. The complete destabilization of these liposomes might be useful for the targeted delivery of drugs such as anticancer agents.[124]

- Polyethylene glycol-coated liposomes containing 3,5-dipentadecyloxybenzamide hydrochloride strongly and selectively bind to subendothelial cells via certain kinds of chondroitin sulfate proteoglycans and have an advantage for use as a specific drug delivery system. Fusogenic liposomes composed of the UV-inactivated Sendai virus effectively and directly deliver their encapsulated contents into the cytoplasm using a fusion mechanism of the Sendai virus, whereas conventional liposomes are taken up by endocytosis.[125]

- To enhance the efficiency of gene delivery by the introduction of molecules directly into the cells, virosomes have been developed by combining liposomes with fusogenic viral envelope proteins.[126,127]

- The liposomal gel-controlled ibuprofen release and dural permeation *in vitro* showed a permeation pattern favorable for maintaining constant drug levels. Therefore, this liposomal polaxamer gel represents a new formulation approach to increase the local epidural availability of ibuprofen.[128]
- A significant breakthrough was achieved in the effectiveness of adriamycin by using its liposomal formulation coated with polyethylele glycol (PEGylation).[129]
- The positively charged liposomal formulation of tropicamide, a mydriatic cycloplegic drug, and liposomes dispersed in polycarbophil were found more effective than those with neutral liposomal dispersion.[130]
- Antitumor activity of mitoxantrone was enhanced by using controlled destabilization of a liposomal drug delivery system. For this drug, programmable fusogenic vehicles with PEG with an 18-carbon acyl chain length were used.[131]
- The ophthalmic drug delivery system consisting of oligolamellar system made up of dipalmitoylphosphatidylcholine-cholesterol-dimethyldioctadecyl glycerol bromide in 7:4:1 molar ratio presented the highest encapsulation capacity and delivered greater amounts of the drug acyclovir into the aqueous humor than saline acyclovir or a physical liposome/drug blend.[132]
- The use of magnetoliposomes (liposomes with entrapped magnetic particles in their bilayers), which are magnetosensitive, may be maneuvered to a given site in the organism. Magnetoliposomes that are strong microwave absorbers can be heated to higher temperatures, which may subsequently lead to a leakage of the entrapped drug. The beneficial effects of glucocorticoids in treating pulmonary inflammatory disorders are complicated by systemic adverse effects. The administration of liposome-entrapped dexamethasone has distinct advantages of enhancing the anti-inflammatory activity of the drug.[133, 134]
- Liposome-infused doxorubicin hydrochloride (DXR), an anthracycline anticancer antibiotic, can be effectively used on murine neuroblastoma and may reduce the incidence of cardiac toxicity as compared to DXR alone.[135,136]
- Since it is known that liposomes are naturally taken up by cells of the mononuclear phagocytic system, liposome-based therapy represents a convenient approach to improving the delivery of anti-HIV agents into infected cells, thereby improving the efficacy of drugs and reducing their adverse side effects. A more specific targeting of HIV-infected cells could be obtained using liposomes bearing surface-attached antibiotics.[137]
- A proniosome-based transdermal drug delivery system of levonorgestrel has been developed, and this system is effective in preventing contraception.[138]

- The analysis of *in vitro* antiproliferative activity on cultured human leukemic K562 cells demonstrated that ionic and neutral liposomes containing chromomycin were 1.5- and 7-fold more effective, respectively, as compared with the free drug.[139]
- Liposomes encapsulating adenosine triphosphate were prepared by sonication, and the liposomes have been evaluated for treatment of ischemic retina.[140]
- The intrahepatic distribution of liposomes containing glycolipid derivatives showed that these were suitable for the selective delivery of liposomes to hepatic parenchymal cells. The authors synthesized branched-type galactoyllipid derivatives for liposome modification for the targeting of asialoglycoprotein receptors on the surface of liver cells. Galactose was coupled to the α- and γ-carboxyl groups of glutamic acid via a triethyleleglycol spacer, and the glutamic moiety bound to the lipid anchor.[141]
- Liver accumulation of liposomes depends on the galactosyl residues. The number of galactosyl residues was more effective for accumulation in the liver than for branching. Niosome-encapsulated ciprofloxacin and norfloxacins were studied, and it was found that intestinal, but not nasal, absorption was significantly higher in comparison with that of nonliposomal parent drugs.[142]
- It is known that a single liposome may carry greater than or equal to 10,000 drug molecules and that the use of PEG-conjugated immunoliposomes increases the drug-carrying capacity of the monoclonal antibody by up to four logarithmic orders in magnitude. Specific OX-26 monoclonal antibody-mediated targeting of daunomycin to the rat brain was achieved by this immunoliposome-based drug delivery system.[143]
- The use of liposome can be helpful in optimizing sustained delivery of glucocorticoids to the lungs via topical administration. The use of triamcinolone acetonide phosphate liposomes as a pulmonary-targeted drug delivery system has been explored.[144]
- Different sugar-coated liposomes were prepared and tested against experimental leishmaniasis *in vivo* using pentamidine isethionate and its methoxy derivative. Both drugs, when encapsulated in sugar-grafted liposomes, were found to be more potent in comparison to normal drug delivery.[145]
- A significant reduction in tumor volume and increased survival time were observed in tumor-bearing mice treated with a combination of hyperthermia and thermosensitive liposome-encapsulated melphalan compared with animals treated with an equivalent dose of free melphalan, with or without hyperthermia. These results suggest that hyperthermia in combination with temperature-sensitive liposome-encapsulated melphalan may serve as a useful targeted drug delivery system for more effective management of melanoma.[146]

- Using virosomes prepared from the P3HR1 strain of Epstein–Barr virus, the authors demonstrated that these particles fused with human hepatocarcinoma cell line Li7A might be used as a drug delivery system to enhance specific macrophagic functions.[147]
- Use of radioprotective drugs in radiotherapy is desirable to protect normal tissues. 2-Mercaptopropionylglycine (MPG) showed promising results in experimental radioprotection. A statistically significant, dose-dependent enhancement of protection by liposome-encapsulated MPG was observed. Liposome-encapsulated MPG, as compared to free MPG, improved the viabilities of spleen and bone marrow cells for different doses of radiation.[148]
- The nuclear enzyme, topoisomerase I, was recently recognized as the target for the anticancer drug, camptothecin (CPT), and its derivatives. This drug was reported to display effective antitumor effects on a variety of human tumor models xenografted in nude mice. The intramuscular administration of liposome-incorporated CPT had considerable potential for the treatment of human neoplastic diseases, especially lymph node metastases.[149]
- The authors developed a lipid-based drug delivery system to provide prolonged levels of gentamicin in local tissues after local administration. Local injection of multivesicular liposome/gentamicin provided sustained drug concentrations in regional tissues, which protected against a massive bacterial challenge for at least 4 days.[150]
- Cytosine arabinoside (Ara-C) was contained in polymer-coated liposomes. Polymers such as dimyristoylphosphatidylcholine, dipalmitoylphosphatidylcholine, and dicetyl phosphate were used and coated with a derivatized polysaccharide. These liposomes were found stable in harsh environments, such as those encountered after oral administration.[151]
- The authors investigated the *in vivo* characteristics of liposomes coated with a polyvinylalcohol having a long alkyl chain as a hydrophobic moiety at the end of the molecule. This moiety reduced uptake in the reticuloendothelial system.[152]
- In the search for an effective immunization against diseases such as cancer, parasitic disease, AIDS, and other viral infections, several peptides and recombinant proteins were synthesized, examined for the ability to induce antibodies and cytotoxic T lymphocytes (CTLs), and tested for binding capability and therapeutic or prophylactic efficacy against the original target cell of the organism. The data suggest that small synthetic peptides, synthesized with or without a lipid tail, or chemically conjugated to the surface liposomes, might serve as effective antigenic epitopes in combination with liposomal lipid A for induction of antibodies and CTLs.[153]
- After intravenous injection in rats, the pharmacokinetics and biodistribution of methotrexate were significantly changed by liposomal incorporation and also by the composition of liposomes. Liposomes

containing a 2:1 ratio of phosphatidylcholine and cholesterol and distereoylphosphatidyl-ethanolamine-N-poly(ethylene glycol) 2000 most effectively prolonged blood circulation and reduced hepato-splenic and kidney uptake of methotrexate.[154]

- Boronphenylalanine-loaded conventional and stabilized liposomes were prepared by the reversed-phase evaporation method to treat liver metastases by boron neutron capture therapy. Conventional vesicles were composed of phosphatidylcholine and cholesterol in a molar ratio of 1:1. To obtain stealth liposomes, polyethylene glycol was included in the lipidic bilayer. Tissue boron concentrations were determined by using inductively coupled plasma-mass spectroscopy. Results indicated that PEG-modified liposomes accumulated boron in therapeutic concentrations in metastatic tissue.[155]
- Spherulites (noncationic multilamellar vectors) composed of phos-phatidylcholine, cholesterol, and polyethylene alcohol, entrapping 125-I protein A, were prepared and biodistribution was studied after IV injection in Wistar rats. Approximately 70% of the radioactivity was found in the liver and about 35% in the spleen. Oral adminis-tration of III-In-NTA in fasting rats showed a significant increase of radioactivity in the blood. This formulation did not show cytotoxicity to human cells and could be used as a drug delivery system.[156]
- Proliposomes in the form of enteric-coated beads using glyburide were prepared. The beads were enteric-coated with Eudragit L-100 by a fluidized bed-coating process using triethyl citrate as a plasti-cizer. The dissolution study of enteric-coated beads exhibited en-hanced dissolution as compared with the pure drug.[157]

VI. Concluding remarks

Liposomes possess a number of favorable properties which, theoretically, may enable them to function as drug delivery systems.[109-113] However, limi-tations exist. First, they are unable to cross the capillary endothelial cells in most organs except the liver,[114] and second, many cell types have a limited capacity to phagocytize particles like liposomes.

Liposomes may seem to be attractive carriers of drugs to macrophages, as has been demonstrated by the successful application of liposomes in the treatment of certain forms of cancer. The use of liposomes also appears to be of significant benefit in the reduction of toxicity of certain anticancer drugs. Potentially important results have also been obtained with the appli-cation of liposomes for the delivery of other drugs.[85,115-119]

Problems concerning large-scale production of liposomes as pharmaceu-tical products, acute and chronic toxicity, and immunogenicity of liposome preparations are certainly important aspects of liposome-based technology and they require careful attention before the clinical application of liposomes as a drug delivery system can be contemplated.[82,120-122] Recently, Klimchak and Lenk have addressed some of these topics.[123] Finally, Roerdink et al.[14] in their review article point out that "despite some early remarkable successes, liposomes are by no means a panacea for pharmacotherapy in general." Their observation still seems to be aptly justified.

References

1. Urquhart, J., Assessing adverse reaction reports on old drugs in new dosage forms. In The Latest Developments in Drug Delivery Systems Conference Proceedings, *Pharm. Tech.*, 11, 32–34, 1987.
2. Urquhart, J. and Nichols, K., Delivery systems and pharmacodynamics in new drug research and development. In The Latest Developments in Drug Delivery Systems Conference Proceedings, *Pharm. Tech.*, 13–16, 1985.
3. Anderson, J.M. and Kim, S.W., Ed., *Advances in Drug Delivery Systems*, Vol. 3, Elsevier, Amsterdam, 1988.
4. Robinson, J.R. and Lee, H.L., Eds., *Controlled Drug Delivery Fundamentals and Applications*, 2nd ed., Marcel Dekker, NY, 1987.
5. Tirrell, D.A., Donaruma, L.G., and Turek, A.B., *Macromolecules as Drugs and as Carriers for Biologically Active Materials*, New York Academy of Sciences, New York, 1985.
6. Bruck, S.D., Ed., *Controlled Drug Delivery*, Vols. 1 and 2, CRC Press, Inc., Boca Raton, FL, 1983.
7. Tyle, P., *Drug Delivery Device Fundamentals and Applications*, Marcel Dekker, New York, 1988.
8. Shacknai, J., Drug delivery systems in light of the new legal situation. In The Latest Developments in Drug Delivery Systems Conference Proceedings, *Pharm. Tech.*, 54–59, 1985.
9. Flynn, G.L., Considerations in controlled release drug delivery system, *Pharm. Tech.*, 6, 33–39, 1982.
10. Tomlinson, E., Biological opportunities for site-specific drug delivery using particulate carriers. In *Drug Delivery Systems: Fundamentals and Techniques*, Johnson, P. and Lloyd-Jones, J.G., Eds., VCH Ellis Horwood Ltd., Chichester, 1987, 32–65.
11. Tomlinson, E., (Patho)physiology and the temporal and spatial aspects of drug delivery. In *Site-Specific Drug Delivery, Cell Biology, Medical and Pharmaceutical Aspects*, Tomlinson, E. and Davis, S.S., Eds., John Wiley & Sons, Chichester, 1986, 1–26.
12. Gregoriadis, G., The liposome drug carrier concept: its development and future. In *Liposomes in Biological Systems*, Gregoriadis, G. and Allison, A.C., Eds., John Wiley & Sons, New York. Also see *Liposome Technology*, Gregoriadis, G. Vol. 1–3, CRC Press, Inc., Boca Raton, FL, 1980.
13. Juliano, R.L., Liposomes as a drug delivery system, *Trends in Pharmacol. Sci.*, 2, 39–41, 1981.
14. Roerdink, F.H., Daemen, T., Bakker-Woudenberg, I.A.J.M., Storm, G., Crommelin, D.J.A., and Schephof, G.L., Therapeutic utility of liposomes. In *Drug Delivery Systems: Fundamentals and Techniques*, Johnson, P. and Lloyd-Jones, J.G., Eds., VCH Horwood Ltd., Chichester, 66–80, 1987.
15. Juliano, R.L. and Layton, D., Liposomes as a drug delivery system. In *Drug Delivery Systems*, Juliano, R.L., Ed., Oxford University Press, 189–236, 1980.

16. Gregoriadis, G., Ed., Liposomes as drug carriers, *Recent Trends and Progress*, John Wiley & Sons, New York, 1988.
17. Papahadjopoulos, D., Liposomes as drug carriers, *Annu. Rep. Med. Chem.* 14, 250–260, 1979.
18. Bassett, J.B., Anderson, R.U., and Tucker, J.R., Use of temperature-sensitive liposomes in the selective delivery of methotrexate and cis-platinum analogues to murine bladder tumor, *J. Urol.*, 135, 612–615, 1986.
19. Magin, R.L. and Niesman, M.R., Temperature-dependent drug release from large unilamellar liposomes, *Cancer Drug Delivery*, 1, 109–117, 1984.
20. Knudsen, R.C, Card, D.M., and Hoffman, W.W., Protection of guinea pigs against local and systemic foot-and-mouth disease after administration of synthetic lipid amine (Avridine) liposomes, *Antiviral Res.*, 6, 123–133, 1986.
21. Gregoroadid, G. and Senior, J., The phospholipid component of small unilamellar liposomes controls the rate of clearance of entrapped solutes from the circulation, *FEBS Lett.*, 119, 43–46, 1980.
22. Kiwada, H., Akimoto, M., Araki, M., Tsuji, M., and Kato, Y., Application of synthetic liposomes based on acyl amino acids or acyl peptides as drug carriers. I. Their preparation and transport of glutathione into the liver, *Chem. Pharm. Bull.*, 35, 2935–2942, 1987.
23. Scherphof, G., Morselt, H., Regts, J., and Wilschut, J., The involvement of the lipid phase transition in the plasma-induced dissolution of multilamellar phosphatidyl-choline vesicles, *Biochem. Biophys. Acta*, 556, 196–207, 1979.
24. Citovsky, V., Blumenthal, R., and Loyter, A., Fusion of Sendai virions with phosphatidyl-choline-cholesterol liposomes reflects the viral activity required for fusion with biological membranes, *FEBS Lett.*, 193, 135–140, 1985.
25. Szoka, F.C. and Papahadjopoulos, D., Comparative properties and methods for preparation of lipid vesicles (Liposomes) *Annu. Rev. Biophys. Bioeng.*, 9, 467–508, 1980.
26. Mayhew, E. and Papahadjoloulos, D., Therapeutic uses of liposomes. In *Liposomes*, Ostro, M., Ed., Marcel Dekker, New York, 1983.
27. Hunt, A.C., Rustum, Y.M., Mayhew, E., and Papahadjopoulos, D., Retention of cytosine arabinoside in mouse lung following intravenous administration in liposomes of different size, *Drug. Metab. Dispo.*, 7, 124–128, 1979.
28. Heath, T.D., Fraley, R.T., and Papahadjopoulos, D., Antibody targeting of liposomes: cell specificity obtained by conjugation of F(ab) to vesicle surface, *Science*, 210, 539–541, 1980.
29. Martin, F.J. and Papahadjopoulos, D., Irreversible coupling of immunoglobulin fragments to preformed vesicles, *J. Biol. Chem.*, 257, 286–288, 1982.
30. Hirano, K., Hunt, C.A., Strubbe, A., and MacGregor, R.D., Lymphatic transport of liposome-encapsulated drugs following intraperitoneal administration-effect of lipid composition, *Pharm. Res.*, 271–278, 1985.
31. Nakatsu, K. and Cameron, D.A., Uptake of liposome-entrapped mannitol by diaphragm, *Can. J. Physiol. Pharmacol.*, 57, 756–759, 1979.
32. Ellens, H., Morselt, H., and Scherphof, G., *In vivo* fate of large multilamellar sphingomyelin-cholesterol liposomes after intraperitoneal and intravenous injection into rats, *Biochem. Biophys. Acta*, 674, 10–18, 1981.
33. Allen, T.M., Murray, L., MacKeigan, S., and Shah, M., Chronic liposome administration in mice: effects on reticuloendothelial function and tissue distribution, *J. Pharmacol. Exp. Ther.*, 229, 267–275, 1984.

34. Roerdink, F.H., Dijkstra, J., Spanjer, H.H., and Scherphof, G.L., *In vivo* and *in vitro* interaction of liposomes with hepatocytes and Kupffer cells, *Biochem. Soc. Trans.*, 12, 335–336, 1984.

35. Nayar, R. and Schroit, A.J., Generation of pH-sensitive liposomes, use of large unilamellar vesicles containing N-succinyldioleoyl-phosphatidylethanolamine, *Biochemistry*, 24, 5967–5971, 1985.

36. Straubinger, R.M., Duzgunes, N., and Papahadjopoulos, D., pH-sensitive liposomes mediate cytoplasmic delivery of encapsulated macromolecules, *FEBS Lett.*, 179, 148–154, 1985.

37. Liburdy, R.P. and Magin, R.L., Microwave-stimulated drug release from liposomes, *Radiat. Res.*, 103, 266–275, 1985.

38. Szoka, F.C. and Mayhew, E., Alteration of liposome disposition *in vivo* by bilayer-situated carbohydrates, *Biochem. Biophys. Res. Commun.*, 110, 140–146, 1983.

39. Singhal, A. and Gupta, C.M., Antibody-mediated targeting of liposomes to red cell *in vivo*, *FEBS Lett.*, 201, 321–326, 1986.

40. Weinstein, J.N., Lesserman, L.D., Henkert, P.A., and Blumenthal, R., Antibody-mediated targeting of liposomes. In *Targeting of Drugs*, Gregoriadis, G., Senior, J. and Trout, A., Eds., Plenum Press, New York, 185–202, 1982.

41. Toonan, P.A.H. and Crommelin, D.J.A., Immunoglobulins as targeting agents for liposome-encapsulated drugs, *Pharm. Weekbl. Sci. Edition*, 269–280, 1983.

42. Connor, J., Sullivan, S., and Huang, L., Monoclonal antibody and liposomes, *Pharm. Ther.*, 28, 341–365, 1985.

43. Rahman, A. et al., Liposomal protection of adriamycin-induced cardiotoxicity in mice, *Cancer Res.*, 40, 1532–1537, 1980.

44. Olson, F., Mayhew, E., Maslow, D., Rustum, Y., and Szoka, F., Characterization, toxicity and therapeutic efficacy of adriamycin encapsulated in liposomes, *Eur. J. Cancer. Clin. Oncol.*, 18, 2, 167–176, 1982.

45. Gabzion, A., Goren, D., Fuks, Z., Meshorer, A., and Barenholtz, Y., Superior therapeutic activity of liposome-associated adriamycin in a murine metastatic tumor model, *Br. J. Cancer*, 51, 681–689, 1985.

46. Weinstein, J.N., Magin, R.L., Yatvin, M.B., and Zaharko, D.S., Liposomes and local hyperthermia: selective delivery of methotrexate to heated tumors, *Science*, 204, 188–191, 1979.

47. Carman-Meakin, B., Kellaway, J.W., and Farr, S.J., A liposomal sustained-release delivery system, International Patent Application No. WO 87/01714, 1986.

48. Trout, A., Increased selectivity of drugs by linking to carriers, *Eur. J. Cancer*, 14, 105, 1978.

49. Gregoriadis, G. and Ryman, B.E., Fate of protein-containing liposomes injected into rats: an approach to the treatment of storage diseases, *Eur. J. Biochem.*, 24, 485–491, 1972.

50. Tyrell, D.A., Heath, T.D., Colley, C.M., and Ryman, B.E., New aspects of liposomes, *Biochim. Biophys. Acta*, 457, 259, 1976.

51. Gregoriadis, G., Senior, J., and Trout, A., Eds., Targeting of drugs, *NATO-ASI Series A*, 47, Plenum Press, New York and London, 1983.

52. Gregoriadis, G., Liposomes in therapeutic and preventive medicine. The development of drug carrier concept, *Ann. N.Y. Acad. Sci.*, 308, 343, 1978.

53. Schroit, E.J., Hart, I.R., Madsen, J., and Fidler, I.J., Selective delivery of drugs encapsulated in liposomes: natural targeting to macrophages involved in various disease states, *J. Biol. Response Modifiers*, 2 ,97–100, 1983.

54. Taylor, R.L., Williams, D.M., Craven, P.C., Graybil, J.R., Drutz, D.J., and Magee, W.E., Amphotericin B in liposomes: a novel therapy for histoplasmosis, *Ann. Rev. Respir. Dis.*, 125, 610–611, 1982.

55. Lopez-Berestein, G., Faibstein, V., Hopfer, R.L., Mehta, K., et al., Liposomal amphotericin B for the treatment of systemic fungal infections in patients with cancer: a preliminary study, *J. Infect. Dis.*, 151, 704–710, 1985.

56. Mehta, R., Lopez-Berestein, G., Hopfer, R.L., Mills, K., and Juliano, R.L., Liposomal amphotericin B is toxic to fungal cells but not to mammalian cells, *Biochim. Biophys. Acta*, 770230–23482, 6, 164–167, 1984.

57. Juliano, R.L. and Lopez-Berestein, G., New lives for old drugs: liposomal drug delivery systems reduce the toxicity but not the potency of certain chemotherapeutic agents, *Pharm. Tech.*, 6, 164–167, 1982.

58. Sunamoto, J., Goto, M., Ida, T., Hara. K., Saito, A., and Tomonaga, A., Unexpected tissue distribution of liposomes coated with amylopectin derivatives and successful use in the treatment of experimental Legionnaires' disease. In *Receptor Mediated Targeting of Drugs*, Gregoriadis, G., Poste, G., Senior, J., and Trout, A., Eds., Plenum Press, New York, 359–371, 1984.

59. Thombre, P.S. and Deodhar, S.D., Inhibition of liver metastases in murine colon adenocarcinoma by liposomes containing human C-reactive protein crude lymphokines, *Cancer Immunol. Immunother.*, 16, 145–150, 1984.

60. Parant, M., Parant, F., Chedid, L., Yapo, A., Petit, J.F., and Lederer, E., Fate of synthetic immunoadjuvant muramyl dipeptide (C-labeled) in the mouse, *Int. J. ImmunoPharmacol.*, 1, 35–47, 1979.

61. Fogler, W.E., Wade, R., Brundish, D.E., and Fidler, I.J., Distribution and fate of free and liposome-encapsulated H nor-muramyl dipeptide and H muramyl tripeptide phosphatidyl ethanolamine in mice, *J. Immunol.*, 135, 1372–1377, 1985.

62. Fidler, I.J., Sone, S., Fogler, W.E., and Barnes, Z.L., Eradication of spontaneous metastases and activation of alveolar macrophages by intravenous injection of liposomes containing muramyl dipeptide, *Proc. Natl. Acad. Sci. USA*, 78, 1680–1684, 1984.

63. Trout, A., Baurain, R., Deprez-De Campeneere, D., Layton, D., and Masquelier, M., DNA, liposomes and proteins as carriers for antitumoral drugs, *Recent Results Cancer Res.*, 75, 229, 1980.

64. Poste, G., Bucana, C., and Fidler, I.J., Stimulation of host response against metastatic tumors by liposome-encapsulated immunomodulators. In *Targeting of Drugs*, Gregoriadis, G., Senior, J., and Trout, A., Eds., Plenum Press, New York, 261–284, 1982.

65. Gregoriadis, G., Neerunjub, D.E., and Hunt, R., Fate of liposome-associated agents injected into normal and tumor-bearing rodents: attempts to improve localization in tumor cells, *Life Sci.*, 21, 357–370, 1972.

66. Proffitt, R.T., Williams, L.E., Presant, C.A., Uliana, J.A., Gamble, R.C., and Baldeschweiler, J.D., Liposomal blockade of the reticuloendothelial system: improved tumor imaging with small unilamellar vesicles, *Science*, 220, 502–505, 1983.

67. Stavridis, J.C., Deliconstantinos, G., Psallidopoulos, M.C., Armenskas, N.A., Hadjiminas, D.J., and Hadjiminas, J., Construction of transferrin-coated liposomes for *in vivo* transport of exogenous DNA to bone marrow erythrocytes in rabbits, *J. Exp. Cell Res.*, 43, 546–550, 1986.

68. Forssen, E.A. and Tokes, Z.A., Improved therapeutic benefits of doxorubicin by entrapment in anionic liposomes, *Cancer Res.*, 43, 546–550, 1983.

69. Gabzion, A., Dagan, A., Goren, D., Barenholz, Y., and Fuks, Z., Liposomes as *in vivo* carriers of adriamycin: reduced cardiac uptake and preserved antitumor activity in mice, *Cancer Res.*, 42, 4734–4739, 1982.
70. Rahman, A., White, G., More, N., and Schein, P.S., Pharmacological, toxicological and therapeutic evaluation in mice of doxorubicin entrapped in cardiolipin liposome, *Cancer Res.*, 45, 796–803, 1985.
71. Van Hoessel, Q.G.C.M., Steerenberg, P.A., Crommelin, D.L.A., Van Djik, A., et al., Reduced cardiotoxicity and nephrotoxicity with preservation of antitumor activity of doxorubicin entrapped in stable liposomes in the LOU/M WsJ rat, *Cancer Res.*, 44, 3698–3705, 1984.
72. Roerdink, F.H., Regts, J., Van Leeuwen, B., and Scherphof, G., Intrahepatic uptake and processing of intravenously injected small unilamellar phospholipid vesicles in rats, *Biochim. Biophys. Acta.*, 770, 195–202, 1984.
73. Krupp, L., Chobanian, A.V., and Brecher, P.J., The *in vivo* transformation of phospholipid vesicles to a particle resembling HDL in the rat, *Biochim. Biophys. Res. Commun.*, 72, 1251–1258, 1976.
74. Scherphof, G., Roerdink, F., Waite, M., and Parks, J., Disintegration of phosphatidylcholine liposomes in plasma as a result of interaction with high-density lipoproteins, *Biochim. Biophys. Acta.*, 542, 296–307, 1978.
75. Weinstein, J.N. and Leserman, L.D., Liposomes as drug carriers in cancer chemotherapy, *Pharmac. Ther.*, 24, 207–233, 1984.
76. Mufson, D., The application of liposome technology to targeted delivery systems. In The Latest Developments in Drug Delivery Systems Conference Proceedings, *Pharm. Tech.*, 16–21, 1985.
77. Pharmaprojects, 1993.
78. Persson, U. et al., *PharmacoEconomics*, 2(6), 500, 1992.
79. Alving, C.R., Steck, E.A., Chapman, W.L., Jr., Waits, V.B., et al., Therapy of leishmaniasis: superior efficacies of liposome-encapsulated drugs, *Proc. Natl. Acad. Sci. USA*, 75, 2959–2963, 1978.
80. Black, C.D.V., Watson, G.J., and Ward, R.J., The use of pentostam liposomes in the chemotherapy of experimental leishmaniasis, *Trans. Roy. Soc. Trop. Med. Hyg.*, 71, 550–552, 1977.
81. New, R.R.C., Chance, M.L., Thomas, S.C., and Peters, W., Antileishmanial activity of antimonials entrapped in liposomes, *Nature*, 272, 55–56, 1978.
82. Gregoriadis, G., Ed., *Liposome Technology*, Vols. 1–3, CRC Press, Boca Raton, FL, 1993.
83. Gregoriadis, G. and Florence, A.T., Liposomes in drug delivery, *Drugs*, 45, 15–28, 1993.
84. Kimura, T., Intestinal absorption of liposomally entrapped drugs, *Sashin Igaku*, 40, 1818–1824, 1985.
85. Kaledin, V.I., Matienko, N.A., Nikolin, V.P., Gruntenko, Y.V., and Budker, V.G., Intralymphatic administration of liposome-encapsulated drugs to mice, *J. Natl. Cancer Inst.*, 66, 881–887, 1961.
86. Payne, N.I., Timmins, P., Ambrose, C.V., Ward, M.D., and Ridgway, F., Proliposomes: a novel solution to an old problem, *J. Pharm. Sci.*, 75, 325, 1986.
87. Chen, C. and Alli, D., Use of fluidized bed in proliposome manufacturing, *J. Pharm. Sci.*, 76, 419, 1987.
88. Klibanov, A.L., Khaw, B.A., Nossiff, N., O'Donnell, S.M., et al., Targeting of macromolecular carriers and liposomes by antibodies to myosin heavy chain, *Am. J. Physiol.*, 261, 60–65, 1991.

89. Artmann, C., Roding, J., Ghyczy, M., and Pratzel, H.G., Liposomes from soya phospholipids as percutaneous drug carriers, *Arzneimittelforschung*, 40, 1365–1368, 1990.

90. Klibanov, A.L., Maruyama, K., Beckerleg, A.M., Torchilin, V.P., and Huang, L., Activity of amphipathic poly(ethylene glycol) 5000 to prolong the circulation time of liposomes depends on the liposome site, *Biochim. Biophys. Acta.*, 1062, 142–148, 1991.

91. Maruyama, K., Holmberg, E., Kennel, S.J., Klibanov, A., Torchilin, V.P., and Huang, L., Characterization of *in vivo* immunoliposomes, *J. Pharm. Sci.*, 79, 978–984, 1990.

92. Singh, M., Ghose, T., Mezei, M., and Belitsky, P., Inhibition of human renal cancer by monoclonal antibody, *Cancer Lett.*, 56, 97–102, 1991.

93. Suzuki, H., Zelphati, O., Hildebrand, G., and Leserman, L., CD4 and CD7 molecules as targets for drug delivery, *Exp. Cell Res.*, 193, 112–119, 1991.

94. Shibata, R., Noguchi, T., Sato, T., Akiyoshi, K., Sunamoto, J., Shiku, J., and Nakayama, E., Induction of *in vitro* and *in vivo* anti-tumor responses, *Int. J. Cancer*, 48, 434–442, 1991.

95. Classen, I., Van Rooijen, N., and Classen, E., A new method for removal of mononuclear phagocytes, *J. Immunol. Methods*, 134, 153–161, 1990.

96. Schwendener, R.A., Trub, T., Schott, H., Langhals, H., Barth, R.F., Groscurth, P., and Hengartner, H., Comparative studies of the preparation of immunoliposomes, *Biochim. Biophys. Acta*, 1026, 69–79, 1990.

97. Matzku, S., Krempel, H., Weckenmann, H., Sinn, H., and Stricker, H., Tumor-targeting with antibody-coupled liposomes, *Cancer Immunol. Immunother.*, 31, 285–291, 1990.

98. Watanabe, M., Pesando, J.M., and Hakomori, S., Effect of liposomes containing sodium butyrate conjugated with anti-CD19, *Cancer Res.*, 50, 3245–3248, 1990.

99. Barenolz, Y. and Haran, G., U.S. Patent 5,192,549.

100. Hayakawa, E., Kato, Y., Watanabe, K., et al., Japanese Patent 04,244,018.

101. Maitani, Y., Asane, S., Takahashi, S., Nakagaki, M., and Nagai, T., Permeability of insulin entrapped in liposomes, *Chem. Pharm. Bull. (Tokyo)*, 40, 1569–1572, 1992.

102. Pajean, M., Huc, A., and Herbage, D., Stabilization of liposomes with collagen, *Int. J. Pharm.*, 77, 31–40, 1991.

103. Patel, H.M., Serum apsonins and liposomes, *Crit. Rev. Ther. Drug Carrier Syst.*, 9, 39–90, 1992.

104. Choi, Y.W. and Rogers, J.A., Characterization of distribution behavior of 2-imidazolines, *J. Pharm. Sci.*, 80, 757–760, 1991.

105. Foldvari, M., Mezei, C., and Mezei, M., Intracellular delivery of drugs by liposomes, *J. Pharm. Sci.*, 80, 1020–1028, 1991.

106. Michel, C., Purmann, T., Mentrup, E., Seiller, E., and Kreuter, J., Effect of liposomes on percutaneous penetration, *Int. J. Pharm. (Amst.)*, 84, 93–105, 1992.

107. Taylor, K.M.G. and Farr, S.J., Liposomes for drug delivery to the respiratory tract, *Drug Dev. Ind. Pharm.*, 19, 123–142, 1993.

108. Waldrep, J.C., Scherer, P.W., Keyhani, K., and Knight, V., Cyclosporin A liposome aerosol particle size and calculated respiratory deposition, *Int. J. Pharm. (Amst.)*, 97, 205–212, 1993.

109. Gregoriadis, G., Liposomes: a tale of drug targeting, *J. Drug Targeting*, 1, 3–6, 1993.

110. Maruyama, K., Unezaki, S., Takahashi, N., and Iwatsuru, M., Enhanced delivery of doxorubicin to tumor, *Biochim. Biophys. Acta*, 1149, 209–216, 1993.

111. Lundberg, B., Hong, K., and Papahadjopoulos, D., Conjugation of apolipoprotein B with liposomes, *Biochim. Biophys. Acta*, 305–312, 1993.

112. Kadir, F., Intramuscular and subcutaneous drug delivery: encapsulation in liposomes and other methods to manipulate drug availability, *Pharm. World Sci.*, 15, 173–175, 1993.

113. Kedar, E., Rutkowski, Y., Braun, E., Emanuel, N., and Barenholz, Y., Delivery of cytokines by liposomes. I. Preparation and characterization of interleukin-2 encapsulated in long-circulating sterically stabilized liposomes, *J. Immunother.*, 16(1), 47–59, 1994.

114. Posete, G., Liposome targeting *in vivo*: problems and opportunities, *Biol. Cell.*, 47, 19–38, 1983.

115. Hopkins, C.R., Site-specific delivery: cellular opportunities and challenges. In *Site-Specific Drug Delivery*, Tomlinson, E. and Davis, S.S., Eds., *Cell Biology Medical and Pharmaceutical Aspects*, John Wiley & Sons, Chichester, 27–48, 1986.

116. Cleland, L.G., Roberts, B.V., Garrett, R., and Allen, T.M., Cortisol palmitate liposomes: enhanced anti-inflammatory effect in rats compared with free cortisol, *Agents Actions*, 12, 348–352, 1982.

117. De Silva, M., Hazelman, B.L., Page-Thomas, D.P., and Wraight, P., Liposomes in arthritis: a new approach, *Lancet*, 1, 1320–1322, 1979.

118. Fehr, K., Velvart, M., Roos, K., et al., *Therapiewoche*, 35, 2986, 1985.

119. Fujiwara, T., Maeta, H., Chida, S., Morita, T., Watabe, Y., and Abe, T., Artificial surfactant therapy in hyaline membrane disease, *Lancet*, 8159, 55–59, 1980.

120. Talsma, H. and Crommelin, D.J.A., Liposomes as drug delivery systems, *Pharm. Tech.*, November 1992, 16, 52–58.

121. Price, C.I. and Horton, J., *Local Liposome Delivery: An Overlooked Application*, CRC Press, Boca Raton, FL, 1994.

122. Huang, L., Ed., *Journal of Liposome Research*, Marcel Dekker, New York, 1993.

123. Klimchak, R.J. and Lenk, R.P., Scale-up of liposome products, *Biopharmacology*, 18, 1988.

124. Hong, M.S., Lim, S.J., Oh, Y.K., et al., pH sensitive, serum-stable and long circulating liposomes as a new drug delivery system, *J. Pharm. Pharmacol.*, 54, 51–58, 2002.

125. Harigai, T., Kondo, M., Isozaki, M., et al., Preferential binding of polyethylene glycol-coated liposomes containing a novel cationic lipid: TRX 20 to human subendothelial via chondroitin sulfate, *Pharm. Res.*, 18, 1284–1290, 2001.

126. Kunisawa, J. and Mayumi, T., Application of novel drug delivery system: fusogenic liposomes for cancer therapy, *Gan To Kagaku Ryoho*, 5, 577–583, 2001.

127. Kaneda, Y., Virosomes: evolution of the liposomes as a targeted drug delivery. *Adv. Drug Del. Rev.*, 43, 197–205, 2000.

128. Paavola, A., Kilpelanien, I., and Ylirussi, J., Controlled-release injectable liposomal gel of ibuprofen for epidural analgesia, *Int. J. Pharm.*, 199, 85–93, 2000.

129. Lewanski, C.R. and Stewart, S., Pegylated liposomal adriamycin: a review of current and future applications, *Pharm. Sci. Technol. Today*, 1461–5347, 12, 473–477, 1999.

130. Nagarsenker, M.S., Londhe, V.Y., and Nadkarni, G.D., Preparation and evaluation of liposomal formulations of tropicamide for ocular delivery, *Int. J. Pharm.*, 190, 63–71, 1999.

131. Adlakha-Hutcheon, G., Bally, M.B., Shew, C.R., et al., Controlled destabilization of a liposomal drug delivery system enhances mitoxantrone antitumor activity, *Nat. Biotechnol.*, 8, 775–779, 1999.

132. Fresta, M., Panico, A.M., Bucolo, C., et al., Characterization and *in vivo* ocular absorption of liposome-encapsulated acyclovir, *J. Pharm. Pharmacol.*, 5, 565–576, 1999.

133. Babincova, M., Targeted and controlled release of drugs using magnetoliposomes, *Cesk Slov. Farm.*, 48, 27–29, 1999.

134. Suntres, Z.E. and Shek, P.N., Liposomes promote pulmonary glucocorticoid delivery, *J. Drug Target*, 6, 175–182, 1998.

135. Nagae, I., Koyanagi, Y., Ito, S., et al., Liposome drug delivery system for murine neuroblastoma, *J. Pediatr. Surg*, 33, 1521–1525, 1998.

136. Desormeux, A. and Bergeron, M.G., Liposomes as a drug delivery system: a strategic approach for the treatment of HIV infection, *J. Drug Target*, 6, 1–15, 1998.

137. Vora, B., Khopade, A.J., and Jain, N.K., Proniosome-based transdermal delivery of levonorgestrel for effective contraception, *J. Control Release*, 54, 149–165, 1998.

138. Cortesi, R., Espisoto, E., Maietti, A., et al., Production and antiproliferative activity of liposomes containing the antitumor drug chromomycin A3, *J. Microencapsul.*, 4, 465–472, 1998.

139. Arakawa, A., Ishiguro, S., Ohki, K., et al., Preparation of liposome-encapsulating adenosine triphosphate, *Tohoku J. Exp. Med.*, 184, 39–47, 1998.

140. Murahashi, N., Ishihara, H., and Sakagami, M., Synthesis and application of neoglycolipids for liposome modification, *Biol. Pharm. Bull.*, 6, 704–707, 1997.

141. Murahashi, N., Ishihara, H., Sasaki, A., et al., Hepatic accumulation of glutamic-acid-branched neogalactosyllipid modified liposomes, *Biol. Pharm. Bull.*, 3, 259–266, 1997.

142. D'Souza, S.A., Ray, J., Pandey, S., et al., Absorption of ciprofloxacin and norfloxacin when administered as niosome-encapsulated inclusion complexes, *J. Pharma. Pharmacol.*, 49, 145–149, 1997.

143. Huwyler, J., Wu, D., and Pardridgr, W.M., Brain drug delivery of small molecules using immunoliposomes, *Proc. Nat. Acad. Sci. USA*, 93, 14164–14169, 1996.

144. Gonzalez-Rothi, R.J., Suarez, S., and Hochhaus, G., Pulmonary targeting of liposomal triamcinolone acetonide phosphate, *Pharm. Res.*, 13, 1699–1703, 1996.

145. Banerjee, G., Nandi, G., Mahato, S.B., et al., Drug delivery system: targeting of pentamidines to specific sites using sugar-grafted liposomes, *J. Antimicrob. Chemother.*, 38, 145–150, 1996.

146. Chelvi, P.T., Jain, S.K., and Ralhan, R., Heat-mediated selective delivery of liposome-associated melphalan in murine melanoma, *Melanoma Res.*, 5, 321–326, 1995.

147. Grimaldi, S., Giuliani, A., Giuliani, A., et al., Engineered liposomes and virosomes for delivery of macromolecules, *Res. Virol.*, 164, 289–293, 1995.

148. Sharan, R.N., Alam, A., and Chakravorty, S., 2-Mercaptopropionylglycine affords enhanced radioprotection after a liposome encapsulation, *J. Radiat. Res.*, 36, 31–37, 1995.

149. Daoud, S.S., Fetouh, M.I., and Giovanella, B.C., Antitumor effect of liposome-incorporated camptothecin in human malignant xenografts, *Anticancer Drugs*, 6, 83–93, 1995.

150. Grayson, L.S., Hansbrough, J.F., Zapata-Sirvent, R., et al., Soft-tissue infection prophylaxis with gentamicin encapsulated in multivesicular liposomes: results from a prospective randomized trial, *Crit. Care Med.*, 23, 84–91, 1995.

151. Sehgal, S. and Rogers, J.A., Polymer-coated liposomes: improved liposome stability and release of cytosine arabinoside (Ara-C), *J. Microencapsul.*, 12, 37–47, 1995.

152. Takeuchi, H., Kojima, H., Yamamoto, H., et al., Polymer coating of liposomes with a modified polyvinyl alcohol and their systemic circulation and RES uptake in rats, *J. Controlled Rel.*, 68, 195–205, 2000.

153. Alving, V.R., Koulchin, V., and Glenn, G.M., Liposomes as carriers of peptide antigens: induction of antibodies and cytotoxic T lymphocytes to conjugated and unconjugated peptides, *Immunol. Rev.*, 145, 5–31, 1995.

154. Hong, M.S., Lim, S.J., and Lee, M.K., Prolonged blood circulation of methotrexate by modulation of liposomal composition, *Drug Deliv.*, 8. 231–237, 2001.

155. Pavanetto, F., Perugini, P., et al., Boron-loaded liposomes in the treatment of hepatic metastases: preliminary investigation by autoradiography analysis., *Drug Deliv.*, 7, 97–103, 2000.

156. Freund, O., Biodistribution and gastrointestinal drug delivery of new lipidic multilamellar vesicles, *Drug Deliv.*, 8, 239–244, 2001.

157. Chrai, S.S., Murari, R., and Ahmad, A., Liposomes: a review, *Pharm. Tech.*, 26, 28–34, 2002.

chapter two

Site-specific drug delivery utilizing monoclonal antibodies*

Contents

I. Introduction

At the beginning of this century, Paul Ehrlich reported the discovery of antibodies.[1] Since that time, many investigators have done extensive work using a wide variety of antibody molecules in immunocytochemistry, radio-immunoassay, and clinical medicine. In 1976, Kohler and Milstein employed a method of somatic-cell hybridization in order to successfully generate a

* Adapted from Ranade, V.V., Drug delivery systems. 2. Site-specific drug delivery utilizing monoclonal antibodies, *J. Clin. Pharmacol.*, 29, 873, 1989. With permission of the *J. Clin. Pharmacol.*, and J.B. Lippincott Publishing Company, Philadelphia, PA.

continuous "hybridoma" cell line capable of producing monoclonal antibody (MAb) of a defined specificity.[2] Subsequently, several MAbs have exhibited specificity for target sites. It is this property of MAbs that makes them excellent candidates as carriers of therapeutic agents for delivery to specific sites.[3,4]

A.   Chemistry

Antibodies are complex proteins, consisting of multiple polypeptide chains that contain a variety of reactive chemical groups, such as amino, carboxyl, hydroxyl, and sulfhydryl. Functionally, MAbs possess a molecular polarity based on the joining of an antigen-binding fragment (Fab) to a complement-fixing fragment (Fc). The Fab fragment is responsible for specific antigen binding, whereas the Fc fragment binds to effector cells, fixes complements, and elicits other *in vivo* biological responses.

In order to obtain a MAb suitable for the treatment of human disease, it is necessary to maintain both the physical and functional properties of the antibody throughout the steps of production, isolation, purification, and modification. Antibody modification, performed to increase theoretical efficacy, can consist of conjugation of the protein to the following: radionuclides (e.g., ^{131}I and ^{111}In), chemotherapeutic drugs (e.g., methotrexate and vinblastine), and polypeptide toxins (e.g., ricin A chain and polkweed antiviral protein [PAP]).

B.   Polyclonals vs. monoclonals

Antibodies can be heterogeneous with respect to size, charge, antigen specificity, and affinity. These factors may be significant when antibodies are used as a drug delivery system, either alone or when conjugated. For example, some antibody molecules may be degraded rapidly and excreted while others may have longer half-lives.[3–5] Earlier researchers used polyclonal antibodies for drug targeting.[6–8] However, polyclonals contain an inherent deficiency due to lack of specificity that is further compounded by the fact that reproducibility within polyclonal antisera was not always obtained. In view of these problems, researchers continued to focus on developing MAbs with their attendant increased specificity.[9]

Polyclonal antibodies may offer potential advantages in drug delivery, such as recognition of more than one specific location at a given target site. However, this can also be achieved by using mixtures of MAbs of desired specificity. A wide range of animal species can be used to produce polyclonal antibodies, which is a distinct advantage. At the present time, production of MAbs is predominantly limited to mice, rats, and, to some extent, humans.[10]

C.   Conjugation of antibodies

Drug targeting and delivery using antibodies has been most useful in the field of chemotherapy[11,12] because this is an area of research in which there is the greatest need for target-site specificity. Anticancer drugs, in particular, often display high toxicity, and they frequently have a low therapeutic index.[2,13,14]

Early work attempting to conjugate polyclonal antibodies with anticancer drugs involved simple covalent-bond coupling. For example, in 1958, Mathe et al.[15] described the conjugation of methotrexate to antimouse leukemic antibodies for drug targeting. Nearly 15 years later, chlorambucil was coupled to polyclonal goat or rabbit antitumor antibodies.[16] Drug-targeting studies followed using rabbit antibodies against a mouse lymphoma coupled to drugs such as chlorambucil, methotrexate, melphalan, daunomycin, and adriamycin. In similar studies, drug-polymeric carrier complexes have also been coupled to an antibody. Researchers working at the Weizmann Institute in Rehovot, Israel devised[17] such polymeric carriers and were successful in coupling methotrexate, cytosine arabinoside, and platinum to polyclonal, as well as MAbs, against both animal and human tumor targets.[18]

During the period between 1980 and 1988, hybridoma technology was developed. Through its use, complex molecules, such as histocompatibility antigens, developmental and differentiation antigens, tumor-specific antigens, serum proteins, hormones, neurotransmitters, and various kinds of receptors, were recognized, isolated, purified, quantified, and biochemically characterized, and their respective antibodies made available for targeting to specific sites.[11,19-21]

II. Production of monoclonal antibodies

Initial success achieved using hybridoma technology led to further expansion of immunoconjugate-based targeting, especially in detecting and treating human cancers.[22] Rowland described a technique for identifying antigens associated with hematological malignancies. He also emphasized that the choice of normal cells and the method of screening are important in the testing of antibodies for therapeutic immunotargeting.[23-26] The widely accepted method for the production of monoclonals for anticancer targeting is that described by Brown and co-workers[27] in which the appropriate type of malignant cell is used as the immunogen. Hybridomas utilizing hybridoma technology are routinely made in stepwise conventional small-scale culture procedures, as is briefly described in the following.[28,29]

1. The antigen, a foreign substance, such as a lung cancer cell, is injected into a mouse. The mouse's immune system recognizes the lung cancer cell as foreign and directs the spleen to produce specific antibodies to attack that antigen. The spleen is then removed, and the antibody-producing cells are collected.
2. Myeloma cells are isolated from a mouse tumor. These cells have the ability to reproduce continuously in the laboratory.
3. Spleen and tumor cells are fused together to form "hybridomas." A drug is added to kill the tumor cells that do not fuse. The surviving hybridomas have the spleen cell's ability to produce antibodies and the tumor cell's ability to reproduce.

4. Each hybridoma is isolated and allowed to grow into a large colony of cells that produce a single MAb.
5. Each MAb is screened for its ability to attack the original cancer cells, and the hybridomas producing the desired antibody are kept.
6. The desired hybridoma cells are injected into a mouse where they form a tumor that produces large amounts of concentrated antibody. The first critical step in generating a therapeutic or diagnostic MAb — after initial isolation — is to produce the antibody product. Damon Biotech of Needham Heights, Massachusetts, has used a microencapsulation process developed to produce significant quantities of therapeutic MAbs. Known as the Encapsel method, this gentle chemical process results in the formation of a semipermeable membrane around a group of hybridoma cells. Within the microcapsule membrane, these cells proliferate rapidly and secrete the MAb. The antibody is harvested from the intracapsular space at the end of a 2- to 3-week culture period.

A.   Continuously proliferating cell lines

Numerous studies have demonstrated that continuously proliferating cell lines can produce human antibodies of predetermined specificity. These lines have been established as a result of infecting peripheral blood lymphocytes with the Epstein–Barr virus (EBV). This approach has proved to be of limited potential use, however, because all EBV-transformed cell lines decline in antibody production over time. Production of rodent MAbs against a wide variety of antigens has recently been reviewed.[28]

B.   Human–human hybridomas

The availability of appropriate human myeloma lines can facilitate production of human hybridoma products, since in these human–human hybrids, repression of human chromosome function is minimal. Intensified research efforts have been made to obtain a drug-sensitive human myeloma cell line capable of fusing with human B-lymphocytes. Olsson and Kaplan have reported the establishment of human–human hybridomas that produce MAbs against the hapten dinitrophenol.[30]

C.   Large-scale production

The need for a successful large-scale MAb production technique is indicated by the growing commercial market for antibody-based products and the increased importance of *in vivo* diagnostic as well as therapeutic applications.[31] According to market research, total sales of *in vivo* and *in vitro* MAb-based products reached approximately \$8 billion in 1993, and this volume is expected to increase in subsequent years. Therefore, significant commercial production of MAbs is emphasized and Cortesis and Proby[32] have described the scale-up production of MAbs. In their procedure, MAb-producing murine hybridomas were cultured in 2-L and 40-L working-volume airlift bioreactors. Batch and semicontinuous culture protocols were used successfully, and ultimate cell density, viability, and monoclonal antibody productivity using these systems were found to compare favorably with results obtained by the conventional small-scale culture method described previously.[33,34]

III. Drug-monoclonal antibody conjugates for drug targeting

A. Principles

Use of MAbs in targeting cytotoxic drugs to specific tissues has been studied for over 20 years.[35-37] Antibodies have been found to have many applications in the management of human carcinomas, including colorectal, gastric, ovarian, endometrial, breast, lung, and pancreatic.[38-40] Schlom, in his articles on cancer therapy, has compiled a list of considerations when assessing the use of MAbs to treat cancer.[41,42] These are summarized as follows: number of antigen molecules per cell surface; number of cells expressing the reactive antigen in the tumor mass; size of the tumor mass; fate of the antigen-antibody complex (stability on cell surface, internalization, capping, shedding); degree of tumor vascularization; degree of tumor mass infiltration and necrosis; presence and reactivity of circulating antigen in the blood; duration of MAb binding to cell surface; isotype of immunoglobulin (IgG subtypes or IgM); species of immunoglobulin (murine, human, or chimeric recombinant); whole immunoglobulin or fragments (Fab, Fab', F(ab')$_2$); clearance of MAb from blood, excretion, or reticuloendothelial system; dose of MAb used; route of inoculation of MAb (intravenous, intraperitoneal, intralymphatic, or intraarterial); and development of a human immune response to the administered MAb.

If a radiolabeled MAb is used, consideration has to be given to factors such as the ability of the MAb to be labeled with specific radionuclide, specific activity of the radiolabeled MAb, affinity of radiolabeled MAb, depth of tumor from body surface (for tumor localization), time of scanning (for tumor localization), choice of radionuclide, method of linkage of radionuclide to MAb (metabolism and catabolism of MAb-radionuclide complex), and dose fractionation of administered MAb.[43]

Widder et al.[44] have enumerated several requirements for an ideal carrier. The essential requirements are illustrated schematically in Figure 2.1.

B. Drug antibody bonding

For drug targeting using antibodies, it is important that the drug and the antibody retain their respective activities and that the conjugate remains stable

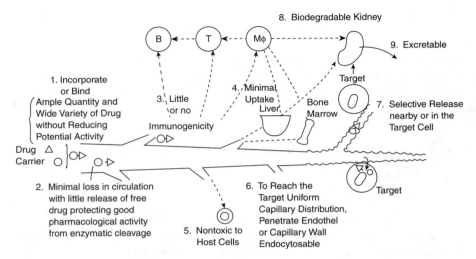

Figure 2.1 Schematic illustration of requirement for drug carriers. (From Bruck, S.D., Ed., *Controlled Drug Delivery*, Vol. II, *Clinical Applications*, CRC Press, Boca Raton, FL, 1983.)

in transit to its target site. In this regard, it is possible that chemical coupling methods may be too drastic or create bonds that are not stable *in vivo*.[26]

Lysine residues occur abundantly in immunoglobulins, with the epsilon amino side chain, the commonly preferred site for drug conjugation.[45] Binding of a drug to the epsilon amino group of the immunoglobulin near its carboxylic acid group forms a carboxamide bond. If the drug's carboxylic acid group is not responsible for its pharmacological action, then conjugation should not affect efficacy. In studies using chlorambucil, the formation of an ionic complex and not a covalent link is also possible. Gallego et al. have reported that a cis-aconityl linkage gives rise to a stable conjugate in the case of daunomycin and amino sugars.[46]

Drawing general conclusions about drug-to-antibody coupling methods when using monoclonals is fraught with difficulties since one monoclonal antibody may behave quite differently from another. This is evident from the studies using an active azide derivative of a vinca alkaloid to produce vindesine-monoclonal antibody conjugates.[47] It has also become clear that when highly homogeneous monoclonal preparations are used in experiments, each antibody needs to be evaluated individually for any particular type of drug-coupling procedure requiring chemical manipulations.[47] Similar conclusions have been reached when attempting to couple cytosine arabinoside to a MAb recognizing a human T cell.[48]

C.   In vitro *and* in vivo *testing*

Research workers in the field of immunoconjugate targeting have predominantly used *in vitro* test systems to evaluate the potential therapeutic value of their preparations. The advantages of *in vitro* test systems are that many variables can be evaluated for drug targeting using small quantities of conjugate over wide ranges, results can be obtained in a short period of time, and many different target cells can be used. It is known that many drug-antibody conjugates, although highly specific, are less potent than the free drug when tested on cells *in vitro*. When tested *in vivo*, loss of potency can be compensated for by a longer target-site residence time. Studies using vinca alkaloids coupled to monoclonals recognizing human tumor-associated antigens clearly demonstrate this point.

The vincas were originally chosen for coupling because of their high molar potency. It appeared likely that if drug potency could be fully retained in immunoconjugates, then effective doses could be delivered even though the site density on the target cell was not high. An extensive study of vindesine conjugated to monoclonal anti-CEA (carcino-embryonic antigen) has been carried out in which nine different human cell lines were examined for target cytotoxicity *in vitro*. In these studies, it was found that free vindesine was considerably more potent than the conjugate. However, it was also found that conjugates did not affect cells lacking the target antigen CEA, whereas free vindesine failed to discriminate between them.[49,50]

Obviously, a major objective of drug delivery using antibodies is *in vivo* therapy. Therefore, it is important to test preparations *in vivo* even if the *in vitro* potency of conjugates appears poor in comparison with the free drug. In this regard, vindesine conjugated to anti-CEA MAb has been found effective in suppressing a human CEA expressing tumor xenograft in athymic mice.[51,52]

The *in vivo* selectivity of vindesine anti-CEA on cells expressing target antigen can be demonstrated in two ways. First, by reduced systemic toxicity giving rise to an improved therapeutic index, and second, by lack of effect on a tumor not expressing CEA. These efforts support the view that targeted site-specific drug delivery has been achieved.[53] However, direct evidence has not been available until recently. To overcome this aspect, a series of experiments was carried out in which the *in vivo* distribution of a radiolabeled drug was determined in tumor-bearing mice using either free vindesine or vindesine conjugated to monoclonal anti-CEA or to an irrelevant monoclonal. The results confirmed that drug delivery was target-site selective when the anti-CEA antibody was used. When tumor- or tissue-to-plasma ratios of a labeled drug were examined, it was found that up to ten times as much drug accumulated in the tumor as normal tissues when delivered in the form of a specific antibody conjugate. In contrast, no selective uptake was observed with either a free drug or a conjugate-involving irrelevant antibody.

Several aspects of these findings are of considerable importance when labeled drugs are used.[54,55] First, the concentration of drug accumulated at the target site remains high for several days. This is probably due to the long biological half-life of the antibody. Second, the high tumor selectivity of the conjugated drug is observed over a wide range of dose levels. From these experiments, it has been possible to calculate the amount of drug delivered to the tumor in its conjugated form as compared to free drug. It appears that increased quantity of drug delivered to the tumor as an antibody conjugate may compensate for apparent loss of potency due to conjugation. According to Rowland,[12] this may explain why the *in vivo*-effective dose levels of free and conjugated drug are more similar than those obtained *in vitro*.

As cited by Rowland in his studies,[12] although the dose of conjugated vindesine that can be administered is considerably higher than that of free drug in studies using human tumor xenografts, it is important to determine the acute toxicity from which an LD_{50} dose can be calculated. In one study, the type of toxicity normally associated with many anticancer drugs, namely bone marrow depression, damage to cells of the gastrointestinal mucosa, or neurotoxicity, was completely absent from mice treated with high doses of conjugated vindesine. This suggests, therefore, that toxicity reduction of many drug-antibody conjugates may be the result of uptake by the reticuloendothelial system (RES).[12] Studies utilizing radiolabeled vindesine-antibody conjugates do indicate an accumulation of drug in the liver and spleen.

Polyclonals and MAbs have been used in radioimmunoimaging in recent years. Ford et al.[56] used a conjugated vindesine and polyclonal sheep anti-CEA preparation that had been shown previously to localize in tumors of patients with gastrointestinal malignancies. This study demonstrated that radiolocalization of the antibody was still possible despite the presence of the conjugated drug. Therefore, it may be possible that an antibody capable of imaging a patient's tumor will also deliver a drug, such as vindesine, to the target site. In one patient with high circulating levels of CEA, tumor biopsy after injection of iodine-labeled antibody conjugate showed nearly five times the radioactivity in the tumor than in surrounding normal tissue. Thus, the presence of circulating CEA did not prevent localization of conjugate.[57]

Antibody toxin conjugates *in vitro* have been found to be highly selective in killing cells bearing the appropriate antigen. For example, Blythman and co-workers have found that murine MAbs of the IgM class directed against the Thy 1.2 differentiation antigen of mouse T cells, when coupled with ricin-A chain, killed mouse leukemia cells carrying the same antigen.[58,59] Cytotoxic activity of the MAb and toxin-subunit conjugate, called immunotoxin, was specific since it did not have an effect against Thy 1.1 cells. Corresponding studies carried out *in vivo* demonstrated prolonged survival time in mice treated with immunotoxin and suggest the potential use of immunotoxin as a highly sensitive test system for studies relating to the treatment of cancer. In the past, several investigators have attempted to use antibodies to target the toxic activity of cytotoxic drugs to tumor cells, but lack of high-titer antibody against specific cell-surface antigens has been a major limiting factor in their use. With these antibodies, it is possible to know which class, subclass, or antibody fragments may be more efficient in promoting the productive internalization of covalently coupled toxin.[60]

Hybridoma antibodies have been used successfully to enhance renal allografts in rats.[61,62] This is the first *in vivo* demonstration whereby passively transferred allo-antibodies against major histocompatibility determinants were fully capable of inducing a state of immunological enhancement.

Cosimi et al.[63] have shown that a MAb to OKT4, an antigen on T inducer cells, had an immunosuppressive effect when given to monkeys and produced prolonged kidney graft survival. Results obtained with conventional antisera have suggested a potential role for antibody therapy, but the success of this approach has been difficult to assess because of the limited quantities of high-titer antibody of appropriate class, affinity, and specificity.[64,65]

Bernstein et al. have used a MAb against a normal differentiation antigen (Thy-1) for the treatment of murine leukemia of spontaneous origin.[66] A MAb-to-rabies virus has been shown to be protective in mice against infection with lethal doses of rabies virus.[66]

Possible application of MAbs in direct therapy against parasites is also under investigation.[67,68] In this respect, two potential kinds of roles can be envisioned for MAbs: first, monoclonal antibody-cytotoxic drug conjugates could be used to carry the drug to the target parasite, thus concentrating the drug's effect. Second, it may be feasible to produce MAbs against parasite antigens that will themselves find and attack the invading parasites, thus intervening in the life cycle of the parasitic organism.

The potential of MAbs in combating malaria has been shown by two research groups.[67,69] One group developed MAbs to surface antigens of *Plasmodium berghei*, which interfered with rodent malaria infection at the sporozoite or marozoite stage. One MAb was of the IgG subclass directed against a protein antigen (Pb44) that is present on the surface membranes of sporozoites. This antibody abolished the infectivity of the parasites in both *in vivo* and *in vitro* studies. Perrin et al. have reported that a monoclonal antibody against *Plasmodium falciparum* can inhibit infection by this parasite in cell cultures of human erythrocytes.[69]

An extensive study of a spectrum of MAbs against *P. falciparum* will help to define antigens required for protection and effective mechanisms of immunity. With the use of these MAbs, it will be possible to purify potentially protective antigens of *P. berghei*, *P. falciparum*, and other parasites. However, because obtaining large quantities of *Plasmodium* antigens is not practical, it may be desirable to utilize recombinant technology to produce defined malarial antigens. In this respect, MAbs will be extremely useful for identifying bacterial colonies secreting the desired antigens. MAbs specific for schistosomal antigens, *Theileria parva*, and *Toxoplasma gondii*, which can be used diagnostically, have also been reported.[69–72]

Table 2.1 presents a partial list of MAb-technology-based research and development firms, their products, and usage.[73]

IV. Recent studies with monoclonal antibodies

A. Highlights of current research

Several investigators have prepared "second-generation" MAbs. In this process, the MAb first evaluated was used to purify the target antigen, which was then used as an immunogen to prepare a new generation of MAbs that

Table 2.1 Monoclonal antibodies

Corporation	Product	Usage
Damon Biotech	Encapsel Technology encapsulating living insulin producing cells	Production of insulin
Monoclonal Antibodies, Inc.	Ophthalmological diagnostic tests	Identification of agents responsible for ocular infections
Ortho Pharmaceutical Co.	Orthoclone OKT3	Prevent rejection of new kidney
Centocor	HA-1A Centoxin endotoxin MAb Myoscint	Gram-negative sepsis Septic shock Detect spread of melanoma, thrombolytic therapy, cardiac imaging
Biogen	CD4 agent	In AIDS
NeoRx	Oncotrac	Detect spread of melanomas
Genentech	CD4 agent Oncogene	In AIDS Breast and ovarian cancer
Cetus	Prolenkin (interleukin-2)	Anticancer
Amgen	Epogen (Erythropoeitin)	Stimulates RBC formation
IDEC	3C9 Murine anti-idiotype inhibitor	In HIV-infected patients
Cytogen	MAbs targeting, breast, colorectal, and ovarian tumors	Anticancer Imaging agents
Xoma	E5 (Xomen) Monoclonal IgM anti-antibody against endotoxin XomaZyme H-65 and 791	Septic shock Gram-negative sepsis for transplant situations and autoimmune diseases
Allergen	Regulatory anti-ALG-991 (Murine MAb)	To modulate allergic disorders (e.g., asthma, allergic rhinitis, poison ivy, and oak allergies) To reverse sensitivity to urushiol in mice
Immunomedics	ImmuRAID-AFP	Detect germ cell tumors
Cell Genesys	Developing technology to produce human–human MAbs in mice	For transferring human genes into mice and to map the human genome
Cantab	LM.CD45	Used in kidney transplants

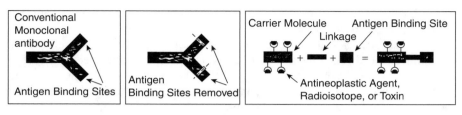

Figure 2.2 Second-generation monoclonal antibodies. (Reprinted with permission from *Drug Topics*, Medical Economics Co., June 2, 1986.)

were reactive with that molecule. However, *a priori* reasons exist for the assumption that the first MAb directed against a given tumor antigen will be the best. Amino acid sequence data obtained from purified antigen of DNA sequences obtained from cloned genes that code for these antigens provide sufficient information for the preparation of synthetic peptides and the subsequent development of MAbs of predefined specificity (see Figure 2.2).

A conjugate of a MAb and the anticancer agent desacetyl vinblastin has been found to recognize lung, colorectal, breast, ovarian, and prostate tumors.[74] MAbs have also been used in trials designed to control the common cold. In this case, the MAbs do not attack the cold virus directly. Instead, they interact with receptors on the surface of the epithelial cells lining the nasal passages. By blocking these receptors, the MAbs prevent viral entry.[75]

Antigenic heterogeneity has been a major consideration in the therapy of solid tumors. Unlike many antigens that are associated with leukemias, lymphomas, and melanomas, many of the oncofetal antigens associated with pancarcinomas are not always expressed in all cells within a given tumor mass. Studies have demonstrated that recombinant α-(clone A), β-ser, and γ-interferons can regulate the expression of certain tumor-associated antigens, such as CEA and TAG-72. These studies have also shown that when cells do not express CEA or TAG-72 — as in the case of normal cells and noncarcinomas, such as melanoma — the exposure of these cells to recombinant interferons does not affect antigen expression.

It has also been reported that interferons can up-regulate tumor targeting of radiolabeled MAbs in an *in vivo* animal model and in clinical trials. Preclinical studies have demonstrated that recombinant interferons can increase both the amount of tumor antigen expressed by a given tumor cell and the percentage of tumor cells that express the antigen. Thus, together with MAb combinations, radionuclides can kill several cell diameters, and the use of recombinant interferons and antigenic heterogeneity of tumor masses can be addressed.[74]

I[125]-labeled MAb B72.3 has been used in radioimmunoguided surgery (RIGS) to localize up to 70% of colorectal carcinoma lesions. Significantly, RIGS also reportedly identified tumors not detected by conventional surgical procedures in 20% of the cases. The RIGS diagnostic procedure also identifies those patients whose tumors are targeted by a given MAb; therefore, the procedure can be used to select patients who are more likely to respond to a specific MAb therapy.[76]

Another drug that has been experimentally piggybacked on MAbs is urokinase, the thrombolytic agent. Urokinase is not a clot-specific agent — it causes the breakdown of fibrinogen, a property that leaves open the possibility of major bleeding problems in patients. Laboratory workers have now succeeded in attaching urokinase to antibodies against fibrin.[77]

The method for dissolving blood clots that cause myocardial infarction is based upon a specially designed MAb that activates clot-dissolving chemicals only at the site of the clot. In theory, the new technique should dissolve blood clots with less risk of bleeding occurring in other parts of the body, as can happen with current clot dissolvers. It also could reduce or even eliminate the use of manufactured clot dissolvers, utilizing instead clot-dissolving substances naturally present in the body.

The basic strategy behind this is to take the antibody that interacts with fibrin and use it to concentrate the natural clot dissolver directly on the clot. One major natural clot dissolver is known as tissue plasminogen activator, or TPA. TPA activates plasminogen that ordinarily lies latent in the blood. Once activated, plasminogen triggers a chemical chain reaction that destroys fibrin and dissolves the blood clot. Current artificially produced versions of the clot dissolvers are infused into the bloodstream where they promote a freer flow of blood throughout the body. However, this is done at the risk of causing hemorrhage, something that should be minimized by the antibody, which should trigger the clot-dissolving reaction only in the vicinity of the clot.[78]

Other examples of studies using MAbs include agents such as immunoabsorbents, hypolipemics, cytokines, porphyrins, antiferritin, and Techniclone (Lym-1). In addition, significant products involving the use of recombinant technology and genetic engineering are: Recombivax HB (a recombinant hepatitis-B vaccine), kidney plasminogen activator, Eminase (anisylated-plasminogen-streptokinase-activator complex), alpha-2 interferon (Intron A), alpha-A interferon (Refron-A), beta interferon (Betaseron), alpha-1 antitrypsin (AAT), and Activase (recombinant version of t-PA).[78]

The IgG murine MAb Alz-50 has been derived from a mouse immunized with homogenates of postmortem ventral forebrain tissue from four patients with Alzheimer's disease. Hybridoma cell-culture supernatants were initially screened based on the comparison of their binding to Alzheimer's brain homogenates immobilized onto polyvinyl plates with identically prepared control homogenates. Alz-50 was described as recognizing an antigen in the affected region of the Alzheimer brain that was elevated 15 to 30 times. Immunocytochemical analysis of the antibody revealed it labeled Alzheimer neurofibrillary tangles, as well as selective neuronal populations.[79]

Many procedures have been reported for coupling anthracycline drugs to an antibody for drug targeting. A recent report describes a new coupling procedure that uses an activated daunorubicin derivative that is later added to the antibody. Utilizing this procedure produced no significant polymerization of the conjugate and a full recovery of pharmacological activity as tested *in vitro* on CEA-producing human colon adenocarcinoma cells. Activated drug was found stable for one week at 25°C, and the coupling procedure is highly reproducible.[80]

Molecules, such as antibodies that bind to cell surfaces, can be used to deliver cytotoxic drugs to selected cells. To be effective, the drug must usually be taken into the cells by endocytosis. Yemul et al. have reported that a T-cell line (CCRF-CEM) was effectively suppressed by liposomes carrying a photosensitizer and bearing the antibody OKT4 (anti-CD4).[81] A procedure has also been described whereby a photosensitizer, benzoporphyrin-derivative monoacid ring (BPD-MA), is covalently linked to a MAb in a manner that is reproducible, quantifiable, and retains both the biological activity of the antibody and the cytotoxicity of the photosensitizer. Preliminary steps involve linking BPD-MA to a modified polyvinyl alcohol (PVA) backbone, followed by conjugation to the antibody using heterobifunctional-linking technology.[82]

Specific binding to human ovarian adenocarcinomas of a drug-antibody conjugate (daunorubicin DNR-OC-125) made from a new analog (PIPP-DNR) of daunorubicin that chemically links the drug to monoclonal antibodies has been studied. Immunofluorescence data show that the DNR-OC-125 conjugate has high affinity and specificity for proliferating malignant cells from human ovarian tumors. The results further demonstrate that the DNR-OC-125 conjugate retains specific binding to CA-125 antigenic sites characteristic of the OC-125 monoclonal antibody moiety. The DNR-OC-125 conjugate selectively binds to CA-125 antigen-positive ovarian cancerous tissue in both cryostat and paraffin-embedded tissue sections. These results indicate that the OC-125 monoclonal antibody can serve as a cancer-targeting carrier for daunorubicin and its analogs.[83]

Bifunctional antibodies (BFA) and enzyme-conjugated antibodies (ECA) can be used to preferentially deliver a hapten or drug to tumor sites for diagnosis and therapy. The authors present here a simple pharmacokinetic model for the two systems by considering only two compartments: the plasma and tumor. The models predict that the longer the time delay between the BFA and hapten or between the ECA and prodrug injections, the higher the tumor-to-plasma-concentration ratio of the hapten drug.[78]

Cis-diamminedichloroplatinum (II) (Cis-Pt) has been complexed to a carboxymethyl dextran-avidin conjugate and targeted to biotin-monoclonal antibody 108(b-MAb108). This MAb recognizes the extracellular domain of the epidermal growth-factor receptor. The results presented in this preliminary investigation suggest that Pt-dex-Av is specifically removed from the circulation by b-MAb108 concentrated at the tumor site.[84]

Antibodies, because of their inherent specificity, appear to be ideal agents for recognizing and destroying malignant cells. However, MAbs, as currently constituted, still have certain inherent limitations. Transfectomas provide an approach to overcoming some of these limitations. Genetically engineered antibodies can be expressed following gene transfection into lymphoid cells.

One of the major advantages of these antibodies is that one is not limited to naturally occurring antibodies. In particular, nonimmunoglobulin sequences can be joined to antibody sequences, thus creating multifunctional chimeric antibodies. In this way, growth factor binding capacity can be joined to a combining specificity, which may be useful in improving targeting therapy to malignant cells and delivering drugs into specific locales in the human body. The presence of the growth factor may also facilitate transcytosis of chimeric antibody across the blood–brain barrier using growth factor receptors. These novel chimeric antibodies may constitute a new family of immunotherapeutic molecules for cancer therapy.[76]

5-Fluorouridine (FUR), an antineoplastic agent, has been conjugated to the carbohydrate moiety of an anticarcinoembryonic antigen (CEA) MAb by using amino-dextran as the intermediate carrier. In the GW-39/nude mouse model, the conjugate remains efficient in targeting the human colonic tumor and possesses greater inhibitory growth effects on this subcutaneous tumor than free FUR or an irrelevant antibody conjugate. In addition, reduced host toxicity of the conjugate may permit its use in a high-dose therapy of this tumor system.[85]

Polyethylene glycol (PEG) modification of the MAb A7 has been found to enhance tumor localization. The F(ab')2 fragment of murine MAb A7 has been covalently bonded. PEG and the conjugate have been compared to the parent F(ab')2 fragment in *in vitro* and *in vivo* studies. PEG-conjugated antibody fragment was found to retain its antigen-binding activity in a competitive radioimmunoassay. The conjugate had a longer half-life and showed increased accumulation in tumors. Although the tumor:blood ratio for the parent F(ab')2 fragment was higher than that for the conjugate, it later showed a higher value than the whole MAb A7. Tissue:blood ratios were kept low with the conjugate, indicating that it was taken up in normal organs to a lesser extent as compared with the parent F(ab')2 fragment. These findings indicate that the PEG-conjugated F(ab')2 fragment may be a promising carrier for use in targeting cancer chemotherapy.[86]

The pharmacokinetics of a disulfide-linked conjugate of a murine monoclonal antibody A7 with neocarcinostatin (A7-NCS) has been studied following its intravenous administration to nude mice. The conjugate was removed from the blood circulation with a half-life of 12 hr, showing nearly the same kinetics as the free antibody. A7-NCS remained stable in the circulation and able to reach the target tumor without releasing significant free NCS.[87]

N-(2-Hydroxypropyl)methacrylamide (HMPA) copolymers have seen extensive development as lysosomotropic drug carriers. They can be used for site-specific drug delivery by incorporation of appropriate targeting groups. Specifically, they have been conjugated to antitumor MAbs murine IgG, antibody 872.3, and its F(ab') and F(ab')2 fragments. Conjugates were synthesized containing an average of 5 copolymer units (MW 20kD) per antibody molecule and achieved prolonged circulation in the bloodstream.[88]

Three novel prodrugs have been designed for use as anticancer agents. Each is a bifunctional alkylating agent that has been protected to form a relatively inactive prodrug. These prodrugs are designed to be activated to their corresponding alkylating agents at a tumor site by prior administration of an antitumor antibody conjugated to the bacterial enzyme carboxypeptidase G2 (CPG2) in a two-phase system called antibody-directed enzyme prodrug therapy (ADEPT). The potential of a tumor-localized bacterial enzyme to activate protected alkylating agents in order to eradicate an established human xenograft has been demonstrated.[89] Murine MAb A7 directed against human colon cancer has been chemically modified using methoxy-polyethylene glycol (MPEG). A high substitution of PEG molecules on MAb A7 produces a progressive reduction in antibody-binding activity. The pharmacokinetic and immunological properties of MPEG-modified MAb A7 and the MPEG-modified F(ab')2 fragment, which retained their antibody-binding activity, have been compared with parent MAb A7 and the F(ab')2 fragment.

Blood clearance of MPEG-modified antibodies appears to be diminished by MPEG modification and fits a two-compartment model. Low MPEG-substituted MAb A7 showed less organ uptake in the liver and spleen and similar uptake in the lung and kidney when compared with the parent MAb A7. Both preparations exhibited less tissue:blood ratios in all respective organs as compared with parent antibodies. Tumor localization was enhanced by MPEG modification of the F(ab')2 fragment, but not by MPEG modification for the whole MAb A7. Multiple intravenous administrations of MPEG-modified antibody to rabbits did not appear to elicit a measurable immune response. In conclusion, MPEG-modified antibodies are promising reagents as drug carriers to the target tumor.[90]

Two murine MAbs have been produced to losartan (DuP 753), a non-peptide angiotensin II receptor antagonist. Using a solid-phase competitive enzyme-linked immunosorbent assay (ELISA), each antibody was examined for its ability to bind to a set of losartan analogs that differ structurally to varying degrees. Both antibodies distinguished fine structural changes in the analogs, particularly at the R5 position of the imidazole ring. No cross-reactivity toward either antibody was observed with the natural ligand angiotensin II, the peptide antagonist saralsin, or the AT2 selective nonpeptide antagonist.[91]

According to Goldenberg,[77] radionuclides, such as I and Tc, are used in antibody imaging. Radioactive antibodies have been found to be safe in over 10,000 patients studied worldwide. On a tumor-site basis, results from 60% to over 90% have been reported, with the highest accuracy rates occurring in MAbs labeled with ^{131}I, ^{123}I, and [99m]Tc. Other selected isotopes for antibody therapy are [90]yttrium, [186]rhenium, [188]rhenium, [67]copper, [211]astatine, and [125]iodine. Tumors as small as 0.5 cm have been identified using ^{99m}Tc-MAbs, especially with emission tomography, but resolution is usually in the range of 1.0 to 2.0 cm. Antibody imaging has revealed tumors missed by other methods, including computed tomography. Antibody imaging can be positive even before the antigen titer in the blood is elevated. Complexation with circulating antigen does not compromise antibody imaging.

Cyclosporin and cyclophosphamide show a significant efficacy in most autoimmune diseases. However, their effects are dependent on continuous drug administration, which can present varied risks of toxicity, such as immunosuppression. Results recently obtained in animal models and discussed by Bach, particularly with anti-CD3 and anti-CD4 monoclonal antibodies, indicate that reestablishment of tolerance to self-antigens is a feasible goal.[92]

Experimental models of autoimmune diseases have demonstrated that such diseases can be prevented or treated by selectively interfering with the activation of any of the following cell types: antigen-presenting cells, autoreactive T cells, and regulatory T cells. Adorini et al. discuss these approaches to selective immunosuppression and examine how similar strategies may become applicable to the treatment of human autoimmune diseases.[93]

MAbs have potential as useful immunosuppressive agents. Short treatment courses with CD4/CD8 MAb can be used to guide the immune system of experimental animals to accept organ grafts and to arrest autoimmunity. This reprogramming has been reviewed by Wildmann and Cobbold, and is accompanied by potent T cell-dependent "infectious" regulatory mechanisms. A goal for therapeutic immunosuppression should be to understand and harness these innate immunoregulatory mechanisms.[94]

Hybridoma technology has enabled rodent MAbs to be created against human pathogens and cells. However, these have limited clinical utility. A strategy to develop effective antibodies for treating infectious disease, autoimmune disease, and cancer involves "humanizing" rodent antibodies. Humanized antibodies have improved pharmacokinetics, reduced immunogenicity, and have been used to clinical advantage.[95]

As mentioned previously, liposomes have a specific liquid-crystalline phase-transition temperature (Tc) at which they release an entrapped drug. Temperature-sensitive liposomes containing adriamycin (TS-Lip-ADM) have been made of dipalmitoylphosphatidylcholine, distearoylphosphatidylcholine, cholesterol, and adriamycin and conjugated with MAbs against human alphafetoprotein. When the liposomal suspension of ADM is immersed in a water bath, the release rate of ADM from TS-Lip-ADM-Ab also increases as the temperature increases from 34 to 42°C.[96]

Following the identification of antibodies as agents of immunity, it was hypothesized that individuals could be both protected against disease by the transfer of unmodified antibody (passive immunization), and cured of established disease by antibody armed with cytotoxic agents (immunotherapy). Although passive immunization has been practiced with great success for many years, successful tissue targeting by systemically delivered immunotoxins in humans has been documented in only a few cases. New modes of drug delivery, engineered for MAb-based products, may enable new applications of passive immunization and may provide improved tissue targeting for immunotherapy.[97]

Liposomes bearing surface-attached antibody (L-Ab) have been prepared to deliver dideoxyinosine triphosphate (ddITP) to human monocyte/macrophages. A mouse MAb (IgG[2a]) was modified using succinimidyl pyridyl dithiopropionate (SPDP) as a heterobifunctional reagent in order to conjugate the antibody to liposomes through a covalent (thioether) bond. Uptake of L-Ab by human monocyte/macrophages was measured as a function of time and compared to liposomes prepared with and without MPB-PE and free ddITP. It was concluded from these studies that the delivery of ddITP could be increased by surface-attached antibody.[74]

Dillman[107] reported on basic concepts and recent developments using monoclonal antibodies. Antibodies can serve as guiding and targeting systems for cytotoxic pharmaceutical products, such as radiolabeled antibodies,[107] for radioimmunodetection and radioimmunotherapy, immunotoxins, chemotherapy/antibody conjugates, cytokine/antibody conjugates, and immune cell/antibody conjugates. Interferon-alpha, interleukin-2 (IL-2), and various hematopoietic growth factors have important significance in biological therapy.

The advances in MAb production encouraged the initial concept of using cancer cell-specific "image bullets." A variety of agents (e.g., toxins, radionuclides, and chemotherapeutic agents) have been conjugated to mouse and human MAbs for selective delivery to neoplastic cells.[108]

Recently, MAbs that block activation of the EGFr and ErbB2 have been developed. These MAbs have shown promising preclinical activity, and "chimeric" and "humanized" MAbs have been produced in order to obviate the problem of host immune reactions.[109]

Trastuzumab, a humanized anti-ErbB2 MAb, was found active and was recently approved in combination with paclitaxel for the therapy of patients with metastatic ErbB2-overexpressing breast cancer. IMC-C225, a chimeric anti-EGFr MAb, demonstrated considerable activity when combined with radiation therapy and was found to reverse resistance to chemotherapy.[110]

Ozogamicin (Mylotarg) employs the antibody-targeted chemotherapy (ATC) strategy and has been approved by the U.S. Food and Drug Administration (FDA) for the treatment of CD33+ acute myeloid leukemia.[111]

Radiolabeled antitumor vascular endothelium monoclonal antibody (TES-23) was assessed in various tumor-bearing animals. This compound accumulated in KMT-17 fibrosarcoma. In meth-A fibrosarcoma, colon-26 adenocarcinoma in BALB/C mice and HT-1080 human tumor tissue in nude mice, radioactivities of 125I-TES-23 were up to 50 times higher than those of control antibody with insiginficant distribution to normal tissues. An immunoconjugate, composed of TES-23 and neocarzinostatin, was tested for its antitumor effect *in vivo*. TES-23-NCS, the immunoconjugate, caused a marked regression of tumor KMT-17 in rats and meth-A in mice.

Using hybridoma fusion, chemical characterization, or molecular biology technology, antibodies with dual specificity can be constructed. The so-called biospecific antibodies (BsAbs) have been used to redirect the cytolytic activity of a variety of immune-effector cells, such as cytotoxic T lymphocytes, natural killer cells, neutrophils, and monocytes/macrophages to tumor cells. Local administration of BsAbs, either alone or in combination with analogous effector cells, has been found highly effective in eradicating tumor cells.[112]

Clinical use of monoclonal antibodies that were produced against the cytokines and adhesion molecules, such as IL-1, IL-6, IG-6R, TNF-alpha, and CD4 molecules, was found effective for the treatment of rheumatoid arthritis. However, these therapeutic agents were also found to exhibit several disadvantages, such as transient efficacy and undesirable side effects.[113]

Takayanagi et al.[114] reported on the "immunogene" system for the targeted delivery of therapeutic genes. In their study, the immunogene system utilizes the EGF receptor-mediated endocytosis. The Fab fragment of MAb B4G7 against human EGF factor was conjugated with polyglycine to form a "Fab-immunoporter," which forms an affinity complex with DNA. The transfection efficiency of Fab immunogene was approximately tenfold higher than the lipofectin. Gene transfer of HSV-tk gene into A431 tumor cells with Fab-immunoporter was successful, and the subsequent treatment with ganciclovir induced remarkable side effects, conferring thousandfold higher drug sensitivity. According to these authors, their data demonstrated that the immunogene system could be useful as a gene transfer vehicle targeting the EGF receptor hyperproducing tumor cells.

Over the years, delivery of monoclonal antibodies has developed some problems, especially in their pharmacokinetic aspects. These include slow elimination of monoclonal antibodies from the blood and poor vascular permeability, low and heterogeneous tumor uptake, cross-reactivity with normal tissues, metabolism of monoclonal antibody conjugates, and immunogenicity of murine forms in humans. Progress has been made in solving these problems (e.g., tumor retention of antibody conjugates may be improved by inhibition of metabolism), and by using stable-linkage chemistry, normal tissue retention may be decreased through the use of metabolizable chemical linkages inserted between the antibody and the conjugated moiety.[115]

V.   Conclusion and basis for future trends

It is becoming apparent that work on the use of MAbs for drug targeting is progressing steadily toward increased clinical use.[98] The applications developed at present have been primarily in cancer chemotherapy, where the greatest need arises for site-specific drug delivery. MAbs are also increasingly used in heart disease, multiple sclerosis, disorders of the immunological defense system, and viral, bacterial, and rickettsial infections. Since each MAb is directed against a single determinant, it attains a finer, more specific recognition of its antigen than conventional antibodies. Investigators have been using MAbs as exquisitely sensitive probes to guide drugs to target cells or organs. As more and more MAbs directed against normal and tumor cells are generated, it will be possible to have a spectrum of these antibodies. Each of these will identify a distinct molecular determinant on the cell surface to better define the stages of lymphoid cell differentiation, for example, as well as a more precise and reliable classification of cell malignancies and immunodeficiencies in humans.[99–101]

MAbs are also being standardized as pure reagents, thereby replacing conventionally made tissue-typing reagents. These MAbs have undoubtedly helped to develop more rational therapeutic strategies for the treatment and prognosis of certain diseases. MAbs by themselves or in combination with surgery have a strong potential for immunotherapy of serum hepatitis, leukemias, etc.

MAbs have opened up new immunodiagnostic markets for identifying various leukemic and lymphoma cell populations, characterization of isoenzymes, hemoglobins, α-1-antitrypsins, lymphokines, hormones, hepatitis-associated antigens, carcinoembryonic antigens, assays for therapeutic drug and drug-abuse monitoring, and specific protein immunoassays. Since they are well-defined chemical reagents, MAbs have great potential for practical applications either by their direct use or through their utilization in drug development.

The production of human monoclonals of predefined human-target site specificity by hybridoma technology has achieved limited success. As anticipated, the immunogenicity of human target structures is different in humans than in other species, and although *in vitro* immunization techniques can work, they have so far failed to produce useful antitumor human monoclonals. It is likely that in the future, modern techniques of molecular gene cloning will be used to produce the required structures. Experiments have been described demonstrating the feasibility of using recombinant DNA technology to produce chimeric antibody molecules in which the antigen-combining site is derived from a mouse myeloma and the constant region of the molecule is derived from human immunoglobulin.[102–104]

Improvements in the supply of immune lymphocytes are feasible, both for immunization protocols and lymphocyte-selection procedures. Of clinical importance are the advances made in *in vitro* immunization procedures. However, a number of factors require extensive investigation before *in vitro* immunization can be fully exploited. These include the source of lymphoid cells, the dose and form of immunogen, the influence of mitogens and adjuvants, the value of growth and differentiation factors, and optimum culture time. The most widely used immortalization procedures have been EBV, transformation and cell fusion, or a combination of these procedures. However, it is possible that these procedures are still far from optimal. Meanwhile, considerable effort has been directed toward improving the levels of antibody secreted by human cell lines and ensuring that high levels of secretion are sustained. This observation may partly be due to improvements in immunization, selection, and immortalization. The most obvious approach has been to frequently enrich antibody-secreting cell lines and pursue a rigorous cloning policy.

A less conventional approach to human MAb production has been the application of gene cloning strategies, but the results have nonetheless been encouraging. So far, complete immunoglobulin molecules have been produced using conventional recombinant procedures employing vectors. Another less sophisticated strategy has been to transfect the antibody-secreting cells. Other advances in this technique for producing antibodies have also indicated considerable potential, and more research and development work in this area should prove valuable.[75,78,105,106]

As summarized by Rowland,[12] it is the specificity conferred by antibody molecules that is now exploited for novel methods of therapy. Without doubt, advances in cellular and molecular biology need to be prudently applied to this area in the years ahead to procure useful site-specific drug delivery systems.

References

1. Ehrlich, P., A general review of the recent work in immunity. In *Collected Papers of Paul Ehrlich*, Vol. 2, *Immunology and Cancer Research 1956*, Pergamon Press, London, 1990, 442.
2. Larson, S.M., Brown, J.P., Wright, P.W., Carrasquillo, J.A., Hellstrom, I., and Hellstrom, K.E., Imaging of melanoma with I-labeled monoclonal antibodies, *J. Nuclear Med.*, 24, 123–129, 1983.
3. Zurawski, V.R., Haber, E., and Black, P.H., Production of antibody to tetanus toxoid by continuous human lymphoblastoid cell lines, *Science*, 199, 1439, 1978.
4. Trout, A., Increased selectivity of drugs by linking to carriers, *Eur. J. Cancer*, 14, 105, 1978.
5. Steinitz, M., Klein, G., Koskimies, S., and Makela, O., EB virus-induced B-lymphocyte cell lines producing specific antibody, *Nature*, 269, 420, 1977.
6. Marguilies, D.H., Kuehl, W.M., and Schraff, M.D., Somatic cell hybridization of mouse myeloma cells, *Cell*, 8, 405, 1976.
7. Kennett, R.H., Denis, K.A., Tung, A.S., and Klinman, N.R., Hybrid plasmacytoma production fusions with adult spleen cells, monoclonal spleen fragments, neonatal spleen cells and human spleen cells, *Curr. Top. Microbiol. Immunol.*, 81, 77, 1978.
8. Kearney, J.F., Redbruck, A., Liesegaug, B., and Rajewskey, K., A new mouse myeloma cell line that has lost immunoglobulin expression but permits the construction of antibody-secreting hybrid cell lines, *J. Immunol.*, 123, 1548, 1979.
9. Birch, J.R., Cells sell, *Chemtech*, 17(6), 378–381, 1987.
10. Schen, W., Chemical aspects of monoclonal antibodies in targeted drug delivery, *Pharm. Tech.*, 32(12), 1988.
11. Rowland, G.F., Davies, D.A.L., O'Neill, G.I., Newman, C.E., and Ford, C.H.J., Specific cancer therapy by drugs synergising with or attached to tumor-specific antibodies: experimental background and clinical results. In *Immunotherapy of Malignant Diseases*, Rainer, H., Ed., Schattauer-Verlag, Stuttgart, 1977, 316–322.
12. Rowland, G.F., Monoclonal antibodies as carriers for drug delivery systems. In *Fundamentals and Techniques*, Johnson, P. and Lloyd-Jones, J.G., Eds., VCH Publishers, Chichester, 1987, 81–94.
13. Brown, J.P., Woodbury, R.G., Hart, C.E., Hellstrom, I., and Hellstrom, K.E., Quantitative analysis of melanoma-associated antigen p97 in normal and neoplastic tissues, *Proc. Nat. Acad. Sci., USA*, 78, 539–543, 1981.

14. Hellstrom, K.E. and Hellstrom, I., Monoclonal antimelanoma antibodies and their possible clinical use. In *Monoclonal Antibodies for Cancer Detection and Therapy*, Baldwin, R.W. and Byerrs, V.S., Eds., Academic Press, London, 1985, 17–51.

15. Mathe, G., Loc, T.B., and Bernard, J., Effet sur la leucemie L1201 de la souris d'une combinaison par diazotation d'A-methopterine et de gamma-globulins de hamsters porteur de cette leucemie par heterogreffe, *Comptes Rendus*, 246, 1626–1628, 1958.

16. Ghose, T., Norwell, S., Guclu, A., Cameron, D., Bodrutha, A., and MacDonald, A.S., Immunotherapy of cancer with chlorambucil-carrying antibody, *Br. Med. J.*, iii, 495, 1972.

17. Hurwitz, E., Maron, R., Bernstein, A., Wilcheck, M., Sela, M., and Arnon, R., The effect *in vivo* of chemotherapeutic drug-antibody conjugates in two murine experimental tumor systems, *Int. J. Cancer*, 21, 747–755, 1978.

18. Hurwitz, E., Maron, R., Wilcheck, M., Arnon, R., and Sela, M., The covalent binding of daunomycin and adriamycin to antibodies with retention of both drug and antibody activities, *Cancer Research*, 35, 1175–1181, 1975.

19. Rowland, G.F., O'Neill, G.I., and Davies, D.A.L., Suppression of tumor growth in mice by a drug-antibody conjugate using a novel approach to linkage, *Nature*, 255, 487–488, 1975.

20. Kadin, S.B. and Otterness, I.G., Antibodies as drug carriers and toxicity-reversal agents, *Ann. Rep. Med. Chem.*, 15, 233–244, 1980.

21. Upselacis, J. and Hinman, L., Chemical modification of antibodies for cancer chemotherapy, *Ann. Rep. Med. Chem.*, 23, 151–160, 1988.

22. Kohler, G. and Milstein, C., Continuous cultures of fused cells secreting antibody of predefined specificity, *Nature*, 256, 495, 1975.

23. Gilliland, D.G., Steplewski, Z., Collier, R.J., Mitchell, K.F., Chang, T.H., and Koprowski, H., Antibody-directed cytotoxic agents: Use of monoclonal antibody to direct the action of toxin A chains to colorectal carcinoma cells, *Proc. Natl. Acad. Sci. USA*, 77, 4539, 1980.

24. Sickle-Santanello, B.J. et al., Radioimmunoguided surgery using monoclonal antibody B72.3 in colorectal tumors, *Dis. Col. Rectum*, 30, 761–764, 1987.

25. Greiner, J.W. et al., Recombinant interferon enhances monoclonal antibody-targeting of carcinoma lesions *in vivo*, *Science*, 235(4791), 895–898, 1987.

26. Rowland, G.F., The use of antibodies and polymer conjugates in drug targeting and synergy. In *Target Drugs*, Goldberg, E., Ed., John Wiley & Sons, New York, 1983, 57–72.

27. Brown, J.P., Noshiyama, K., Hellstrom, I., and Hellstrom, K.E., Structural characterization of human melanoma-associated antigen p97 with monoclonal antibodies, *J. Immunol.*, 127, 539–546, 1981.

28. Jarvis, A.P. Jr., Producing monoclonal antibodies for clinical investigations. In The Latest Developments in Drug Delivery Systems, Conference Proceedings, *Pharm. Tech.*, 11, 48–53, 1987.

29. Holyoke, E.D. and Petrelli, N.J., Tumor markers and monoclonal antibodies: An update, *Medical Times*, 57–63, 1987.

30. Olsson, L. and Kaplan, H., Human-human hybridomas producing monoclonal antibodies of predefined antigenic specificity, *Proc. Nat. Acad. Sci. USA*, 77, 5429, 1980.

31. Kennett, R.H., McKearn, T.J., and Bechtol K.B., Eds., *Monoclonal Antibodies*, Plenum Press, Inc., New York, 1980.

32. Cortesis, G.P. and Proby, C.M., Airlift bioreactors for production of monoclonal antibodies, *Biopharm*, Nov. 1987, 30.
33. Lebherz III, W.B., Batch production of monoclonal antibody by large-scale suspension culture, *Biopharm*, Feb. 1988, 22.
34. Familletti, P.G., Gel-immobilized cell culture for monoclonal antibody production, *Biopharm*, Nov. 1987, 48.
35. Koprowski, G., Steplewski, Z., Herlyn, D., and Herlyn, M., Study of antibodies against human melanoma produced by somatic cell hybrids, *Proc. Nat. Acad. Sci. USA*, 75, 3405, 1978.
36. Carrel, S., Accolla, R.S., Gross, N. and Mach, J.P., Human melanoma-associated antigens identified by monoclonal antibodies. In *Monoclonal S4Antibodies and T-Cell Hybridoma Perspectives and Technological Advances*, Hammerling, G.J., Hammerling, Y., and Kearney, J.F., Eds., Elsevier, Amsterdam, 1981, 174.
37. Imai, K., Wilson, B.S., Kay, N.E. and Ferrone, S., Monoclonal antibodies to human melanoma cells comparison of serological results of several laboratories and molecular profile of melanoma-associated antigens. In *Monoclonal S4Antibodies and T-Cell Hybridoma Perspectives and Technological Advances*, Hammerling, G.J., Hammerling, Y., and Kearney, J.F., Eds., Elsevier, Amsterdam, 1981, 183.
38. Herlyn, M., Steplewski, Z., Herlyn, D., and Koprowski, H., Colorectal carcinoma-specific antigen detection by means of monoclonal antibodies, *Proc. Nat. Acad. Sci. USA*, 76, 1438, 1979.
39. Hellstrom, I., Hellstrom, K.E., Brown, J.P., and Woodbury, R.G., Antigens of human tumors, particularly melanomas, as studied with the monoclonal antibody technique. In *Monoclonal Antibodies and T-Cell Hybridoma Perspectives and Technological Advances*, Hammerling, G.J., Hammerling, Y. and Kearney, J.F., Eds., Elsevier, Amsterdam, 1981, 191.
40. Kennett, R.H. and Gilbert, F., Hybrid myelomas producing antibodies against a human neuroblastoma antigen present on fetal brain, *Science*, 203, 1120, 1979.
41. Schlom, J., Monoclonal antibodies in cancer therapy: the present and the future, *Biopharm*, Sept. 1988, 44–48. (Also see *Pharm. Tech.*, Sept. 1988, 56–60.)
42. Schlom, J. and Weeks, M.O., Potential clinical utility of monoclonal antibodies. In *The Management of Human Carcinomas in Important Advances in Oncology*, DeVita, V., Hellman, S., and Rosenberg, S., Eds., J.B. Lippincott, Philadelphia, 1984, 170–192.
43. Order, S.E., Analysis, results and future prospective of the therapeutic use of radiolabelled antibody in cancer therapy. In *Monoclonal Antibodies for Cancer Detection and Therapy*, Baldwin R.W. and Byers, V.S., Eds., Academic Press, London, 1985, 304–306.
44. Widder, K.J., Senyei, A.E., and Ranney, D.F., Magnetically responsive microspheres and other carriers for the biophysical targeting of antitumor agents, *Adv. Pharmacol. Chemotherapy*, 16, 213, 1979.
45. O'Neill, G.J., The use of antibodies as drug carriers. In *Drug Carriers in Biology and Medicine*, Gregoriadis, G., Ed., Academic Press, Inc., London, 1979, 23–41.
46. Gallego, J., Price, M.R., and Baldwin, R.W., Preparation of four daunomycin-monoclonal antibody 791T/36 conjugates with anti-tumor activity, *Int. J. Cancer*, 33, 737–744, 1984.
47. Rowland, G.F., Use of antibodies to target drugs to tumor cells, *Clinics in Allergy and Immunology*, 8, 2, 235–257, 1983.

48. Arnon, R. and Hurwitz, E., Monoclonal antibodies as carriers for immuno-targeting of drugs. In *Monoclonal Antibodies for Cancer Detection and Therapy*, Baldwin R.W. and Byers, V.S., Eds., Academic Press, London, 1985, 367–383.

49. Hockey, M.S., Stokes, H.J., Thompson, H., Woodhouse, C.S., MacDonald, F., Fielding, J.W.I., and Ford, C.H.I., Carcinoembryonic antigen (CEA) expression and heterogeneity in primary and autologous metastatic gastric tumors demonstrated by a monoclonal antibody, *Br. J. Cancer*, 49, 192–233, 1984.

50. Philpott, G.W., Grass, E.H., and Parker, C.W., Affinity cytotoxicity with an alcohol dehydrogenase-antibody conjugate and allyl alcohol, *Cancer Res.*, 39, 2084, 1979.

51. Rowland, G.F., Corvalan, J.R.F., Axton, C.A., Gore, V.A., Marsden, C.H., Smith, W., and Simmonds, R.G., Suppression of growth of a human colorectal tumor in nude mice by vindesine-monoclonal anti-CEA conjugates, *Protides Biol. Fluids*, 31, 783–786, 1984.

52. Rowland G.F., Axton, C.A., Baldwin, R.W., Brown, J.P., et al., Antitumor properties of vindesine-monoclonal antibody conjugates, *Cancer Immunol. Immunother.*, 19, 1–7, 1988.

53. Rowland, G.F., Simmonds, R.G., Gore, V.A., Marsden, C.H., and Smith, W., Drug localization and growth-inhibition studies of vindesine-monoclonal anti-CEA conjugates in a human tumor xenograft, *Cancer Immunol. Immunother.*, 21, 183–187, 1986.

54. Levy, R. and Dilley, J., Rescue of immunoglobulin secretion from human neoplastic lymphoid cells by somatic cell hybridization, *Proc. Nat. Acad. Sci. USA*, 75, 2411, 1978.

55. Vaughan, A.T.M., Bradwell, A.R., Dykes, P.W. and Anderson, P., Illusions of tumor killing using radiolabelled antibodies, *Lancet*, 1492, 1986.

56. Ford, C.H.J., Newman, C.E., Johnson, J.R., Woodhouse, C.S., et al., Localization and toxicity study of a vindesine-anti-CEA conjugate in patients with advanced cancer, *Br. J. Cancer*, 47, 35–42, 1983.

57. Dykes, P.W., Hine, K.G., Bradwell, A.R., Blackburn, J.C., et al., Localization of tumor deposits by external scanning after injection of radiolabelled anti-carcinoembryonic antigen, *Br. Med. J.*, 280, 220–222, 1980.

58. Jansen, F.K., Blythman, H.E., Carrierre, D., Casellas, P., et al., Assembly and activity of conjugates between monoclonal antibodies and the toxic subunit of ricin (immunotoxins) in monoclonal antibodies, *Proc. Nat. Acad. Sci. USA*, 76, 229, 1979.

59. Blythman, H.E., Casellas, P., Gross, O., Gross, P., et al., Immunotoxins: Hybrid molecules of monoclonal antibodies and a toxin subunit specifically kill tumor cells, *Nature* (London), 290, 145, 1981.

60. McKearn, T.J., Weiss, A., Stuart, F.F., and Fitch, F.W., Eds., Selective suppression of humoral and cell-mediated immune responses to rat alloantibodies by monoclonal antibodies produced by hybridoma cell lines, *Transplant Proc.*, 11, 932, 1979.

61. Melchers, F., Potter, M., and Warnen, N.L., Eds., Lymphocyte hybridomas, *Curr. Top. Microbiol. Immunol.*, 81, 246, 1978.

62. D'Eustachio, P. and Ruddle, F.H., *Current Topics in Developmental Biology*, Vol. 14, Frieldlander, M., Ed., Academic Press, New York, 1980, 59.

63. Cosimi, A.B., Burton, R.C., Kung, P.C., Colvin, R., et al., Evaluation in primate renal allograft recipients of monoclonal antibody to human T-cell, *Transplant Proc.*, 13, 499, 1981.

64. Potocnjak, P., Yoshida, N., Nussenzweig, R.S., and Nussenzweig, V., Monovalent fragments (Fab) of monoclonal antibodies to a sporozoite surface antigen (Pb44) protect mice against malarial infection, *J. Exp. Med.*, 151, 1564, 1980.

65. Witkor, T.J. and Koprowski, H., Monoclonal antibodies against rabies virus produced by somatic cell hybridization: Detection of antigenic variants, *Proc. Nat. Acad. Sci. USA*, 75, 3938, 1978.

66. Bernstein, I.D., Tam, M.R., and Nowinski, R.C., Mouse leukemia therapy with monoclonal antibodies against a thymus differentiation antigen, *Science*, 207, 68, 1980.

67. Tung, A.S., Monoclonal antibodies, *Ann. Rep. Med. Chem.*, 16, 243–255, 1981.

68. Ferrone, S. and Dietrich, M.P., Eds., *Handbook of Monoclonal Antibodies: Applications in Biology and Medicine*, 1985, 477.

69. Perrin, C.H., Ramirez, E., Lambert, P.H., and Miescher, P.A., Inhibition of *P. falciparum* growth in human erythrocytes by monoclonal antibodies, *Nature* (London), 289, 301, 1981.

70. Freeman, R.R., Trejdosiewicz, A.J., and Cross, G.A.M., Protective monoclonal antibodies recognizing stage-specific merozoite antigens of a rodent malaria parasite, *Nature* (London), 284, 366, 1980.

71. Verwaere, C., Grzch, J.M., Bazin, H., Capron, M., and Capron, A., Production d'anticorps monoclonaux anti Schistosoma monsoni Etude preliminaire de Leurs activites biologiques, *CR Acad. Sci. Ser. D.*, 289, 725, 1979.

72. Mitchell, C.F., Cruise, K.M., Chapman, C.B., Anders, R.F., and Howard, M.C., Hybridoma antibody immunoassays for the detection of parasitic infection: Development of a model system using a larval cestode infection in mice, *Aust. J. Exp. Biol. Med. Sci.*, 57, 287, 1979.

73. Pharmaprojects, 1993.

74. Betageri, G.V., Jenkins, S.A., and Ravis, W.R., Drug delivery using antibody-liposome conjugates, *Drug Dev. Ind. Pharm.*, 19/16, 2109–2116, 1993.

75. Goding, J.W., *Monoclonal Antibodies: Principles and Practice*, Academic Press, San Diego, CA, 1986, 315.

76. Shin, S.U., Chimeric antibody: potential applications for drug delivery and immunotherapy, *Biotherapy*, 3, 43–53, 1991.

77. Goldenberg, D.M, New developments in monoclonal antibodies for cancer detection and therapy, *CA Cancer J. Clin.* (U.S.), 44, 43–64, 1994.

78. Oates, K.K., Therapeutic and drug delivery application of monoclonal antibodies, *Targeted Diagn. Ther.*, 3, 99–118, 1990.

79. Wolozin, B.L., Pruchnicki, A., Dickson, D.W., and Davies, P., A neuronal antigen in the brains of Alzheimer patients, *Science*, 232(4750), 648–650, 1986.

80. Page, M., Thibeault, D., Noel, C., and Dumas, L., Coupling a preactivated daunorubicin to antibody, *Anticancer Res.*, 10, 353–357, 1990.

81. Yemul, S., Berger, C., Katz, M. Estabrook, A., et al., Phototoxic liposomes coupled to an antibody, *Cancer Immunol. Immunother.*, 30, 317–322, 1990.

82. Jiang, F.N., Jiang, S., Liu, D., Richter, A., and Levy, J.G., Development of technology for linking photosensitizers, *J. Immunol. Methods*, 134, 139–149, 1990.

83. Dezso, B., Torok, I., Rosik, L.O., and Sweet, F., Human ovarian cancers specifically bind daunorubicin-OC-125 conjugate, *Gynecol. Oncol.*, 39, 60–64, 1990.

84. Schechter, B., Arnon, R., Wilchek, M., Schlessinger, J., et al., Indirect immunotargeting of cis-Pt to human epidermoid carcinoma KB using the avidin-biotin system, *Int. J. Cancer*, 48, 167–172, 1991.

85. Shih, L.B., Xuan, H., Sharkey, R.M., and Goldenberg, D.M., A fluorouri-dine-anti-CEA immunoconjugate is therapeutically effective in a human co-lonic xenograft model, *Int. J. Cancer*, 46, 1101–1106, 1990.

86. Kitamura, K., Takahashi, T., Takahashi, K., Yamagucbi, T., et al., Polyethylene glycol modification of the monoclonal antibody A7 enhances its tumor local-ization, *Biochem. Biophys. Res. Commun.*, 171, 1387–1394, 1990.

87. Kitamura, K., Takahashi, T., Noguchi, A., Tsurumi, H., et al., Pharmacokinetic analysis of the monoclonal antibody A7 neo-carzinostatin conjugate admin-istered to nude mice, *Tohoku J. Exp. Med.*, 164, 203–211, 1991.

88. Seymour, L.W., Flanagan, P.A., al-Shamkhani, A., Subr, V., et al., Synthetic polymers conjugated to monoclonal antibodies: Vehicles for tumor-targeted drug delivery, *Sel. Cancer Ther.*, 7, 59–73, 1991.

89. Springer, C.J., Bagshawe, K.D., Sharma, S.K., Searle, F., et al., Ablation of human choriocarcinoma xenografts in nude mice by antibody-directed en-zyme pro-drug therapy with three novel compounds, *Eur. J. Cancer*, 27, 1361–1366, 1991.

90. Kitamura, K., Takahashi, T., Yamaguchi, T., Noguchi, A., et al., Chemical engineering of the monoclonal antibody A7 by polyethylele glycol, *Cancer Res.*, 51, 4310–4315, 1991.

91. Reilly, T.M., Christ, D.D., Duncia, J.V, Pierce, S.K., and Timmermans, P.B, Monoclonal antibodies to the nonpeptide angiotensin II receptor antagonist, losartan, *Eur. J. Pharmacol.* (Netherlands), 226, 179–182, 1992.

92. Bach, J., Immunosuppressive therapy of autoimmune diseases, *Trends Phar-macol. Sci.* (U.K.), 14, 213–216, 1993.

93. Adorini, L., Guery, J., Rodriguez-Tarduchy, G., and Trembleau, S., Selective immunosuppression, *Trends Pharmacol. Sci.* (U.K.), 14, 178–182, 1993.

94. Wildmann, H. and Cobbold, S., The use of monoclonal antibodies to achieve immunological tolerance, *Trends Pharmacol. Sci.* (U.K.), 14, 143–148, 1993.

95. Winter, G. and Harris, W., Humanized antibodies, *Trends Pharmacol. Sci.* (U.K.), 14, 139–143, 1993.

96. Shibata, S., Kumai, K., Takahashi, T., Murayama, Y., et al., Targeting cancer chemotherapy using temperature-sensitive liposomes containing adriamycin conjugated with monoclonal antibodies, *Gan To Kagaku Ryoho* (Japan), 19 (Suppl. 10), 1671–1674, 1992.

97. Saltzman, W.M., Antibodies for treating and preventing disease: the potential role of polymeric controlled release, *Crit. Rev. Ther. Drug Carrier Syst.* (U.S.), 10, 111–142, 1993.

98. Brown, J., Ed., *Human Monoclonal Antibodies: Current Techniques and Future Perspectives*, IRL, Oxford, 1987.

99. Cohn, M., Langman, R., and Geckler, W. In *Progress in Immunology*, Vol. 4, Fougereau, M., Dausset, J., Eds., Academic Press, New York, 1980, 153.

100. Dennis, K., Kennett, R.H., Klinman, N.R., Molinaro, C., and Sherman. L. In *Monoclonal Antibodies*, Kennett, R.H., McKearn, T.J., and Bechtol, K.B., Eds., Plenum Press, New York, 1980, 49.

101. Solomon, E. and Jones, E.A. In *Monoclonal Antibodies*, Kennett, R.H., McKearn, T.J., and Bechtol, K.B., Eds., Plenum Press, New York, 1980, 75.

102. Handman, E. and Remington, J.S., Monoclonal antibodies diagnostic and therapeutic use. In *Tumor and Transplantation*, Chatterjee, S.N., Ed., PSG Pub-lishing Co., Littleton, MA, 1985.

103. Pinder, M. and Hewerr, R.S., Monoclonal antibodies detect antigenic diversity in *Theileria parva* parasites, *J. Immunol.*, 124, 1000, 1980.
104. Handman, E. and Remington, J.S., Serological and immunochemical characterization of monoclonal antibodies of *Toxoplasma gondii*, *Immunology*, 40, 4, 1980.
105. Begent, R.H., Pedley, R.B., and Begent, J., Monoclonal antibody administration, current clinical pharmacokinetic status and future trends, *Clin. Pharmacokinet.* (New Zealand), 23, 85–89, 1992.
106. Liddell, J.E. and Cryer, A. In *A Practical Guide to Monoclonal Antibodies*, John Wiley & Sons, Chichester, 1991, 206.
107. Dillman, R.O., Monoclonal antibodies in the treatment of malignancy: basic concepts and recent developments, *Cancer Invest.*, 19, 833–841, 2002.
108. Bodey, B., Genetically engineered antibodies for direct antineoplastic treatment and systemic delivery of various therapeutic agents to cancer cells, *Expert Opinons Biol. Ther.*, 1, 603–617, 2002.
109. Mendelsonh, J. and Baselga, J., The EGF receptor family as targets for cancer therapy, *Oncogene*, 19, 6550–6565, 2000.
110. Williams, J.P. and Handler, H.L., Antibody-targeted chemotherapy for the treatment of relapsed acute myeloid leukemia, *Am. J. Manag. Care*, 6(Suppl. 18), S975–S985, 2000.
111. Tsunoda, S., Tsutsumi, Y., et al., Targeting therapy using a monoclonal antibody against tumor vascular endothelium, *Yakugaku Zasshi*, 120, 256–264, 2000.
112. Molema, G., Kroesen, B.J., et al., The use of bispecific antibodies in tumor cell- and tumor vasculature-directed immunotherapy, *J. Control Rel.*, 64, 229–239, 2000.
113. Abe, T. and Takeuchi, T., Monoclonal antibodies as an immunotherapy of rheumatoid arthritis, *Nippon Rinsho*, 56, 776–781, 1998.
114. Takayanagi, A., Chen, J., et al., Targeting delivery of therapeutic genes using monoclonal antibody; immunogene approach, *Nippon Rinsho*, 56, 731–736, 1998.
115. Reilly, R.M., Sandhu, J., et al., Problems of delivery of monoclonal antibodies, pharmaceutical and pharmacokinetic solutions, *Clin Pharmacokin.*, 28, 126–42, 1995.

Polymers, implantable drug delivery

chapter three

Role of polymers in drug delivery*

Contents

* Adapted from Ranade, V.V., Drug delivery systems. 3A. Role of polymers in drug delivery, *J. Clin. Pharmacol.*, 30, 10, 1990; and 3B. Role of polymers in drug delivery, *J. Clin. Pharmacol.*, 30, 107, 1990. With permission of *J. Clin. Pharmacol.* and J.B. Lippincott Publishing Company, Philadelphia, PA.

I.   Introduction

The usefulness of polymers in drug delivery systems is well established. Continued improvement and accelerating research and development in polymeric materials has played a vital role in the progress of most controlled-release technologies. In the past 25 years, there has been a considerable increase in interest in this technology, as is shown by the increasing number of publications and patents in the area of controlled drug-release systems using synthetic as well as naturally occurring polymeric materials.[1–5]

II.   Currently available polymers

Currently available polymers for controlled release can be classified into four major categories: (1) diffusion-controlled systems, (2) solvent-activated systems, (3) chemically controlled systems, and (4) magnetically controlled systems.

A.   Diffusion-controlled systems

Diffusion-controlled systems involve two types: reservoir and matrix. A reservoir is generally spherical, cylindrical, or disc-like in shape and consists of a drug core in powdered or liquid form. A layer of nonbiodegradable polymeric material, through which the drug slowly diffuses, surrounds the core. The properties of the drug and the polymer govern the diffusion rate of the drug and its release rate into the bloodstream. In order to maintain uniformity of drug delivery, the thickness of the polymer must be consistent. One of the problems with the reservoir system is that such a system must be removed from the body after the drug is depleted because the polymer remains intact. Another potential problem is that if the reservoir membrane accidentally ruptures, a large amount of drug may be suddenly released into the bloodstream (known as "drug dumping").

In the matrix type of diffusion-control system, the drug is uniformly distributed throughout the polymer matrix and is released from the matrix at a uniform rate as drug particles dislodge from the polymer network. In such a system, unlike the reservoir, there is no danger of drug dumping in case of an accidental rupture of the membrane.

B.   Solvent-activated systems

Solvent-activated systems are also of two types: osmotically controlled systems and swelling-controlled systems. In the osmotically controlled system, an external fluid containing a low concentration of a drug moves across a semipermeable membrane to a region inside the device, where the drug is in high concentration. Osmotic pressure tends to decrease the concentration gradient between one side of the membrane and the other. The inward movement of fluid forces the dissolved drug out of the device through a small orifice.

In the swelling-controlled systems, the polymer holds a large quantity of water without dissolving. The system consists of hydrophilic macromolecules cross-linked to form a three-dimensional network. A characteristic of such systems is their permeability, for low molecular weight solutes, at a controlled rate as the polymer swells.

C.   Chemically controlled systems

Chemically controlled systems also have two classes: the "pendant-chain" system and the bioerodible, or biodegradable, system. A "pendant chain system" is one in which the drug molecule is chemically linked to the backbone of the polymer. In the body, in the presence of enzymes and biological fluids, chemical hydrolysis, or enzymatic cleavage, occurs with concomitant release of the drug at a controlled rate. The drug may be linked directly to the polymer or via a "spacer group."

In the bioerodible system, the controlled release of the drug involves polymers that gradually decompose. The drug is dispersed uniformly throughout the polymer and is slowly released as the polymer disintegrates. Two major advantages of erodible systems are (1) polymers do not have to be removed from the body after the drug supply is exhausted, and (2) the drug does not have to be water-soluble. In fact, because of these factors, future use of bioerodible polymers is likely to increase more than any other type of polymer in the future.

D.   Magnetically controlled systems

Selective targeting of antitumor agents, while minimizing toxic effects, has been a major goal in cancer chemotherapy. Conventionally used systemic antineoplastic agents are unable to achieve ideal tumor specificity. Magnetically responsive drug carrier systems, composed of albumin and magnetic microspheres, have been developed for use in cancer chemotherapy. Because of their magnetic characteristics, these microspheres are theoretically capable of enhanced area-specific localization. This carrier system is capable of accommodating a wide variety of drugs. Two major advantages of the magnetically responsive carrier system over other drug delivery systems are its high efficiency for *in vivo* targeting and its controllable release of a drug at the microvascular level.

Due to rapid advances in recent years, the application of polymers to drug delivery has grown considerably. In order to provide a better understanding of the relationships and factors affecting various polymers, we have divided research and development into the following areas:

1. Soluble polymers
2. Biodegradable or bioerodible polymers
3. Mucoadhesive polymers

III.   Soluble polymers as drug carriers

A.   Pinocytosis

Soluble synthetic polymers are emerging as drug delivery vehicles of great promise. They appear to be more versatile than microparticulate carriers because of a greater number of potential target sites in the body.[6]

Biological membranes are effective barriers to macromolecules. The plasma membrane of the cell prevents the loss of enzymes from the cytoplasm, while intracellular membranes delineate functionally distinct subcellular compartments. Mechanisms for translocation of macromolecules across membranes exist, but these are often specific and sophisticated (e.g., pinocytosis).

Ideal characteristics for a macromolecular drug carrier include adequate drug-loading capacity; retention of water solubility when drug-loaded; molecular weight high enough to permit glomerular filtration, but low enough to reach all cell types; unmodified carrier not captured by adsorptive pinocytosis; a stable carrier-drug linkage in body fluids, but degradable in lysosomes; a slowly biodegradable carrier in the extracellular compartment or degraded in lysosomes; nontoxic; nonimmunogenic; and generally biocompatible.

During pinocytosis, the cell membrane invaginates to form a membrane-bound vesicle that contains extracellular fluid, solutes, and sometimes substances adhering to the cell surface. After "pinching off" from the plasma membrane, the pinocytotic vesicle migrates into the cytoplasm, fusing with other incoming vesicles and ultimately fusing with lysosomes to form what is known as a secondary lysosome. Normally, all macromolecules entering the secondary lysosome are susceptible to the organelles' degradative activity. The monomeric constituents liberated during hydrolysis can usually pass through the lysosomal membrane for reutilization in anabolic metabolism or, alternatively, are lost from the cell.

Large macromolecule-drug conjugates normally do not pass through cell membranes, but usually enter by pinocytosis. Drug conjugates that accumulate in lysosomes are termed "lysosomotropic." Coupling to a macromolecule automatically alters drug distribution. If the conjugate is passively captured solely as a solute, body distribution will depend on the rate of pinocytosis of individual cell types, as well as accessibility of the conjugate to each cell type. However, in those instances in which the conjugate has affinity for cell-surface receptors, and is therefore captured by adsorptive pinocytosis, the rate of uptake is dependent upon binding capacity. It is the latter carrier-mediated uptake that holds promise for targeting drug-carriers. To date, a number of cell-specific, receptor-mediated uptake processes have been identified. Many of these depend upon the interaction of specific carbohydrate moieties of a polymer with unique membrane receptors. If this type of approach, or other possible targeting systems (e.g., cell-specific antibodies), can be incorporated as a homing device into the carrier vehicle, there is a real possibility of achieving selective targeting (see Figure 3.1).

Although pinocytosis of polymers is somewhat affected by the molecular weight of the polymer-conjugate, its rate of penetration into a cell may be

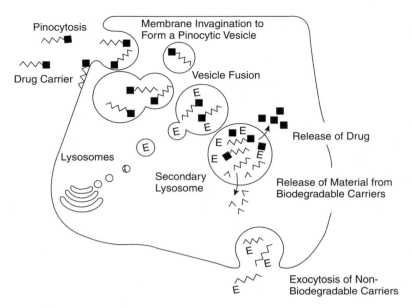

Figure 3.1 Intracellular fate of macromolecular drug conjugates. (From Anderson, J.M. and Kim, S.W., Eds., *Recent Advances in Drug Delivery Systems*, Plenum Publ. Corp., NY, 1984, 10. With permission.)

increased to some extent by the incorporation of hydrophobic units, (e.g., binding tyramine or tyrosinamide to water-soluble polymers). Both approaches, however, lack specificity. The targeting of polymers requires either binding of specific antibodies or binding of saccharide units able to interact with receptors on the surface of certain cells. The binding of saccharide units on synthetic polymers is based on the fact that a small change in the structure of glycoproteins leads to changes in the fate of modified glycoproteins in the organism. It is possible to facilitate the transport of both natural and synthetic polymers into liver hepatocytes, Kupffer cells, fibroblasts, or macrophages.

B.   Ideal soluble polymers

According to Duncan and Lloyd,[6] the ideal drug carrier should possess the following features: polymer-drug linkages that display controlled biodegradability, a suitable molecular weight range, possibility for incorporation of residues that will facilitate direction to and efficient pinocytotic capture by the target cells, absence of any deleterious toxic effects, and nonpersistence in the body.

With the exception of biodegradability, synthetic polymers have advantages over their natural counterparts. Perhaps the most exciting feature of synthetic polymers is the wide choice that is available. In addition to homo-polymers, which consist of chains of identical repeating units, there are many types of copolymers. Two or three different monomers may be copolymerized in a defined ratio. The resultant copolymer may have its component monomers arranged randomly or as regularly repeating dimers or trimers. Block copolymers consist of pieces of two homopolymers joined end-to-end. There is also the possibility of attaching several polymer chains together by cross-links, although this process frequently leads to loss of water solubility.

A useful polymer is one that adheres specifically to cells. Many authors have reported that polymers with a high density of positive charges, such as polylysine and polyornithine, bind tightly to cell membranes. Even a small change in charge density has profound effects. For example, a copolymer composed of 93% vinylpyrrolidone units and 7% (cationic) vinylamine adheres to mammalian cell surfaces, whereas the homopolymer polyvinylpyrrolidone does not. Conversely, a synthetic polyanion, pyran copolymer, has been found to adsorb to rat peritoneal macrophages and to enter these cells by pinocytosis 100 times more rapidly than polyvinylpyrrolidone.[7] Polyhydroxypropylmethacrylamide (polyHPMA) does not adsorb to cell membranes, but its rate of pinocytosis increases dramatically if 10 to 20% of the monomer residues are substituted with a phenolic residue.[8,9] Similarly, the incorporation of 10 to 20% phenolic side-chains greatly increases the cell-binding of another polymer, polyhydroxyethyl-aspartamide.[10]

Polymers that bind to cell surfaces are also likely to bind to plasma proteins. This fact will inevitably alter their interactions with cells and, *in vivo*, may lead to intravascular aggregate formation. A block copolymer composed of a hydrophilic portion, polyethyleneoxide, and a hydrophobic polylysine, whose ε-amino group was substituted to 50% with palmitoyl residues, has been synthesized.[11] Its rate of pinocytosis by rat peritoneal macrophages is similar to that of the homopolymer polyethyleneoxide, indicating that the major hydrophobic domain was without significant effect. This appears to be due to the fact that in an aqueous environment the copolymer forms a unimolecular micelle, and that the cell sees only its hydrophilic portion.

Thus far, the best molecules that have been developed are polyvinylpyrrolidone and polyHPMA, with the latter preferred because of the ease of adding substituent groups. Derivatization of polyHPMA with low percentages of oligopeptides or phenolic residues is possible without causing adherence to cells.[12] Both polymers are water-soluble, even at high degrees of polymerization, but nonspecific cell adherence is seen with both at high molecular weights, thereby offering an advantage.[13,14] Another advantage of these two polymers is their biocompatibility. Both homopolymers polyVP and polyHPMA may be potential plasma expanders.

Using polyHPMA, investigators have been able to demonstrate both targeting and intracellular drug delivery. Targeting has been accomplished by derivatizing polyHPMA with glycylglycylgalactosamine.[15,16] This moiety appears to be recognized by the asialoglycoprotein receptor on hepatocytes. The polymer, when injected into the rat bloodstream, is efficiently removed by the liver's parenchymal cells and taken into their lysosomes.

It has been reported that an enzyme mix from rat liver lysosomes can, under appropriate circumstances, cleave p-nitroaniline from polyHPMA conjugates. The crucial factor is the size and nature of the spacer moiety linking the ligand to the polymer. p-Nitroaniline conjugated directly by an amide-linkage to methacryloyl moieties is not released, while interposition of a suitable oligopeptide renders the distal amide-linkage susceptible to cleavage.[17-19]

Oligopeptides can also be used as lysosomally digestible components of cross-links between polymer chains. Short lengths of polyHPMA can be linked by di(oligopeptidyl)diamines to yield a larger macromolecule. If such cross-linked molecules were used for targeted delivery of a cytotoxic drug, intralysosomal processing would not only release the drug, but also degrade the cross-links. The polymer fragments released from the target cell, upon its demise, would be small enough to enter the glomerular filtrate, thus preventing the accumulation of nondegradable polymer within the body. Degradation of oligopeptide-containing cross-links by lysosomal enzymes has been demonstrated.[14,20] A drug carrier must not release its drug prematurely. This means that the drug-spacer linkage must not be susceptible to degradation in body fluids. Although amidases are active in the bloodstream, it is possible to design oligopeptide spacers that retain the drug during transit through the bloodstream, but release it under the influence of the lysosomal enzymes.[21]

IV. Biodegradable or bioerodible polymers

Pioneering studies in the field of controlled subdermal drug delivery began in the 1960s and used biostable commercial polymers, such as polyethylene and silicon rubber.[22-24] The rate of release of the drug from the polymeric matrix, or reservoir device, was determined solely by diffusion. Biodegradation of the polymer was thought to represent a less well-defined and unnecessary experimental variable. Subsequently, interest in biodegradable polymers developed for two reasons. First, as the field expanded from research to application, it was recognized that surgical removal of a drug-depleted delivery system was difficult, leaving nondegradable foreign materials in the body for an indefinite time period, which constituted an undesirable toxicological hazard. Second, while diffusion-controlled release is an excellent means of achieving predefined rates of drug delivery, it is limited by polymer permeability and the characteristics of the drug.[25-27]

The development of polymers containing hydrolytically or enzymatically labile bonds has been an ongoing process, principally in connection with the search for improved absorbable sutures. Although absorbable sutures were originally derived almost exclusively from various forms of collagen, and evolved to the modern-day catgut, there has also been an increasing emphasis on developing synthetic materials that would hydrolyze to yield natural metabolites. As a result of these efforts, two materials have emerged: poly(lactic acid) and poly(glycolic acid).

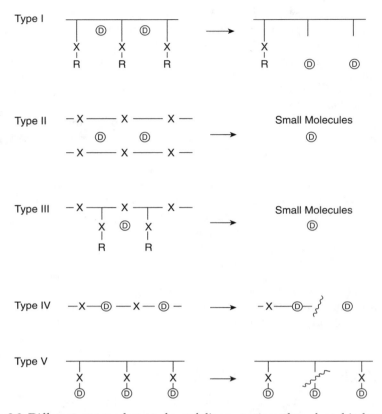

Figure 3.2 Different approaches to drug delivery systems based on biodegradable polymers (X is a bio-labile linkage; D is a drug molecule). (From Bruck, S.D., Ed., *Controlled Drug Delivery*, Vol. 1, CRC Press, Boca Raton, FL, 1983, 56.)

The first disclosure of the use of a synthetic biodegradable polymer for the systemic delivery of a therapeutic agent was made in 1970 by Yolles and Sartori.[43] Since that time, a substantial body of literature on drug release from bioerodible polymers has been generated as attention turned to custom-synthesized biodegradable polymers. Three basic approaches have evolved:[28–35] (1) erosion of the polymer surface with concomitant release of physically entrapped drug; (2) cleavage of covalent bonds between the polymer and drug, occurring in the polymer bulk or at the surface, followed by drug diffusion; and (3) diffusion-controlled release of the physically entrapped drug, with bioabsorption of the polymer delayed until after drug depletion. The third approach avoids any irreproducibility of the bioerosion rate and the difficulty of trying to synchronize the diffusion and bioerosion processes to achieve a specified delivery rate (see Figure 3.2).

A polymer that is to be used in a biodegradable delivery system must be tailored to meet a number of requirements, the most important of which are permeability, biodegradability, biocompatibility, and tensile strength.

These properties are interdependent to some degree, and modification of a polymer to optimize one property will have an effect on the other three. Commercial polymers rarely meet all desired specifications, and custom synthesis is therefore advantageous.

A number of potentially biodegradable polymer systems are used based on the known susceptibility of their monomer analogues to undergo cleavage under mild hydrolytic conditions. These include activated carbon-carbon polymers; polyamides and polyurethanes; polyesters and polycarbonates; polyacetals, polyketals, and polyorthoesters; and inorganic polymers. To this list can be added natural polymers subject to enzymatic attack, examples of which are polypeptides and polysaccharides. Until recently, there have been no proven examples of synthetic polymers that undergo enzymatic degradation.

The preceding chemical classes cannot be ranked in order of susceptibility to hydrolytic or enzymatic attack because, in practice, the degree of substitution of the polymer morphology and the physical form (e.g., surface-to-volume ratio) of the implanted polymer all contribute to the observed degradation rate.

Specific physical properties that contribute to the rate of polymer degradation are as follows:

1. Water permeability and water solubility, a reflection of the free volume of the polymer and its hydrophilicity, will determine the rate of hydrolysis and whether bulk or surface hydrolytic degradation occurs. Autocatalysis of the degradation process is possible if acidic or basic groups are produced by the polymer breakdown, as in the case of polyesters and ortho-esters.
2. Crystallinity of the polymer; only the amorphous phase of the polymer is accessible to permeants (i.e., water, drug) and to enzymatic attack.
3. Glass-transition temperature; the glassy or rubbery nature of the polymer will be reflected in its permeability and molecular chain mobility. The chain mobility appears to be an important factor in determining the susceptibility to enzymatic attack. In addition, the inability of cleaved fragments to diffuse out of a glassy polymer will magnify an autocatalytic hydrolytic process. This may contribute to the rate of degradation of polymers such as polylactic and polyglycolic acid.
4. Physical dimensions (e.g., size and surface-to-volume ratio); these appear to become significant in the advanced stages of biodegradation, when phagocytosis may come into play.

Biodegradable polymers can be defined as polymers that are degradable *in vivo*, either enzymatically or nonenzymatically, to produce biocompatible or nontoxic by-products. These polymers can be metabolized and excreted via normal physiological pathways. They are classified into three groups, namely natural, semisynthetic, and synthetic, based on their sources. Examples of commonly used natural biodegradable polymers are gelatin, alginate,

Table 3.1 Biodegradable *in situ* solid-forming delivery systems

Delivery system	Common problems	Common components
Thermoplastic pastes	High temperature at the time of injection	PLA, PLGA, PCL; alcohols as initiator
In situ cross-linked systems; thermosets	Unacceptable level of heat released during reaction Burst in drug release Toxicity of unreacted monomers	Stannous octoate as catalyst; oligomers of PLA, PDLLA, PCL, polyols as initiator and peroxides as curing agent
Photo-cross-linked gels	Shrinkage and brittleness of the polymer due to high degree of cross-linking	PGA, PLA, PEG, initiators such as eosin dye, light source (e.g., UV or laser)
Ion-mediated gelatin	Low shelf life Burst in drug release Long degradation time	Alginate with Ca^{2+} as gelling agent
In situ polymer precipitation; solvent removal	Burst in drug release Burst in drug release	PDLLA, PCL, PLA, solvents such as DMSO or NMP
Precipitation	Application of organic solvents	
Thermally induced sol-gel transition	Stability of oils and purity of waxes	NIPAAM, PEG, PLA, PLGA, chitosan, pluronics
Organogels	Lack of toxicity data Phase separation	Oils, such as peanut oil and labrafil, waxes (e.g., beeswax and pericerol)

Source: From Elsevier, *J. Control Rel.*, 80, 9–28, 2002. With permission.

albumin, collagen, starch, dextran, chitosan, and chitin, whereas examples of synthetic biodegradable polymers are polylactic acid, polyglycoloc acid, poly(lactide-co-glycolide), poly(orthoester), polyhydroxybutyrate, polyhydroxyvalerate, and polyanhydride. Modifications can be made to naturally occurring biodegradable polymers, such as chitosan, alginate, and hyaluronic acid, to produce semisynthetic biodegradable polymers. These modifications can result in altered physicochemical properties, such as thermogelling properties, mechanical strength, and degradation rates. Synthetic polymers are composed of repeating monomeric units, which are linked together by covalent bonds in the main chain backbone. Polymerization can be achieved by addition and condensation reactions, and these contain monomeric units. Synthetic biodegradable polymers are preferable to the natural biodegradable polymers because they are presumed to be free of immunogenicity and their physicochemical properties are more predictable and reproducible. Polydioxanone, polyphosphazone, pseudopoly(amino acids), water-soluble SELPs protein polymers (based on silk-like and elastin-like amino acid blocks), diblock polymers, and multiblock copolymers are examples of synthetic biodegradable polymers. These have been prepared to afford a multi-

Table 3.2 Hydrogel material

Based on natural materials
Collagen
Starch
Chitosans
Gelatin
Alginates
Dextrans

Based on synthetic polymers
N-vinylpyrrolidone
Poly(vinyl alcohol)
Polyphosphazenes
Poly(ethylene oxide-b-poly(propylene oxide)
Copolymers
PL(G)A/PEO/PL(G)A copolymers
PVA-g-PLGA graft-polymers
PEGT-PBT copolymers (PolyActive)
MA-oligolactide-PEO-oligolactide-MA

Responsive polymers
Methacrylates (pH-dependent swelling)
Poly(N-isopropylacrylamide) (LCST)
PEO-PPO-PEO (Pluronics)
PEO-PPO-PAA graft-copolymer (LCST)
PLGA-PEO-PLGA (LCST)

Source: From Advanstar, *Pharm. Tech.*, March 2002, 144. With permission.

Table 3.3 Commercially available biodegradable drug delivery systems

Name of product	Dosage form	Active ingredient	Biodegradable polymer[a,b]
Lupron Depot	Microspheres	Leuprolide	PLGA
Sandostatin LAR	Microspheres	Octreotide	PLGA
Neutropin Depot	Microspheres	Somatropin	PLGA
Trelstar Depot	Microspheres	Triptorelin	PLGA
Gliadel	Waffer	Cumustin	Polyanhydride
Zoladex	Rod	Goserelin	PLGA
Atridox	Gel	Doxycycline	PLGA

[a] PLGA: poly(lactic-co-glycolic acid)

[b] Polyanhydride: poly[bis(p-carboxyphenoxy) propane: sebacic acid] in a 20:80 molar ratio

Source: From Russell Publ., *Am. Pharm. Rev.*, 4, 4, 25, 2001. With permission.

tude of polymers with diverse properties, such as degradation rates, mechanical strength, porosity, diffusivity, and inherent viscosity.

According to Sun and Watts,[178] the factors that affect the degradation rate of the polymer involve chemical properties such as structure of monomers, which can affect the lability of the cleavable bonds and composition

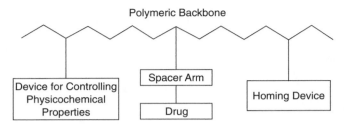

Figure 3.3 Ringsdorf's model of polymeric pro-drugs. (From Ringsdorf, H., in *Polymeric Delivery Systems*, Kostelnik, R.J., Ed., Gordon & Breach Publishers, New York, 1978, 197. With permission.)

of the monomers; physical properties, such as hydrophilicity and crystallinity, which are controlled by the chemical composition of the monomers and process conditions; molecular weight of the polymers; geometric factors of the polymer devices, such as size, shape, and surface area; and additives and environmental factors, such as pH and ionic strength. Biodegradation of polymer devices or drug delivery systems usually undergoes four steps: hydration, mechanical strength loss, integrity loss, and mass loss. The hydration step is critical and is determined by the hydrophilicity/hydrophobicity or crystallinity of the polymer.[179,180] Natural biodegradable polymers (see Figures 3.4 and 3.5), such as human serum albumin and collagen, are hydrophilic and undergo degradation by hydrolysis, whereas most of the synthetic biodegradable polymers are hydrophobic. Polymers are never 100% crystalline, and amorphous regions separate crystalline domains. The degradation of biodegradable polymers is sensitive to the pH of the environment (e.g., poly(lactide-co-glycolide) degrades faster in a highly alkaline buffer than in

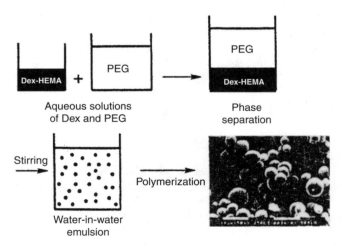

Figure 3.4 Schematic representation of the microsphere preparation process. (With permission, Advanstar, *Pharm. Tech.*, Oct. 2001, 110.)

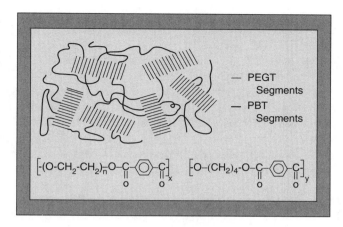

Figure 3.5 Schematic representation of the morphology of PEGT-PBT copolymers. The PBT segments form hydrophobic domains in the hydrophilic PEG matrix, thereby creating a physically cross-linked network. (With permission, Advanstar, *Pharm. Tech.*, Oct. 2001, 110.)

acidic and physiological buffers, polyanhydrides degrade faster in basic conditions, and hydrolysis of poly(orthoester) is catalyzed by acid).[181] Biodegradable polymers (see Figure 3.6) that are hydrophobic can undergo surface degradation (i.e., degradation occurs on the outer layer exposed to the aqueous body fluid). Environmentally catalyzed biodegradation normally involves naturally occurring biodegradable polymers, such as polysaccharides, proteins, and poly(beta-hydroxy acids). For synthetic biodegradable polymers, degradation involves enzymes only at certain stages of physical conditions. Insignificant enzyme involvement is expected in the early stages for polymers in the glassy state. However, as erosion or fragmentation occurs, enzymes can play an important role in the degradation of polymer (see Figures 3.7–3.9).[182–184]

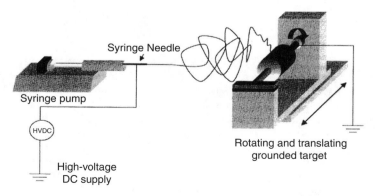

Figure 3.6 Schematic of electrospinning system. (With permission, Elsevier, *J. Control Rel.*, 81, 57–64, 2002.)

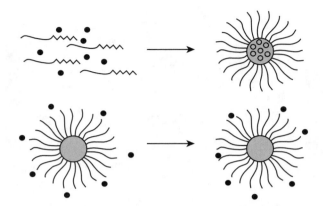

Figure 3.7 Process of drug incorporation to polymeric micelles. Preformed micelles have no ability to incorporate ADR. (With permission, Elsevier, *J. Control Rel.*, 78, 155–163, 2002.)

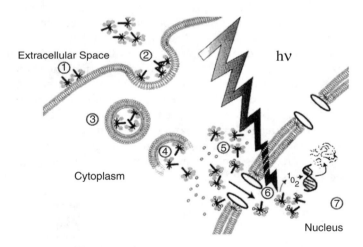

Figure 3.8 Proposed cellular import mechanism of Ce6-loligomer. Loligomers are represented as branched structures, and chlorine e_6 groups are represented as gray ovals. Ce6-loligomers bind to cell surfaces via their cationic CTS sequences (step 1). This triggers membrane invagination (step 2), followed by the internalization of the Ce6-loligomer molecules into vesicular compartments (step 3) in a process referred to as absorptive endocytosis. A fraction of the Ce6-loligomers escape from these vesicles (step 4), and their NLS sequences are recognized by cytosolic carrier proteins (small open ovals in the diagram) (step 5), enabling import into the nucleus (step 6). A light burst from outside the cell (hv), results in activation of the Ce6 molecules and production of singlet oxygen species ($^1O_2$) in the nucleus, leading to efficient DNA damage (step 7). This damage eventually results in apoptosis and cell death. (With permission, Elsevier, *J. Control Rel.*, 78, 115–123, 2002.)

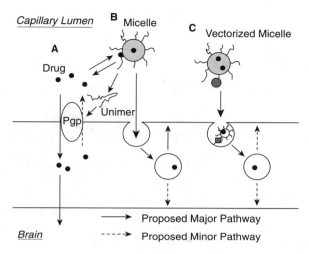

Figure 3.9 Proposed mechanism of drug transport in brain's microvessel endothelial cells with Pluronic® block copolymers: (A) inhibition of Pgp results in increased flux of drug from blood to brain, (B) solubilization of drugs in micelles decelerates drug transport across BBB, micelles undergo fluid phase endocytosis, and (C) conjugation of micelles with insulin vector enhances drug transport through adsorptive endocytosis. (With permission, Elsevier, *J. Control Rel.*, 82, 189–212, 2002.)

A.   Drug release by matrix solubilization

Materials in this category include currently used enteric coatings, which can generally be classified as polyacids.[36] In their un-ionized form, they are water-insoluble, but upon ionization of their carboxylic acid groups, they become more water-soluble. Some of the most widely studied systems are partially esterified copolymers of methyl vinyl ether and maleic anhydride or partially esterified copolymers of ethylene and maleic anhydride.[37–39] In a constant pH environment, esterified polymers undergo a controlled dissolution process and are, therefore, useful materials for the controlled release of therapeutic agents dispersed within them.

B.   Erodible diffusional systems

Erodible diffusional systems combine the attributes of a rate-controlling polymer membrane, which provides a constant rate of drug release from a reservoir-type device, with erodibility, which results in bioerosion and makes surgical removal of the drug-depleted device unnecessary. Because consistency of drug release requires that the bioerodible polymer membrane remain essentially unchanged during the delivery regimen, significant bioerosion must not occur until after drug delivery has been completed. Major emphasis for the development of erodible diffusional systems has centered on devices that release contraceptive steroids or narcotic antagonists. The polymer systems most extensively investigated in the form of subdermal capsules for the release of levonorgestrel are various aliphatic polysters, in particular, poly(ε-caprolactone).[40]

C.   Monolithic systems

In monolithic systems, the drug is physically incorporated into a polymer matrix and is released to the surrounding environment as the polymer bioerodes. In describing drug release from such systems, it is necessary to consider both polymer erosion and drug diffusion. If mobility of the drug in the matrix is such that rapid diffusional release is possible, its release kinetics will be first order. Zero-order release requires that the erosion process be confined to the surface of the solid device and that the drug be highly immobilized in the matrix. Although surface erosion is difficult to achieve, such systems have several significant advantages. Among these are the ability to control drug delivery rate by simply varying drug loading within the matrix, controlling lifetime of the device, varying the physical dimension of the device, and the ability of one matrix to deliver a variety of therapeutic agents.

Narcotic antagonists have been incorporated into poly(L (+) lactic acid) in the form of films implanted in rats.[41-43] The release of narcotic antagonists from composites in particle form has also been investigated *in vitro* and *in vivo*. For cyclazocine and naltrexone, *in vitro* release rates were faster than *in vivo* release rates, whereas for naloxone, both the rates were similar.[44,45] The large difference in the *in vitro* release rates was ascribed to the excess of extractant present.

Poly(L+-lactic acid) has also been used for the controlled release of progesterone, β-estradiol, and dexamethasone. Devices have been fabricated by dissolving the drug and the polymer in dichloromethane. The solvent is evaporated under reduced pressure and the solid residue melt-pressed.[43,46] The release of d-norgestrel from cylindrical implants fabricated from various homopolymers and copolymer of L(+) lactic acid, DL-lactic acid, and glycolic acid has also been studied. Because poly(L+ lactic acid) is highly crystalline, chain segments have restricted mobility and release of d-norgestrel is low. However, the introduction of either DL-lactic acid or glycolic acid into a poly(L+ lactic acid) chain disrupts the crystalline nature of the polymer, and chain mobility is increased.[47-49] Because crystalline regions are highly hydrophobic and prevent access of water to the labile ester linkages, a decrease of crystallinity will also result in increased rates of matrix hydrolysis.

The release of cyclophosphamide, doxorubicin, and cis-dichloro diamine platinum from poly(L+ lactic acid) has been evaluated.[50] Although *in vitro* and *in vivo* release of these agents has been poorly characterized, this methodology may offer advantages in lowering drug toxicity while increasing the number of "cures" relative to single-dose administration. Poly(L+ lactic acid) or copolymers of lactic and glycolic acids have also been evaluated as injectable controlled-release systems for the antimalarial drugs quinazoline derivative (WR-158122) and sulfadiazine. Using WR-158122 and a copolymer prepared from 25 wt% DL-lactic acid and 75 wt% glycolic acid, sustained release through 14 weeks was demonstrated by means of radioactivity measurements of excreted urine.[51] Using the rodent malaria *Plasmodium berghei*, no parasitemia was detected for several weeks, and some animals survived through 14 weeks. Copolymers of gluconic acid and (γ-ethyl-L-glutamate have also been used in the development of bioerodible monolithic devices. Unlike poly(lactic acid) and poly(glycolic acid), which were originally developed as biodegradable surgical sutures and were not intended to be used as bioerodible monolithic devices for controlled drug release, poly(orthoesters) were specifically designed as monolithic matrixes capable of undergoing a surface-erosion process.

In recent years, there have been major advances in genetic engineering and, consequently, the production of many interesting and pharmacologically active polypeptides.[52] There have also been concurrent improvements in procedures for total chemical synthesis of lower molecular weight peptides, such as Zoladex (ICI-118630), which is a highly potent, synthetic analog of luteinizing hormone-releasing hormone (LHRH). However, the therapeutic and commercial potential of this and other polypeptide drugs will only be fully realized if these advances are accompanied by improvements in the design of dosage forms, leading to practical and effective formulations.

Polypeptides are ineffective by the oral route since they are rapidly degraded and deactivated by the acidic pH and proteolytic enzymes in the alimentary tract. Even if stable to enzymatic digestion, their relatively high molecular weights prevent facile translocation through the intestinal wall. Other routes of administration, including intranasal, buccal, intravaginal, and rectal, have been used, but these are associated with low and variable bioavailability, and none of these rates offers a general solution applicable to all polypeptides. Consequently, polypeptides and proteins are best administered parenterally. Since these drugs have short elimination half-lives, frequent injections are required to produce an effective therapy.

For polypeptide hormones, in which the pharmacology of the agent is compatible with sustained release, the most appropriate dosage form is one that is capable of releasing a drug continuously at a controlled rate over a period of weeks or even months. If such release is from a polymer, then it is preferred that the polymer be biodegradable. Experience with homo- and copolymers of lactic and glycolic acids has shown that these materials are inert and biocompatible in the physiological environment of the body and degrade to toxicologically acceptable products. Consequently, these polymers are invariably the materials of choice in the initial design of parenteral sustained-delivery systems using a biodegradable carrier, particularly when release over many weeks is required.[53–59]

V.   Mucoadhesive polymers

Bioadhesive polymers have been employed in both surgery and dentistry for many years.[60] Such polymers include the well-documented "super glues," the esters of cyanoacrylates, which have found applications ranging from repair of osteochondral fractures to capping extraction wounds in dentistry. Other synthetic bone-glue candidates have included polyurethanes, epoxy resins, acrylate, and polystyrene. Often, the mechanism of bonding for these bioadhesive polymers involves the formation of covalent bonds with the target tissue in order to provide a permanent or semipermanent linkage.[61,62]

In the development of oral controlled-release dosage forms, considerable benefits may ensue from the use of bioadhesive polymers providing relatively short-term adhesion between the drug delivery system and the mucus or epithelial cell surface of the gastrointestinal tract.[63,64] Binding will therefore involve secondary forces, such as hydrogen bonds or van der Waals forces. Mucoadhesives may, therefore, be regarded as a specific class of bioadhesives. Polymer candidates need to be nontoxic and nonabsorbable, adhere rapidly to wet tissues, and release the incorporated drug in a controlled manner.

The ability to localize a drug delivery system in a selected region of the GI tract could conceivably lead to improved bioavailability, especially for drugs exhibiting narrow windows of absorption or instability in certain sectors of the tract. Intimate contact with the target absorption membrane should lead to optimization of both the extent and rate of drug absorption. Alternative mechanisms for the control of GI transit of the dosage form, for example, through manipulation of particle size and density, together with the use of fibrous materials, have not, in general, been successful.[65]

A material may adhere to a mucosal surface in two ways: by binding to the tissue itself or by associating with the mucus coat that is ultimately associated with the tissue surface. The gastric mucosa is the primary target in the development of a mucoadhesive-based sustained release action since gastric retention will be the main mechanism in delaying the rapid absorption that occurs once the formulation reaches the specialized absorptive areas of the small intestine.[66,67]

Throughout the GI tract, the mucosal surface is comprised of columnar epithelial cells, the morphology of which changes as the tract is descended. In the stomach, specific mucus-secreting glands are in the cardiac and pyloric region, which serve to coat incoming food boli and hence reduce possible abrasive action. Mucus-secreting cells are also found in the necks and depths of the acid-secreting gastric pits, where they form a protective buffer zone around the stream of acid. The surface columnar epithelial cells maintain the mucus coating over the rest of the stomach surface, and secretion is stimulated by mechanical and chemical irritation. The mucus layer also serves to protect the gastric epithelium from the action of secreted acid and proteolytic enzymes. The layer is usually continuous, but can be disrupted under the action of certain irritant substances, and an ineffective mucus layer is usually associated with conditions of gastric ulceration.[68,69]

Particles that are small enough to be buried in the surface of the mucus will be securely held due to the relatively high storage capacity of the gel.

However, as mucus is continually secreted, such particles will be pushed farther from the mucosal surface to a point where they are sheared away, either under the weight of the gel itself, or due to mechanical abrasion of the luminal contents. Larger particles, for which there is a favorable interface interaction with the mucus gel, may, nevertheless, be pulled from the mucosal surface due to their weight or because they are more easily dislodged by the peristaltic action of the stomach. One method of prolonging mucosal association can be to use a hydrophilic polymer in a dry powder or granule, from which, after embedding in the mucus, will slowly hydrate and take up water at the expense of the mucus gel. This will compensate for the continued gel secretion by increasing the elasticity or storage capacity of the gel, thereby enabling a more substantial erosion of the polymer surface.[70–76]

Although the mucus gel presents only a limited barrier to small molecules, due to the low microviscosity of the interstices, the diffusion of macromolecules is more severely restricted because of physical obstruction.[77] Thus, molecularly dispersed polymers can interact with the mucus gel at the surface via a combination of secondary bonds. Diffusional resistance of the mucus gel can prevent a total mixing of mucin and polymer on the mucosa and lead to a stiffening of the mucus gel, such as that observed under selected *in vitro* conditions. However, a limited degree of chain presence at the adhesive-mucus interface will be essential for effective mucoadhesion.

The most effective mucoadhesives are linear or lightly cross-linked polymers, which differ considerably in structure to mucus glycoproteins. Consequently, it is unlikely that they adhere to the gel through interactions similar to the mucin–mucin interaction that is so important to inherent gel structure. Interestingly, one common factor in effective mucoadhesives is the presence of carboxylate groups that have no significant role in the purely mucin–mucin interaction. Likely points of interaction for these polymers are the oligosaccharide side-chains on the mucin that are aligned normal to the linear axis of the protein backbone of the glucosylated subunit. If penetration of this glycosylated coat is a prerequisite to the formation of a viable interaction, then the "free ends" of the interacting polymers need be no more than several monomer units long. However, as there seems to be a relation between the molecular weight of a polymer and its supposed mucoadhesive properties, it could be that interdigitation between the whole mucin subunits is of greater relevance in the polymer–mucin interaction. The polymers considered to date lack characteristics that promote an interaction with hydrophobic regions of the glycoprotein, such as the globular protein unit or the numerous esterified fatty acid residues.[78–81]

The development of mucoadhesive polymers may be traced back as far as 1947, when gum tragacanth and dental adhesive powders were combined to form a vehicle for applying penicillin to the oral mucosa. An improvement in this system resulted when carboxymethyl cellulose and petrolatum were combined to form the vehicle. The development of Orahesive® followed, leading to trials of Orabase® in 1959. Orahesive is a mixture of finely ground sodium carboxymethyl cellulose (SCMC), pectin, and gelatin, while Orabase is a blend of these in a polymethylene/mineral oil base. After several trials, it was found that dry polymer powders would form better mucoadhesive agents since such formulations would be capable of absorbing a greater amount of water and, hence, adhere more strongly to the tissue substrate than when blended with the polymer carrier. A further development was the blending of SCMC with poly(isobutylene) (PIB) and laminating this mixture onto a polyethylene sheet. This system benefited from both wet-surface and dry-surface adhesion, with the added bonus of being protected from physical interference (e.g., from the tongue, by the polyethylene-sheet backing).[82-84]

An extensive range of such systems, whereby a water-soluble polymer and PIB are blended together and laminated with a polyethylene film, was tested by Chen and Cyr.[85] The polymers identified as exhibiting the best adhesion were sodium alginate, SCMC, guar gum, hydroxyethylcellulose (HEC), Karya gum, methylcellulose (MeC), polyethylene glycol, Retene, and Tragacanth. Acrylic polymers were soon recognized as useful mucoadhesive materials, and the early 1980s saw a plethora of patents in which hydroxypropylcellulose, or MeC and poly(acrylic acid), were blended together to form mucoadhesive preparations. By far the most-studied mucoadhesive polymers through the 1980s have been poly(acrylic acid), hydroxypropylcellulose, and SCMC. Some polymers used have been standard pharmaceutical materials, such as MeC, HEC, and sodium alginate, and others have been specifically synthesized to achieve optimal results, such as 2-ethyl hexyl acrylate-lauryl methacrylate-vinyl stearate copolymer and isooctyl acrylate-methoxy poly (ethylene oxide) acrylate-acrylic acid polymer.

The work of Chen and Cyr,[85] together with Park[64] and Smart et al.,[80] involved the investigation of a range of polymers of varying molecular character. These studies appeared to arrive at similar conclusions as to the molecular characteristics required for mucoadhesion. The properties exhibited by such a molecule, described by Peppas and Buri,[79] may be summarized as follows: (1) strong H-bonding groups (-- OH; -- COOH); (2) strong anionic charges; (3) sufficient flexibility to penetrate the mucus network or tissue crevices; (4) surface tension characteristics suitable for wetting mucus/mucosal tissue surfaces; and (5) high molecular weight.

In accordance with the theory that secondary bond formation is the principal source of mucoadhesion, those polymers with carboxyl groups present are, without exception, all mucoadhesive. The carboxyl group in its un-ionized form is capable of strong H-bond formation and in its ionized form can interact electrostatically. However, the functional groups on the polymer backbone should not be in such proximity that they interfere with each other (e.g., by intramolecular H-bonding). As the carboxyl concentration along a polymer chain decreases, for example, in moving from sodium alginate to Karya gum to gelatin, the mucoadhesive strength also decreases.

The effect of other secondary bond-forming groups (e.g., hydroxyl, ether, oxygen, amine) on the mucoadhesive properties of the polymers previously mentioned is not as clearly defined as that for the carboxyl group.

The cellulosic polymers have an abundance of hydroxyl and ether groups along their length, yet their mucoadhesion exhibits little relationship to this characteristic.

Another important feature of a mucoadhesive molecule is believed to be the ability to form physical bonds, principally by entanglement with the substrate molecules. This is illustrated by polyethylene oxide (PEO), a linear, flexible molecule with minimal secondary bond-forming capacity. At high molecular weights, this molecule exhibits a mucoadhesive strength comparable to MeC and sodium alginate, whose secondary bond-formation is far greater. This may be due to the fact that the segmental mobility of PEO is extremely high since ether linkages make for a flexible backbone and, hence, penetration into substrate networks is deep and relatively rapid. The effective depth is, however, affected by molecular chain length (i.e., molecular weight) since a short-chain molecule can form fewer entanglements and penetrate to a lesser degree than a larger molecule. The interaction between the polymer adhesive and mucus or mucosal tissue is primarily a surface-tension phenomenon. Therefore, the lower the contact angle between the adhesive and the mucus/mucosa, the better the chances of interaction.

The ideal mucoadhesive polymer is composed of a combination of various carefully balanced properties. It must be a polymer of high molecular weight to maximize adhesion through entanglements and van der Waal's forces. The segmental mobility of the polymer chain should be high to facilitate rapid and deep penetration into the substrate. The repeating unit of the polymer should contain carboxyl groups and other secondary bond-forming groups, principally primary hydroxyl groups and short-chain ethers. This would ensure the potential for adhesion via as many modes as possible. For further discussion of structural features of mucoadhesive polymers, see Hunt et al.[60]

VI. Polymers containing pendant bioactive substituents

A major approach to increasing the therapeutic efficiency of bioactive agents while decreasing their toxicity has involved their bonding to synthetic or naturally occurring macromolecules.[86] Thus, various agents have been bound via degradable linkages to many different polymeric systems. The original rationale behind this approach was that systems could be designed that would undergo hydrolysis or enzyme-catalyzed cleavages when placed in the body in order to release the agent at a predetermined rate. Since the rate of excretion of high-molecular weight polymers is extremely slow, it was felt that agent/polymer adducts could function as depots for extended periods of time. Early work in this area led to the hope that perhaps polymeric systems could also be modified (e.g., by the attachment of a tumor-specific antibody) in order to display high specificity for target organisms, such as tumors. In this case, the modified polymer was to carry the active agent to a specific site of action and then release it. In effect, the systems were to function as target-seeking guided missiles.[87–89]

With the exception of some substituted polyethyleneglycols, large macromolecules cannot readily enter the body via the GI tract or by cutaneous absorption. In fact, a molecular weight of 5,000 to 10,000 is considered high enough to prevent any appreciable absorption through skin or mucosal tissues. Thus, adducts that are taken orally or administered topically can only function as depots. However, such systems can still offer considerable advantages for localized treatments of the GI tract or the eye, mouth, skin, vagina, etc. In these cases, a high molecular weight, biostable polymeric carrier is preferred. Since topically administered systems experience such mild conditions, the agent should be attached to the polymer via a linkage that is extremely susceptible to hydrolysis. For treatment of the GI tract, it is likely that the system would have to be protected with an enteric coating to prevent premature hydrolysis from occurring in the stomach.[90,91]

A dextromethorphan-polymer complex (dextromethorphan is an antitussive) can be coated with a semipermeable outer coating of varying thickness. The drug is released only when ions in the GI tract cross the outer coating and displace the active drug. Since ion concentration in the GI tract is quite stable, drug release is precise, controlled, and unaffected by variations in pH, temperature, or volume of contents in the stomach or intestine. The system releases its active agent at an effective level for 12 h.[90]

Since most synthetic polymers with molecular weights above 60,000 to 80,000 cannot be excreted via renal glomerular filtration, biodegradable systems are usually preferred for implantation of parenteral administration. It has been claimed that the body can eliminate high-molecular weight, biostable polymers via the liver and its biliary system into the intestine. However, the rate of excretion by this route is normally quite slow. The main result of an uptake of a biostable polymer is lysosome and cellular overloading, which can lead to toxic effects. Large macromolecules can cause erythrocyte aggregation and changes in platelet or leukocyte distribution. Since these high molecular weight species can be present in polymers with relatively low average molecular weights, samples may require fractionation to remove high molecular weight species. Unfortunately, physiological interactions can even result in the complete retention of polymers with molecular weights below the limit of glomerular filtration. Biostable polymers are, in general, more likely to function as antigens than are biodegradable systems. Olefin polymers have produced immunological responses in rabbits at levels of 10 g per animal. A notable exception is a series of biostable, sulfoxide-containing polymers with molecular weights as high as 172,000 that are claimed to be nontoxic and excretable. Of course, if an injected polymeric adduct is expected to reach a specific target via the bloodstream, it should be water-soluble. Regardless of the method of administration, both the polymer and the adduct must not produce any toxic or immunogenic response.[92-94]

Trout has divided the potential sites of action of targeted systems into three major areas:[89] extracellular, pericellular (i.e., cell surfaces), and intracellular. Active agents that might be directed toward extracellular targets include antibiotics acting on extracellular bacteria or parasites; inhibitors that block the deleterious effects of enzymes released by inflammation, shock, or rheumatoid arthritis; enzymes like asparginase and urease; and anticoagulants. In the preceding cases, a form of targeting can be achieved if the active agent is maintained in the extracellular space at a desired level and for an extended period of time. Thus, a system might be targeted by manipulating its molecular weight so that it is high enough to retard the permeation of the adduct through membrane capillaries but low enough to minimize its uptake by the endocytizing cells of the RES system. Cations might also be distributed along the backbone to maximize the interaction of the adduct with negatively charged blood proteins. The carrier could also be designed to shield the bound agent in order to decrease its immunogenicity and decrease its reactivity with free or cell-bound antibodies. However, the primary function of the retained adduct polymer complex would be to act as a drug depot.

The targeting of agents that have pericellular and intracellular receptor sites is somewhat similar because, for an adduct to reach the latter, absorption must also occur on the cell surface. In the first case, it would be highly desirable for the complex to release the drug upon contact with the cell surface. This could be achieved if the drug-polymer linkage was susceptible to hydrolysis induced by enzymes in the plasma membrane or by an enzyme secreted by the target cell and having a short range of action. For example, Trout[89] suggests that systems might be designed to release anti-inflammatory or antirheumatoid agents upon contact with the neutral proteases or collagenases secreted by cells involved in the initiation and development of inflammation (e.g., rheumatoid arthritis).

Agents released as previously described, could be directed against targets located inside the cell. As mentioned, intracellular sites can also be reached via endocytosis of pinocytotic vesicles. Since endocytosis occurs at different rates with different polymer types and different cells, adducts can be prepared that will be preferentially taken up by certain cells. However, attempts to prepare systems that are only endocytized by specific cells other than those of the RES system are plagued by the high endocytic activity of the latter. A side benefit of this approach is that some agents that are normally unable to penetrate the plasma membrane may enter the cell via the endocytic route.

Although a level of selectivity for intracellular sites is provided by the fact that cells differ in their endocytic activity, a much higher degree of selectivity can be attained, at least *in vitro*, by attaching "homing molecules" to the adduct that interact with specific cell types. For example, considerable work has been done with antibodies that interact with specific tumor-associated antigens.[95–97] Other targeting moieties that have been used to target proteins to specific cell receptors include peptide hormones, viral components, and carbohydrates, such as galactose, mannose, fucose, and N-acetylglucosamine. Acetylation of the side chains of proteins can also dramatically change their cellular-uptake patterns. For example, acetylation of low-density lipoprotein with acetic anhydride stops its uptake by fibroblasts while stimulating its uptake by peritoneal macrophages. Several polymers can function as both the carrier and the homing molecule. Antibodies and abrin, ricin, and diphtheria toxins have been investigated as inherent targeting carriers. Lectin carriers, such as concanavalin A, also give evidence of tumor-specific association.[98–101]

Although there have been many reports of successful agent targeting *in vitro*, there have been few successes *in vivo*. Goldberg et al.[102] have listed the following problems that occur with antibody-targeting systems:

1.   Circulatory antigen and antigen–antibody complexes
2.   Metabolic/biochemical changes in adducts with loss of activity
3.   Transport kinetics to tumor tissue versus competitive binding and metabolism
4.   Changing and cross-reactive antigenicity
5.   Masking or interiorization of tumor-cell-specific antigens

Various approaches to overcoming these problems include:

1.   Complexing or removing
2.   Use of (Fab′) portion of the immunoglobulin to avoid F-complement binding and reduce molecular size
3.   Therapy with intratumor and IV injections of antibody adducts
4.   Surgical or radiation reduction of primary lesion tumor burden coupled with systemic administration of the antibody adducts for elimination of metastasis

Another approach to targeting agent polymer adducts involves the direct injection and retention of soluble or insoluble systems into a specific site, such as a tumor. Insoluble adducts will, of course, be retained by physical immobilization. Various approaches to retaining soluble systems include the use of targeting moieties, as discussed previously, and the introduction of pendant functional groups along the polymer backbone that can form covalent bonds with tissue carbonyl groups. Nonspecific electrostatic bonding between negatively charged cells and cationic adducts has also been used.[102]

Rowland et al.[103] have successfully attached a p-phenylene-diamine mustard (PDM) and an immunoglobulin (I) from a rabbit antiserum against mouse lymphoma cells (EL4) to polyglutamic acid (PGA). Goldberg and coworkers have investigated the use of lectin adducts in intratumor immunochemotherapy. For example, mitomycin C (MC) and adriamycin (AD) have been attached to the lectin concanavalin A (Con A). Goldberg points out that several processes may explain the favorable intratumor activity of these adducts.[102] These include cell-surface binding via lectin receptors, antimetabolic and cytotoxic activity of intact adduct, capping of endocytic receptors favoring cell uptake and lysosomal cleavage, and release of free MC locally.

VII. Matrix systems

Within the scope of this general term, there are a variety of controlled-release devices.[104] Included among these are dissolved systems that are prepared from a matrix containing a drug at or below the saturation solubility of the drug in the polymer and dispersed systems that contain the drug within a matrix at a concentration that greatly exceeds the saturation solubility of the drug in the polymer. In this case, it is assumed that the drug is present as discrete solid particles. This implies that upon leaching of the drug, macroscopic channels or pores within the polymer matrix do not exist. Other controlled-release devices include reservoir-dispersed matrix systems, which are analogous to the dispersed system except that a barrier layer is present at the surface of the device that is of lower permeability to a drug than the bulk polymer matrix, and porous matrix systems, which are prepared from a dispersion of drug particles and preformed polymer. In porous matrix systems, it is assumed that upon leaching of the drug, continuous macroscopic pores or channels arise from the displacement of drug by solvent.

One of the major advantages of matrix devices relative to other types of controlled-release drug delivery systems (e.g., reservoir devices) is the ease of manufacture. In general, matrix devices can be prepared by mixing the drug as a finely divided powder with the prepolymer. This mixture is then placed in an appropriate mold and allowed to cure. This technique is especially useful for dispersed-type matrix devices, provided that the initial drug load is below the saturation solubility of the drug in the cured polymer. The preparation of reservoir-matrix devices is more complicated due to the need to incorporate the barrier layer onto the matrix.

Most often, dispersed-type matrix devices have been prepared from polydimethyl siloxane. This polymer has a number of advantages for controlled-release systems, including: (1) it is an elastomer with good mechanical properties; (2) it is highly permeable to hydrophobic solutes; (3) it is nontoxic; (4) it is molded into a wide variety of shapes and is polymerized with simple techniques; and (5) its permeability is not affected via prolonged contact with biological fluids. Its major disadvantages are (1) it is not permeable to highly water-soluble solutes, especially charged species; (2) it evokes a moderate foreign-tissue response upon subdermal implantation; and (3) the permeability of the polymer is not easily varied by alterations in polymer composition.[105–110]

Because of the disadvantages associated with polydimethyl siloxane, a number of investigators have utilized polymers prepared from various derivatives of hydroxyalkyl methacrylates. These polymers offer a number of advantages, including: (1) they are not toxic; (2) they evoke a minimal foreign-tissue response; (3) they are highly permeable to both hydrophobic and water-soluble solutes, including charged species; and (4) they are of variable permeability to drugs, depending upon copolymer composition and cross-link density. Copolymers of the hydroxyalkyl methacrylates and methyl methacrylate have also been utilized. Such copolymers offer the advantage of increased mechanical strength and may offer some advantage relative to blood and tissue compatibility. Other authors have utilized a variety of polymers, including ethylene vinyl acetate, polyacrylamide, polyvinyl acetate, polyethylene, and polyether urethanes.[111–118]

The release of drugs from matrix devices is governed by the diffusion of solute within the matrix phase. The development of the appropriate form of the release-rate equation is generated via Ficks' first or second laws of diffusion. In general, three limiting factors exist. First, when the initial drug load is equal to or less than the saturation solubility of the drug, the rate of release is dependent upon the diffusion coefficient of the drug in the polymer and upon the initial drug load. The diffusion coefficient, in turn, is dependent upon the properties of the drug and the polymer matrix. Such systems can be described as a homogeneous matrix. Second, when the initial drug load is greater than the saturation point, but small relative to the total volume of the polymer (e.g., less than 10% w/w), drug-release rates will also be dependent upon the diffusion coefficient of the drug within the polymer matrix and the initial drug load. However, in such systems, an additional variable becomes important, namely, the saturation solubility of the drug in the polymer. Such systems should be described as a heterogeneous matrix. Third, when the initial drug load is increased beyond 10% w/w, a point is reached when the solid drug particles begin to form continuous pores or channels within the matrix. Under these circumstances, the path of least resistance for the drug is diffusion within channels formed where the drug has previously leached from the matrix. In this case, the rate of release is governed by diffusion within these channels, the diffusional characteristics of which are governed by the elution medium. Such systems are termed "porous" or "granular" matrices.

The previous classifications must be taken to represent general guidelines. It is apparent, for example, that as the initial drug load is increased, the matrix will become more porous as drug is leached from the polymer. In effect, the free volume for diffusion increases as a result of the voids created by the leached drug. This increase in void volume will be reflected by changes in the "effective" diffusion coefficient of drug in the matrix phase.

In addition to effects arising from the initial drug load, the release characteristics of a polymer matrix are also a function of the geometry of the matrix. This fact arises due to variations in the nature of the concentration gradient within the drug depletion zone of the matrix. For example, in a heterogeneous polymer matrix containing dispersed drug, a zone of depletion is formed as the drug is released from the matrix. For devices (e.g., cylinders or spheres) in which the area of the receding drug boundary decreases with time, the flux of the drug will again follow a path that is perpendicular to the receding boundary. However, the volume of the depletion zone will increase radially from the surface, and the concentration gradient is nonlinear within the zone of depletion. As a consequence, release-rate equations are dependent upon the geometry of the device.[119–121]

VIII. Heparin-releasing polymers

The pioneering work in heparin-controlled release materials was accidentally initiated by Gott et al.[122] At that time, these investigators were evaluating numerous materials for thromboresistance by venous implantation, and
colloidal graphite gave the best results. These investigators first thought the
thromboresistance was due to the extreme smoothness imparted to surfaces
following graphite coating and the chemically inert nature of the colloidal
graphite. These materials were sterilized by soaking in a benzalkonium-sul-
fate solution. Further studies showed that these graphite-benzalkonium-hep-
arin (GBH) surfaces retained significant quantities of heparin even after three
months of implantation in the venous system.[123]

A major disadvantage of the GBH surfaces is that the graphite can only
be coated to rigid materials because any flexing would result in a disruption
in the integrity of the graphite coating with possible "flaking off" of the
GBH coating. To circumvent this problem, Leininger et al.[124] chemically
modified numerous polymer surfaces by forming permanent surface-asso-
ciated quaternary ammonium groups, thus eliminating the need for prior
adsorption of a cationic surfactant onto a hydrophobic surface, such as
graphite. Depending upon the polymer, three surface treatments were used:
(1) chloromethylation of styrene followed by quaternization with dimethyl
aniline; (2) radiation grafting of vinyl pyridine to numerous polymers followed by quaternization with methyl iodide or benzyl chloride; and (3)
incorporation of quaternizable monomers, such as vinyl pyridine, into
copolymer formulations.

After quaternization, the surfaces were placed in a heparin solution and
heparin was ionically bound to the ammonium groups. Following contact
with fibrinogen, γ-globulin, and albumin solutions, Zeta potential measurements indicated that the surfaces were progressively becoming less negatively charged, which can be attributed to plasma protein adsorption. From
these studies, the authors attributed the nonthrombogenic nature of the
heparinized surfaces to alterations in the plasma protein adsorption properties of the heparinized materials relative to the starting materials, rather
than to heparin release.

In an attempt to provide heparinized cellulose membranes that could
be utilized in kidney dialysis applications, Merrill et al.[125] ionically bound
heparin to cellulose membranes via an ethyleneimine intermediate. Various
procedures were used to couple ethyleneimine to the hydroxyl groups on
cellulose. Of those procedures, pretreatment with ethylene oxide vapor to
convert secondary cellulose hydroxyl groups into primary hydroxyl groups
was followed by reacting ethyleneimine in toluene-produced aminated surfaces, which could then ionically bind heparin to the greatest extent. Plasma
exposed to these materials demonstrated prolonged clotting times.

Hufnagel et al.[126] were first to incorporate heparin into either silicone
rubber or a combination of silicone rubber plus colloidal graphite. A novel
approach to the controlled release of heparin from polymer matrixes has

been provided by Ebert et al.[127,128] It is known that heparin can adversely interact with platelets, thereby resulting in aggregation and potentiation of aggregation and release reactions caused by exogenous agents. Prostaglandins (e.g., PGE_1, PGI_2, PGD_2), on the other hand, are agents known to prevent platelet aggregation and degranulation by stimulating membrane-bound adenylate cyclase, resulting in increased intracellular cAMP levels. By combining both heparin and prostaglandin into controlled-release polymer matrixes, both intrinsic coagulation and adverse platelet interactions may be controlled.

A disadvantage of ionically bound and physically dispersed heparin/polymer systems is that heparin is continually depleted with time, thereby limiting the effective anticoagulant duration of such materials. Numerous investigators have covalently bound heparin to polymer surfaces to provide long-term heparinized materials. For example, a procedure for radiation-grafting polystyrene to various polymeric materials has been described. The resultant polystyrene surfaces are chloromethylated and subsequently treated with an ammonia/alcohol solution to form benzylamine groups. These polystyrene/benzyl-amine surfaces are then heparinized via a peratin/cyanuric chloride adduct.

Salyer and Weesner[129] have blended heparin into epoxy resins. Although these authors initially thought the nonthrombogenicity of these materials was due to the slow leaching out of heparin into the blood, later studies showed that when heparin was combined with epoxy resins and urethane monomers, polymerization resulted in covalent incorporation of heparin into the copolymer composition and heparin did not leach out. Epoxy and urethane polymers with chemically incorporated heparin demonstrated vastly increased whole-blood clotting times relative to control polymers. Merrill et al.[125] covalently coupled heparin to polyvinyl alcohol via glutaraldehyde cross-linking in the presence of an acid catalyst through hydroxyl groups on heparin and polyvinyl alcohol. Using S-labeled heparin covalently coupled to polyvinyl alcohol, numerous clotting tests were conducted, including thrombin time, partial thromboplastin time, activated partial thromboplastin time, prothrombin time, and whole-blood clotting time.[35]

IX. Ionic polymers

Ionic polymers used as drug carriers include soluble as well as insoluble (cross-linked) polymer systems.[130] However, of the different ionic macromolecules, ion-exchange resins have been investigated most extensively. Although constant rate (zero-order) kinetics is not necessarily achievable by these systems, it is likely that future developments in this field may utilize ionic polymers as drug carriers in controlled delivery.

The use of ion-exchange resins to prolong the effect of drugs is based on the principle that positively or negatively charged drugs combined with appropriate resins yield insoluble poly-salt resinates. The slow release of drugs from ion-exchange resins was recognized early by Saunders and

Srivastava as a suitable approach to the design of sustained-release prepa-rations.[131] A major route of administration of such resinate formulations is via the oral route. Ion exchangers administered orally are likely to spend approximately two hours in the stomach in contact with an acidic pH (1–2). They will then pass to the intestine, where, for six hours or more, they will be in contact with a fluid of slightly basic pH and an ion strength equivalent to that of 0.1 N sodium chloride. The drug can then be slowly liberated by exchange with ions such as sodium or chloride present in the GI fluid.

Drugs to be used in prolonged-action dosage forms, and particularly in resinate formulations, must meet certain conditions. Obviously, only drugs having acidic or basic groups in their chemical structure can be considered. The biological half-life ($t\,^1/_2$) of drugs to be formulated should be 2 to 6 h. There is probably no rational reason for preparing long-acting preparations for oral use of drugs having a $t\,^1/_2$ of 8 or more hours. Active ingredients having a $t\,^1/_2$ of 1 h or less are difficult to be formulated into this type of dosage form if their usual single dose is high (e.g., more than 100 mg). It is necessary to know whether the drug candidate is absorbed from all regions of the GI tract. In the case of a limited absorption zone, the bioavailability of such a drug will be insufficient. The drug should also be sufficiently stable in the gastric juice; otherwise its therapeutic effectiveness will decrease drastically.

Ion-exchange materials are basically insoluble ionic materials possessing acidic or basic groups, covalently bound, and placed in repeating positions on the resin chain. These charged groups are associated with other ions of opposite charge. Depending on whether the mobile counter ion is a cation or anion, it is possible to distinguish between cationic and anionic ion-exchange resins. The matrix carries ionic groups, such as $-SO_3^\ominus$, $-COO^\ominus$, and $-PO_3^{2-}$ (in cationic exchangers), and $-NH_3^\oplus$, $-NH_2^\oplus$, and $-N^-{}^\oplus$ (in anionic exchangers). The resin matrix determines its physical properties, its behavior toward biological substances, and, to a certain extent, its capacity. The matrix may be based on inorganic compounds, polysaccharides, or organic synthetic resins. The most important ion exchangers are the synthetic organic-ion exchangers. Carboxylic acid-type exchangers are prepared mostly by poly-merization of organic acids, such as acrylic or methacrylic acid in the pres-ence of a cross-linking agent (e.g., a diacrylate or divinyl benzene [DVB] to yield cross-linked networks).

Copolymers of styrene and maleic anhydride cross-linked with DVB, as well as cross-linked methacrylate terpolymers, have been described for spe-cific therapeutic purposes. The majority of cationic resins used for preparing drug resinates are sulfonic acid exchangers. They are, in general, cross-linked polystyrenes with sulfonic acid groups that have been introduced after poly-merization by treatment with sulfuric acid or chlorosulfonic acid.

As a rule, DVB is used as a cross-linker.[132] Ion-exchange resins should be insoluble and able to swell to a limited extent. Swelling is attained by the substitution of ionic groups on the hydrophobic hydrocarbon chain. The extent of swelling depends on the degree of cross-linking. By varying the

DVB content, cross-linking and swelling can be adjusted. The DVB content is used to indicate the degree of cross-linking. Commercial products usually contain 40 to 55% DVB-isomers and 45 to 60% ethylstyrene.

The major anion-exchange resins are made from cross-linked polystyrene "pearl" polymers.[133,134] The basic groups can be introduced by a number of different procedures. Most anion exchangers are produced by chloromethylation of polystyrene beads with subsequent treatment with ammonia, or primary, secondary, or tertiary amines.

Ion exchangers based on polysaccharides (e.g., sephadex, sepharose, or cellulose) have found only a limited use in therapeutic applications. The capacity of an ion exchanger is a quantitative measure of its ability to take up exchangeable counter-ions and is, therefore, of major importance. In general, commercial exchangers specify the total capacity. The actual capacity obtainable under specific experimental conditions depends on the accessibility of the functional groups for the drug of interest. The so-called "available capacity" will be related to the drug properties and, as a rule, will be inferior to the total capacity.[135,136]

Another fundamental property is the type of the charged groups which, in turn, determines the type and the strength of the ion exchanger. The acid or base strength of an exchanger is dependent on the various ionogenic groups incorporated into the resin. Resins containing sulfonic, phosphoric, or carboxylic acid-exchange groups have approximate pK_A values of <1, 2–3, and 4–6, respectively. Anion exchangers with quaternary, tertiary, or secondary ammonium groups have apparent pK_A values of >13, 7–9, and 5–9, respectively. The pK_A value of the resin has a significant influence on the rate at which the drug is released from the resinate in gastric fluids.

A number of chemical and physical properties of ion-exchange resins can be varied by modifying particle size and cross-linkage. The rate of an ion-exchange reaction will depend on the size of the particles. Decreasing the size of a resin particle significantly decreases the time required for the reaction to reach equilibrium with a surrounding solution.[137,138]

Rates of ion-exchange reactions and the limiting size of ions that can penetrate into a resin matrix depend strongly on its porosity. In the broadest sense, porosity is defined as the ratio of the volume of interstices of the material to the volume of its mass. Various physical methods have been developed for measuring pore volume, pore diameter, and the internal surface. With the older ion-exchange resins, one was dealing with homogeneous single-phase gels. Later, macroporous resins were produced. They consist of conglomerations of quasispherical particles with interconnecting cavities. The active centers are located both on the surface of the microspherical particles and within them. In contrast to small organic ions, penetration of large organic ions in the resin phase is slow, and capacities are limited to those sites exposed to the macroporous cavities. The diameter of the resin pores through which a molecule must pass for exchange to take place markedly affects the uptake and release of large molecules for which the resin can exhibit a sieve effect. The porosity of an ion exchanger depends not only on the amount of cross-linking substance used in polymerization, but also on the polymerization procedure.

The structural parameters discussed previously will significantly influence the swelling behavior of a resin and consequently have a marked effect on the release characteristics of drug resinates. The interaction between resins, solvents, solutes, and electrolytes has been discussed by Samsonov and Pasechnik.[139] Cation exchangers, in the salt form, brought in contact with acid were reported to shrink. A reduction of pore diameter can lead to the entrapment of large ions.

Since drug-resin combinations contain 60% or more of the resin, it is necessary to establish the toxicity of the ion-exchange resins themselves. Administration of large quantities of ion-exchange resin can disturb the ion strength in body fluids and cause harmful side effects. McChesney et al.[140] have found that administration of sulfonic and carboxylic acid anionic exchangers results in a reduced potassium level in the blood. Macaulay and Watson treated young children with Katonium®, a sulfonic acid exchanger.[141] After prolonged use, symptoms of tetany were manifested as a result of reduced calcium levels.

Synthetic as well as natural polysaccharide-based ion-exchange resins have been used with good results for diagnostic determinations (e.g., gastric acidity). They have also found applications as adsorbents of toxins, as antacids, and as bile-acid binding agents. Among other therapeutic applications, they have been successfully utilized for treatment of liver diseases, renal insufficiency, urolithic disease, and occupational skin diseases. However, with chronic use, the risk of disturbing the ionic strength in the GI fluids should be considered.[142] Despite the numerous positive results reported in the literature, the validity of drug resinates as prolonged-release dosage forms has been questioned. Berg and Ostrup,[143] for example, have made a critical study of the use of resinate formulations.

It should also be recognized that the duration of action of a resinate administered orally may vary considerably from one patient to another. The transport of a solid dosage form through the GI tract is not a standardized process. It depends on many variables, including stomach-emptying time, composition of the alimentary fluid, and peristaltic effects. The constituents of gastric and intestinal secretions in diseased patients may also vary from that of healthy persons. Furthermore, the acid content in the stomach differs with age.

Soluble polyelectrolytes, such as polyacrylic and methacrylic acids, sulfonated or phosphorylated poly(vinyl alcohol), or polysaccharides and polyuronic derivatives, are frequently used as additives in drug formulations (e.g., as suspending agents or tablet disintegrants). Their viscosity-enhancing effect, due to swelling in GI fluids, in addition to their ability to form poorly soluble salts with appropriate drugs, has been utilized in novel drug delivery systems to change the release profile of a drug.

According to Miller and Holland, different salts of the same drug rarely differ pharmacologically.[144] Variations are usually based on their physical properties. Although the nature of the biological response may not differ appreciably, the intensities of the responses may differ markedly. The salt form, in general, and the poly-salt, in particular, are known to influence a number of physiochemical properties of the parent drug, including stability, hygroscopy, solubility, and dissolution rate. These properties, in turn, affect the bioavailability of the drug.

The release process of a drug from a polymeric salt after oral administration can be divided in various stages: (1) penetration of the dissolving medium in the dosage form with simultaneous liberation of a small quantity of drug; (2) swelling of the polymer with formation of a gel barrier; (3) release of the drug ion by exchange with penetrating ions and subsequent diffusion through the gel matrix; and (4) eventual dissolution of the polymeric matrix with liberation of the drug by an ion-exchange process between the polymeric salt and the surrounding medium. If a slow dissolution of the drug-polymer system occurs in the gastric juice as well as in the intestinal fluids, the final result will be a prolonged release. However, ionic polymers having weak acid ionic groups are poorly soluble in gastric juice, and a major release of the drug will occur in the intestine. Delivery systems of this type act as delayed-action dosage forms.

The first long-acting preparations were based on the formation of macromolecular salts. They were combinations of antibiotics with polyacids, such as poly(acrylic acid), sulfonic or phosphorylated polysaccharides, carboxymethyl starch, and poly(uronic acids). Malek et al.[145] showed that parenteral administration of these compounds produced low blood levels of the antibiotics for long periods, while high concentration levels were attained in lymph. In comparison, drug sulfates gave high blood levels but low levels in lymph. The high uptake of the poly-salt in lymph, attributed to the high affinity of the lymphatic system for macromolecules, caused a prolonged passage through the body since the lymphatic circulation is quite slow.

Streptomycin alginates have been prepared by El-Shibini et al. and shown to be effective in prolonged-release preparations.[146] Ozawa et al. report that streptomycin dextran sulfate injected in rabbits gradually releases the antibiotic over a period of approximately 48 h.[147] This prolonged effect may, nevertheless, be due to storage of the poly-salt in the lymphatic system. This phenomenon, first reported by Malek et al., demonstrates the ability of poly-salts to alter the transport of drugs in the body and, hence, modify the intensity and duration of the therapeutic response.[145]

Cavallito and Jewell[148] prepared polygalacturonates of several therapeutic amines in which the polygalacturonates served as agents for influencing the rate of release of the amines. Dialysis experiments showed that poly-galacturonates can reduce the rate of release of therapeutically effective amines. This finding has applications for the preparation of oral repository drug formulations. Poly(galacturonic acid) has also been used to prepare poorly soluble quinidine salts, which have been reported to be four times less toxic orally than the sulfate salts. This reduction in toxicity is attributed to slow release of quinidine from the polygalacturonate.

A remarkable example of a long-acting polymer-drug salt is pilocarpine alginate. When dispersed in sterile water and dried to a solid gel, this preparation was found to possess long duration of action for ophthalmic application. While liquid preparations of alginate or hydrochloride salts had a similar miotic activity, the solid pilocarpine alginate preparations were found to significantly increase the duration of miosis. In contrast to eye drops, which release pilocarpine immediately to the conjunctival fluid, the solid dose of pilocarpine diffuses slowly through the gel matrix and is available more uniformly.

Klaudianos has prepared long-acting preparations based on alginic acid according to a simple and economical method.[149] Sodium alginate was mixed with calcium phosphate and a therapeutic amine and compounded into tablets. Upon oral administration, GI fluids diffuse into the tablet, and the soluble sodium alginate is transformed by cation exchange into an insoluble but swellable calcium alginate. The resulting hydrogel acts as a depot from which the drug slowly diffuses. In the approach of Klaudianos, it is not the drug, but a polyvalent metal ion that causes cross-linking of the polyacid. Salib et al.[150] used an analogous procedure to obtain long-acting chloramphenicol dosage forms based on carboxymethylcellulose to which aluminum sulfate was added as the gel-forming agent.

It has been shown that on precipitation of polyacids by the addition of cationic drugs, considerable amounts of drug are physically entrapped. Goodman and Banker[151] developed a system of molecular-scale drug entrapment by flocculation of highly concentrated colloidal dispersions of acrylic copolymers in the presence of cationic drugs (e.g., methapyrilene). Studies of effectiveness in rats indicated a significantly increased duration of action and reduced acute toxicity of methapyrilene in the entrapped form.

Drug entrapment by polymeric flocculation as an approach to slow-release dosage forms was further studied by Rhodes et al.[152] and Elgindy.[153] It was shown that polymer–drug interactions in flocculates are complex processes that cannot be explained by ionic effects. Hydrogen bonding, as well as hydrophobic drug–drug and drug–polymer interactions, may be involved. This confirmed earlier reports of Kennon and Higuchi,[154] who studied the interaction of cationic drugs with the sodium salt of anionic polyelectrolytes and concluded that drug entrapment appeared to take place by coacervation of oppositely charged ions, additional intermolecular force phenomenon, or replacement of bound sodium by organic cations.

In summary, combining drugs with appropriate ionic polymers is a relatively simple means of altering their physiochemical and biological characteristics. Polymers can contribute to improved drug therapy, particularly in reducing drug toxicity, and influencing the release profile of novel dosage forms. Several sympathomimetics, antitussives, antihistamines, anticholinergics, anthelmintics, antibacterials, and miscellaneous compounds, such as morphine, gentisic acid, and salycylic acid, have been developed by utilizing the drug–resin combination approach.

X. Oligomers

The use of oligomeric instead of high molecular weight matrices to prepare derivatives of drugs can lead to products with considerably prolonged pharmacological activity.[155] In the case of oral, and possibly intradermal administration, the oligomeric matrix is often able to transfer the active principles across physiological barriers, thus facilitating absorption and increasing bioavailability.

Broadly speaking, the preparation of oligomeric or polymeric derivatives of drugs may be achieved in two ways: the preparation of a polymerizable derivative of the drug and the preparation of oligomeric or polymeric matrices carrying chemical functions able to react selectively with some constituent present in the drug molecule. The latter is more convenient, as a rule, since a single matrix can be used to prepare derivatives of a number of drugs. Furthermore, in many cases, drug moieties contain chemical functions that can interfere with the polymerization processes. An interesting variation to these techniques is to use the drugs themselves, leading to polymeric or oligomeric products that are degradable in body fluids reverting to the parent monomers.[156,157] Ferruti et al. have reported on the various possible oligomers and polymers as drug carriers.[155]

XI. Miscellaneous

The following polymers or polymeric materials have been investigated for their use in sustained-release medications:

1. Ethylcellulose and methyl stearate mixtures
2. Hydrated hydroxyalkyl cellulose
3. Salts of polymeric carboxylates
4. Chelated hydrogels
5. Water-insoluble hydrophilic copolymers
6. Cellulose ether compositions
7. Partial esters of acrylate-unsaturated anhydride copolymer
8. Water-soluble coating resins
9. Polymers with oxacycloalkane units
10. Polymers and copolymers of arylene-substitutes orthoesters
11. Polymers with alkoxy or oxacycloalkane substituents
12. Polyglycolic acid polyester condensates
13. Partial esters of polycarboxylic acids
14. Ionene-modified polymeric beads
15. Ethylene-vinyl acetate copolymers
16. Silicone polymer matrix having microsealed compartments
17. Gelatin nanoparticles
18. Serum albumin spherules
19. Phospholipid dispersion
20. Polyglycolic acid sutures and films

21. Polylactides
22. Dacron sutures
23. Caprolactone polymers and copolymers
24. Polysiloxane with N-vinylpyrrolidone
25. Hydrophilic acrylates or methacrylate polymers
26. Siloxane rubbers
27. Hydrocolloids
28. Amine-modified polyanhydrides
29. Polyelectrolytes or gelatin
30. Hydrophobic polycarboxylic acids
31. Metal cation cross-linked polyelectrolytes
32. Polymer–prostaglandin anticoagulant
33. Propranolol spheroids
34. Polymeric macrolides
35. Aspirin–polysiloxane-cellulose derivative matrix
36. Aspirin–pectin combinations
37. Iron compounds with natural resins
38. Polyacrylic alkali metal salts
39. Iron preparation with carboxylic polymers
40. Micronized insoluble cellulose
41. Furosemide–polystyrene
42. Glassy hydrophobic hydrogels
43. Beads containing acetaminophen
44. Acetaminophen using microcrystalline cellulose/wax formulations
45. Polyethylene glycol-derivatized superoxide dismutase
46. Poly(β-hydroxybutyrate), a copolymer with hydroxy valearate
47. Ibuprofen with acrylic polymers
48. Catecholamines using poly-(DL-Lactide-CO-glycolide)
49. Fenvalerate-poly-urea
50. Caffeine release using polyacrylate-methacrylate
51. Release of niclosamide and pituitary hormones using polymers
52. Theophylline and cimetidine using bioadhesive polymers
53. N-(2-hydroxypropyl) methacrylate copolymers
54. Alloys of hydrophilic-balanced coploymers
55. Collagen-poly hydroxyethylmethacrylate hydrogels
56. Ethylene vinyl acetate matrices
57. Hydroxyproline polyesters
58. Indomethacin in biodegradable polymers
59. Pluronic F-127, polaxamer
60. Pesticide chlordimeform in polymeric systems
61. Silicone–cellulose dispersions
62. Progesterone, testosterone, propranolol, and indomethacin from silicone matrices
63. Biodegradable fibers and tetracycline
64. Polymeric-pellet delivery systems for aquatic herbicides (e.g., fluridone)

65. Ethyl cellulose and ranitidine hydrochloride
66. Cyclodextrins for controlled release of insecticides, microbiocides, fungicides, pesticides, and polyorthoesters
67. Cellulose acetate trimellitate and phthalate
68. Hydropropyl methyl cellulose phthalate
69. N-(2-hydroxypropyl) methacrylamide
70. Ethylene-CO vinyl acetate
71. Glucoside monomers
72. Maleic anhydride/mono-methoxyoligoethylene glycol vinyl ether copolymers
73. Oligo(N-isopropylacrylamide)
74. N,N-dimethyl acrylamide

In veterinary products:

1. Enteric-coated swine vaccines
2. Rumen stable pellets (e.g., terpolymers of alkanolamine acrylates) polyamides of piperizine derivatives, and imidazoline-modified styrene-acrylonitrile copolymers

XII. Recent advances

Aqueous polymeric dispersions for controlled drug delivery have been prepared by the Wurster process. Methods of producing sustained-release products from small-coated particles have been reported. The feasibility of obtaining aqueous polymer-coated bead formulations using Aquacoat® and Surelease® dispersions of propranolol as the model drug have been investigated.[158,159]

A delivery system using "Medisorb" bioresorbable polymers has been created by microencapsulating a drug in a polymer. These microcapsules are usually about 50 microns in diameter, which is small enough to be injected through a syringe. Microcapsules can be created in two configurations. As the polymer of a monolithic delivery system breaks down, minute doses of drug are continuously released into the body. The second form delivers a burst of medication in the body. Combining the two capsule forms in one injection creates a comprehensive treatment profile that is particularly useful in the administration of antibiotics. The speed at which the polymer dissolves is regulated by choosing lactide, glycolide, or a copolymer of the two. Copolymer blends can be formulated in varying ratios to yield drug-release times ranging from 7 days to 1 year.[160]

Biodegradable and bioabsorbable polymers have been synthesized, which may be used as a temporary scaffold for tissue regeneration, as a transient barrier, or in controlled drug delivery systems. The copolymers consist of polyester segments creating hard, crystalline blocks of the copolymer and flexible polyether glycols forming the soft blocks of the segmented chains.[161]

A biodegradable polymer has been developed by the Massachusetts Institute of Technology. It is implanted at tumor sites in the brain following

Table 3.4 Commercial preparation of drug–polymer combinations

Corporation	Drug	Polymer as a matrix
Scios Nova & MIT	Gentamicin and carmustine	BIODEL delivery system (Polifeprosan)
DynaGen	Vaccine, immunogens	Sleeper system
KabiPharmacia & Berol Nobel	Drugs for blood disorders	Bioadhesive thermogel
Fidia	Antibiotics, antiseptics, and anti-inflammatories	HYAFF series (modified hyaluronic acids)
TheraTech	Systemic drug administration	BHHA, biodegradable hydrogel
	Wide variety of drugs	HIPN (heterogeneous interpenetrating polymer network)
Verex	Propranolol	POLiM (polymers liquid hydrogel matrix)
Searle/Monsanto	Misoprostol	OLipHEX and pHEMS Polymer delivery system
Advanced Polymer Systems & Rhone-Poulenc Rorer	5-FU 2,4, (1H, 3H)-Pyrimidine-delivery system dione-5-fluoro	Microsponge-based
Biosearch	Piloplex, a derivative of pilocarpine	Polymeric complex
Allelix & Glaxo	Corticosteroids	ALX 25 corticosteroid binding globulin (CBG)
(Alkermes)Enzytech	Therapeutic proteins OraLease, ProLease	Polymer-based delivery system

surgery. Once in place, it slowly releases drug or antibodies, thereby enabling delivery of drug doses hundreds of times greater than is normally possible. Eventually, the polymer implant dissolves. Alza Laboratories manufactures a "bioerodible" polymer called Alzamer that releases drugs at a controlled rate. Possible applications include delivery of drugs or hormones to treat chronic diseases, to provide contraception, or for topical therapy.[162]

Proteins — such as antibodies and lipoproteins, liposomes, synthetic polymers — and polysaccharides — such as dextran and insulin — are various types of macromolecules used as drug delivery systems. Polymers have been used extensively in these systems, including nanoparticles, microcapsules, laminates, matrices, and microporous powders. In all these delivery systems, the drug is merely dispersed or incorporated into the system without the formation of a covalent bond between the drug and polymer. Because the molecular weight of a polymeric drug delivery system is so high, such systems are often referred to as macromolecular carrier systems. Although the majority of polymer-drug conjugate systems have no biological activity, all such systems release the conjugated drug *in vivo*. A schematic diagram of Ringsdorf's model is given in Figure 3.3.

The system has a polymer backbone, which can be a homopolymer or a heteropolymer, depending on the constituents of the carrier polymer. Dextran and insulin are two polysaccharides that have been widely used. Sparer et al.[163] propose using glycosaminoglycans as drug carriers. Cellulose and polyarabogalactans have also been studied as possible drug carriers by these investigators Grolleman et al.[164] prepared a polymer pro-drug of naproxen with polyphosphazene, using a spacer molecule. Gros et al.[165] have synthesized a polymeric conjugate of poly(glutamic acid) and p-phenylenediamine, using immunoglobulin as a homing device. The polymer's immunogenicity, hemolytic activity, pyrogenicity, osmotic properties, and its interaction with plasma components must be studied before the polymer can be used in a drug delivery system. For example, even endogenous polymers, such as chondroitin sulfate, might show toxic effects after prolonged use at very high doses. Until recently, a polymeric pro-drug system has been used only in intravenous administration, but as in the case of phosphazene, such a system can now be used as a bioerodible implant. Localized effects, as in the case of gastrointestinal delivery, can be used effectively.[164,166]

Sustained-release tablets using an inert, compressed plastic matrix have become increasingly used clinically since their introduction several years ago. With these tablets, drug release is delayed because the dissolving drug must diffuse through a network of channels between the compacted polymer particles. The rate of release of a drug from a polymeric matrix can be controlled by altering the porosity or surface area of the matrix, thereby changing the solubility of the drug or its diffusion coefficient, or by adding other compounds that speed up or delay the release of the drug.

Rhodes et al.[152] have demonstrated that tablet matrices containing mixtures of two or more substances might be superior to the individual matrices currently available. The materials used in the study by Chang et al.[167] included polycaprolactone and cellulose propionate.

Because of cost, stringent environmental regulations, and the safety hazards associated with the use of organic solvents in coating processes, the pharmaceutical industry has been moving away from the use of organic solvent- based film-coating systems. Increasingly, the industry is relying on water-based coating formulations. New aqueous polymeric dispersions have also been developed, and intensive research is being conducted to maximize the use of water-dispersible colloidal particles in formulations for coating. Development of controlled-release dosage forms in which the mechanism of release is diffusion through a polymeric membrane formed via film coating requires the optimization of several processing and formulation variables to ensure reproducibility of the release rate.

When polymeric-coating systems composed of a latex or pseudo-latex are used to coat pellets or tablets, film deposition on the substrate must be followed by a curing stage in which the spherical submicron polymeric particles coalesce to form a continuous film. One procedure for curing involves storing the coated material at high temperatures for various periods of time, depending on the formulation. However, this procedure often leads to problems with product handling because the film softens, causing tackiness. Although the tackiness eventually subsides after the temperature is lowered, the possibility of the film rupturing is always present, and this could have a detrimental effect on dissolution properties.[169]

Synthetic hydrogels are used in drug delivery systems primarily because their permeability can be controlled for aqueous solutes and they exhibit favorable swelling pressures and generally good biocompatibility. The hydrogels currently in use are based on covalently cross-linked hydrophilic polymers. This concept, which is more than 30 years old, has several inherent limitations. A new concept for hydrogels was developed over the past several years based on the use of multiblock copolymers containing hydrophilic and hydrophobic blocks. The hydrophobic blocks separate in the presence of water, and the hydrophobic domains formed in this manner can replace covalent cross-linking. The most advanced of these multiblock copolymers are the hydrogels with polyacrylonitrile blocks, which form crystalline domains of exceptional stability. This new concept allows processing by conventional methods and provides high degrees of strength even at a high level of water content.[170]

A wide variety of polymeric materials have been used in the fabrication and development of transdermal drug delivery systems. These materials have taken the form of components for devices, as well as polymeric materials that are mixed with drugs to slow down or enhance delivery. In reservoir-type transdermal devices, polymers have been used within the contents of the reservoir and in the rate-limiting membranes to regulate the passage of drug across the skin. In matrix transdermal systems, polymers have been used to form the device as well as to mediate drug absorption across the skin. In adhesive-type systems, polymers have been used as adhesives and have been mixed with the drug or used in the device.[171]

Amantadine has been modified by direct acylation with succinic and glutaric anhydrides and a covalent bond formed with substituted aspartamide (PHEA). The amount of amantadine in the copolymers was evaluated by hydrolysis of the conjugates. Binding of PHEA-succinylamantadine to surfactant micelles appeared to be stronger than that shown by PHEA-glutarylamantadine.[172]

A polymer carrier system has been developed to reduce the bitterness of erythromycin and its 6-O-methyl derivative, clarithromycin, by absorption to Carbopol.® The mechanism involves ionic bonding of the amine macrolide to high molecular weight polyacrylic acid, thereby removing the drug from the solution phase in an ion-free suspension. The macrolide-Carbopol complexes were prepared by dissolving or slurring predetermined ratios of drug and polymer in water or hydroalcoholic mixtures. Human bioavailability studies demonstrated that the microencapsulated Carbopol absorbates of erythromycin and clarithromycin give blood levels comparable to those from conventional solid formulations.[173]

Medical College of Ohio, Bowling Green State University, and Lilly have developed an azo cross-linked polymer coating for use in the delivery of peptide drugs to the large intestine. The coating protects the peptides from stomach acid and digestive enzymes in the small intestine until bacteria in the large intestine break down the coating, releasing the peptides. Other potential applications are to deliver drugs such as heparin, peptide contraceptives, analgesics, anticancer, anti-inflammatory drugs, and the Sabin polio vaccine.

Biocompatible polymers have been tested as potential delivery systems for therapeutic antibodies and antibody fragments. The researchers incorporated antibodies and antibody fragments directed against a pregnancy hormone; human chorionic gonadotropin; into poly(ethylene-CO-vinyl) acetate, which is stable in biological environments; and a biodegradable polyanhydride copolymer of stearic acid dimer and sebacic acid. Saltzman and co-workers found that the antibodies released slowly from both polymers during 30 days of continuous immersion in buffered saline and retained their ability to bind antigens.[162]

The authors examined enantioselective release of controlled-delivery granules based on molecularly imprinted polymers (MIPs) for various racemic drugs (e.g., S-ibuprofen, S-ketoprofen, and R-propranolol). These were prepared using a multistep swelling and thermal polymerization method. The release profile of MIP granules exhibited differential release of enantiomers. The enantioselective release appeared to depend on polymer loading and medium pH. The drug/polymer ratio of 1:25 showed the best enantioselective release with initial enantiomeric excess of 100%.[185]

Polylactide-co-glycolide and polylactide polymer particles entrapping immunoreactive tetanus toxoid (TT) were prepared in order to study single-shot controlled-release vaccine formulation.[186] The results indicated the significance of protecting the immunoreactivity of TT during formation of polymer particles for sustained and improved antibody response.

Polyisobutylcyanoacrylate nanocapsules (PIBCA-NC) of pilocarpine were prepared by interfacial polymerization. Physicochemical characterization of the colloidal dispersion of pilocarpine was performed by measuring drug loading, particle-size analysis, and scanning electron microscopy.[187] It was found that Pluronic F127 gel delivery system increases the contact time of pilocarpine with the absorbing tissue in the eye, thereby improving ocular bioavailability of such hydrophobic drugs. Spray-dried powders of poly(D-L lactic acid) (PLA) or poly-epsilon-caprolactone (PepsilonC) from colloidal suspensions containing indomethacin using benzyl benzoate in nanocapsules or micelles were prepared by nanoprecipitation. After one month, the formulations with highest drug content (2.0mg/ml) showed a decline of total quantity of indomethacin.

Saito et al. investigated biodegradable poly-D-L-lactic acid-polyethylene glycol block copolymers as a bone morphogenetic protein (BMP) delivery system for inducing bone formation. According to the authors, in combination with biomaterials, these proteins can be used in a clinical setting as bone-graft substitutes to promote bone repair. Most recently, synthetic biodegradable polymers were tested as a delivery vehicle for osteoinductive agents. In their earlier studies, these authors noted that polylactic acid homopolymers and poly-D-L-lactic acid polyethylene glycol block copolymers could be used as BMP delivery systems. These polymers were implanted into the dorsal muscle of mice to evaluate their capacity to elicit new bone formation.[188]

XIII. Conclusion

Recently, it has been stated that,[174] as in the past, when certain ages were characterized by the discovery of major materials (e.g., the Stone Age or the Bronze Age) the current period could be called the Polymer or Plastic Age. Most notably in the area of pharmaceutical applications, the rapid expansion of scientific work and intense interest in the development of new drug delivery systems have provided strong motivation for the creation of polymers and new polymeric materials.[167]

In state-of-the-art research and drug delivery system design, involving these entities in particular, the following topics have undergone extensive investigation: soluble synthetic polymers, oligomers, copolymers, bioerodible and biodegradable polymers, polymer-coated liposomes, encapsulated drugs for cancer, colloid carrier systems, albumin and gelatin microspheres, magnetic microspheres and magnetically modulated systems, microsealed drug delivery systems, matrix devices, swellable polymers and pseudo-latex dispersions, polymer-bioactive agent (or pro-drug) complexes, hydrogels, insulin delivery, and polymeric implants, liquid crystalline photoreactive, and performance polymers.

Currently, continuing significant advances in drug delivery devices composed of polymers and polymeric materials have occurred primarily with osmotic pumps, implants, and dermal and oral drug delivery systems. Exciting research in the area of polymers undoubtedly promises the development of new drug delivery systems. These systems will be designed for specific targeting and capable of providing precise and predictable systemic drug release with greater efficacy and minimal side effects. In the near future, the multidisciplinary efforts of leading researchers dealing with polymers will certainly result in the development of novel delivery systems in this rapidly expanding field.[175–177]

References

1. Wise, D.L., *Biopolymeric Controlled Release Systems*, Vol. 1, CRC Press, Inc., Boca Raton, FL, 1984.
2. Guiot, *Polymeric Nanoparticles and Microspheres*, CRC Press, Inc., Boca Raton, FL.
3. Langer, R.S., *Medical Applications of Controlled Release*, Vol. 1, CRC Press, Inc., Boca Raton, FL.
4. Tirrel, D.A., *Macromolecules as Drugs and as Carriers for Biologically Active Materials*, Vol. 446, The New York Academy of Sciences, New York, 1985.

5. Illum, L. and Davis, S.S., *Polymers in Controlled Drug Delivery*, Wright, Bristol, England, 1987.
6. Lloyd, J.B., Soluble polymers as targetable drug carriers. In *Drug Delivery Systems, Fundamentals and Techniques*, Horwood, E., Ed., VCH Publishers, England, 1987. Also see Duncan, R. and Lloyd, J.B., Biological evaluation of soluble synthetic polymers as drug carriers. In *Recent Advances in Drug Delivery Systems*, Anderson, J.M. and Kim, S.W., Eds., Plenum Press, New York, 1983, 9–22.
7. Prattern, M.K., Duncan, R., Cable, H.C., Schnee, R., et al., Pinocytotic uptake of divinyl ether-maleic anhydride (pyran copolymer) and its failure to stimulate pinocytosis, *Chem. Biol. Interactions*, 35, 319–330, 1981.
8. Duncan, R., Cable, H.C., Rejmanova, P., Kopecek, J., and Lloyd, J.B., Tyrosinamide residues enhance pinocytic capture of N-(2-hydroxypropyl)methacrylamide copolymers, *Biochem. Biophys. Acta*, 799, 1–8, 1984.
9. Duncan, R., Starling, D., Rypacek, F., Drobnik, J., and Lloyd, J.B., Pinocytosis of poly(α,β-(N-2-hydroxyethyl)-DL-aspartamide and a tyramine derivative by rat visceral yolk sacs cultured *in vitro*, ability of phenolic residues to enhance the rate of pincocytic capture of a macromolecule, *Biochem. Biophys. Acta*, 717, 248–254, 1982.
10. Duncan, R., Cable, H.C., Rypavek, F., Drobnik, J., and Lloyd, J.B., Characterization of the adsorptive pinocytic capture of a polyaspartamide modified by the incorporation of tyramine residues, *Biochem Biophys. Acta*, 840, 291–293, 1985.
11. Prattern, M.K., Lloyd, J.B., Horel, G,. and Ringsdorf, H., Micelle-forming block copolymers; pinocytosis by macrophages and interaction with model membranes, *Macromol. Chem.*, 186, 725–733, 1985.
12. Duncan, R.D., Rejmanova, P., Kopacek, J., and Lloyd, J.B., Pinocytic uptake and intracellular degradation of N-(2-hydroxypropyl)methacrylamide copolymers, *Biochem. Biophys. Acta*, 678, 143–150, 1981.
13. Duncan, R., Pattern, M.K., Cable, H.C., Ringsdorf, H., and Lloyd, J.B., Effect of molecular size of I-labelled poly(vinylpyrrolidone) on its pinocytosis by rat visceral yolk sacs and rat peritoneal macrophages, *Biochem. J.*, 196, 49–55, 1981.
14. Cartlidge, S.A., Duncan, R., Lloyd, J.B., Rejmanova, P., and Kopacek, J., Soluble, cross-linked N-(2)hydroxypropyl methacrylamide copolymers as potential drug carriers, 1. Pincocytosis by rat visceral yolk sacs and rat intestine cultured *in vitro*, effect of molecular weight on uptake and intracellular degradation, *J. Controlled Release*, 3, 55–66, 1986.
15. Duncan, R., Kopacek, J., Rejmanova, P., and Lloyd, J.B., Targeting of N-(2-hydroxypropyl)methacrylamide copolymers to liver by incorporation of galactose residues, *Biochem. Biophys. Acta*, 755, 518–521, 1983.
16. Duncan, R., Seymour, L.C.W., Scarlett, L., Lloyd, J.B., et al., Fate of N-(2-hydroxypropyl)methacrylamide copolymers with pendent galactosamine residues after intravenous administration to rats, *Biochem. Biophys. Acta*, 880, 62–71, 1986.
17. Duncan, R., Lloyd, J.B., and Kopacek, J., Degradation of side chains of N-(2-hydroxypropyl)methacrylamide copolymers by lysosomal enzymes, *Biochem. Biophys. Res. Comm.*, 94, 284–290, 1980.
18. Duncan, R., Cable, H.C., Lloyd, J.B., Rejmanova, P., and Kopacek, J., Degradation of side-chains of N-(2-hydroxypropyl)methacrylamide copolymers by lysosomal thiol-proteinases, *Bioscience Reports*, 2, 1041–1046, 1982.

19. Duncan, R., Cable, H.C., Lloyd, J.B., Rejmanova, P., and Kopecek, J., Polymers containing enzymatically degradable bonds, 7, Design of oligopeptides side-chains in poly N-(2-hydroxypropyl)methacrylamide copolymers to promote efficient degradation by lysosomal enzymes, *Macromol. Chem.*, 184, 1997–2008, 1983.

20. Rejmanova, P., Kopecek, J., Pohl, J., Baudys, M., and Kostka, V., Polymers containing enzymatically degradable bonds, 8, Degradation of oligopeptide sequences in N-(2-hydroxypropyl)methacrylamide copolymers by bovine spleen cathepsin, B. *Macromol. Chem.*, 184, 2009–2020, 1983.

21. Rejmanova, P., Kopacek, J., Duncan, R., and Lloyd, J.B., Stability in rat plasma and serum of lysosomally degradable oligopeptide sequences in N-(2-hydroxy propyl)methacrylamide copolymers, *Biomaterials*, 6, 45–48, 1985.

22. Pitt, C.G. and Schindler, A., Biodegradation of polymers. In *Controlled Drug Delivery*, Vol. 1, Basic Concepts, CRC Press, Inc., Boca Raton, FL, 1983, 53-81.

23. Desai, S.J., Simonelli, A.P., and Higuchi, W.L., Investigation of factors influencing release of solid drug dispersed in inert matrices, *J. Pharm. Sci*, 54, 1459, 1965.

24. Folkman, J. and Long, D.M., The use of silicone rubber as a carrier for prolonged drug therapy, *J. Surg. Res.*, 4, 139, 1964.

25. Baker, R.W. and Lonsdale, H.K., *Controlled Release: Mechanism and Rates in Controlled Release of Biologically Active Agents*, Vol. 47, Tarquasy, A.C. and Lacey, R.E., Eds., Plenum Press, New York, 15, 1974.

26. Rogers, C.E., Solubility and diffusivity, In *Physics and Chemistry of the Organic Solid State*, Vol. 2, Fox, D., Labes, M.M., and Weissberger, A., Eds., Wiley Interscience, New York, 1965.

27. Crank, J. and Park, G.S., Eds., *Diffusion in Polymers*, Academic Press, London, 1968.

28. Langer, R.S. and Peppas, N.A., Present and future applications of biomaterials in controlled drug delivery, *Biomaterials*, 2, 201, 1981.

29. Heller, J., Controlled release of biologically active compounds from bioerodible polymers, *Biomaterials*, 1, 51, 1980.

30. Benagiano, G. and Gabelnick, H., Biodegradable systems for the sustained release of fertility-regulating agents, *J. Steroid Biochem.*, 11, 449, 1979.

31. Pitt, C.G. and Schindler, A., The design of controlled drug delivery systems based on biodegradable polymers. In *Biodegradables and Delivery Systems for Contraception*, Vol. 1, Hafez, E.S.E. and van Os, W.A.A., Eds., MTP Press, Ltd., Lancaster, U.K., 17, 1980.

32. Pitt, C.G., Marks, A., and Schindler, A., Biodegradable drug delivery systems based on aliphatic polyesters; application to contraceptives and narcotic antagonists. In *Controlled Release of Bioactive Materials*, Baker, R., Ed., Academic Press, New York, 19–43, 1980.

33. Graham, N.B., Polymeric inserts and implants for the controlled release of drugs, *Br. Polym. J.*, 10, 260, 1978.

34. Kim, S.W., Petersen, R.V., and Feijen, J., *Polymeric Drug Delivery Systems in Drug Design*, Vol. 10, Ariens, E.J., Ed., Academic Press, New York, 1980.

35. Schindler, A., Jeffcoat, R., Kimmel, G.L., Pitt, C.G., et al., Biodegradable polymers for sustained drug delivery. In *Contemporary Topics in Polymer Science*, Vol. 2, Pearce, E.M. and Schaefgen, J.R., Eds., Plenum Press, New York, 251, 1977.

36. Heller, J., Zero-order drug release from bioerodible polymers. In *Recent Advances in Drug Delivery Systems*, Anderson, J.M. and Kim, S.W., Eds., Plenum Press, New York, 101–121, 1983.

37. Lappas, L.C. and McKeehan, W., Synthetic polymers as potential enteric and sustained-release coatings, *J. Pharm. Sci.*, 51, 808, 1962.
38. Lappas, L.C. and McKeehan, W., Polymeric pharmaceutical coatings materials, I. Preparation and properties, *J. Pharm. Sci.*, 54, 176, 1965.
39. Lappas, L.C. and McKeehan, W., Polymeric pharmaceutical coating materials, II. *In vivo* evaluation as enteric coatings, *J. Pharm. Sci.*, 56, 1257, 1967.
40. Heller, J., Baker, R.W., Gale, R.M., and Rodin, J.O., Controlled drug release by polymer dissolution, I. Partial esters of maleic anhydride copolymers, properties and theory, *J. Appl. Polymer Sci.*, 22, 1991, 1978.
41. Heller, J., *Bioerodible Systems 69–101 Medical Applications of Controlled Release*, Vol. 1, Langer, R.S. and Wise, D.L., Eds., CRC Press, Inc., Boca Raton, FL, 1984.
42. Woodland, J.H.R., Yolles, S., Blake, D.A., Helrich, M., and Meyer, F.J., Long-acting delivery systems for narcotic antagonists, I. *J. Med. Chem.*, 16, 897, 1973.
43. Yolles, S. and Sartori, M.F., Degradable polymers for sustained drug release. In *Drug Delivery Systems*, Juliano, R.L., Ed., Oxford University Press, New York, 1980.
44. Yolles, S., Eldridge, J., Leafe, T., Woodland, J.H.R., et al., Long-acting delivery systems for narcotic antagonists. In *Controlled Release of Biologically Active Agents*, Tanquary, A.C. and Lacey, R.E., Eds., Plenum Press, New York, 1974.
45. Yolles, S., Controlled release of biologically active agents. In *Polymers in Medicine and Surgery*, Kronenthal, R.L., Oser, Z., and Martin, E., Eds., Plenum Press, New York, 1975.
46. Yolles, S., Leafe, T., Sartori, M., Torkelson, M., et al., Controlled release of biologically active agents. In *Controlled Release Polymeric Formulations*, Paul, D.R. and Harris, F.W., Eds., American Chemical Society, Washington, D.C., 1976.
47. Gresser, J.D., Wise, D.L., Beck, L.R., and Howes, J.F., Larger animal testing of an injectable sustained-release fertility control system, *Contraception*, 17, 253, 1978.
48. Wise, D.L., Gregory, J.B., Newberne, D.M., Bartholow, L.C., and Stanbury, J.B., Results on biodegradable cylindrical subdermal implants for fertility control. In *Polymeric Delivery Systems*, Kostelink, R.J., Ed., Gordon & Breach, New York, 1978.
49. Kulkarni, R.K., Moore, E.G., Hegyeli, A.F., and Leonard, F., Biodegradable poly-(lactic acid) polymers, *J. Biomed. Mater. Res.*, 5, 169, 1971.
50. Yolles, S., Leafe, T.D., and Myer, F.J., Timed-release depot for anticancer agent, *J. Pharm. Sci.*, 64, 115, 1975.
51. Wise, D.L., McCormick, G.L., Willet, G.P., and Anderson, L.C., Sustained release of an antimalarial drug using a copolymer of glycolic/lactic acid, *Life Sci.*, 19, 867, 1976.
52. Hutchinson, F.G. and Furr, B.J.A., Design of biodegradable polymers for controlled release. In *Drug Delivery Systems, Fundamentals and Techniques*, Johnson, P. and Lloyd-Jones, J.G., Eds., VCH Publishers, Ellis Horwood, U.K., 106–119, 1987.
53. Anik, S.T., Sanders, L.M., Chaplin, M.D., Kushinsky, S., and Nerenberg, C., Delivery systems of LHRH and analogs. In *LHRH and Its Analogs: Contraceptive and Therapeutic Applications*, Vickery, B.H., Nestor, Jr., J.J., and Hafez, E.S.E., Eds., MTP Press, Ltd., Boston, MA, 421–435, 1984.
54. Petri, W., Seidel, R., and Sandow, J., Pharmaceutical approach to long-term therapy with peptides, *Int. Cong. Series — Excerpta Medica*, 656, 63–76, 1984.

55. Anders, R., Merkle, H.P., Schurr, W., and Ziegler, R., Buccal absorption of protirelin: An effective way to stimulate thyrotropin and prolactin, *J. Pharm. Sci.*, 72, 1481–1483, 1983.
56. Okado, H., Zamazaki, I., Ogava, Y., Hirai, S., et al., Vaginal absorption of a potent leutenizing hormone-releasing hormone analog (Leuprolide) in rats, I. Absorption by various routes and absorption enhancement, *J. Phar. Sci.*, 71, 1367–1371, 1982.
57. Okado, H., Zamazaki, I., Yashiki, T., and Mima, H., Vaginal absorption of a potent leutenizing hormone-releasing hormone analog (Leuprolide) in rats, II. Mechanism of absorption enhancement with organic acids, *J. Pharm. Sci.*, 72, 75–78, 1983.
58. Okado, H., Yashiki, T., and Mima, H., Vaginal absorption of a potent leutenizing hormone-releasing hormone analog (Leuprolide) in rats, III. Effect of estrous cycle on vaginal absorption of hydrophilic model compounds, *J. Pharm. Sci.*, 72, 173–176, 1983.
59. Okado, H., Zamazaki, I., Yashiki, T., Shimamoto, T., and Mima, H., Vaginal absorption of a potent leutenizing hormone-releasing hormone analog (Leuprolide) in rats, IV. Evaluation of the vaginal absorption and gonadotrophin responses by radioimmunoassay, *J. Pharm. Sci.*, 73, 298–302, 1982.
60. Hunt, G., Kearney, P., and Kellaway, I.W., Mucoadhesive polymers in drug delivery systems. In *Drug Delivery Systems, Fundamentals and Techniques*, Johnson, P. and Lloyd-Jones, J.G., Eds., VCH Publishers, Ellis Horwood, U.K., 180–199, 1987.
61. Mungiu, C., Gogalniceanu, D., Leibovici, M., and Negulescu, I., On the medical use of cyanoacrylate esters:tonicity of pure n-butyl-cyanoacrylate, *J. Polym. Sci. Polym. Symp.*, 66, 189–193, 1979.
62. Vezin, W.R. and Florence, A.T., *In vitro* heterogeneous degradation of poly(n-alkyl-cyanoacrylates), *J. Biomed. Mater. Res.*, 14, 93–106, 1980.
63. Meyer, G., Muster, D., Schmitt, D., Jung, P., and Jaeger, J.H., Bone bonding through bioadhesives: present status, *Biomat. Med. Dev. Art. Org.* 7, 55–71, 1979.
64. Park, J.B., Acrylic bone cement: *in vitro* and *in vivo* property-structural relationship: a selective review, *Ann. Biomed. Eng.*, 11, 297–312, 1983.
65. Bechgaard, H. and Ladefoged, K., Distribution of pellets in the gastrointestinal tract. The influence on transit time exerted by the density or diameter of pellets. *J. Pharm. Pharmacol.*, 30, 690-692, 1978.
66. Florey, H., Mucin and the protectin of the body, *Proc. R. Soc. B.*, 143, 147–155, 1955.
67. Davenport, H.W., *Physiology of the Digestive Tract*, Year Book Publishers, Inc., Chicago, IL, 1977.
68. Allen, A., Bell, A., Mantle, M., and Pearson, J.P., The structure and physiology of gastrointestinal mucus. In *Mucus in Health and Disease*, Vol. 2, Chantler, E.N., Elder, J.B., and Elstein, M., Eds., Plenum Press, New York, 115–133, 1982.
69. Parke, D.V., Pharmacology of mucus, *Brit. Med. Bull.*, 34, 89–94, 1978.
70. Kulenkampff, H., The structural basis of intestinal absorption. In *Pharmacology of Intestinal Absorption: Gastrointestinal Absorption of Drugs*, Forth, W. and Rummel, W., Eds., Pergamon Press, London, 1–70, 1975.
71. Neutra, M.R., Grand, R.J., and Trier, J.S., Glycoprotein synthesis, transport and secretion by epithelial cells of human rectal mucosa: normal and cystic fibrosis, *Lab. Invest.*, 36, 535–536, 1977.

72. Silberberg, A. and Meyer, F.A., Structure and function of mucus. In *Mucus in Health and Disease*, Vol. 2, Chantler, E.N., Elder, J.B., and Elstein, M., Eds, Plenum Press, NY, 35–74, 1982.

73. Bickel, M. and Kauffman, G.L., Gastric gel mucus thickness: Effect of distension 16, 16-dimethyl prostaglandin E_2 and carbenoxolone, *Gastroenterology*, 80, 770–775, 1981.

74. Allen, A., The structure of gastrointestinal mucus glycoproteins and the viscous and gel-formimg properties of mucus, *Brit. Med. Bull.*, 34, 28–33, 1978.

75. Allen, A., Pain, R.H., and Roberts, T.R., Model for the structure of gastric mucus gel, *Nature*, 264, 88–89, 1976.

76. Meyer, F.A., King, M., and Gelman, R.A., On the role of sialic acid in the rheological properties of mucus, *Biochim. Biophys. Acta.*, 392, 223–232, 1975.

77. Kearney, P., Kellaway, I.W., Evans, J.C., and Rowlands, C., Probing the mucus barrier with spin labels, *J. Pharm. Pharmacol.*, 36, 26, 1984.

78. Allen, A., Foster, S.N.E., and Pearson, J.P., Interaction of polyacrylate, carbomer, with gastric mucus and pepsin, *Brit. J. Pharmacol.*, 87, 126, 1986.

79. Peppas, N.A. and Buri, P.A., Surface, interfacial and molecular aspects of polymer bioadhesion on soft tissues, *J. Cont. Rel.*, 2, 257–275, 1985.

80. Smart, J.D., Kellaway, I.W., and Worthington, H.E.C., An *in vitro* investigation of mucosa-adhesive materials for use in controlled drug delivery, *J. Pharm. Pharmacol.*, 36, 295–299, 1984.

81. Slomiany, A., Slomiany, B.L., Witas, H., Aono, M., and Newman, L.J., Isolation of fatty acids covalently bound to the gastric mucus glycoprotein of normal and cystic fibrosis patients, *Biochim. Biophys. Res. Commun.*, 113, 286–293, 1983.

82. Scrivener, C.A. and Schantz, C.W., Penicillin: new methods for its use in dentistry, *J. Am. Dental Assoc.*, 35, 644–647, 1947.

83. Rothner, J.T., Cobe, H.M., Rosenthal, S.L., and Bailin, J., Adhesive penicillin ointment for topical application, *J. Dent. Res.*, 28, 544–548, 1949.

84. Keutscher, A.H., Zegarelli, E.V., Beube, F.E., Chiton, N.W., et al., A new vehicle (Orabase) for the application of drugs to the oral mucus membranes, *Oral Surg., Oral Med., Oral Pathol.*, 12, 1080–1089, 1959.

85. Chen, J.L. and Cyr, G.N., Compositions producing adhesion through hydration. In *Adhesion in Biological Systems*, Manly, R.S., Ed., Academic Press, New York, 163–167, 1970.

86. Harris, F.W., Controlled release from polymers containing pendent bioactive substituents. In *Medical Applications of Controlled Release*, Vol. 1, Langer, R.S. and Wise, D.L., Eds., CRC Press, Inc., Boca Raton, FL, 103–128, 1984.

87. Ringsdorf, H., Structure and properties of pharmacologically active polymers, *J. Polym. Sci. Polym. Symp.*, 51, 135, 1975.

88. Ringsdorf, H., Synthetic polymeric drugs. In *Polymeric Delivery Systems*, *Midl. Macromol. Monogr.*, No. 5, Kostelnik, R.J., Ed., Gordon & Breach, New York, 197, 1978.

89. Trout, A., Carriers for bioactive materials. In *Polymeric Delivery Systems*, *Midl. Macromol. Monogr.*, No. 5, Kostelnik, R.J., Ed., Gordon & Breach, New York, 157, 1978.

90. Goldberg, E.P., Polymeric affinity drugs. In *Polymeric Delivery Systems*, *Midl. Macromol. Monogr.*, No. 5, Kostelnik, R.J., Ed., Gordon & Breach, New York, 197, 1978.

91. deDuve, C., deBarsy, T., Poole, B., Trout, A., et al., Lysosomotropic agents, *Biochem. Pharmacol.*, 23, 2495, 1974.

92. Zaffaroni, A. and Bonsen, P., Controlled chemotherapy through macromolecules. In *Polymeric Drugs*, Donaruma, L.G. and Vogl, O., Eds., Academic Press, Inc., New York, 1978.

93. Regelson, W., Thrombocyclopenic and related physiological effects of heparin and heparinoids: Macromolecular-induced syndrome, *Hematol. Rev.*, 193, 1968.

94. Kalal, J., Drobnik, J., Kopecek, J., and Exner, J., Synthetic polymers in chemotherapy: general problems. In *Polymeric Drugs*, Donaruma, L.G. and Vogl, O., Eds., Academic Press, New York, 1978.

95. Ghose, T. and Blair, A.H., Antibody-linked cytotoxic agents in the treatment of cancer: Current status and future prospects, *J. Natl. Cancer Inst.*, 61, 657, 1978.

96. Sinkula, A.A., Methods to achieve sustained drug delivery: The chemical approach. In *Sustained and Controlled Release Drug Delivery Systems*, Robinson, J.R., Ed., Mercel Dekker, New York, 1978.

97. Thorpe, P.E., Edwards, D.C., Davies, A.J.S., and Ross, W.C.J., Monoclonal antibody-toxin conjugates: Aiming the magic bullet. In *Monoclonal Antibodies in Clinical Medicine*, Fabre, J.W. and McMichael, A.J., Eds., Academic Press, New York, 1982.

98. Goldstein, J.L., Ho, Y.K., Basu, S.K., and Brown, M.S., Binding site on macrophages that mediates uptake and degradation of acylated low-density lipoprotein producing massive cholesterol deposition, *Proc. Natl. Acad. Sci.* (USA), 76, 333, 1979.

99. Mahley, R.W., Weisgraber, K.H., Innerarity, T.L., and Windmueller, H.G., Accelerated clearance of low-density and high-density lipoproteins and retarded clearance of E apoprotein-containing lipoproteins from the plasma of rats after modification of lysine residues, *Proc. Natl. Acad. Sci.* (USA), 76, 1746, 1979.

100. Bradley, S.G., Marecki, N.M., Bond, J.S., Munson, A.E., and John, D.T., Enhanced cytotoxicity in mice of combinations of concanavalin A and selected antitumor drugs, *Adv. Exp. Med. Biol.*, 55, 291, 1975.

101. Lin, J.Y., Li, J.S., and Tung, T.C., Lectin derivatives of methotroxate and chlorambucil as chemotherapeutic agents, *J. Natl. Cancer Inst.*, 66, 523, 1981.

102. Goldberg, E.P., Iwata, H., Terry, R.N., Longo, W.E., et al., Polymeric-affinity drugs for targeted chemotherapy: Use of specific and non-specific cell-binding ligands. In *Affinity Chromatography and Related Techniques*, Gribnau, T.C.J., Vesser, J., and Nivard, R.J.F., Eds., Elsevier/North-Holland, Amsterdam, 375, 1982.

103. Rowland, G.F., O'Neill, G.J., and Davies, D.A., Suppression of tumor growth in mice by a drug-antibody conjugate using a novel approach to linkage, *Nature* (London), 255, 487, 1975.

104. Cardinal, J.R., *Matrix Systems Medical Applications of Controlled Release*, Vol. 1, Langer, R.S. and Wise, D.L., Eds., CRC Press Inc., Boca Raton, FL, 41–67, 1984.

105. Roseman, T.J., Monolithic polymer devices. In *Controlled Release Technologies: Methods, Theory and Applications*, Vol. 1, Kydonieus, A.F., Ed., CRC Press, Inc., Boca Raton, FL, 1980.

106. Leininger, R.I., Polymers as surgical implants. In *CRC Crit. Rev. Bio.*, Fleming, D.G., Ed., CRC Press, Boca Raton, FL, 333, 1972.

107. Zentner, G.M., Cardinal, J.R., and Kim, S.W., Progestin permeation through polymer membranes, I. Diffusion studies on plasma-soaked membranes, *J. Pharm. Sci.*, 67, 1347, 1978.

108. Ermini, M., Carpino, F., Russo, M., and Nengiano, G., Studies on sustained contraceptive effects with subcutaneous polydimethylsiloxane implants, III. Factors affecting steroid diffusion *in vivo* and *in vitro*, *Acta Endocrinol.*, 73, 360, 1973.

109. Jeyaseelan, S., Tukkar, D., Bhuyan, U.N., Laumas, K.R., and Hingorani, V., Local tissue response to silastic implant containing norethindrone acetate in women, *Contraception*, 15, 39, 1977.

110. Anderson, J.M., Niven, H., Pelagalli, J., Olanoff, L.S., and Jones, R.D., The role of the fibrous capsule in the function of the implanted drug-polymer sustained release systems, *J. Biomed. Mater. Res.*, 15, 889, 1981.

111. Abrahams, R.A. and Ronel, S.H., Biocompatible implants for the sustained zero-order release of narcotic antagonists, *J. Biomed. Mater. Res.*, 9, 355, 1975.

112. Anderson, J.M., Koinis, T., Nelson, T., Horst, M., and Love, D.S., The slow release of hydrocortisone sodium succinate from poly(2-hydroxyethyl acrylate)membrabes. In *Hydrogels for Medical and Related Applications*, Andrade, J.D., Ed., American Chemical Society, Washington, D.C., 167, 1976.

113. Cowsar, D.R., Tarwater, O.R., and Tanquary, A.C., Controlled release of fluoride from hydrogels for dental applications. In *Hydrogels for Medical and Related Applications*, Andrade, J.D., Ed., American Chemical Society, Washington, D.C., 180, 1976.

114. Halpern, B.D., Solomon, O., Kopec, L., Korostoff, E., and Ackerman, J.L., Release of inorganic fluoride ion from rigid polymer matrices. In *Controlled Release Polymeric Formulations*, Paul, D.R. and Harris, F.W., Eds., American Chemical Society, Washington, D.C., 135, 1976.

115. Cardinal, J.R., Kim, S.W., Song, S.Z., Lee, E.S., and Kim, S.H., Controlled-release drug delivery systems from hydrogels: Progesterone release from monolithic reservoir, combined reservoir-monolithic and monolithic devices with rate controlling barriers. In *AIChE Symp. Series No. 206, Controlled Release Systems*, Vol. 77, Chandrasekaran, S.K., Ed., Am. Inst. Chem. Eng., New York, 52, 1981.

116. Wood, J.M., Attwood, D., and Collett, J.H., The swelling properties of poly(2-hydroxyethyl methacrylate) hydrogels polymerized by gamma-radiation and chemical initiation, *Int. J. Pharm.*, 7, 189, 1981.

117. Refojo, M.F., Natchair, G., Liu, H.S., Lahav, M., and Tolentino, R.I., New hydrophilic implant for scheral buckling, *Ann. Ophthalmol.*, 12, 88, 1980.

118. Tuttle, M.F., Baker, R.W., and Laufe, L.E., Slow-release aprotinin delivery for control of intrauterine-device-induced hemmorrhage, *Membr. Sci.*, 7, 351, 1980.

119. Kalkwarf, D.R., Sikov, M.R., Smith, L., and Gordon, R., Release of progesterone from polyethylene devices *in vitro* and in experimental animals, *Contraception*, 6, 423, 1972.

120. McRae, J.C. and Kim, S.W., Characterization of controlled release of prostaglandin from polymer matrixes for thrombus prevention, *Trans. Am. Soc. Artif. Intern. Organs*, 24, 746, 1978.

121. Baker, R.E., Tuttle, M.E., Longsdale, H.K., and Ayres, J.W., Development of an estradiol-releasing intrauterine device, *J. Pharm. Sci.*, 68, 20, 1979.

122. Gott, V.L., Whiffen, J.D., and Datton, R.C., Heparin bonding on colloidal graphite surfaces, *Science*, 142, 1297, 1963.

123. Whiffen, J.D. and Beeckler, D.C., The fate of the surface heparin of GBH-coated plastics after exposure to the bloodstream, *J. Thorac. Cardiovasc. Surg.*, 52, 121, 1966.

124. Leininger, R.I., Cooper, C.W., Falb, R.D., and Grode, G.A., Nonthrombogenic plastic surfaces, *Science*, 152, 1625, 1966.
125. Merrill, E.W., Salzman, E.W., Lipps, B.J., Gilliland, E.R., Austen, W.G., and Joison, J., Antithrombogenic cellulose membranes for blood dialysis, *Trans. Am. Soc. Artif. Intern. Organs*, 12, 139, 1966.
126. Hufnagel, C.A., Conrad, P.W., Gillespie, J.F., Pifarre, R., et al., Characteristics of materials for intravascular applications, *Ann. N.Y. Acad. Sci.*, 146, 262, 1968.
127. Ebert, C.D., McRea, J.C., and Kim, S.W., Controlled release of antithrombotic agents from polymer-matrices. In *Controlled Release of Bioactive Materials*, Baker, J., Ed., Academic Press, New York, 107, 1980.
128. Ebert, C.D. and Kim, S.W., Polymers for the prevention of thrombosis. In *Medical Applications of Controlled Release*, Vol. 2, CRC Press, Inc., Boca Raton, FL, 77–106, 1984.
129. Salyer, I.O. and Weesner, W.E., Materials and components for circulatory assist devices. In *Artificial Heart Program Conf. Proc.*, National Institute of Health, U.S. Department of Health, Education and Welfare, Washington, D.C., June 9–13, 59, 1969.
130. Schscht, E.H., Ionic polymers as drug carriers. In *Controlled Drug Delivery*, Vol. 1, Basic Concepts, Bruck, S.D., Ed., CRC Press, Inc., Boca Raton, FL, 149–173, 1983.
131. Saunders, L. and Srivastava, R., The absorption of quinine by a carboxylic acid ion-exchange resin, *J. Chem. Soc.*, 2915, 1950.
132. Hwa, J. and Loeffler, D., Therapeutic ion-exchange resins, *German Off.*, 1, 070, 381, 1959.
133. Mathur, N., Narang, C., and Williams, R., *Polymers as Aids in Organic Chemistry*, Academic Press, New York, 1980.
134. Hodge, P. and Sherrington, D., Polymer-Supported Reactions in Organic Synthesis, Wiley Interscience, New York, 1980.
135. Determann, H., Meyer, N., and Wieland, T., Ion exchanger from pearl-shaped cellulose gel, *Nature* (London), 223, 499, 1969.
136. James, K. and Stanworth, D., Chromatography of human serum proteins on diethylaminoethyl cellulose, *J. Chrom.*, 15, 324, 1964.
137. Helfferich, F., *Ion Exchange*, McGraw-Hill, New York, 87, 1962.
138. Boyd, G.E., Adamson, A.W., and Myers, L.S. Jr., The exchange adsorption of ions from aqueous solutions by organic zeolites, II. Kinetics, *J. Am. Chem. Soc.*, 69, 2836, 1947.
139. Samsonov, G.V. and Pasechnik, V.A., Ion exchange and the swelling of ion-exchangers, *Russ. Chem. Rev.*, 38(7), 547, 1969.
140. McChesney, E.W., Nachod, F.C., and Tainter, M.L., Aspects of cation-exchange resins as therapeutic agents for sodium removal, *Ann. N.Y. Acad. Sci.*, 57, 252, 1954.
141. Macaulay, D. and Watson, G.H., Tetany following cation-exchange resin therapy, *Lancet*, 2, 70, 1954.
142. Kamp, W., Application of ion-exchange resins in medicine, *Pharm. Weekblad.*, 97, 141, 1962.
143. Berg, P.R. and Ostrup, P., Ion-exchange resins as carriers for oral medications in order to achieve sustained release, parts I and II, *Dansk. Tidsskr. Farm.*, 40, 33, 55, 1966.
144. Miller, L.C. and Holland, A.H., Physical and chemical considerations in choice of drugs, *Mod. Med.*, 28, 312, 1960.

145. Malek, P., Kolc, J., Herold, M., and Hoffman, J., Problems of aimed penetration of antibiotics into the lymphatic system, III. Antibiolymphins and the lymphatic system. In *Antibiotics Annual* 1957–1958, Medical Encyclopedia, New York, 564, 1958.

146. El-Shibini, H.A.M., Abdel-Nasser, M., and Motawi, M.M., Streptomycin alginate as potential long-acting preparation, *Pharmazie*, 26(10), 630, 1971.

147. Ozawa, H., Ozeki, E., Shimizu, H., and Nishio, S., Gradually releasing drugs, *Japan Kokai*, 75, 24, 429; *Chem. Abstr.*, 83, 103292q, 1975.

148. Cavallito, C.J. and Jewell, R., Modification of rates of gastrointestinal absorption of drugs, I. Amines, *J. Am. Pharm. Assoc.*, 47, 165, 1958.

149. Klaudianos, S., Verfahren zur Herstellung von Retard-Tabletten auf Alginsaure Basis und Untersuchung der Wirkstoff-Freigabe, *Pharm. Ind.*, 33(5), 296, 1971.

150. Salib, N.N., El-Menshawy, M.E., and Ismail, A.A., Polysalt flocculates as a physicochemical approach in the development of controlled-release oral pharmaceuticals, *Pharmazie*, 31, 12, 1976.

151. Goodman, H. and Banker, G.S., Molecular-scale drug entrapment as a precise method of controlled drug release, I. Entrapment of cationic drugs by polymeric flocculation, *J. Pharm. Sci.*, 59(8), 1131, 1970.

152. Rhodes, C., Wai, K., and Banker, G.S., Molecular-scale drug entrapment as a precise method of controlled drug release, II. Facilated drug entrapment to polymeric colloidal dispersions, *J. Pharm. Sci.*, 59, 1578, 1581, 1970.

153. Elgindy, N.A., Molecular entrapment of cationic drugs by Carbopol 934, *Can. J. Pharm. Sci.*, 11(1), 32, 1976.

154. Kennon, L. and Higuchi, T., Interaction studies of cationic drugs with anionic polyelectrolytes, II. Polyacrylic and styrene polymers, *J. Am. Pharm. Assoc.*, 46, 21, 1957.

155. Ferruti, P., Angeloni, A.S., Scapini, G., and Tarisi, M.C., New oligomers and polymers as drug carriers. In *Recent Advances in Drug Delivery Systems*, Anderson, J.M. and Kim, S.W., Eds., Plenum Press, New York, 63–76, 1983.

156. Weiner, B.Z., Zilkha, A., Porah, G., and Grundfeld, Y., *Eur. J. Med. Chem.-Chim. Ther.*, 11, 525, 1976.

157. Pinazzi, C., Benoit, J.P., Rabadeux, J.C., and Pleurdeau, A., *Eur. Polym. J.*, 15, 1069, 1979.

158. Rekhi, G.S., Mendes, R.W., Porter, S.C., and Jambhekar, S.S., Aqueous polymeric dispersions for controlled drug delivery — Wurster process, *Pharm. Tech.*, 13(3), 112–125, 1989.

159. Harris, M.R., Ghebre-Sellasie, I., and Nesbitt, R.U., A water-based coating process for sustained release, *Pharm. Tech.*, 102, 1986.

160. Magda, A. et al., In *Polymeric Delivery Systems: Properties and Applications*, ACS Symposium Series Nos. 520, 408, 1993.

161. Tsuruta, T. et al., In *Biomedical Applications of Polymeric Materials*, CRC Press, Inc., Boca Raton, FL, 1993.

162. Saltzman et al., *Chem. Eng. News*, November 30, 1992 (Ref., *Bio/Technology*, 10, 1446, 1992).

163. Sparer, R.V., Ekwuribe, N., and Walton, A.G., Controlled release from glycosamino glycan drug complexes. In *Controlled Release Delivery Systems*, Roseman, T.J. and Mansdorf, S.Z., Eds., Marcel Dekker, New York, 107–119, 1983.

164. Grolleman, C.W.J., deVisser, A.C., Wolke, J.G.C., vanDer Goot, H., and Timmerman, H., Studies on a bioerodible drug carrier system based on a polyphosphazine, Part II, Experiments *in vitro*, *J. Controlled Release*, 4(2), 119–131, 1986.

165. Gros, L., Ringsdorf, H., and Schupp, H., Polymeric antitumor agents on a molecular and cellular basis, *Angew. Chem.*, 93(4), 311–332, 1981.

166. Friend, D.R. and Pangburn, S., Site-specific drug delivery, *Med. Res. Rev.*, 7(1), 53–106, 1987.

167. Chang, R., Price, J.C., and Whitworth, C.W., Control of drug-release rates through the use of mixtures of polycaprolactone and cellulose propionate polymers, *Pharm. Tech.*, 24, 1986.

168. Mollica, J.A., Technical considerations for advanced drug delivery systems. In *Recent Advances in Drug Delivery Systems*, Anderson, J.M. and Kim, S.W., Eds., Plenum Press, New York, 343–348, 1984.

169. Rosoff, M., *Controlled Release of Drugs*, VCH Publishers, New York, 1989.

170. Darby, T.D., Safety evaluation of polymeric materials, *Ann. Rev. Pharmacol. Toxicol.*, 27, 157–167, 1987.

171. Peppas, N.A., *Hydrogels in Medicine and Pharmacy*, Vol. 1, Fundamentals; Vol. 2; Vol. 3, Properties and applications, CRC Press, Inc., Boca Raton, FL, 1986.

172. Giammona, G., Carlisi, B., Pitarresi, G., Cavallaro, G., and Liveri, V.T., Water-soluble copolymers of an antiviral agent, synthesis and their interaction with a biomembrane model, *J. Control. Rel.*, 22, 197–204, 1992.

173. Fu Lu, M.-Y., Borodkin, S., Woodward, L., Li, P., et al., Polymer carrier system for taste masking of macrolide antibiotics, *Pharm. Res.*, 8, 706–712, 1991.

174. Lewin, M., Ed., *Polymers for Advanced Technologies*, VCH Publishers, New York, 1988.

175. Sheskey, P.J. and Cabelka, T.D., Reworkability of sustained-release tablet formulations containing HPMC polymers, *Pharm. Tech.*, 16, 60–74, 1992.

176. Dunn, R.L. and Ottenbrite, R.M., Eds., *Polymeric Drugs and Drug Delivery Systems*, ACS Symposium Series Nos. 469, 314, 1991.

177. Gebelein, C.G., Ed., *Biotechnological Polymers: Medical, Pharmaceutical and Industrial Applications (A Conference in Print)*, Technomic Publishing, Lancaster, PA, 224, 1993.

178. Sun, Y. and Watts, D.C., Biodegradable polymers and their degradation mechanisms, *Am. Pharm. Rev.*, 4, 8–18, 2001.

179. Kurita, K. et al., Nonnatural branch polysaccharides, synthesis and properties of chitin and chitosan having alpha mannoside branches, *Macromolecules*, 31, 4764–4769, 1998.

180. Denuziere, A. et al., Chitosan-chondroitin sulfate and chitosan hyaluronate polyelectrolyte complexes, biological properties, *Biomaterials*, 19, 1275–1285, 1998.

181. Wang, X. et al., Structural characterization of phosphorylated chitosan and their applications as effective additives of calcium phosphate cements, *Biomaterials*, 22, 2247–2255, 2001.

182. Bulpitt, P. and Aeschlmann, D., New strategy for chemical modification of hyaluronic acids: preparation of functionalized derivatives and their use in the formation of novel biocompatible hydrogels, *J. Biomed. Mater. Res.*, 47, 152–169, 1999.

183. Luo, Y. and Prestwich, G.D., Synthesis and selective cytotoxicity of a hyaluronic acid-antitumor bioconjugate, *Bioconjug. Chem.*, 10, 755–763, 1999.

184. Pelletier, S. et al., Amphiphilic derivatives of sodium alginate and hylauronate for cartilage repair, rheological properties, *Biomed. Mater. Res.*, 54, 102–108, 2001.

185. Suedee, R., Enantioselective release of controlled delivery granules based on molecularly imprinted polymers, *Drug Deliv.*, 9, 19–30, 2002.

186. Raghuvanshi, R.S. et al., Formulation and characterization of immunoreactive tetanus toxoid biodegradable polymer particles, *Drug Deliv.*, 8, 99–106, 2002.

187. Desai, S.D. and Blanchard, J., Pluronic F127-based ocular delivery system containing biodegradable polyisobutylcyanoacrylate nanocapsules of pilocarpine, *Drug Deliv.*, 7, 201–207, 2000.

188. Saito, N. et al., Biodegradable poly-D,L-lactic acid-polyethylene glycol block copolymers as a BMP delivery system for inducing bone, *J. Bone Joint Surg. Am.*, 83-A Suppl. 1(Pt. 2)S92–S98, 2001.

chapter four

Implants in drug delivery*

Contents

I.   Introduction

Although most current controlled drug delivery systems are designed for transdermal, subcutaneous, or intramuscular uses, others (e.g., implants) can also deliver drugs into the bloodstream. This approach to drug delivery has become quite appealing for a number of classes of drugs, particularly those that cannot be given via the oral route.[1] Implantable drug delivery

* Adapted from Ranade, V.V., Drug delivery systems. 4. Implants in drug delivery, *J. Clin. Pharmacol.*, 30, 871, 1990. With permission of *J. Clin. Pharmacol.* and J.B. Lippincott Publishing Company, Philadelphia, PA.

systems are designed to transmit drugs and fluids into the bloodstream without the repeated insertion of needles. These systems are particularly well suited to the drug delivery requirements of insulin, steroids, chemotherapeutics, antibiotics, analgesics, total parenteral nutrition, and heparin.

Implantable drug delivery systems are placed completely under the skin — usually in a convenient but inconspicuous location. The patient is aware of only a small bump under the skin. Because the device is completely subcutaneous, with no opening in the skin, there is little chance of infection or interference with daily activities. Some of the critical questions for ongoing research on implants have been concerned with the reproducibility of erodibility, irritation/carcinogenicity, dose dumping, duration, and pulses.

While it is possible to surgically implant and remove drug-concentrating devices or polymeric matrices, the requirement for such intervention could have a significant negative impact on the acceptability of a product candidate. Two approaches to this problem seem possible. The first is the use of implanted electrically driven pumps which can be refilled by simple injection of the drug through a septum into the pump reservoir. An advantage of such pumps is that the pumping rate can be regulated by microprocessor control (it can be reliably programmed and altered via radio signals). The major disadvantages are the large size of the devices and the need for surgical implantation with the possibility of infection. The second approach is the use of erodible implants. Here, the requirements are for a system that will be safe and whose erosion rate can be sufficiently well controlled to give a reproducible and precise drug-release rate over the entire lifetime of the implant.

The desire to build into polymers precise zero-order surface erosion, without alteration of the structural integrity of the inner structures, has been difficult to achieve. Thus, although surface erosion can account for a significant portion of the release process, diffusion of the drug out of the device or solvent into the polymer ultimately contributes to the drug-release process and causes unpredictable changes in release rate, some of which may not be desirable. The future use of polymeric systems as implants requires greater input from polymer chemistry and related fields.[2]

Polymers that are used in medicine can be divided into two groups: those that are introduced for a chronic period of time and polymers whose presence is transient. The first case includes the use of polymeric materials in cardiovascular surgery, orthopedics, plastic surgery, and otolaryngology. Such applications impose high demands on the stability of the materials used. An implant must retain the properties necessary for its functioning throughout its lifetime, and the structure is chosen so that degradative changes are minimal.

To be able to fully assess the biological properties of polymers, it is necessary to know their chemical composition, ingredients, and fabrication methodologies. All too often, it is the additives or fabrication parameters that influence the behavior of material in contact with blood. Blood-contacting applications pose severe requirements on materials. While clotting and thrombosis are the most obvious evidences of blood incompatibility, they are only the end products of a complex series of events when materials come in contact with blood.

Most, if not all, synthetic materials adversely affect plasma proteins, enzymes, and clotting factors, as well as formed blood elements, namely platelets, erythrocytes, and leukocytes. To what extent these processes can cause serious problems in the body will be influenced by the relative surface area to which blood is exposed, the duration of implantation, and the individual physiological and biochemical responses elicited by the implant. Prolonged periods of implantation may conceivably lead to carcinogenesis induced by chemical or physical mechanisms. Materials in contact with blood should not cause thrombus formation, either on the surface of foreign materials or embolization elsewhere in the circulatory system, or at distant organ sites as the result of endothelial damage and platelet injury.

In addition to not producing thrombosis, there are a number of other requirements that polymeric implants must meet for clinical applications. First, they must not cause injury or sensitization to any of the formed blood elements leading to hemolysis and aggregation of leukocytes in the microvasculature. Second, they must neither alter plasma proteins to any considerable extent, nor cause adverse responses by the activation of either the classical or alternate pathways of the complement system. In addition, they must not cause cancer. Finally, polymeric implants must be sterilizable without degradation or changes in their surface properties.

Implantable polymeric miniature pumps have made contributions to numerous areas of biomedical research, in particular, to drug delivery systems. The examples that will be reviewed in this chapter deal with the process of drug scheduling, toxicology, targeted delivery, and patterned administration.

II.   Insulin delivery as a model implant pump system

Conventional controlled-release formulations are designed to deliver drugs at a predetermined, preferably constant, rate. Only under special circumstances are these formulations modified to provide variable-rate delivery. Some clinical situations, however, necessitate either external control of the drug delivery rate or a volume of drug that is beyond the capabilities of existing controlled-release formulations. Implantable drug delivery pumps have been devised to meet these situations.

A pump can be distinguished from other controlled-release dosage forms in that the primary driving force for delivery by a pump is not the concentration difference of the drug between the formulation and the surrounding tissue, but, rather, a pressure difference. This pressure difference can be generated by pressurizing a drug reservoir, by osmotic action, or by direct mechanical actuation.

The primary impetus for the development of such pumps has been the experience of electromechanical devices for the control of hyperglycemia in insulin-dependent diabetes — the "artificial pancreas." The limitations of the miniaturized syringe or peristaltic pumps that are currently used to deliver insulin to diabetics in clinical trials are becoming apparent, which is generating an interest in implantable devices. While some implantable pumps have been used for other applications, it is the difficulty of delivering insulin that has received the most attention and has underscored the problems and limitations of such devices.

Sefton[3] has summarized the characteristics for the ideal pump. The pump must deliver a drug within a range of prescribed rates for extended periods of time. It should include features such as reliability; chemical, physical, and biological stability; and be compatible with drugs. The pump must be non-inflammatory, nonantigenic, noncarcinogenic, nonthrombogenic, and have overdose protection. The pump must be convenient to use by both the patient and the health professional, have long reservoir and battery life, easy programmability, and be implantable under local anesthesia. There must also be a simple means to monitor the status and performance of the pump, and both the interior and exterior of the pump must be sterilizable.[4,5]

Implantable pumps are expected to reliably deliver a drug at a prescribed rate for extended periods of time. The delivery-rate range of the pump must be sufficiently wide to provide both basal and enhanced delivery of the drug as dictated by the clinical situation. Alternately, there must be a capability for providing bolus injection of a drug in addition to basal delivery. A wide range of delivery rates is also needed to meet the expected patient-to-patient variability in demand for a drug and the individual patient's changes in drug need during the course of therapy.

Accuracy and precision of delivery must be maintained over extended periods of time. To justify the surgery associated with the implantation of a pump, this period must be at least 2 years or, preferably, 5 years. This implies a reliability for both the pump and (implanted) electrical components since neither is easily replaceable. Sufficient biological, physical, and chemical stability of the drug within the pump are also required.

The goal of an implantable pump is to improve existing therapeutic methods of drug delivery and not be a lifesaving measure. However, the device also must be safe. In addition to the normal concerns of an implant, the implantation of a large quantity of a drug poses the additional danger of "dose dumping." While in some situations, delivery of less than the required amount of a drug on the prescribed schedule can be considered dangerous, this can be corrected for by reverting to conventional therapy. Overdoses, however, are not as easily correctible. An insulin overdose, for example, could result in severe hypoglycemia, coma, and death if not corrected with a rapid administration of glucose.

An overdose can occur in a number of ways when drug delivery is by an implantable pump. For example, the life of a peristaltic pump is typically limited by the life of the tubing, which is repeatedly compressed. Splitting of the tube can result in contamination of nonhermatically sealed electrical components, electrical failure of the pump, and a drug overdose if there is a leak in the pump housing. This restriction is particularly severe in implantable pumps since it is not possible to change the tubing routinely, as in the case of portable devices. Mechanical trauma may pierce the reservoir, also resulting in drug overdose if the pump is not sufficiently well protected. Mechanical failure of a pump, particularly one that uses valves to regulate an otherwise high delivery rate, can result in delivery at a higher than desirable rate. Thus, mechanical failure is an important consideration because it not only affects the performance of the pump, but also is a safety concern.

The presence of a finite reservoir life, a finite battery life, patient-to-patient variability in drug demand, or long-term changes in an individual patient's drug demand require that the implantable device be convenient to use. This is in addition to any requirement for a simple means to adjust the delivery rate in accordance with the physiological effects of the drug.

The reservoir of an implantable pump should be as large as possible. The total volume of a pump that can be implanted at a single site is limited to approximately 200 to 300 cm,^{3} of which a maximum of 50 cm^3 can be set aside for the drug reservoir. Reservoir life is determined by the drug requirement and the maximum concentration of the drug that can be used, as dictated by the constraints of viscosity, drug stability, or availability. In the event that reservoir life is less than 2 to 5 years, then a simple means to refill the reservoir is required.[6,7]

Battery life should also be more than the 2- to 5-year pump life. This means that pump energy requirements should be within the range of the available battery systems. Alternatively, rechargeable batteries or a transcutaneous energy-transmission system can be used to supply the required power. These alternatives must obviously be designed with the safety and convenience of the user in mind.

The pump must also be easily programmable. Simple methods are required for initial programming of the pump in order to meet the delivery needs of the individual patient and for choosing among various delivery profiles during the course of therapy. Also, initial programming should allow for adjusting the delivery profiles to the changing needs of the patient.

The location for the pump can be the anterior subcutaneous tissue of the chest or abdomen, depending on the route of administration, since these sites are well protected and the implant is well concealed under the clothing. The abdomen is the preferred site for i.p. delivery since placement of the delivery catheter requires only limited dissection.[8]

Implicit in meeting the stated criteria is a need for a means of continuous monitoring of the current status and performance of the implanted device. Parameters may include current delivery rate, accumulated drug delivered, and amount of drug remaining in the reservoir. Warning indicators need to be developed in the event of too low or too high a delivery rate, low battery power, low reservoir content, or any mechanical or electrical failure.[9,10]

The difficulty of sterilizing complex electromechanical devices should not be overlooked. Since the patient could ultimately be exposed to microorganisms inside the pump, conventional sterilization methods may be inadequate if only the outside of the device is sterilized. Furthermore, the effect of sterilization on the materials used within the pump should be considered since the associated changes in these materials may be serious.[11,12]

Implantation of a pump introduces design constraints that are not present in corresponding portable devices. Refilling or replacing the reservoir and recharging the battery are matters of convenience in a portable device, while reservoir and battery life assume more importance in an implanted device, which has restricted access. A drug reservoir should be able to deliver a reasonably large volume of drug if implanted. However, now the potential of leakage of the drug becomes a significant safety concern that is not present in a portable device. Similarly, the design of the transcutaneous energy-transmission system to drive the pump or to recharge the implanted batteries is a necessity for smaller size and biocompatible materials.[13,14]

Although pumps based on a conventional peristaltic mechanism have been implanted in humans, many implantable pumps based on unusual or unconventional driving mechanisms have also been described. These include fluorocarbon propellant, osmotic pressure, piezoelectric disk benders, or the combination of a concentration gradient with an oscillating piston.

A.   *Peristaltic pumps*

Sandia National Laboratories has developed[15] a rotary, solenoid-driven peristaltic pump, which has been implanted in diabetics. It is based on the principle of a portable pump. Each electrical pulse to the motor produces 10 rotations of the pump head, with delivery of 2.1 µl against a pressure head of up to 30 psi. While not as efficient as DC motors, rotary or stepper motors cease operation as soon as the power is removed, thus making them capable of more accurate delivery in stop-and-start situations. They are also safer since no drug can be delivered in a case of electrical malfunction.[16]

Although originally housed in a 0.7-mm-thick, type-304, stainless-steel casing, a laser-welded titanium chamber is currently used to house the pump, electronics, and battery in order to provide a hermatic seal. The housing is further coated with silastic for enhanced biocompatibility. Internal components are either nickel-plated or made from corrosion-resistant materials. Flat silicone rubber pouches are used as reservoirs. The 0.5-mm-thick walls can withstand more than 60 psi without rupture. These reservoirs are percutaneously refilled through a silicone rubber septum in a refill port made from 2-mm-thick polypropylene. Polypropylene prevents the needle from puncturing the wall of the reservoir. Silicone rubber tubing is used to connect the reservoir to the pump, and a silicone rubber Codman Hydrocephalus shunt is used as the catheter for i.p. delivery of insulin, for example. The wall of this catheter is reinforced with a stainless-steel helix to prevent kinking and has a low-pressure valve at the distal end to prevent retrograde flow of peritoneal tissue into the catheter.[17]

The flow controller is carried externally, and two-way communication is achieved by induction coupling at 30 kHz. The operator of the pump can define delivery rates, initiate bolus or basal delivery, or initiate an audible signal to check on battery voltage and pump operation.[18,19] Protection from external electrical noise is provided. Readout capability on the external module includes program data, accumulated dose, remaining dose to be delivered, and whether the unit is operating in basal or augmented delivery mode.

Summers[20] has prepared an implantable prototype version of their Promedos El portable pump. The implantable dosing unit consists of the stepper motor-driven peristaltic pump, lithium battery, control electronics for regulating a 10-ml insulin reservoir, and a septum for percutaneous refilling of the insulin reservoir. All components are hermatically encapsulated in a titanium pacemaker casing, which is at a lower pressure than the exterior to minimize the effect of a pump, reservoir, or septum leak.

An implantable, three-roller, peristaltic pump that is driven by a rotatable magnet located outside the body has also been described by Summers.[20] A visual signaling system has been incorporated into the implanted unit. An implanted light source is energized during each revolution of the pump rotor to indicate that the pump is operating and to provide a measure of the administered dose. The pump delivers a drug from a percutaneously refillable, silastic bladder lined with an impervious layer of latex rubber.

The most sophisticated of the emerging implant delivery technologies is the noninvasively programmable drug administration device (DAD, Medtronic, Minneapolis, Minnesota). The device's titanium housing contains a 20-cm^3 refillable reservoir, an electronic control module, an integral battery, and a peristaltic drive pump that provides drug delivery with an accuracy of ±15%. A catheter routed to the site of administration is secured to the device. As with venous access ports, the reservoir is refilled or evacuated by percutaneous insertion of a syringe-mounted hypodermic needle through the device's self-sealing septum. The inert properties of the titanium and silicone DAD containment and drug delivery surfaces allow the use of a wide variety of drugs (see Figure 4.1).

The DAD contains an audible alarm system that alerts the patient and physician to low battery power, low reservoir volume, or memory error. For most applications, the entire system is implanted using only local anesthesia. The procedure is performed on an outpatient basis.

The DAD can deliver continuous infusion rates ranging from 0.025 to 0.9 ml/h or single or multiple boli. The physician can reset the rate at any time using an office-based programming system. Communication between the DAD and the program is accomplished by a radio wave-like telemetry link. Automatic security codes are exchanged between the implanted electronics and the programmer system to verify that proper and appropriate transfer of information has taken place. In addition, programming can be accomplished only in the presence of a strong magnetic field produced by the programming wand. These security measures ensure that spurious environmental signals or other causes do not inadvertently reprogram the DAD.

The DAD's delivery capabilities allow considerable clinical flexibility. Dosage titration and schedule revision can be accomplished conveniently

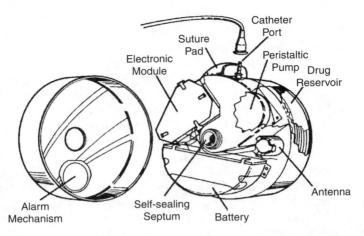

Figure 4.1 Cross-sectional view of the DAD showing key components. (From *Pharm. Technol.*, The Latest Developments in Drug Delivery Systems, Conf. Proc., 1987, 20. With permission.)

without reformulating the drug concentrations or exchanging the device for another with a different flow rate. The peristaltic drive pump, with its delivery accuracy, enables potent substances or agents with narrow therapeutic indices to be delivered precisely. The risk of infection is reduced since the entire system is fully implanted. One model of the DAD contains a bioretentive filter in the reservoir fluid outlet path. This filter enables substances to be delivered directly to the intrathecal space and to the brain, effectively bypassing the blood–brain barrier. Thus, the DAD is the first fully implanted system that provides convenient chronic, site-targeted, rate- and pattern-controlled drug delivery.

B.   *Fluorocarbon propellant-driven pumps*

Blackshear et al.[21–23] have devised a unique "no external energy," constant-rate, implantable pump that, appropriately modified, has also been used for variable-rate insulin delivery. The basic constant-rate pump (Infusaid) consists of a hollow titanium disk that is divided into two chambers by freely moveable titanium bellows. The inner chamber contains the drug solution, while the outer chamber contains a fluorocarbon liquid that exerts a vapor pressure well above atmospheric pressure at 37°C. The inner drug chamber is refilled through percutaneous injection by means of a self-sealing silicone rubber and Teflon septum. The pressure of the injection causes expansion of the inner chamber and compression of the fluorocarbon. Once filled, the fluorocarbon vaporizes and compresses the inner chamber. The drug solution is then forced through fine-bore Teflon capillary tubing, which acts as a flow regulator, and subsequently through an intravascularly located silicone-delivery catheter. Bacterial filters are included in the refill and delivery lines.[24,25]

Flow rate can be modified by changing the length of the capillary tubing or by changing the viscosity of the drug solution (e.g., high-molecular-weight dextran). According to the Poiseuille equation, flow through the pump is inversely related to the capillary length or solution viscosity. These pumps can deliver insulin or heparin solutions at constant flow rates in the 1 to 5 ml/day range. Drug delivery rate is altered by adjusting drug concentration. The primary advantage of this type of device is the absence of any need for external power. It has been found to be reliable in long-term animal studies as well as in human clinical trials.

The fluorocarbon-driven pump has been modified for insulin delivery at two infusion rates by connecting a three-way valve to the pump assembly so that a portion of the flow-restricting capillary can be bypassed when the valve is opened. A 15-fold increase in flow rate can be obtained since flow is shunted through 1/10 the length of the capillary tubing. The flow is directed through the remaining 9/10 of the capillary when the valve is closed. The valve has been modified so that it can be actuated by placing a small permanent magnet outside the body at a distance of 2 to 3 cm from the valve. The delivery rate can be maintained between maximum and minimum rates by cycling the valve on and off to provide an intermediate rate determined by the fraction time that the magnet is held near the valve and the valve is open.

In newer designs, the valve is housed in a module attached to the side of a pump along with an infusion regulator to compensate for the effects of changes in ambient pressure and temperature; it also has an auxiliary injection port and associated check valve to provide direct access to the cannula. A pressure transducer and transmitter can also be incorporated to make pressure data available for flow rate and reservoir-volume computation. In this design, machine-grooved capillaries replace the Teflon tubing restrictor. The external magnetic controller consists of an electronic timer that rotates a permanent magnet over the pump site to cycle the valve on and off.[26]

Without the infusion regulator, these pumps are sensitive to changes in ambient temperature and pressure since they are implanted near the skin. The vapor pressure of the fluorocarbon liquid increases and the viscosity of the infused fluid decreases with increasing temperature. This is important in febrile conditions or if there are significant changes in the skin temperature. Similarly, the lowering of ambient pressure causes a similar decrease in delivery rate.

In humans, the pump has been implanted in a subcutaneous pocket under the infraclavicular fossa and sutured to the underlying fascia for heparin therapy or in a subcutaneous pocket in the abdominal wall for chemotherapy. For heparin administration, the cannulae are threaded through a tributary of the subclavian vein into the superior vena cava. Cannula plugging due to thrombosis has been noted in nine of the clinically implanted pumps and generally occurs after one year of heparin infusion when the heparin is replaced with bacteriostatic water. A check valve is also incorporated at the end of the catheter to prevent the backflow of blood.[27]

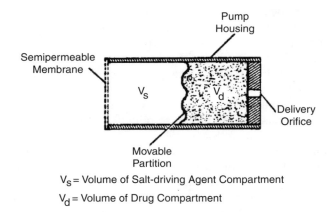

Figure 4.2 Schematic representation of a generic osmotic pump. (From *Pharm. Tech.*, June 1987, 98. With permission.)

C.   Osmotic pumps

The Alza osmotic minipump (Alzet) has been used in a wide variety of experimental situations for constant-rate delivery and preprogrammed delivery of a biological agent.[28,29] This minipump consists of a flexible, impermeable diaphragm surrounded by a sealed layer containing an osmotic agent at a particular concentration, which, in turn, is contained within a cellulose ester semipermeable membrane. A stainless steel tube or a polyethylene catheter is inserted into the innermost chamber for delivery. When the filled pump is placed in an aqueous environment, water diffuses into the osmotic agent chamber at a rate determined by the permeability of the surrounding membrane and the concentration of the agent. The absorbed water generates a hydrostatic pressure that acts on the flexible lining to force drug through the pump outlet. The pump is filled with sterile solution with a separate filling tube; the pump itself is presterilized (see Figures 4.2 and 4.3).

An osmotic-pressure actuated, constant-rate pump has also been described with a freely moveable piston rather than a rubber diaphragm. The piston is used to maintain a constant pressure in a low osmotic pressure solution reservoir, which is separated from the high osmotic pressure fluid by a semipermeable membrane. Movement of solvent across the membrane increases the pressure on that side of the membrane, forcing drug solution out of a chamber, which is separated from the high osmotic pressure solution by a second freely moving piston. The freely moving piston on the low osmotic pressure side moves to lower the volume of that reservoir as the solvent moves across the membrane. It is assumed that the piston is exposed to a source of atmospheric pressure on its other side. A device conforming to these requirements has been made from two concentric tubes, one inserted part way into the other.[30, 31]

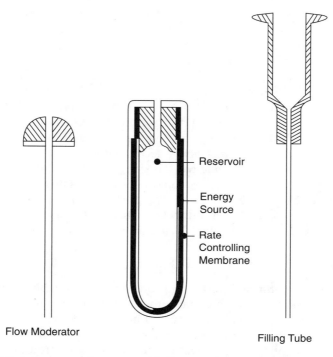

Reservoir

Energy
Source

Rate
Controlling
Membrane

Flow Moderator

Filling Tube

Figure 4.3 Miniature osmotic pump with flow moderator. (From *Pharm. Tech.*, June 1987, 98. With permission.)

D. Miniosmotic pumps: systemic delivery

The work of Nau and his colleagues exemplifies the value of using osmotic pumps as subcutaneous drug delivery devices in toxicology.[32] Nau studied the effects of the antiepileptic drug valproic acid on fetal development in pregnant mice. Nau compared the effects of giving the dose by two different administration regimens: a once-daily subcutaneous injection and a constant subcutaneous infusion from an osmotic pump.[33,34] With constant infusion, an order of magnitude higher total dose was required to produce fetal resorptions and encephaly comparable to that obtained with the once-daily injection bolus regimen. Despite the large difference between mouse and man in the half-life of valproate, miniosmotic pumps can produce plasma concentrations in mice that are bioequivalent to concentrations achieved by conventional dosing in man.[35,36]

Another pattern of drug dynamics is illustrated by the work of Sikic et al. with bleomycin.[37] This antineoplastic drug was administered for one week to tumor-bearing mice by three different dosing schedules: twice-daily injections, an injection on the first and third day, and a continuous infusion by osmotic pump. Over the course of all three schedules, the same total dose was administered. Efficacy was measured by reductions in tumor size, and toxicity was measured by hydroxyproline content of the lung, an indicator of pulmonary fibrosis. Therapeutic doses given by infusion achieved significantly greater reductions in tumor size than identical doses given by either of the injection schedules. In contrast, at a given dose, the infusion regimen resulted in significantly less pulmonary fibrosis than either of the injection schedules. Thus, bleomycin appears to be a drug in which the infusion dose-response curve for one effect is shifted to the left, while the infusion dose-response curve for another effect is shifted to the right. These concomitant shifts have the net effect of widening the therapeutic index of bleomycin.

Bleomycin is thus safe and more effective when given by infusion in this model. Such pharmacodynamic work is drug-specific. Constant drug delivery is not *a priori* the superior regimen. For example, it appears that gentamicin and cyclophosphamide are drugs that are better given by injection rather than by infusion. It has been advocated that both injection and infusion regimens should be investigated during drug screening programs.

E.   *Miniosmotic pumps: local delivery*

A catheter can be attached to the exit port of an implantable osmotic pump to perfuse a discrete location distant from the site of implantation.[38] In this manner, drug solutions may be delivered into solid tissue or against arterial pressures without measurable reduction of flow. The miniature osmotic pump is capable of changing local drug concentrations around the catheter tip without influencing the rest of the body. Flows of 0.5 to 1.0 µl/hr appear to be low enough that hydraulic damage or edema is minimal in the microperfused region.

Sendelbeck and Urquhart[39] have investigated the spatial distribution of the polar drugs (relatively non-lipid-soluble)[14]C-dopamine hydrochloride (DA), ^{3}H-sodium methotrexate (MTX), and the lipid-soluble drug ^{14}C-antipyrine (AP) during continuous intracerebral microperfusion. Following microperfusion, DA and MTX remained concentrated in brain tissue whereas the more lipid-soluble AP escaped across the blood–brain barrier and was removed by the circulation. From a therapeutic perspective, these results indicate that brain tissue can sequester polar drugs directed from a catheter while minimizing drug levels elsewhere. Such targeted administration might maximize local effects and limit side effects in adjacent tissues or other areas of the body.

Another example of targeted administration has been reported in the studies by Ruers et al.[40] Their work indicates that continuously infused prednisolone (an immunosuppressant) to kidney-transplant patients is superior to bolus treatment in prolongation of survival time and kidney function. The longer survival of allografts with continuously infused versus bolus-injected intraperitoneal prednisolone confirms the earlier results of Proovst et al.[41] in studies on cardiac allograft survival. Continuously infused prednisolone has superior immunosuppressive action, dose for dose, compared to bolus-injected prednisolone.

F.   Miniosmotic pumps: patterned delivery

Although miniosmotic pumps operate at a constant rate, they can be readily adapted to deliver drugs according to a variable time schedule. Time-varied drug administration is accomplished by coupling the miniosmotic pump to a catheter displacement tube containing a predetermined program of sequential drug infusions. The pump is filled with an inert liquid, and the displacement catheter containing the drug sequence can be thermoformed into a tight coil around the pump, thereby forming a compact package that is readily implanted.

If the catheter is loaded with a sequence of drug solution segments, alternating with segments of an inert drug-free spacer solution (which is immiscible with the drug solution), a time-based, on-off sequence is created. Thus, a linear array of alternating segments of drug solution and drug-free spacer solution in the catheter creates a pulsatile sequence of drug infusions. Other patterns of administration may be achieved by varying the concentration of drug in the segments or the length of the drug segments or spacers. More complexity is achieved if multiple drugs or multiple drug concentrations are used in the segments.

Adaptation for time-varied drug administration allows for investigation of the pharmacodynamics of time-varied drug administration patterns and the generation of synthetic circadian rhythms. Cronan et al.[42] used this time-varied method of drug administration to mimic the effects of human drug use patterns in rats. Lynch et al.[43] have investigated the artificial induction of circadian melatonin rhythm in pinealectomized rats. Temporally programmed delivery has also been used in reproductive studies. Lasley and Wing[44] successfully stimulated ovarian function in several exotic female carnivores with pulses of gonadotropin-releasing hormone (GnRH).

Miniosmotic pumps, although preprogrammed at discrete volumetric rates, allow the researcher freedom in the selection of drug and drug delivery rate. Although osmotic pumps deliver drugs by volume displacement, they deliver at low flow rates that allow undisturbed targeted tissue or organ perfusion. Catheter attachments to such pumps can be loaded with varying patterns of drugs for patterned drug delivery. Such systems appear to have unique value for polypeptide drug delivery.[45]

G.   Positive-displacement pumps

Bessman and Layne[46] have described one of the early developments of an implantable, positive-displacement, insulin pump made from piezoelectric disk benders. Two 1-in. diameter thin wafers of piezoelectric material, bonded to brass, were glued to a ring of Lexan tubing. Upon applying a voltage, the piezoelectric wafers, unable to shrink or expand in diameter because of the brass disk, bend in the middle to form spherical surfaces (bellows). The bender-bellows are connected via a three-way, solenoid-driven valve to a drug reservoir. Using an appropriately shaped voltage signal, the valve can be opened and closed in sequence with the flexing inward or outward of the disk benders-bellows. Flexing outward causes suction of drug through the valve into the bellows, while a voltage signal of the opposite polarity causes flexing inward, forcing drug through the valve and delivery catheter. Control of the pulse train results in control of the delivery rate.

Another early piezoelectric bellows pump has been prepared with piezoelectric valves. Piezoelectric disks epoxied to two titanium disks are used as valves in a modified diaphragm pump driven by a propellant gas.[47,48] The piezoelectric disks lie on either side of a ceramic disk to close off a hole separating a pressurized insulin reservoir from the body. Activation of the reservoir-side piezoelectric disk causes fluid to move from the reservoir into the space between the ceramic and piezoelectric disk because of the displacement of the piezoelectric disk. Deactivation of that disk, and activation of the piezoelectric disk on the other side of the ceramic disk, draws fluid through the hole in the ceramic disk and into the body. A 24-hour clock and control package are designed to operate from a 5-V power supply and are contained, along with a refillable reservoir, in a hermatically sealed can.

Andros, Inc. has designed a solenoid-driven, positive-displacement, diaphragm pump. When the solenoid is energized, the insulin in the pump chamber is pressurized by a rubber diaphragm driven by the solenoid. Fluid pressure opens the multiple, redundant-outlet valves to the delivery catheter, while an inlet valve prevents backflow into the reservoir. The reservoir is refillable through a self-sealing septum. Another implantable positive-displacement pump utilizes fail-safe pneumatic valves under microprocessor control to assure delivery safety. Other positive-displacement pumps for insulin delivery are under development elsewhere (St. Jude/Coratomic).

H.   Controlled-release micropump

An implantable pump has been developed utilizing diffusion across a rate-controlling membrane for basal delivery, which can be augmented by a rapidly oscillating piston acting on a compressible disk of foam.[49] Without an external power source, the concentration difference between the drug reservoir and the delivery site is sufficient to cause diffusion of the drug to the delivery site (basal delivery). Augmented delivery is achieved without valves by repeated compression of the foam disk by a coated piston. The piston is the core of a solenoid, and compression is affected when current is applied to the solenoid coil (see Figure 4.4). Interruption of the current causes the membrane to relax, drawing more drug into the foam disk for the next compression cycle. The basal rate is determined by the magnitude of the concentration or pressure difference and by the permeability of the rate-controlling membrane and other diffusion resistances between the reservoir and the outlet. The augmented rate is a function of the elastic properties of the foam, the force applied by the solenoid piston, and the frequency of compression.

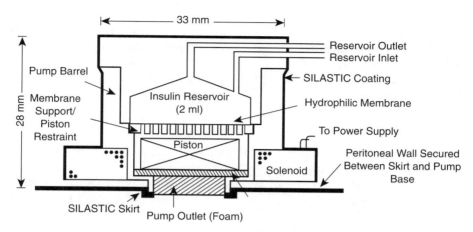

Figure 4.4 Schematic illustration of prototype VIII of the controlled-release micropump (CRM) with a solid piston. (From Anderson, J.M. and Kim, S.W., Eds., *Recent Advances in Drug Delivery Systems*, Plenum Publ. Corp., New York, 1984, 351. With permission.)

The actual mechanism of augmented delivery is unclear, since there are no valves to impose a preferred direction for augmented delivery. It is presumed that augmentation arises from a pressure difference superimposed during piston movement on the basal-concentration gradient or from a mixing effect associated with piston movement. In short-term experiments performed to date with insulin and hydrophilic membranes, no problem with deposition has been noted. This is in distinct contrast to the experience with hydrophobic membranes used in an earlier prototype in which delivery rate decreased within 2 to 3 h of operation due to deposition of insulin crystals.

Although the capability for operation with high-concentration/low-volume reservoirs is the primary advantage of the controlled-release micropump (CRM), two inherent fail-safe mechanisms are also important. Augmented delivery is achieved without valves. Therefore, the mechanical unreliability associated with the inadvertent opening and sticking of valves with complex motors or with the peristaltic action of a rotating metal component on a soft plastic tube is avoided. The long-term stability of the foam membrane after repeated compression is also important. *In vitro* results indicate that a life of one year can be expected under normal use. In the CRM, basal delivery is not achieved by regulating a large flow rate, as is done in valve-operated systems. Failure of the CRM, therefore, cannot result in uncontrolled delivery at the maximum rate and cause an inadvertent insulin overdose, for example. Furthermore, the presence of a membrane in the CRM eliminates the effect of sudden acceleration or deceleration, which can result in overdoses in other pumps.

The need to minimize diffusion resistance limits the location of the implant to the delivery site. This introduces greater emphasis on the biocompatibility of the pump exterior, particularly, the pump outlet. The development of a fibrotic capsule, for example, can change tissue perfusion and interfere with the absorption and subsequent distribution of any drug from the delivery site. Furthermore, the fibrotic capsule can act as an uncontrollable diffusion-resistance factor and adversely affect the performance characteristics of the pump. The tissue-implant interface is a major focus of current animal studies.[50]

I.   Other devices

Various electrochemical methodologies have been proposed for implantable pumps, particularly for the delivery of insulin.[51,52] An electrolytic pump, utilizing the pressure of gases evolved at the electrodes of an electrolytic cell, has been described. However, it is not clear how the evolved gases will be collected, vented, or recombined to cause the driving pressure to be reduced and to slow the pump.[53] Another group of investigators has proposed using electroosmosis to drive water across a cation-exchange membrane to pressurize an appropriate drug reservoir. Although aqueous flows of the appropriate magnitude for insulin delivery have been developed in repeated fashion over long periods of time, and with little power consumption, the necessary valve and reservoir arrangements have not yet been devised. Such devices are of interest because of their low power and particularly low voltage requirements. Whether they can ultimately be powered with a glucose fuel cell in a closed-loop fashion or not still remains to be explored.[54,55]

III.   Implants for contraception

A.   Biodegradable

Biodegradable polymers are the most recent developments in contraceptive drug delivery systems. They appear to be an excellent contraceptive strategy since they can provide a programmed rate of release of steroids, thereby possibly eliminating menstrual abnormalities associated with constant steroid levels. Following implantation or injection, the devices can be used for three months and longer.

The primary mechanisms of steroid release are erosion, diffusion, cleavage of covalent linkage, or a combination of these processes. The most investigated polymer materials are poly(lactic acid), poly(glycolic acid), and poly-(ε-caprolactone). The steroids used are primarily norethisterone and levonorgestrel. The mode of action at high blood levels may involve central inhibition of ovulation, while at low levels, it may involve alterations in cervical mucus, sperm migration, ovum transport, and implantation.[56,57]

Little human clinical work has been reported in this area. The most extensively examined system is composed of norethisterone in microcrystals of DL-poly(lactide-co-glycolide) or DL-poly(lactic acid). A saline suspension of microspheres — 25% w/w norethisterone in DL-poly(lactic acid) — was injected intramuscularly at a dose of either 200 mg or 400 mg. The release of steroid occurred over 6 months. The treatment was well tolerated with no adverse effects except spotting and irregular menstrual cycles. It was concluded that doses of 1.33 to 3.45 mg/kg are necessary to inhibit ovulation for six months. Due to a problem of DL-poly(lactic acid) accumulation with continuous injections, the release of norethisterone from a copolymer DL-poly(lactide-co-glycolide) was examined. This copolymer was reported to have similar kinetics of steroid release, but degrades at a faster rate than DL-poly(lactic acid).[58,59]

Several other methods of steroid release from biodegradable polymers are also currently under examination. Poly(ε-caprolactone), which is permeable to levonorgestrel, is believed to release the drug for at least a year at a constant diffusion-controlled rate, after which the device erodes. Subdermal implantation of poly(ε-caprolactone) capsules containing levonorgestrel into the lateral hip suppressed ovulation in all subjects without any serious adverse effects.[60,61]

Norethisterone has been prepared as compressed pellets with cholesterol. It has been covalently bonded to polyN-(3-hydroxypropyl)-L-glutamine to produce an implant that erodes rather than relying on diffusion. Another approach involves the use of a poly(orthoester) known as Chromoner as a matrix for a suspension of norethisterone and levonorgestrel with a stabilizing buffer. This product has been shown to release norethisterone in a fairly constant manner until the 32nd week after implantation.

B.   Nonbiodegradable

One of the methods of steroid release involves the use of a nondegradable polymer, silastic. The polymer is shaped into capsules or rods, which are implanted subdermally. The advantages of these devices are that their effectiveness does not depend on patient compliance, the duration of action is longer, and the effects can be terminated by removing the implant. The usefulness of such implants, however, may be limited by the occurrence of menstrual abnormalities and systemic side effects. A primary disadvantage with their use is the need for medical personnel to implant and remove them. Additional concerns are the possibility of the implants migrating, thus making retrieval difficult. Possible toxicological effects of the polymers also represent a concern.[62]

The Norplant device has been the most extensively examined implant. It consists of medical-grade silastic capsules 34 mm long containing levonorgestrel. Six capsules are placed subdermally into the inner aspect of the upper arm in a fan shape through a 5-mm incision within 1 week of the onset of menses. The implant is designed to be used for approximately 5 years.

This device operates by interfering with ovulation or luteal function. The rate of anovulation ranges from 25 to 80%, being highest in the first year of treatment. In a 3-year study, Norplant was found to have excellent contraceptive effectiveness and demonstrated a significantly lower pregnancy rate than the TCu 200 IUD. Menstrual abnormalities occur with both devices, but patients using the implant show higher blood hemoglobin levels. In Norplant users, the dominant medical complaints leading to removal are those associated with progestational contraceptive agents (primarily bleeding irregularities). Capsule migration was found to be minimal.[63]

Other steroids that have been used within implants are estradiol and ST 1435 (a 19-norprogesterone derivative) that is seven times more potent as an ovulation inhibitor than levonorgestrel.[64]

IV. Delivery of chemotherapeutic agents using implants

The size of a potential market often drives drug development; the larger the market, the greater the competition. Hypertension, diabetes, cancer, and arthritis markets, for example, have attracted a number of companies because of the number of patients in these market populations.[65–67] Diabetes and cancer have been identified by companies involved in a myriad of different technologies. Both implantable and external ambulatory infusion devices are currently in use, providing controlled delivery of insulin and chemotherapeutic agents via various types of catheters and access devices.[68–70]

Work has progressed in several laboratories around the world in which implanted insulin-infusion pumps are used. The objective is to establish a safe and effective approach to "open-loop" insulin delivery from an implanted system. Open-loop means that the pump itself does not sense blood glucose; rather, the patient must monitor blood glucose and, in some way, signal the pump with a command describing when and how much insulin to infuse.

The Programmable Implantable Medication System (PIMS) was developed at The Johns Hopkins University Applied Physics Laboratory.[71] The implanted unit is a disk approximately 3 inches in diameter and 0.78 inches thick, surgically placed beneath the skin in the left side of the abdomen. It delivers pulses of insulin via a catheter, the tip of which is placed deep in the peritoneal cavity. The pump spaces its pulses to deliver a basal release rate, which is programmable and recycles every 24 h. The patient then uses an external transmitting unit (a box about 6 × 4 × 2 in.) to command the pump to deliver any of a variety of insulin doses.

A major step in the future will be the development of a continuous glucose sensor. This has been a difficult problem over the years. The ideal sensor should have long life, be sensitive to small changes in glucose, be rapid in its response rate, remain in contact with either blood or a body fluid that reflects blood glucose, and, above all, be reliable.

Insulin, like other medications, can be bound to various polymers and implanted as a pellet under the skin. It can then slowly leach off the pellet and find its way into the bloodstream. This relatively simple approach would be of limited use, however, because it would require repeated implantations of the pellet and would provide only a continuous infusion of insulin and would not give physiologic variations needed to control both between-meal and after-meal changes in blood glucose. More elegant approaches are under development that could allow modification of the rate of insulin release from insulin products, such as proinsulin, for example, by an external device that alters an electrical field.[72,73]

The capabilities of the programmable drug administration device (DAD) make it a useful device for chronotherapy.[74,75] Chronotherapy is based on the fact that the efficacy of a drug can change when administered at different times during the circadian cycle. This fact, explored for more than three decades, has been demonstrated in laboratory and clinical trials. For commonly used cancer chemotherapeutic drugs, animal studies have shown that both efficacy and toxicity to the host are related to the time of administration. The susceptibility of normal tissues to these powerful drugs varies rhythmically, with tumor cells displaying a different time-related response. Therefore, the timing of drug delivery via a DAD can be important in achieving therapeutic specificity.

The preferred objective is to deliver the chemotherapeutic agent when normal cells are least susceptible and when cancer cells are more susceptible. Chronic evaluation of these principles is difficult in large numbers of patients because of the complex, nonlinear dosing patterns required for rhythm-based chronotherapy. Current medical practice cannot readily and consistently achieve the dosing patterns on either an inpatient or outpatient basis. The DAD, however, may be capable of implementing these protocols automatically and over an extended period of time.

The DAD has been used clinically in several patients in three primary application areas: terminal cancer pain management, intractable spasticity management, and cancer chemotherapy. The DAD's longevity is a function of the capacity of the power source and the dispensing rate of the drug. Depletion of the power source is affected principally by the cumulative amount of drug administered by the pump. The expected longevity of an implanted pump is 3 to 5 years, depending on the application and the amount of drug delivered.[76]

In cancer pain management, clinically effective relief of intractable cancer pain has been obtained with the DAD using morphine sulfate delivered intrathecally in 60 patients for whom oral medications had failed. The majority of the patients judged pain relief to be good to excellent. Respiratory depression was not a problem. In comparison to previous methods of administration, the patients were more alert and active and did not experience many of the secondary complications of chronic narcotic administration, such as lethargy, confusion, and constipation.[77] Although the development of tolerance is a concern during intrathecal administration, it was not an overwhelming clinical problem with programmable delivery. According to Penn et al.,[78] only 2 out of 43 patients with implanted pumps developed significant tolerance. Its ability to alter dosage noninvasively makes the DAD a convenient system for meeting patients' changing needs. The DAD also conveniently accommodates a broad patient range of initial dosage levels.

Spasticity caused by spinal cord trauma or multiple sclerosis is often treated with oral baclofen (an analog of the inhibitory neurotransmitter gamma aminobutyric acid). The goal is to reduce muscle tone to normal levels and to suppress spasms. The major side effects of the drug are drowsiness and, in some cases, confusion. The DAD has been used to administer baclofen intrathecally to patients with severe spasticity who are refractory to oral baclofen.[79] As with pain patients, noninvasive programmability is clinically useful for initial-dose titration and for accommodating changes in dosage requirements. No drowsiness, confusion, or weakness was experienced at dosage levels adequate to suppress symptoms.

As noted previously, studies have demonstrated that drug toxicity, side effects, and therapeutic results are affected by the timing of cancer chemotherapy drug delivery during the circadian cycle. However, the nonequal dosing regimens needed to obtain chronotherapeutic results simply do not readily lend themselves to conventional therapy. The use of the DAD in cancer chemotherapy by Hrushesky[75] illustrates the therapeutic effect of implanted programmable drug infusion. In one series of patients with carcinoma of the kidney, constant-rate intravenous infusion of floxuridine (FUDR) was compared with time-modified administration. The time-modified schedule consisted of four dosage intervals: low-level administration in the early morning quadrant, a stepwise dosage increase from late morning into early afternoon (second quadrant), peak delivery rates from late afternoon into early evening, and a decrease in dosage to second quadrant levels in the final interval. Results of this study were encouraging and support the usefulness of DAD. Oncologists currently believe that the amount of drug administered, as well as adherence to monthly treatment schedules, are important to the ultimate success of chemotherapy. In the intravenous FUDR groups studied, 40% of the patients receiving constant-rate infusion required treatment delays compared to 6% of the time-modified group. Reductions in dosage were necessary in 60% of the former group, while only 12% of the time-modified patients required reduction because of drug-related symptoms.[80,81]

In conclusion, programmable implantable drug delivery is an emerging technology. Its clinical benefits include improved drug efficacy, dynamic dosing, noninvasive prescription modification, reduced side effects, improved quality of life, and cost-effectiveness compared to traditional in-hospital therapies. These benefits accrue principally from ambulatory targeted delivery and from programmability — particularly as it relates to complex dosing patterns. This and similar systems are expected to be used in the delivery of genetically engineered substances, which have inherent problems in delivery.

V.   Recent advances in implants and related devices (excluding inserts)

In veterinary applications, implants are commercially available for estrus synchronization via delivery of hormones. COMPUDOSE is a polymeric controlled-release device for the delivery of estradiol to improve both growth rate and feed efficiency in beef cattle. The product is composed of a non-medicated silicone rubber core coated with a thin layer of medicated silicone rubber containing estradiol. COMPUDOSE is implanted subcutaneously in the ear of beef cattle.[82]

For peptides contained in film-coated implants, degradation can occur inside the implant while crossing the rate-limiting membrane or in the bathing solution. As part of a program using coated implants to deliver peptides, it has been found that conjugated peptides ranging in molecular weight from 1200 Daltons through 30,000 Daltons were degrading during *in vitro* testing.[82]

Ouabain-induced ventricular tachycardia in the dog has been converted to normal sinus rhythm via controlled release drug delivery of lidocaine from a polymeric matrix directly into the ventricular myocardium. This therapeutic effect was achieved as rapidly as an intravenous bolus, but with comparatively lower plasma levels. Antiarrhythmic drug delivery implants may prove to be a useful approach to optimize efficacy while minimizing untoward effects.[82]

The development of inexpensive, biocompatible, subcutaneous implants for the controlled delivery of peptides has been undertaken. The release of peptides from Eudragit NE30D coated implants using an incubating medium was studied. *In vivo*, the implants containing LHRH have been used to induce ovulation and mating in anestrus sheep.[82]

Studies have been carried out in an effort to develop implants for the controlled delivery of a synthetic growth hormone-releasing peptide (His-D-Trp-Ala-Trp-D-Phe-Lys-NH) for sustained periods to ruminants. Various polymeric materials have been employed as coating agents to modify the surface area of the implants, thereby affecting the release profile. Formulation and surface area modifications were combined to obtain the desired uniform release rates and optimum release period. *In vivo* release profiles were obtained for several sets of implants, which correlated well with the *in vitro* profiles.[82]

An elastomer matrix implant providing release for a period in excess of one year of an agonistic analogue of leutenizing hormone-releasing hormone (LH-RH) has been developed. The compound is a decapeptide, and the system was targeted for reversible suppression of estrus, reversible chemical castration, and treatment of sex-hormone-dependent conditions in companion animals. The system is biocompatible and nondegradable. At the end of one year of therapy, or when it is otherwise desired to discontinue the therapy, the implant may be removed via a minor surgical procedure. A new device may be implanted at this time and therapy continued. Formulation factors are critical to both rate and duration of delivery of the compound, and their appropriate manipulation allows design of this extremely prolonged release system.[82]

The feasibility of incorporating insulin into an osmotic pump whose pumping rate is dependent on blood glucose has been evaluated.[83] Such a pump could contain insulin in virtually any liquid or semisolid form, and its release rate would be independent of the formulation. The approach has been to develop a semipermeable membrane whose aqueous permeability increases with blood glucose concentration. The membrane consists of two layers: the first layer contains immobilized glucose oxidase, which converts glucose to gluconic acid, thereby lowering the local pH, while the second layer consists of a cross-linked, hydrophobic, polybasic hydrogel. This hydrogel absorbs little water at physiologic pH, but becomes quite hydrated as pH is lowered.

Bioerodible implants have been investigated using polylactides, caprolactone polymers or copolymers, solid solutions in polylactic acid, and cyclazocine, norethidrone, and d-norgestrel, respectively.[83] Permeable implants have also been studied using polysiloxane grafted with N-vinyl-pyrrolidone, hydrophilic acrylate or methacrylate polymers and ACTH hormone, and norethandrolone (Nilevar), respectively.[83]

Dedrick et al.[84] have developed a device called a diffusion cell for release of methotrexate, while Schopflin[85] used silicone rubbers and norethisterone acetate as the medicinal agent.

An implanted apparatus that dispenses a drug over a prolonged period of time has been developed by Ellinwood.[86] A self-powered dispensing device stores one or more substances in powdered, liquid, or other dispensable form and uses a compressible container (i.e., bellows, for withdrawing substances from the reservoir and dispensing to the body). The dispensing operation may be on a fixed schedule or may be controlled by monitoring single or multiple sensors implanted in the body and evaluating the sensed data in order to control the conditions under which dispensing takes place, as well as the kind of dispensing. Dual dispensers and dual medication also may be used. The types of application used with evaluation of biological signals according to this process include chemical transducers and feedback, such as detection of glucose and pH, as well as ionic change detection; temperature, pressure, or mechanical transduced changes (e.g., blood pressure, blood flow, gut motility); and electrical activity, as might be measured in an electrocardiogram or electroencephalogram.

An implantable dosing device composed of a medication reservoir, a propellant chamber, and flow control has been described by Kuhl and Luft.[87] The release of the medication to the body can be controlled or regulated and thus adapted to demand at any time. This is achieved by providing an electroosmotic regulatory control valve with an ion-exchange diaphragm arranged between two porous electrodes for flow control. In such a valve, liquid is transported through the electrodes and through the ion-exchange diaphragm when current flows. For example, negative charges are fixed at the pore walls of the ion-exchange diaphragm, and the mobile positive ions, which are necessary for reasons of electroneutrality, then travel in the electric field and take along the liquid by friction.

In addition to the advantage that this implantable dosing device can be controlled or regulated, the device is also uninfluenced by changes of body temperature insofar as its operation and effectiveness are concerned. This is because the transport of the medication, due to the gas pressure of a propellant in the propellant chamber, is superimposed (i.e., regulated by the amount of liquid passing through the ion).

In the process described by Wichterle,[88] long-term tubular outlets through the skin are replaced by an implant introduced into a subcuticular ligament immediately below the skin. The implant is generally in the shape of a capsule or pouch and formed of a wall construction that substantially retains its shape both when filled and empty. This defines a hollow interior cavity of substantially constant volume in which the liquid may be stored and is easily filled through injection with a hypodermic needle. The capsule is provided with at least one channel, which may be connected to an implanted tube leading to the body organ or organ substitute, even though it may be remote from the skin or the location of the capsule.

Wichterle[88] has also developed an implant for infusion consisting of a hollow body with one wall formed by a thin, permeable membrane with a chamber inside the body, the chamber being connected by at least one channel with the outside. This system enables essentially unidirectional diffusion of the active substance directly to the affected tissue and maintenance of arbitrary changes of the concentration of the active agent. This device is useful for directing drugs into the location of nonoperable tumor diseases.

A self-powered, vapor-pressure delivery device for the controlled and continuous dispensing of an active agent has been developed by Michaels et al.[89] This device uses vapor pressure as the motive force, and it may be used for administering drugs internally in the body of an animal or human. Michaels and colleagues have also described a device comprising an expandable laminate surrounding a collapsible container filled with drug and positioned in a rigid housing chamber. When in operation, the device releases a drug in response to the laminate imbibing fluid and expands, thereby exerting pressure on the container, which then collapses and delivers a drug from the device.[89]

Epicardially implanted D-sotalol polyurethane composite matrices for preventing ischemic ventricular arrhythmias have been studied in open-chest dogs. D-sotalol was combined with a polyureapolyurethane (3:7) in solvent-cast films, which were characterized *in vitro* for their drug release. Placement of 200-mg D-sotalol matrices in the nonischemic zone was ineffective for significantly reducing the occurrence of ventricular arrhythmias. Furthermore, D-sotalol controlled-release matrices were ineffective for preventing ventricular fibrillation (VF) regardless of dose or placement site. It was concluded that epicardial D-sotalol controlled-release matrices inhibited ischemic ventricular arrhythmias, but not VF, if placed in the left ventricular ischemic zone during repeated left anterior descending coronary artery (LAD) occlusions.[90]

Novel biodegradable implants have been designed for extended delivery of effective levels of the growth-promoting agent17-β estradiol to steers. The initial burst of release from poorly entrapped drug on the surface of the implant was found to be minimized by reducing the drug loading in the terminal active compacts, which tend to contribute disproportionately to the initial surface area of the device. Prolonged dissolution testing on single compacts and composite implants facilitated selection of implant designs that showed the desired increase in active release.[91]

A microcapsule for implantation that reduces immune response has been described. Active material was encapsulated within a semipermeable barrier, the outermost layer of which contained an alginate substantially composed of alpha1-guluronic acid. Islets of Langerhans from rats were suspended in a concentrated aqueous solution of the acid and then injected into aqueous calcium chloride to form cross-linked microcapsules. Capsules were subsequently soaked in sodium alginate solution to form an outer alginate membrane.[92]

Schindler and Hollomon[93] have prepared random copolymers of caprolactone containing 5 to 25 mol% trimethylene carbonate. Copolymers can be shaped into tubular containers and used for sustained drug delivery after subcutaneous implantation. In one preparation, they dissolved trimethylene carbonate and stannous octoate in caprolactone and then heated it to 140°C. They cast the resulting copolymer as a thin film from chloroform and rolled it at 80°C. The resulting tube was shaped into capsules and filled with levonorgestrel for testing.

French researchers have developed a cellular implant-based targeted delivery system that may have potential in the treatment of cancer. Although cytokines are of increasing interest in the treatment of cancer, they are rapidly broken down in the body, and a more targeted approach is needed. Several research teams have tried using genetically modified cancer cells to secrete IL-2 locally in mice. The implants stimulate the immune system in two ways: they are histocompatible, and the IL-2 they secrete activates natural killer cells. To make the method more lasting and specific, the plan is to insert into the implants other genes coding for specific tumor antigens as well as the IL-2 gene. This approach could be a viable alternative to the use of viral or retroviral vectors.[94]

Alza's tetracycline peridontal implant, developed in conjunction with On-Site Therapeutics, Inc., has been targeted for a potentially large market. A survey in the mid-1980s conducted by the National Institute for Dental Research indicated that as many as eight out of ten Americans have some form of periodonitis. Therefore, this product could be well recognized in oral care as well as in the area of dental consumer products.

Biodegradable materials have been successfully utilized for guided tissue regeneration (GTR) and local delivery systems as they are biocompatible, less cytotoxic, and do not require removal. The regenerative effect of 25%

doxycycline-loaded biodegradable GTR membrane was evaluated in dogs. The results suggested that doxycycline-loaded membrane might have beneficial effect on osteogenesis to favor peridontal regeneration. Repeated estrus synchronization of beef cows with intravaginal progesterone implants and the effects of a GnRH agonist buserelin following implant insertion was investigated.[98]

The release characteristics of antibiotics from *in vivo*- and *in vitro*-processed morselized cancellous bone have been compared. The results indicate that this bone can act as a carrier of antibiotics. The elution profiles of netilmicin-, vancomycin-, clindamycin-, and rifampicin-impregnated cancellous bone were similar.

Ceramic hydroxyapatite implants have been used in dentistry for their unique compatibility with alveolar bone. Bisphosphonates may be beneficial in preventing alveolar bone destruction associated with natural and experimental periodontal disease. It also prevents resorption of alveolar bone following mucoperiosteal flap surgery. Effects of highly bisphosphonate-complexed hydroxyapatite implants on osteoconduction and repair in rat tibiae were investigated, and it was found that normal osteoconduction and repair did occur on and around the tibiae.[99]

The controlled delivery of toremifene citrate from subcutaneously implanted silica xerogel carrier has been evaluated. Toremifene citrate was incorporated into hydrolyzed silica sol, and the implants were tested *in vivo* and *in vitro* in mice. The silica xerogel discs showed a sustained release of toremifene citrate over 42 days, and toremifene-related changes in the uterus were detectable at all studied time points. These findings suggest that silica xerogel is a promising carrier material for implantable controlled drug delivery systems.[100]

The effect of bone morphogenic protein (BMP) on the bond strength of titanium implants at the bone-implant interface was evaluated. It was concluded from this study that the use of BMP-atelopeptide type I collagen mixture is an effective means of obtaining greater bond strength at the bone-implant interface within a shorter time period than the titanium implants without BMP.[101]

Resistance of antibiotics, such as rifampicin-, vancomycin-, and gentamicin-bonded gelatin-coated polymer meshes to *Staphylococcus aureus* in a rabbit subcutaneous pouch model, was studied. At the time of explanation, none of the antibiotics-soaked meshes were infected, while all of the untreated meshes were infected. These results indicate that antibiotic soaking evidently prevents perioperative infection of gelatin-coated knitted polymer meshes in this experimental model.[102]

Bioprosthetic heat valves made from glutaraldehyde-fixed porcine aortic valves or bovine pericardium have been shown to have some advantages over mechanical valves. However, their durability is low due to calcification and immunological rejection. Studies on immunogenicity play an important role in understanding the biocompatibility of materials. For example, the effect of polyethylene glycol on pericardial calcification has been investigated. The authors studied the complement activation potential and the contribution of complement factors on the calcification of polyethylene glycol (PEG)-grafted pericardium samples and compared the results with standard glutaraldehyde-treated pericardium samples. Based on the results, the authors selected activated PEG-grafted bovine pericardium using glutaraldehyde and carbodimde for further studies.[103,104]

VI.   Future prospects

Among implants, ambulatory drug delivery technology represents one of the fastest growing areas in the health care market. Vascular access ports are particularly important because of their compatibility with current economic trends aimed at reducing the length of hospital stays and moving adaptable therapies to more profitable settings in the hospital, such as the outpatient surgery unit, outpatient clinic, or home health department.[95]

Perhaps the most promising market segment for ambulatory long-term infusion therapy is chemotherapy. This segment alone is projected to increase at a rate of 30 to 40% annually during the next decade. In addition, other relatively new markets for these devices, such as long-term antibiotic therapy, total parenteral nutrition, and pain management, will expand greatly as infusion therapy is moved to ambulatory settings, such as the outpatient clinic, the home, and the physician's office. In the near future, pediatric and epidural venous access systems will undoubtedly be introduced, and additional products serving the dual lumen market will probably be developed. But the most interesting opportunities for growth lie in the area of dedicated port and pump systems.[83,96,97]

Based upon the established work on implantable delivery vehicles, it is probable that these or related devices may well be in widespread clinical use within the next 10 to 20 years. Availability of devices that can provide not only insulin infusion, but also delivery of chemotherapeutic agents, is not too far in the future. It would be highly desirable to combine an insulin-delivery device with a totally implanted glucose sensor, thereby achieving the development of a completely "closed-loop" implantable artificial beta cell. Although sensor development has been under study for 15 to 20 years, there still appears to be none ready for combination with an insulin-delivery device to make a completely "closed-loop" artificial beta cell. Several serious problems in sensor technology, including electrode drift and problems with standardization in a totally implanted device, as well as changes in sensor function with overgrowth of tissue cells, have made this an extremely difficult problem to solve. Whatever the eventual outcome, it seems clear that the next two decades will be an active time for research into insulin-delivery devices of all kinds and their clinical evaluation. Most important, these future implantable delivery systems will perhaps offer the patient greater freedom and thus improved quality of life.

References

1. Bruck, S.D., Evaluation of blood compatibility of polymeric implants. In *Controlled Drug Delivery*, Vol. 2, Clinical Applications, Bruck, S.D., Ed., CRC Press, Inc., Boca Raton, FL, 45–64, 1983.
2. Lawrence, W.H., Acute and chronic evaluations of implanted polymeric materials. In *Controlled Drug Delivery*, Vol. 2, Clinical Applications, Bruck, S.D., Ed., CRC Press, Inc., Boca Raton, FL, 1–44, 1983.
3. Sefton, M.V., *Implantable Pumps in Medical Applications of Controlled Release*, Vol. 1, Langer, R.S. and Wise, D.L., Eds., CRC Press, Inc., Boca Raton, FL, 129–158, 1984.
4. Hsieh, D.S.T., Langer, R., and Folkman, J., Magnetic modulation of release of macromolecules from polymers, *Proc. Natl. Acad. Sci.*, 78, 1863, 1981.
5. Merrill, E.W., U.S. Patent 3,608,540, 1981.
6. Leininger, R.I., Polymers as surgical implants, *CRC Crit. Rev. Bioeng.*, 1, 1973.
7. Williams, D.F., Ed., *Biocompatibility of Clinical Implant Materials*, Vols. 1 and 2, CRC Press, Inc., Boca Raton, FL, 1981.
8. Schade, D.S. et al., Future therapy of the insulin-dependent diabetic patient — the implantable insulin-delivery system, *Diabetes Care*, 4, 319, 1981.
9. Soeldner, J.S., Treatment of diabetes mellitus by devices, *JAMA*, 70, 183, 1981.
10. Blackshear, P.J. et al., Control of blood glucose in experimental diabetes by means of totally implantable insulin-infusion device, *Diabetes*, 28, 634, 1979.
11. Marliss, E.B., Caron, D., Albisser, A.M., and Zinman, B., Present and future expectations regarding insulin-infusion systems, *Diabetes Care*, 4, 325, 1981.
12. Buchwald, H. et al., Intraarterial infusion chemotherapy for hepatic carcinoma using a totally implantable infusion pump, *Cancer*, 45, 866, 1980.
13. Ellinwood, E.H., U.S. Patent 3,923,060, 1975.
14. Spencer, W.J., A review of preprogrammed insulin-delivery systems, *Trans. Biomed. Eng.*, BME28, 237, 1981.
15. Schade, D.S., Eaton, R.P., Edwards, W.S., Doberneck, R.C., et al., Successful short-term implantation of a remotely programmable insulin-delivery system in man, *JAMA*, 247, 1848, 1982.
16. Carlson, G.A. et al., A new low-power high-reliability infusion pump., *Proc. Seventh N. Engl. Bioeng. Conf.*, Ostrander, L.E., Ed., 193, 1979.
17. Carlson, G.A. et al., Development of an artificial beta cell suitable for animal implantation, *Trans. Am. Soc. Artif. Intern. Organs*, 26, 523, 1980.
18. Love, J.T. and Goana, J.L., An implantable insulin-delivery system. In *Frontiers of Engineering in Health Care*, Cohen, B.A., Ed., 51, 1981.
19. Spencer, W.J. et al., Some engineering aspects of insulin-delivery systems, *Diabetes Care*, 3, 345, 1980.
20. Summers, G.D., U.S. Patent 3,527,220, 1970.
21. Blackshear, P.J., Dorman, F.D., Blackshear, P.L., Varco, R.L., and Buchwald, H., The design and initial testing of an implantable infusion pump, *Surg. Gynaecol. Obstet.*, 134, 51, 1972.
22. Blackshear, P.J., Dorman, F.D., Blackshear, P.L., Buchwald, H., and Varco, R.L., U.S. Patent 3,731,681, 1973.
23. Blackshear, P.J., Rohde, T.D., Varco, R.L., and Buchwald, H., One year of continuous heparinization in the dog using a totally implantable infusion pump, *Surg. Gynaecol. Obstet.*, 141, 176, 1975.

24. Perkins, P.R. et al., Design and initial testing of a totally implantable trans-
    cutaneously controllable insulin-delivery device, *Trans. Am. Soc. Artif. Intern.
    Organs*, 24, 229, 1978.

25. Buchwald, H. et al., A totally implantable drug-infusion device: Laboratory
    and clinical experience using a model with single flow rate and new design
    for modulated insulin infusion, *Diabetes Care*, 3, 351, 1980.

26. Rohde, T.D., Blackshear, P.J., Varco, R.L., and Buchwald, H., Chronic heparin
    anticoagulant in dogs by continuous infusion with a totally implantable
    pump, *Trans. Am. Soc. Artif. Intern. Organs*, 216, 510, 1975.

27. Loughheed, W. and Albisser, A.M., Insulin delivery and the artificial beta cell:
    Luminal obstruction in capillary conduits, *Int. J. Artif. Org.*, 3, 50, 1980.

28. Alzet miniosmotic pump bibliography, Alza Corporation, Palo Alto, CA,
    1981.

29. Lynch, H.J., Rivest, R.W., and Wurtman, R.J., Artificial induction of melatonin
    rhythms by programmed microinfusion, *Neuroendocrinology*, 31, 106, 1980.

30. Theeuwes, F., Elementary osmotic pump, *J. Pharm. Sci.*, 64, 1987, 1975.

31. Stolzenberg, S.J. and Linkenhermer, W.H., U.S. Patent, 3,604,417, 1971.

32. Nau, H., Trotz, M., and Wenger, C., Controlled-rate drug administration in
    testing for toxicity, in particular, teratogenicity, towards interspecies bioequiv-
    alance. In *Topics in Pharmaceutical Sciences*, Breimer, D.D. and Speiser, P., Eds.
    Elsevier Press, Inc., New York, 143–157, 1985.

33. Nau, H., Zierer, R., Spielmann, H., Neubert, D., and Gansau, C.H., A new
    model for embryotoxicity testing: teratogenicity and pharmacokinetics of val-
    proic acid following constant-rate administration in the mouse using human
    therapeutic drug and metabolic concentrations, *Life Sci.*, 29, 2803–2814, 1981.

34. Nau, H., Teratogenic valproic acid concentrations: infusion by implanted
    minipumps versus conventional injection regimen in the mouse, *Toxicol. Appl.
    Pharmacol.*, 80, 243–250, 1985.

35. Ray, N. and Theeuwes, F., Implantable osmotically powered drug delivery
    systems. In *Drug Delivery Systems, Fundamentals and Techniques*, Johnson, P.
    and Lloyd-Jones, J.G., Eds., Ellis Horwood, VCH Publishers, Chichester,
    120–138, 1987.

36. Theeuwes, F. and Yum, S.I., Principles of the design and operation of generic
    osmotic pumps for the delivery of semisolid or liquid drug formulations,
    Ann. Biomed. Eng., 4, 343–353, 1976.

37. Sikic, B.I., Collins, J.M., Mimnaugh, E.G., and Gram, T.E., Improved thera-
    peutic index of bleomycin when administered by continuous infusion in mice,
    Cancer Treat. Rep., 62, 2011–2017, 1978.

38. Urquhart, J., Fara, J., and Willis, K.L., Rate-controlled delivery systems in
    drug and hormone research, *Ann. Rev. Pharmacol. Toxicol.*, 24, 199–236, 1984.

39. Sendelbeck, S.L. and Urquhart, J., Spatial distribution of dopamine, methotr-
    exate, and antipyrine during continuous intracerebral microperfusion, *Brain
    Res.*, 328, 251–258, 1985.

40. Ruers, T.J.M. et al., Local treatment of renal allografts, a promising way to
    reduce the dosage of immunosuppressive drugs, *Transplantation*, 41, 156–161,
    1986.

41. Proovst, A.P., de Keyzer, M.H., Kort, W.L., and Wolff, E.D., Superiority of
    continuous infusion of prednisolone over daily injections in the prolongation
    of heart allograft survival in rats, *Transplantation*, 34, 221–222, 1982.

42. Cronan, T., Conrad, J., and Bryson, R., Effects of chronically administered nicotine and saline on motor activity in rats, *Pharmacol. Biochem. Behav.*, 22, 897–899, 1985.

43. Lynch, H.J., Rivest, R.W., and Wurtman, R.J., Artificial induction of melatonin rhythms by programmed microinfusion, *Neuroendocrinology*, 31, 106–111, 1980.

44. Lasley, B.L. and Wing, A., Stimulating ovarian function in exotic carnivores with pulses of GnRH, *Ann. Proc. Amer. Assoc. Zoo. Vet.*, 14–14, 1983.

45. Phillips, J.A., Alexander, N., Karesh, W.B., Millar, R., and Lasley, B.L., Stimulating male sexual behavior with repetitive pulses of GnRH in female green iguanas Iguana-Iguana, *J. Exper. Zool.*, 234, 481–484, 1985.

46. Bessman, J.P. and Layne, E.C., Implantation of a closed-loop artificial beta cell, *Abstr. Am. Soc. Artif. Intern. Organs*, 67, 1981.

47. Schubert, W., Baurschmidt, P., Nagel, J., Thull, R., and Schaldach, M., An implantable artificial pancreas, *Med. Biol. Eng. Comput.*, 18, 527, 1980.

48. Schapiro, G.A., Implantable insulin-delivery system, *Med. Electron.*, 55, 1979.

49. Sefton, M.V. and Burns, K.J., Controlled-release micropumping of insulin at variable rates, *Ind. Eng. Chem. Prod. Res. Dev.*, 20, 1, 1981.

50. Anderson, J.M., Niven, H., Pelagalli, J., Olanoff, L.S., and Jones, R.D., The role of the fibrous capsules in the function of implanted drug-polymer sustained-release systems, *J. Biomed. Mater. Res.*, 15, 889, 1981.

51. Nalecz, M., Lewadonski, J., Werynski, A., and Zawicki, I., Bioengineering aspects of the artificial pancreas, *Artif. Org.*, 2, 305, 1978.

52. Uhlig, E.L.P., Graydon, W.F., and Zingg, W., The electroosmotic activation of implantable insulin micropumps, *J. Biomed. Mater. Res.*, 17, 931, 1983.

53. Lougheed, W.D., Woulfe-Flanagan, H., Clement, J.R., and Albisser, A.M., Insulin aggregation in artificial delivery systems, *Diabetologica*, 19, 1, 1980.

54. Schade, D.S., Eaton, R.P., and Spencer, W., Implantation of an artificial pancreas, *JAMA*, 245, 709, 1981.

55. Sefton, M.V., Allen, D.G., Horvath, V., and Zingg, W., Insulin delivery at variable rates from a controlled-release micropump. In *Recent Advances in Drug Delivery Systems*, Anderson, J.M. and Kim, S.W., Eds., Plenum Publishing Corp., New York, 349–365, 1984.

56. Benagiano, G. and Gabelnick, H.L., Biodegradable systems for the sustained release of fertility-regulating agents, *J. Steroid Biochem.*, 11,449–455, 1979.

57. Bengiano, G., Ermini, M., and Gabelnick, H.L., *Hormonal Factors in Fertility, Infertility, and Contraception*, Vander Molen, H.J., Klopper, A., Lunefeld, B.L., Neves e Castro, M., Sciarro, F., and Vermeulen, A., Eds., Excerpta Medica, 141–147, 1982.

58. Beck, L.R. et al., Clinical evaluation of injectable biodegradable contraceptive systems, *Am. J. Obstet. Gynecol.*, 140, 799–806, 1981.

59. Beck, L.R. et al., Poly(DL-lactide-co-glycolide)/norethinsterone microcapsules: an injectable biodegradable contraceptive capsule, *Biol. Reprod.*, 28, 186–195, 1983.

60. Pitt, C.G., Marks, T.A., and Schlinder, A., *Natl. Inst. Drug Abuse Res. Monogr. Ser.*, 28, 232–252, 1980.

61. Ory, S.J., Hammond, C.B., Yancy, S.G., Hendern, R.W., and Pitt, C.G., The effect of a biodegradable contraceptive capsule (Capronor) containing levo-norgestrel on gonadotropin, estrogen, and progesterone levels, *Am. J. Obstet. Gynecol.*, 145, 600–605, 1983.

62. Croxatto, H.B., Diaz, S., Pavez, M., Miranda, P., and Brandeis, A., Plasma progesterone levels during long-term treatment with levo-norgestrel silastic implants, *Acta. Endocrinol*, 101, 307–311, 1982.

63. Sivan, I. et al., Three-year experience with Norplant subdermal contraception, *J. Fertil. Steril.*, 39, 799–808, 1983.

64. Faundes, A., deMejias, V.B., Leon, P., Robertson, D., and Alvarez, F., First-year clinical experience with six levo-norgestrol rods as subdermal contraception, *Contraception*, 20, 167–175, 1979.

65. Blackshear, P.J., Implantable pumps for insulin delivery: current clinical status. In *Drug Delivery Systems, Fundamentals and Techniques*, Johnson, P. and Lloyd-Jones, J.G., Eds., Ellis Horwood, VCH Publishers, Chichester, 139–149, 1987.

66. Blackshear, P.J., Rohde, T.D., Prosl, F., and Buchwald, H., The implantable infusion pump: A new concept in drug delivery, *Med. Prog. Technol.*, 6, 149–161, 1979.

67. Blackshear, P.J., Implantable drug-delivery systems, *Sci. Am.*, 241, 66–73, 1979.

68. Blackshear, P.J. and Rohde, T.D., Artificial devices for insulin infusion in the treatment of patients with diabetes mellitus. In *Controlled Drug Delivery*, Vol. 2, Bruck, S.D., Ed., CRC Press, Inc., Boca Raton FL, 111–147, 1984.

69. Blackshear, P.J., Implantable infusion pumps: Clinical applications. In *Methods in Enzymology*, Vol. 112, Colowick, S.P. and Kaplan, N.O., Eds., Academic Press, Inc., New York, 520–530, 1985.

70. Blackshear, P.J., Wigness, B.D., Roussell, A.M., and Cohen, A.M., Implantable infusion pumps: Practical aspects. In *Methods in Enzymology*, Vol. 112, Colowick, S.P. and Kaplan, N.O., Eds., Academic Press, Inc., New York, 530–545, 1985.

71. Fischell, R.E. et al., A programmable implantable system (PIMS) for the treatment of diabetes, *Artif. Organs*, 7A, 82, 1983.

72. Blackshear, P.J., Rupp, W.M., Rohde, T.D., and Buchwald, H., A totally implantable constant-rate insulin-infusion device: Preliminary studies in Type II diabetic subjects. In *Artificial Systems for Insulin Delivery*, Brunnetti, P., Alberti, K.G.M.M., Albisser, A.M., Heff, K.D., and Mussin Benedetti, M., Eds., Raven Press, New York, 131–139, 1983.

73. Citron, P., Benefits of programmable implanted drug administration. In *The Latest Developments in Drug Delivery Systems, Conf. Proc. Pharm. Tech.*, 20–22, 1987.

74. Halberg, F. et al., Toward a chronotherapy of neoplasis: tolerance of treatment depends upon host rhythms, *Experientia*, 29, 909–934, 1973.

75. Hrushesky, W., Circadian timing of cancer chemotherapy, *Science*, 228, 73–75, 1985.

76. Levi, F. et al., in *Chronobiology: Principles and Applications to Shifts in Schedules*, Scheving, L.E. and Halberg, F., Eds., Sijthoff and Noordhoff, The Netherlands, 481–511, 1980.

77. Roemeling, R.V. et al., Time of day modified continuous FUDR infusion, using an implanted programmable pump, improves therapeutic index. Abstract from *ASCO Proceedings, 1986.*

78. Penn, R.D. et al., Cancer pain relief using chronic morphine infusions: early experience with a programmable implanted drug pump, *J. Neurosurg.*, 61, 302–306, 1984.

79. Penn, R.D., Drug pumps for treatment of neurological diseases and pain, *Neurologic Clinics*, 3, 439–451, 1985.
80. Penn, R.D. and Kroin, J.S., Long-term baclofen infusion for treatment of spastcity, *J. Neurosurg.*, 66,181–185, 1987.
81. Roemeling, R.V. and Hrushesky, W., Circadian shaping of FUDR infusion reduces toxicity even at high-dose intensity, Abstract from *ASCO Proceedings*, 1987.
82. Lee, P.I. and Leonhardt, B.A., *Proc. 14th Int. Symp. Control. Rel. Bioact. Mater.*, August 2–5, 1987, Toronto, Canada.
83. *Program and Abstracts of the 15th Int. Symp. Control. Rel. Bioact. Mater.*, August 15–19, 1988, Basel, Switzerland.
84. Dedrick, R.L., Lutz, R.J., and Zaharko, D.S., U.S. Patent 3,946,734, 1976.
85. Schopflin, G., U.S. Patent 4,012,497, 1977.
86. Ellinwood, E.H. Jr., U.S. Patent 4,003,379, 1977.
87. Kuhl, D. and Luft, G., U.S. Patent 4,140,122, 1979.
88. Wichterle, O., U.S. Patents 3,971,378, 1976 and 3,896,806, 1975.
89. Michaels, A.S., Bashwa, J.D., and Zaffaroni, A., U.S. Patent 3,901,232, 1975; Michaels, A.S., U.S. Patent 3,788,322, 1974.
90. Labhasetwar, V., Kadish, A., Underwood, T., Sirinek, M., and Levy, R.J., The efficacy of controlled-release D-sotalol-polyurethane epicardial implants for ventricular arrhythmias due to acute ischemia in dogs, *J. Control. Rel.*, 23/1, 74, 1993.
91. Deasy, P.B., Finan, M.P., Klatt, P.R., and Hornkiewytsch, T., Design and evaluation of a biodegradable implant for improved delivery of oestradiol-17 beta to steers, *Int. J. Pharmaceut.*, 89, 251–259, 1993.
92. Skjak-Barek, G. et al., Canadian Patent CA 2,034,641.
93. Shindler, A. and Hollomon, M., PCT Int. Appl. (WO)91 16, 887, *Pharm. Technol.*, March 1993, 178.
94. SCRIP No. 1841, July 27th, 1993, 23.
95. Eckenhoff, B., Theeuwes, F., and Urquhart, J., Osmotically actuated dosage forms for rate-controlled drug delivery, *Pharm. Technol.*, June 1987, 96–102.
96. Theeuwes, F. and Bayne, W., Dosage form index, an objective criterion for evaluation of controlled-release drug delivery systems, *J. Pharm. Sci.*, 66, 1388–1392, 1977.
97. Urquhart, J., Methods of drug administration. In *Proc. National Academy of Sciences,* Institute of Medicine, Conf. on Pharmaceuticals for Developing Countries, 329–348, 1979.
98. Chang, C.Y. and Yamada, S., Evaluation of the regenerative effect of a 25% doxycycline-loaded biodegradable membrane for guided tissue regeneration, *J. Periodontal.*, 71, 1086–93, 2000.
99. Denissen, H. et al., Normal osteoconduction and repair in and around submerged highly bisphosphonate-complexed hydroxyapatite implants in rat tibiae, *J. Periodontal.*, 71, 272–8, 2002.
100. Kortesue, P. et al., Silica xerogel as an implantable carrier for controlled drug delivery: Evaluation and tissue effects after implantation, *Biomaterials*, 21, 193–8, 2000.
101. Bessho, K. and Carnes, D.L., BMP stimulation of bone response adjacent to titanium implant *in vivo*, *Clin. Oral Implants Res.*, 10, 212–8, 1999.

102. Goeau-Brissonniere, O. et al., Resistance of antibiotic-bonded gelatin-coated polymer meshes to *Staphyloccus aureus* in a rabbit subcutaneous pouch model, *Biomaterials*, 20, 229–32, 1999.
103. Aravind, S. et al., Polyethylene glycol (PEG)-modified bovine pericardium as a biomaterial: A comparative study on immunogemicity, *J. Biomater. Appl.*, 13, 158–65, 1998.
104. Witso, E. et al., Cancellous bone as an antibiotic carrier, *Acta. Orthop. Scand.*, 71, 80–4, 2000.

section three

Oral drug delivery

chapter five

Oral drug delivery*

Contents

* Adapted from Ranade, V.V., Drug delivery systems. 5A. Oral drug delivery, *J. Clin. Pharmacol.*, 31, 2, 1991 and 5B. Oral drug delivery, *J. Clin. Pharmacol.*, 31, 98, 1991. With permission of *J. Clin. Pharmacol.* and J.B. Lippincott Publishing Company, Philadelphia, PA.

I. Introduction

Historically, the most convenient and commonly employed route of drug delivery has been by oral ingestion. The original controlled release of pharmaceuticals was through coated pills, which dates back over 1000 years. Coating technology advanced in the mid- to late 1800s with the discovery of gelatin and sugar coatings. A major development in coating technology was the concept of coating drug-containing beads with combinations of fats and waxes. Since the mid-1900s, hundreds of publications and nearly 1000 patents have appeared on various oral-delivery approaches encompassing delayed, prolonged, sustained, and, most recently, controlled release of the active substance.[1]

The first truly effective oral drug delivery system, the "Spansule," was introduced in the 1950s. This prolonged-release system was marketed by Smith Kline & French Laboratories and consisted of small coated beads placed in a capsule. The 50 to 100 or more beads per capsule were designed to release at a different rate.[2]

In the mid- to late 1960s, the term "controlled drug delivery" came into being to describe new concepts of dosage-form design. These concepts usually involved controlling drug dissolution, but also had additional objectives. The primary objectives of a controlled-release system have been to enhance safety and extend duration of action. Today, we also have controlled-release systems designed to produce more reliable absorption and to improve bioavailability and efficiency of delivery.

An illustration of a controlled-release product designed to enhance solubility, absorption rate, and bioavailability is the antifungal drug griseofulvin. Dorsey has marketed a product called Gris-Peg, which is a molecular dispersion of griseofulvin in polyethylene glycol. This molecular dispersion has such enhanced-solubility properties that the dose of griseofulvin can be reduced by 50% over previously existing micronized powder forms of the drug. And, due to the higher blood levels produced, less frequent dosing of the drug is also possible.

An even newer concept of controlled release is that of site-specific release. New technology is also being developed that utilizes drug delivery systems capable of prolonged retention in the stomach or other body cavities, using bioadhesion and other factors to control not only rates of release, but also sites of release. In the 1970s, another concept of drug product design and administration has appeared: the therapeutic system. The objective of the therapeutic system is to optimize drug therapy by the design of a product that incorporates an advanced engineering systems-control approach.[3]

The modern controlled-release system is capable of producing not only sustained release, but also controlled release (i.e., a release rate that is not greatly influenced by the gastrointestinal environment). The oral controlled-release system is usually made of polymers, and the mechanisms of release are generally regulated by diffusion, bioerosion or degradation, and swelling or generation of osmotic pressure. Diffusion occurs when the drug–polymer mixture is exposed to the gastrointestinal fluid, resulting in release of the drug from the tablet or capsule. Bioerosion or degradation occurs with certain polymer–drug complexes when they pass through the gastrointestinal tract. Swelling or generation of osmotic pressure occurs with certain polymer–drug formulations when they are exposed to the gastrointestinal fluid, resulting in the release or expulsion of the drug.

The advantages of oral controlled-release products are as follows: decreased fluctuation of serum concentrations resulting in reduced toxicity and sustained efficacy; and decreased frequency of dosing resulting in improved patient compliance, reduced patient care time, and possibly reduced total amount of drug used. The disadvantages of oral controlled-release products are: longer time to achieve therapeutic blood concentrations, possible increased variation in bioavailability after oral administration, enhanced first-pass effect, dose dumping, sustained concentration in overdose cases (after oral administration), lack of dosage flexibility, and, usually, greater expense.[4]

When evaluating different proprietary controlled-release drug products, one will find that the absorption characteristics of each product are likely to be different from one another due to different mechanisms of release. Controlled-release preparations should generally not be considered bioequivalent or be substituted for one another, even though each product may contain a similar amount of an identical drug and meet the bioavailability requirements of the FDA. This consideration is especially important for drugs with narrow therapeutic ratios (e.g., antiarrhythmics, theophylline products, anti convulsants). However, if two drug products have similar bioavailability in addition to pharmacodynamics (i.e., therapeutic effect), substitution of such products should not cause any problem. Properties of drugs not suitable for controlled-release formulations are: very short or very long half-life, significant first-pass metabolism, poor absorption throughout the gastrointestinal tract, low solubility, and drug concentration not related to pharmacologic or therapeutic effect.

A controlled-release system is designed to produce a sustained concentration of a drug in the body. Many such products are now available, and following their introduction, oral drug delivery technology has enjoyed commercial success, with domestic sales approaching $1 billion. During the 1980s, more than two-thirds of the $20 billion U.S. drug market consisted of orally administered drugs, and more than 85% of that market was in the form of solid oral dosage forms. At present, a great opportunity lies in converting solid oral dosage formulations to controlled-release forms.[5]

Within the profitable and large solid oral drug market, major opportunities exist for marketing controlled-release formulations of several categories of drugs. Drugs that are taken on a chronic or extended basis — cardiovascular, arthritic, respiratory, and analgesic products — often have the most potential for controlled-release delivery improvements. The oral controlled-release drug delivery market is currently small, but growing rapidly, with total sales of more than $500 million. This market segment is fueled by an emerging trend in the drug industry favoring controlled-release products and improved drug delivery systems.

In order to gain a better understanding of the factors involved in developing controlled-release oral drugs, it is worthwhile to understand some of the basic elements of gastrointestinal (GI) physiology, particularly as they pertain to the mechanisms and factors influencing drug absorption and GI transit time.

These factors have had a profound influence on the design of oral controlled drug delivery. As our understanding of GI physiology increases, it should be possible to develop strategies for controlled drug delivery on the molecular or cellular events that are critical in overcoming the limitations of this technology.[6]

II.   Features of the GI tract

While a number of drugs are in sustained-release form and have an intended site of action in a local region of the GI tract, the overwhelming majority of oral drugs are targeted to act elsewhere in the body. Thus, the GI tract is usually a conduit to get the drug to the bloodstream. For oral dosage forms, it can, therefore, be assumed that the focus is primarily on the temporal aspects of drug release.

It is assumed that a constant level of drug in the blood for a specified period of time is a desired end point. This is most easily accomplished by direct administration of a drug by IV drip, where the rate of drug administered is adjusted, based on the pharmacokinetic properties of the drug, to achieve an invariant, steady-state level. In the simplest concept, the rate of drug administration is computed on the basis of replacement. Thus, the rate of drug elimination is the same as the rate of drug administration, which, in turn, is the product of the desired blood level of the drug. An assumption is usually made that drug levels in the bloodstream parallel the apparent volume of distribution of the drug and the first-order elimination-rate constant for the drug.[7]

For routes involving drug absorption, such as the oral route, an absorption phase is introduced prior to appearance in the blood. However, this does not change the approach used in computing the desired rate of release of drug from the dosage form to achieve a constant level in the blood. Thus, the rate constant of drug release from an oral sustained-release dosage form will be computed in exactly the same manner as previously mentioned. However, since a lag time has been introduced in getting the drug to the blood (i.e., the absorption phase) it is necessary to make some adjustments in computing the total amount of the drug that will be contained in the dosage form. It is therefore common to see a sustained-release oral system composed of two parts: an immediately available dose used to establish therapeutic levels of the drug quickly, and a reserve portion that is intended to slowly release the drug for eventual absorption and maintenance of constant blood levels. The total drug, therefore, is the sum of immediate and reserve forms. It is also clear that a zero-order rate of drug release will commonly be used to sustain levels of the drug. Thus, the total amount of reserve drug will be equal to the zero-order release-rate constant multiplied by the total number of hours of sustained effect desired.[8]

It should be pointed out that there are a number of constraints on the design of oral controlled drug delivery systems: dose size, drug molecular size, charge and pKa, aqueous solubility, partition coefficient, stability, absorption, metabolism, half-life, margin of safety, toxicity, and clinical response.[9]

III. Targeting of drugs in the GI tract

The GI tract is the preferred site of absorption for most therapeutic agents as seen from the standpoints of convenience of administration, patient compliance, and cost. The majority of oral dosage forms consist of tablets and capsules, which are often provided as instant-release systems designed to disintegrate rapidly in the stomach.[10] The dissolved drug substance is usually absorbed from the small intestine. The efficiency of these processes of release and uptake is dependent upon the physicochemical characteristics of the drug (e.g., solubility, stability in acid and alkaline environments, permeability through GI membranes) as well as physiological variables, such as GI transit time.[11]

Briefly, the approach has been to consider the distance a dispersed drug has to pass down the small intestine before the total available dose is absorbed. Mathematical analysis has shown that the more efficient the dissolution and absorption processes, the greater the reserve length. Whether the small intestine alone should be taken as the predominant absorption site is debatable. The opinions presented in the literature suggest that absorption of drugs from the large bowel is often poor and erratic. However, recent studies conducted on beta blockers indicate that the large intestine may have a more significant contribution to total absorption than hitherto realized.[12]

Controlled-release dosage forms are gaining rapid popularity in clinical medicine. The more sophisticated systems are used to alter the pharmaco-kinetic behavior of drugs in order to provide twice- or once-a-day dosage. Other applications include enteric coatings for the protection of drugs from degradation within the GI tract or the protection of the stomach from the irritating effects of the drug, and the delivery of drugs to so-called absorption windows or specific targets within the GI tract, particularly the colon.

Much about the performance of a system can be learned from *in vitro*-release studies using conventional and modified dissolution meth-ods. However, an essential stage in development must also be a subsequent evaluation *in vivo*. Davis has used the noninvasive technique of gamma-scin-tigraphy to follow the GI transit and release characteristics of a variety of pharmaceutical dosage forms in human subjects. Such studies not only pro-vide insight into the fate of a dosage form and its integrity, but also allow a correlation to be made between the position of a system in the GI tract and resultant pharmacokinetic profiles. Davis has also studied methods for the evaluation of the fate and performance of orally administered dosage forms:[10] radiology (x-ray), endoscopy, radiotelemetry, epigastric impedence, gamma-scintigraphy, and deconvolution of pharmacokinetic data.

GI motility presents a major impediment to the development of devices necessary for site-specific drug release. This is most easily overcome in the large intestine, where conditions are most predictable and quiescent. Target-ing delivery to the stomach is technically more difficult due to the power of gastric movement during both the digestive and interdigestive phases. Buoy-ancy, dimensional change, mucosal adhesives, and drugs such as propan-theline and fatty excipients have all been suggested as methods of ensuring gastric retention of small formulations. The carcinogenic nature of nitro-samines derived from the interaction of nitrates in food with secondary or tertiary amines in both food and drugs has prompted the delivery of N-nitroso-blocking agents to the stomach.[13]

The "hydrodynamically balanced system," for example, derives its effect from hydration and swelling, which entrap significant quantities of air and confer a density that is less than that of gastric fluid. This buoyancy is claimed to greatly extend residence time in the stomach, thereby allowing the N-nitroso blockers to diffuse. More specific targets for delivery within the small intestine include the duodenum, for the preferential absorption of peptides and proteins, by exploiting known facilitated transport mechanisms for dipeptides and tripeptides, as well as the delivery of antigens and aller-gens to M-cells residing in the Peyer's Patch regions.[14]

There is growing interest in the specific delivery of drugs to the colon, either for local treatment, such as that of ulcerative colitis and irritable bowel syndrome, or for the systemic delivery of compounds that are normally not well absorbed from the GI tract by exploitation of the long residence time in the colon.[15] It is possible to modify the absorption characteristics of the colon using a variety of absorption enhancers, including mixed micelles. Clearly for such applications, sophisticated delivery systems will need to be developed that will allow site-specific delivery of not only the drug, but also the absorption enhancer.

IV. Mathematical models for controlled-release kinetics

The controlled release of drugs can be achieved by incorporating solutes, either in dissolved or in dispersed form, in polymers. During the design stage of these formulations, it is desirable to develop and use simple yet sophisticated mathematical models to describe release kinetics. From a mathematical modeling point of view, controlled-release systems can be classified according to the physical mechanisms of the release of the incorporated solute. Mathematical modeling of the release kinetics of specific classes of controlled-release systems may be used to predict solute release rates from and solute diffusion behavior through polymers and to elucidate the physical mechanisms of solute transport by simply comparing the release data to mathematical models.

Peppas[16] has discussed diffusion-controlled, osmotically controlled, and chemically controlled systems. Diffusion-controlled systems contain a reservoir, matrix, and porous membrane. In chemically controlled systems, shrinking core models provide the most accurate description. Hopfenberg[17] has derived expressions for solute release from erodible slabs, cylinders, and spheres. Mathematical models exist for erodible systems in which solute release from the surface is also important. These have recently been discussed by Lee.[18]

V. Design and fabrication of oral delivery systems

The overwhelming majority of controlled-release systems rely on dissolution, diffusion, or a combination of dissolution and diffusion to generate slow release of a drug. Starting with limited data on a drug candidate for a sustained-release system, such as dose, rate constants for absorption and elimination, and some elements of metabolism, one can compute a desired release-rate for the dosage form, and the amount of drug required.[19-21]

While the desirability of having a correlation between *in vivo* bioavailability and *in vitro* release is obvious, many, if not most, sustained-release products do not show such a correlation unless one varies *in vitro* experimental conditions. Thus, when a correlation is found for a particular drug in a particular dosage form, it cannot be applied to another drug or dosage form. The correlation becomes better when the *in vitro* test is done in a pH gradient rather than distilled water. Furthermore, optimization of test conditions can also help minimize variations. A number of such systems have been described and utilized.[22-24]

Within the scope of this review, a variety of controlled-release systems are discussed. Included among these are the following:

1. Dissolution-controlled release
2. Osmotically controlled release
3. Diffusion-controlled release
4. Chemically controlled release
5. Miscellaneous controlled release

A. Dissolution-controlled release

The most important attribute of membrane-controlled drug delivery systems is their ability to maintain a constant rate of drug delivery over a reasonably long period of time. The duration of constant drug delivery must be compatible with physiologic constraints and the route of administration. For example, while a duration of several weeks may be appropriate for a membrane-controlled implant, it is much too long a time frame to consider for an oral dosage form. Clearly, the selection of a membrane system or its duration of action must be based on an appropriate set of conditions. It may well be that a constant input rate of a drug provides little real advantage over well-controlled, first-order mechanisms under certain biopharmaceutic conditions. On the other hand, there are certainly situations that call for membrane-controlled systems that provide constant rate input for time frames ranging from several hours to several months.[25]

The oral route of drug administration presents its own unique set of problems and constraints. The time frame, or "window," for absorption is limited to the total GI residence time. Even this time may be an overestimate if the drug in question is absorbed only in certain segments of the GI tract. Moreover, individual differences in residence time and motility patterns are generally quite large. Taking into account gastric emptying and small and large intestine transit time, it would seem that a reasonable duration in the GI tract is approximately 24 hours. The absorption, distribution, and elimination of drugs are normally simplified by considering them all to be simple first-order processes. Given the average 24-hour residence time and high individual variability in the GI tract, only drugs with relatively short elimination half-lives should be considered for membrane-controlled reservoir systems.

In sustained-release formulations employing dissolution as the rate-limiting step, drug release is controlled by dissolution of a polymer or by a chemical reaction with a soluble subunit. Individual particles or granules containing a drug can be uniformly dispersed in the matrix or coated with varying thicknesses of coating material resulting in dissolution and release of the drug over extended periods of time. If the dissolution process is assumed to be diffusion-layer controlled, in which the rate of diffusion from the solid surface to the bulk solution is rate-limiting, the flux is the product of the diffusion coefficient and the concentration gradient from the solid surface to the bulk solution side. Flux can also be defined as the flow rate of material through a unit area.

With encapsulated dissolution control, the drug may be coated with slowly dissolving polymeric materials. Once the polymeric membrane has dissolved, all the drug inside the membrane is immediately available for dissolution and absorption. Thus, drug release can be controlled by adjusting the thickness and the dissolution rate of the polymeric membrane. If only a few different thicknesses of the membrane are used, usually three or four, the drug will be released at different, predetermined times ("pulses"). If a spectrum of different thicknesses is employed, a more uniformed sustained release can be obtained.[26]

Membrane-coated particles can be directly compressed into tablets or placed in capsules. If the particles are compressed into a tablet, fracture of some of the surfaces generally occurs, with a resultant increase in release rate. It is a common practice to employ $1/4$ or $1/3$ of the particles in nonsustained form (i.e., particles without a barrier membrane) to provide for immediate release of the drug. Alternatively, a portion of the drug can be placed in a rapidly dissolving coating membrane to quickly establish therapeutic levels. One of the principal methods of coating a drug is microencapsulation, wherein the drug solution or crystal is encapsulated with a coating substance. The most common approach for microencapsulation is coacervation, which involves the addition of a hydrophilic substance to a solution of colloid. Whether a drug is water-sensitive or not, it can be microencapsulated if the drug is protected from the aqueous environment by coating with polymers, such as ethylcellulose, cellulose acetate phthalate, or carnauba wax prior to microencapsulation.

The thickness of the coat can be adjusted from 1 to 200 μm by changing the amount of coating material from 3 to 30%. Microencapsulation has the additional advantage that sustained drug release can be achieved with taste abatement and better GI tolerability of microencapsulations. Good examples are microencapsulated aspirin and potassium chloride. In both cases, drug effects from the microencapsulated dosage forms are more prolonged and less irritating than the same amount taken as ordinary tablets. Both formulations show the same total drug absorbed, as calculated from the area under the curve. One of the disadvantages in employing microencapsulation is that no single process can be applied to all core-material candidates. Moreover, incomplete or discontinuous coatings can cause unstable and irregular release characteristics.[27]

Sears[28] applied synthetic phospholipids as a coating material to obtain sustained release from microcapsules. The synthetic phospholipids, when the polar moiety of the phosphatidylcholine head group was altered, showed a decreased rate of hydrolysis by phosphorylase C. These compounds have been employed as surfactants and encapsulation agents for drugs such as insulin, which require protection from hydrolysis in the stomach. Microorganisms have also been used as microcapsules. Yeast, molds, or other fungi that synthesize fat within themselves can absorb fat-soluble drugs and prolong their potency.[29]

With matrix dissolution control, the two general methods of preparing drug–polymer particles are congealing and aqueous-dispersion methods. In the congealing method, the drug is mixed with polymeric substances or waxes. The wax- or polymer–drug material can be cooled and put through a sieve to obtain the correct particle size, or it can be spray-congealed. Kawashima et al.[30] used a modified spherical agglomeration technique as an alternative to the spray-congealing method. In the aqueous-dispersion method, the drug–polymer mixture is sprayed or placed in water and then collected. Usually, the aqueous-dispersion method shows a higher release rate than wax congealing or spraying, probably due to the increased area and entrapment of water.

Recently, Heller and Trescony[31] synthesized a methyl vinyl ether-maleic anhydride copolymer that has extraordinary sensitivity to the surrounding pH. These polymer systems have a characteristic pH, above which they are completely soluble and below which they are completely insoluble. The specific pH depends on the size of the alkyl group in the copolymer ester. The polymer dissolution and drug release can be strictly controlled to fit any desired pH environment. These systems have the potential, therefore, to be used in oral controlled drug delivery cases in which absorption at a specific site in the GI tract is desired.

Zero-order release at a particular site in the GI tract can be achieved by maintaining the pH of the system. Theeuwes and Higuchi[32] prepared sustained-release procainamide in matrix forms and compared the release rate to that of IV dosing. The rate of absorption *in vivo* correlated well with *in vitro* dissolution. A variety of slowly dissolving coatings, based upon various combinations of carbohydrate sugars and cellulose, polymeric materials and wax, are also available.

B.   Osmotically controlled release

In addition to the mechanism of solution diffusion, drug release from a membrane-reservoir device can also take place through a membrane via an osmotic pumping mechanism. In this case, a semipermeable membrane, such as cellulose acetate, is utilized to regulate osmotic permeation of water. With constant reservoir volume, this type of device delivers a volume of drug solution equal to the volume of osmotic water uptake within any given time interval. The rate of osmotic water influx, and therefore the rate of drug delivery by the system, will be constant as long as a constant thermodynamic activity gradient is maintained across the membrane. However, the rate declines parabolically once the reservoir concentration falls below saturation. Such an osmotic delivery system is capable of providing not only a prolonged zero-order release, but also a delivery rate much higher than that achievable by the solution-diffusion mechanism. Osmotically controlled release is also applicable to drugs with a wide range of molecular weight and chemical composition, which are normally difficult to deliver by the solution-diffusion mechanism.

There are basically two types of osmotic delivery devices, namely, the miniosmotic pump and the elementary osmotic pump. In the miniosmotic pump delivery system, the drug reservoir is separated from the osmotic agent compartment by a movable partition. At the other end of the osmotic compartment is a semipermeable membrane, and a rigid impermeable material forms the remaining three sides of the pump, with a delivery orifice at the front. In contrast, the elementary osmotic pump consists of an osmotic core containing the drug, surrounded by a semipermeable membrane with a delivery orifice. The delivery rate from these devices is regulated by the osmotic pressure of both the osmotic agent of the core formulation and by the water permeability of the semipermeable membrane.[33]

Unlike the solution-diffusion mechanism, the osmotic delivery system involves a volume flux of water across a semipermeable membrane. In the miniosmotic pump system, as long as a large enough reservoir is present, the delivery of dissolved drug at any concentration can be zero-order because of the separate compartmental design. In the elementary osmotic pump, since the core formulation is also the osmotic driving agent, the delivery rate is constant as long as excess solid is present within the drug reservoir.

Osmotically controlled drug release requires only osmotic pressure to be effective, and is essentially independent of the environment. As a consequence, this should be an excellent sustained-release system for oral dosage forms. Thus, the drug delivery rate for an oral osmotic therapeutic system can be precisely predetermined regardless of pH change. In fact, the delivery rate of sodium phenobarbital from this system into artificial gastric juice at pH 2 and intestinal fluid at pH 7.5 (containing no enzymes) was shown to be pH-independent.[34]

The development of an OROS system refers to the quality of a therapeutic system designed to control pharmacologic effects through control of plasma concentrations. This can be judged through the constancy of drug concentrations during its use. The flatness of plasma-concentration curves can be expressed by the ratio of maximum to minimum concentration within one dosing interval at a steady state for repetitive injections. For plasma concentrations obtained following the administration of a therapeutic system, this ratio is, in addition to pharmacokinetic constants and dosing interval, a function of the system's design parameters and is called the dosage form index, or DI.[35]

During selection of a drug substance for delivery via the OROS system (developed by Alza Corporation), one also needs to consider the site of entry and factors that can modify the rate and extent of drug absorption en route from that site to the target tissue. Considering that the OROS system is a solid, tablet-sized object, it will pass through the GI tract within the transit time of foodstuff. To reduce drug plasma-concentration fluctuations on repetitive administration of an OROS system, it is also necessary to consider the half-life associated with the distribution phase. Some drugs, such as lithium, are rapidly absorbed but are distributed slowly in the tissues, giving rise to sharp absorption peaks following administration. For lithium and many other drugs, such peaks are associated with side effects that can be prevented by administration in a controlled-delivery dosage form (see Figure 5.1).

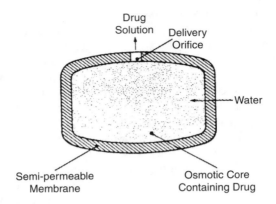

Figure 5.1 Cross-sectional diagram of an OROS system. (Reprinted with permission from *Annual Reports in Medicinal Chemistry,* Vol. 15, Academic Press, New York, 1980, 308 and Alza Corporation, Palo Alto, CA.)

Theophylline is a drug that has the desired attributes for delivery via the OROS system. It is used primarily for the treatment of obstructive airway disease (e.g., asthma). Its pharmacokinetics and pharmacodynamics in man have been well documented. In particular, its pharmacology has been studied over a wide range of plasma concentrations during intravenous administration of aminophylline (a form of theophylline).[36] These and other studies have shown that the OROS system allows safe and effective delivery of theophylline and creates less need for individual dose adjustment than a system with a higher DI.

A currently marketed over-the-counter (OTC) appetite suppressant, Acutrim®, incorporates Alza's OROS system. In Acutrim, the active ingredient (phenylpropanolamine) is released at a controlled rate. Another benefit of controlled rate delivery of Acutrim is that, in this form, phenylpropanolamine does not produce the adrenergic-like side effects that are normally seen in other conventional formulations.

For insoluble or extremely soluble drugs, Alza Corporation has designed another system, the "push-pull" OROS. This system has two compartments, one containing an osmotic agent and the other containing the drug. A semipermeable membrane surrounds both. In the GI tract, water enters each compartment through the membrane at a different rate. In the drug compartment, soluble drugs are formulated into solutions and insoluble ones into suspensions. As water enters the other compartment, it expands and pushes against the drug compartment. This causes the drug solution or suspension to be released at a controlled rate through the orifice in the membrane surrounding the drug compartment.

Elan Corporation of Ireland has developed its own osmotic pressure system called MODAS. MODAS stands for Multi-Directional Oral Absorption System. MODAS is similar to OROS in some respects, yet quite different from it in others. Like OROS, this system consists of a tablet core surrounded by a semipermeable membrane. However, unlike OROS, MODAS has a multitude of small pores through which the drug solution can exit. The rate of drug-solution release can be controlled by the composition of the membrane. Since the drug release is multidirectional, concentration of the drug in any one area of the GI tract is avoided. Elan has identified a number of drugs that are suitable for MODAS, including alphamethyldopa, ibuprofen, theophylline, quinidine, indomethacin, potassium chloride, and naproxen.

C.   Diffusion-controlled release

The most commonly used type of membrane material in drug delivery systems is homogeneous films of amorphous and semicrystalline polymers above their glass transition temperatures. Drug transport occurs by dissolution in the membrane at one interface, followed by diffusion down a concentration gradient across the membrane and, finally, release from the second interface into the external medium. Such a solution-diffusion membrane is typically observed in hydrophobic membrane materials, such as silicone rubber and ethylene vinyl acetate copolymer. A similar mechanism is also responsible for drug permeation through most swollen hydrogel membranes.[16]

The rate of drug permeation through solution-diffusion membranes is directly proportional to the product of the drug-diffusion coefficient in the polymer and the polymer/solution partition coefficient. The former is a kinetic or nonequilibrium transport parameter, while the latter is an equilibrium thermodynamic property. Despite progress in estimating diffusion and partition coefficients of simple gases in polymers, no reliable method is presently available for the quantitative prediction of both the diffusion and partition coefficients of more complicated organic molecules in polymers. Nevertheless, various trends can be identified based on accumulated experimental evidence in the literature.

Above the polymer glass transition temperature, drug diffusion coefficients in a polymeric medium generally decrease with increasing drug molecular weight, molecular size, crystallinity of the polymer, and the amount of filler in the polymer. On the other hand, the drug-diffusion coefficient will increase with more plasticizer content and solvent swelling in the polymer. Other parameters, such as copolymerization, cross-linking, and grafting, as well as the distribution and orientation of crystallites, may either increase or decrease the observed drug-diffusion coefficient. In some instances, the concentration dependence of the diffusion coefficient may further complicate the situation.[37]

With regard to solubility and partitioning effects, one generally observes that a drug will be more soluble in the polymer phase as the difference in the solubility parameters of the drug polymer becomes smaller. Michaels et al.[38] have demonstrated that steroid permeability in polymers can be correlated with thermodynamic parameters, such as the melting temperature of the steroid and the solubility parameters of the steroid and polymer. The

Table 5.1 Different types of commercially available osmotic systems

(I) Osmotic pumps for experimental research	
ALZET (Durect Corp., USA)	Miniature, implantable osmotic pumps for laboratory animals. Commonly implanted subcutaneously or intraperitoneally, but, with the help of a catheter, can be used for intracerebral, intraveneous, and intraarterial infusion. Different models having delivery rates from 0.25 to 10 µl/h and durations from 1 day to 4 weeks available. Delivery profile independent of drug formulation.
OSMET (Durect Corp.)	Used as experimental tools for human pharmacological studies and can be used for oral, rectal, or vaginal administration. Delivery profile independent of drug formulation, and it is available with release rates ranging from 8 to 20 µl/h.
(II) Osmotic pumps for humans	
Oral	
Elementary osmotic pump (Alza Corp., USA)	Single-layer tablet for delivery of drugs having moderate water solubility. Can be utilized for zero-order delivery as well as pulsed release.
Push–pull osmotic pump (Alza Corp.)	Bilayer tablet used to deliver drugs having low to high water solubility. Products such as Ditropan XL (oxybutynin chloride), Procardia XL (nifedipine), and Glucotrol XL (glipizide) are based on this technology. Number of modifications available, such as delayed push–pull system, multilayer push–pull system, and push–stick system.
L-OROS (Alza Corp.)	Designed to deliver lipophilic liquid formulations and is suitable for delivery of insoluble drugs.
OROS-CT (Alza Corp.)	For targeted delivery to colon; can be used for local or systemic therapy.
Portab System (Andrx Pharmaceuticals, USA)	Tablet core consists of soluble agent, which expands and creates microporous channels for drug release.
SCOT (single composition osmotic tablet, Andrx Pharmaceuticals)	Utilized various osmotic modulating agents and polymer coatings to provide zero-order release.
ENSOTROL drug delivery system (Shire Labs, Inc., USA)	Utilized various solubilizing and wicking agents for delivery of poorly water-soluble drugs.
Zero-Os tablet technology (ADD Drug Delivery Technologies AG, Switzerland)	Specifically for delivery of lipophilic compounds. Consists of gel-forming agents in the core that forms gel after coming in contact with water, and drug is released as a fine dispersion.

Table 5.1 Different types of commercially available osmotic systems (Continued)

Implantable	
DUROS (Durect Corp.)	Miniature (4×45 mm), implantable osmotic pumps for long-term, parenteral, zero-order delivery of potent therapeutic agents. Delivers drugs at a precisely controlled and constant rate within therapeutic range for long periods. Viadur (leuprolide acetate), a successful product in the market, delivers leuprolide continuously at a nominal rate of 125 µg/day over 1 year for palliative treatment of prostate cancer. DUROS sufentanil (3 months continuous delivery for treatment of chronic pain) and DUROS hydromorphone (for continuous delivery to the spine) are in various developmental phases.
(III) Osmotic pumps for veterinary use	
VITS (veterinary implantable therapeutic system, Alza Corp.)	Designed to deliver drugs at a controlled rate in animals for a period of 1 day to 1 year, and can be implanted subcutaneously or intraperitoneally in any ruminant, nonruminant, companion, or production animals. Available in various sizes (2–10 mm in diameter) and can be designed to give delivery rates from µg/day to mg/day. Drug is kept isolated from body fluids and thus can be used to deliver water-labile compounds (e.g., proteins and peptides).
RUTS (ruminal therapeutic system, Alza Corp.)	For controlled delivery of drugs up to one year in the rumen of cattle and sheep. Up to 10 g of drug can be administered. Generally, 2–3 cm in diameter and up to 10 cm in length, but larger dimensions are possible, depending upon application. Can be designed for zero-order delivery of up to g/day. Ivomec SR (ivermectin) and Dura SE (sodium selenite) available commercially.

Source: With permission, Elsevier, *J. Control Rel.*, 79, 7–27, 2002.

partition coefficient, defined as the ratio of the drug concentration in the external solvent medium, may also be concentration-dependent.

Many of the partition coefficients reported in the literature have been measured in saturated drug solutions and subsequently used in situations where the drug concentration may deviate from saturation considerably. Depending on the nonlinearity involved in the absorption isotherm, such practice can lead to appreciable error in the determination of permeation parameters. Therefore, for the design of a specific membrane-reservoir drug delivery system, it is necessary to determine both the drug diffusion and partition coefficients experimentally. Preferably, one should also carry out selected experiments over the entire concentration range of interest so that any concentration dependence can also be established.

Being cross-linked and hydrophilic, hydrogel polymers are unique in that they are quite glassy in the dry state, whereas in the presence of water they can swell significantly to form an elastic gel. In addition to having good biocompatibility, their ability to release drug in aqueous media and the ease of regulating such drug release by controlling the water swelling and cross-link density make hydrogels particularly suitable as carrier matrices or rate-controlling membranes in the controlled release of pharmaceuticals.

A typical hydrogel membrane device usually consists of either a solid core of drug or a slightly cross-linked hydrogel matrix containing dissolved or dispersed drug, and a surrounding rate-controlling hydrogel membrane. In both cases, the membrane can be either prefabricated or coated and subsequently polymerized. When a hydrogel matrix is used as a drug reservoir, a rate-controlling membrane can also be formed by a newly developed interpenetrating network (IPN) technique. In this case, the surface layer of the matrix is first treated with heat or UV irradiation or via *in situ* olycondensation generated by immersion in a second reactant solution producing a less permeable, rate-controlling membrane layer.[39–41]

For other, specific purposes, hydrogel-membrane devices may be stored in either dry or hydrated states. The release of water-soluble drugs from initially dry hydrogel membrane devices generally involves the swelling of the membrane and subsequent dissolution or swelling of the core. In the case of a membrane originally saturated with a drug, a simultaneous absorption of water and release of a drug via a swelling-controlled diffusion mechanism is also observed. Thus, as water penetrates a glassy hydrogel membrane device, the polymer swells and its glass transition temperature is lowered. At the same time, the dissolved drug diffuses through this swollen flexible region into the external releasing medium.[42,43]

Yasuda et al.[44] have derived a theoretical expression relating the solute diffusion coefficient in a water-soluble polymeric membrane to the free volume and degree of hydration in the membrane. Conformity of experimental results to the theory suggests that the permeation of solute occurs predominately through the porous regions of the network. As pointed out by Yasuda et al., these porous, water-filled regions through which the transport of permeant can occur may only be conceived as fluctuating pores or channels of the polymer matrix, which are not fixed either in size or location.

Zentner et al.[45] have studied the effect of a cross-linking agent on progesterone permeation through swollen hydrogel membranes. In addition to the decrease in progesterone-diffusion coefficient with increasing cross-linker, they found that at low concentrations of the cross-linker, the chain length of the cross-linker did not affect the "fluctuating-pore" permeation mechanism. However, at high concentrations of cross-linker, the diffusion coefficient of progesterone in the system with a shorter cross-linker, ethylene glycol dimethacrylate, was relatively independent of the cross-linker concentration. This was rationalized as a change in permeation mechanism to that of a solution-diffusion-controlled process. A transition from porous to solution-diffusion transport is consistent with the water permeation results previously reported by Chen[46] and Wisniewski et al.[47]

The resistance to mass transfer in the stagnant fluid layer adjacent to a membrane surface is an inescapable consequence of the membrane-permeation process. Thus, during drug release from a membrane-reservoir device, drug concentration in the upstream diffusion boundary layer can be much lower than that in the adjacent drug reservoir due to the fast transport of drug across the membrane. Similarly, drug concentration in the downstream diffusion boundary layer can become much higher than the concentration in the releasing medium due to an insufficient drug removal rate. Boundary-layer effects can alter the rate, or even the kinetics, of drug release from drug delivery devices, depending on the type of device and the environment of use. The frequently observed discrepancy between *in vitro* and *in vivo* release rates can generally be attributed to this type of phenomenon. The influence of the boundary layer on the release kinetics of monolithic devices has been analyzed by Higuchi,[48,49] who used a pseudo-steady-state approach.

In the case of membrane-reservoir systems, the boundary layers offer additional resistance to mass transfer across the membrane, as if the effective membrane thickness has been increased. The steady-state release rate from such a membrane device with a saturated reservoir would therefore be reduced. Similar reduction in release rates are also expected in membrane devices with nonconstant reservoir concentration. Several approaches have been proposed in the literature, mostly in the area of membrane dialysis, to elucidate the mechanism of this boundary-layer effect and to make quantitative calculations of the true intrinsic membrane transport parameters. These proposals suggest a reduction or elimination of the boundary layer by increasing fluid turbulence (e.g., by stirring) or an estimation of the boundary-layer resistance by performing transport experiments at different membrane thicknesses or stirring speeds.

The less permeable polymer or drug selected should still provide sufficient drug-release rate to meet the therapeutic requirement. In practice, sometimes this can be difficult to achieve due to a large release-rate requirement. In this situation, compromises in membrane permeability, thickness, and area would have to be made in order to minimize the contribution of a boundary-layer effect and still maintain the desired rate of release. Aside from the material and system parameters discussed previously, other factors, such as temperature and membrane porosity, may also affect the rate of drug release.

In diffusion-controlled release systems, the transport of solute through the polymer is achieved by molecular diffusion due to concentration gradients. Depending on the molecular structure of the polymer, these systems may be classified as porous or nonporous. Porous controlled-release systems contain pores of large enough size so that diffusion of the solute is accomplished through water, which has filled the pores of the polymer. These pores are usually in the range of 200 to 500 Å. At the lower limit of this range, hindered diffusion may occur. Therefore, correction of the solute-diffusion coefficient may have to be made to account for pore wall effects.[50,51]

Molecular diffusion occurs effectively through the whole polymer, and the solute-diffusion coefficient refers to the polymer phase. The macromolecular structure of the polymer affects solute diffusion according to theoretical analyses. Some of the polymer parameters controlling the solute-diffusion coefficient are degree of crystallinity and size of crystallites, degree of cross-linking and swelling, and the molecular weight of the polymer. Many swollen, porous polymer systems retain the main characteristics of the porous structure, so that solute diffusion occurs simultaneously through water-filled pores and through the swollen polymer per se.

In reservoir (membrane) systems, the bioactive agent is usually enclosed at relatively high concentrations between two semipermeable membranes and placed in contact with a dissolution medium (water or other biological fluid). The bioactive agent may be solvent-free or in the form of a concentrated solution. The partition coefficient describes thermodynamic rather than structural characteristics of the solute/polymer/solvent system. It is rather easy to determine experimentally, and it is a measure of solute solubility in a swollen polymer. A rigorous derivation of the partition (distribution) coefficient is presented by Lightfoot.[52]

In matrix (monolithic) systems, the bioactive agent is incorporated in the polymer phase either in dissolved or in dispersed form. Therefore, the solubility of the solute in the polymer becomes a controlling factor in the mathematical modeling of these systems. When the initial solute loading is below the solubility limit, release is achieved by simple molecular diffusion through the polymer. However, when solute loading is above the solubility limit, dissolution of the solute in the polymer becomes the limiting factor in the release process. Park et al.[37] have listed examples of diffusion-controlled reservoir and matrix devices.

D.   *Chemically controlled release*

Chemically controlled systems include all polymeric formulations in which solute diffusion is controlled by a chemical reaction, such as the dissolution of the polymer matrix or cleavage of the drug from a polymer backbone. In most chemically controlled systems, solute release is controlled by the geometric shape of the device. Depending on the type of degradation reaction, these systems may be classified as chemically degradable (e.g., by hydrolysis) or biodegradable (e.g., by enzymatic reaction) controlled-release systems.

In chemically controlled drug delivery systems, the release of a pharmacologically active agent usually takes place in the aqueous environment by one or more of the following types of mechanisms: gradual biodegradation of a drug-containing polymer matrix, biodegradation of unstable bonds by which the drug is coupled to the polymer matrix, and diffusion of a drug from injectable and biodegradable microbeads. In contrast to mechanical and osmotic devices, the main advantages of such biodegradable systems are the elimination of the need for their surgical removal, their small size, and potential low cost. On the other hand, all biodegradable products, as well as their metabolites, must be nontoxic, noncarcinogenic, and nonteratogenic. These requirements are not easily met and must be subject to careful scrutiny.[53]

In a system of the first type, the drug is either dispersed in the biodegradable polymer matrix or encapsulated in it, from which it is released into the surrounding biological environment by controlled rates. The particular kinetic behavior depends on the chemical composition of the polymer, the solubility of the drug in the polymer, and preparative aspects of the polymer matrix. Gradual degradation of the polymer can be facilitated by either converting an otherwise water-soluble polymer into a water-insoluble one by cross-links that are nevertheless hydrolytically or enzymatically unstable, or by using polymers that can undergo main-chain cleavage by hydrolytic or enzymatic actions. As noted previously, it is essential that none of the biodegradation products be toxic. Furthermore, all degradation products must be fully metabolized and excreted without excessive or permanent accumulation in the body. These requirements pose formidable challenges, especially when they must be combined with drug-release parameters.

E. Miscellaneous forms of controlled release

1. Ion-exchange resins

Resins are water-insoluble materials containing salt-forming groups in repeating positions on the resin chain. Ion-exchange resins have been used as drug carriers for preparing prolonged and sustained delivery by releasing the drug from the complex over approximately 8 to 12 h into the GI tract. Drug release from the complex depends on the ionic environment, such as pH or electrolyte concentration, within the GI tract as well as properties of the resin. Resin-drug complex can also increase stability of the drug by protecting the drug from hydrolysis or degradative enzymes. It also improves palatability of the formulation.

A drug-resin complex is prepared by mixing the resin with a drug solution, either by repeated exposure of the resin to the drug in a chromatographic column or by prolonged contact of the resin with the drug in a container. The drug-resin complex is then washed and dried. Drug molecules attached to the resin are exchanged by appropriately charged ions in contact with the ion-exchange groups, and the released drug molecule diffuses out of the resin. The rate of diffusion is controlled by the area of diffusion, diffusional path length, and the amount of cross-linking agent (i.e., the rigidity of the resin). Thus, the rate of drug release can be controlled during formulation.

The release rate can be further modified by coating the drug-resin complex. Coating on the resin-drug complex can be achieved by a microencapsulation process. Different coating materials alter the release of the organic anion from the anion-resin complex, and a dramatic difference in release rate is observed with different waxes. The amount of wax covering the surface of the drug–resin complex appears to depend on the polar character of the wax. Coated and uncoated drug-resin complexes can be mixed and filled into capsules with excipients or suspended in a palatable, flavored vehicle containing suitable suspending agents. The release of drug from uncoated resin beads is expected to begin immediately, while release from the coated form begins slowly, depending on the type and thickness of coat. Mixing the coated and uncoated drug-resin complexes in suitable ratios is a reliable technique for obtaining desired release profiles.

Based on the observation that amines are released slowly from ion-exchange resins, polystyrol resins have been tried for oral depot preparations of alkaloids, such as ephedrine and amphetamine. The release rate is best prolonged if only partly alkaline exchange resins are used and if a mixture of alkaloid base and an alkaloid salt is employed. Thus, the initial phase is reduced and the continuing release of the drug is prolonged. However, the release rate depends upon pH and electrolyte concentration in the GI tract, which is higher in the stomach and declines during transit through the small intestine. Both cationic exchangers, as well as anionic exchangers for alkaline and acidic compounds, respectively, are used. Resinates and resin salts are soluble in water or in intestinal fluids and are not degraded by intestinal enzymes. Although the drug is released according to the ionic environment, it is difficult to regulate the rate of release. Disadvantages of ion-exchange resins for depot preparations are that only ionized drugs can be used and binding capacity is limited. Thus, only relatively small amounts of drugs can be bound per tablet.

2.   Altered density: Drug-coated micropellets

Empty globular shells, which have an apparent density lower than that of gastric juice, can be used as carriers of drugs for sustained-release purposes. Conventional gelatin capsules, polystyrol, and poprice are all candidates as carriers. The surface of one of the empty shells is undercoated with a polymeric material, such as cellulose acetate phthalate, acrylic and methacrylic copolymer, or sugar. This undercoated shell is further coated with a drug–polymer mixture and any polymeric material that shows dissolution-controlled drug release (e.g., ethylcellulose, hydroxypropylcellulose, or cornstarch).[54]

This type of carrier floats on the gastric juice for an extended period while slowly releasing the drug. This same principle can be applied to formulate buoyant capsules. The particles of a drug–hydrocolloid mixture will swell to form a soft gelatinous mass on the surface when in contact with gastric juice. This somewhat enlarged particle has a density less than one and floats on stomach chyme, where it releases the drug. *In vitro* dissolution studies with this formulation show a good correlation with plasma concentration levels for chlordiazepoxide. Hydrocolloids that are suitable for this purpose are alginate, hydroxyalkylcellulose, carboxymethylcellulose, carrageenan, guar gum, agar, gum arabic, gum karaya, gum tragacanth, locust bean gum, pectin, and the like.

It has been reported that multiple-unit formulations have an advantage over single-unit preparations in that subunits of the multiple-unit formulation are distributed throughout the GI tract, and their transport is less affected by transit time of food. Specific density of the subunits of the multiple-unit dose is reported to significantly influence the average transit time of the subunits through the GI tract. An increase in density from 1.0 to 1.6 extended the average transit time from 7 to 25 h. The pellets are dispersed throughout the small intestine at a rate that depends predominantly on their density. Barium sulfate, zinc oxide, titanium dioxide, and iron powder are the substances used to increase pellet density. Density of the pellets must exceed that of the normal stomach contents and should therefore be at least 1.4. Moreover, a diameter of 1.5 mm is considered maximal for a true multiple-unit formulation. The drug can be coated on a heavy core or mixed with heavy inert materials, and the weighted pellet can be covered with a diffusion-controlling membrane.[55]

3. pH-independent formulations

When a drug formulation is administered orally, it encounters several pH environments until absorbed or excreted. If the formulation is chewed, the first environment will be pH 7. The drug will then be exposed to a pH of 1 to 4 in the stomach, depending on the amount and type of food, followed by a pH of 5 to 7 in the intestine. Many reports show a pH dependency of drug release from a sustained-release formulation. For example, the release of papaverine[56] from a commercial sustained-release preparation is significantly affected by pH of the dissolution media. Most of the drug is released in the stomach from this preparation and little is released in the intestine due to low solubility in the small bowel. Release of the drug from polymeric films has also been shown to depend on external fluid pH and not film thickness.

To achieve pH-independent drug release, buffers can be added to the drug to help maintain a constant pH. Salts of phosphoric acid, phthalic acid, citric acid, tartaric acid, or amino acids are preferred because of physiological acceptability. The rate of availability of propoxyphene after administration of a buffered controlled-release formulation showed significantly increased reproducibility, probably due to lower sensitivity of its release rate to the surrounding pH.[57]

4. Pro-drugs

A pro-drug is a compound resulting from chemical modification of a pharmacologically active compound, which will liberate the active compound *in vivo* due to enzymatic or hydrolytic cleavage. The primary purpose of employing a pro-drug is to increase intestinal absorption or to reduce local side effects (e.g., aspirin irritation). On this basis, one does not generally classify a pro-drug as a sustained-release mechanism. However, the ability to reversibly modify the physicochemical properties of a drug allows better intestinal transport properties and, hence, influences the blood–drug concentration-time profile. Thus, pro-drugs can be used to improve strategies for controlled release and, in a limited sense, can be sustaining in their own right.

A water-soluble derivative of a water-insoluble drug can be developed to be a substrate for enzymes in the surface coat of the brush border region of the microvillus membrane. The water-soluble derivative becomes insoluble with a high membrane-water partition coefficient just prior to reaching the membrane. Improved blood levels by orders of magnitude for water-insoluble drugs have been reported.[57,58]

If a pro-drug has less water solubility, and hence a slower dissolution rate in aqueous fluid than the parent drug, appearance of the parent drug in the body is slowed because the dissolution process would be rate-limiting. In fact, the dissolution rate of 7,7'-succinylditheophylline is 35 times slower than that of theophylline under the same conditions, and its dissolution rate is independent of pH within the physiological pH range. Many derivatives of aspirin have been made to reduce gastric irritation, rather than to increase its absorption.

5.   Barrier coating

The barrier-coating principle can be applied to beads, granules, or a whole tablet. If barrier-coated beads or granules are used, one portion is usually left uncoated for the immediate dosage form, while others are coated differentially in order to acquire different release patterns. Release of drug depends upon degradation or moisture-induced permeability of the coat, which is dependent on its composition and thickness. If coated granules are used for compression, care must be taken that the coating does not fracture during compression. The release mechanism is generally by dialysis, since water-insoluble but permeable plastics are used for coatings. Only in rare cases does release follow degradation. This occurs where waxes, such as beeswax, or fats and fatty acid esters, such as glycerine monostearate, are used. Within this group, the technique of microencapsulation also belongs.

Previously used film-forming or coating materials often lacked programmable release characteristics since they frequently disintegrated or dissolved upon exposure to GI fluids. The development of lacquer materials of well-defined permeability, based on methacrylate, has led to the development of suitable barrier-coating dosage forms. The barrier-coating principle can only be employed for water-soluble drugs.[59]

When plastic material, which is insoluble and undigestible in GI fluids, is used, release of drug depends on the solubility of the drug, the size and number of pores in the membrane, and the thickness of the membrane. A constant release of drug can be expected when water forms a saturated solution within the tablet, leading to drug dissolution. The tablet case, filled with water, will pass through the intestinal tract unchanged and will finally be eliminated in the feces.

By varying the functional groups of acrylic resins (Eudragit L, Eudragit S), coatings are obtained with solubility and permeability characteristics independent of pH (2 to 8). These resins possess identical properties for the pH range found in the GI tract. Thus, drug release of the active ingredient is independent of the position of the drug in the tract. Following a short period of swelling, drug liberation follows zero-order kinetics until 80–90% of the drug is released.[60]

Prolonged action of oral dosage forms based on the barrier-coating principle can be prepared by the following methods: simple film-coating of the tablet, simple film-coating of pellets or granules and filling into gelatin capsules, and compression to tablets of approximately 80% of total volume of the tablet or barrier-coated particles with approximately 20% of a filler. Even if the coatings are opened by cracks during compression, new diffusing cells are formed by fusion of the remaining film-coated particles.[61]

6.   Embedment in slowly eroding matrix

In embedding, the active ingredients are dissolved or suspended in a mixture of fats and waxes, such as beeswax, carnauba wax, hydrated fats, synthetic waxes, butyl stearate, stearic acid, saccharose monostearate, saccharose distearate, or in mixtures of glycerine monostearate, castor oil, etc. The melt is either dispersed by spray congealing, or the solidified drug-vehicle mass is ground or milled to a proper particle size. The granules obtained are either filled into hard gelatin capsules or compressed to tablets. For retard preparations, one part of the active ingredient is formed in a normal granulate with a vehicle that disintegrates rapidly, and the rest of the active ingredient is embedded into the fat vehicle. The two different types of granules are then mixed and filled into capsules or compressed. It is also possible to form a sandwich-like tablet by compressing the embedment granules into one layer and the rapid-disintegrating granulate into a second layer on the top of the first.

Liberation of the drug from its embedment depot is by gradual erosion of the fat granules. Enzymes and pH can be of great influence by hydrolyzing the fatty acid esters, depending on the type of vehicle substance. If the esters are hydrolyzable, drug release from fat-embedded dosage forms runs parallel to the hydrolysis of the glycerides. If digestible or partly digestible fats and waxes are used, individual variations in drug release from fat-embedment dosage forms can be assumed to be high due to individual differences in pH and enzyme patterns.[62,63]

7.   Embedment in plastic matrix

Skeleton-type preparations are made by granulating the active ingredients with inert plastic material. Several possibilities exist, including: the drug powder can be mixed and kneaded with a solution of the same plastic material in an organic solvent and then granulated or a solid–solid solution of the drug in plastic particles may be produced by dissolving the drug in the plastic-containing organic solvent and granulating it. After the solvent evaporates, a solid–solid solution of the drug in plastic particles is produced. The granules are then compressed into tablets.

Liberation of the active ingredient from this dosage form is by leaching from the inert plastic skeleton or matrix. Only water-soluble or fairly soluble drugs can therefore be used for this procedure. The plastic skeleton retains its shape throughout transit through the GI tract and is excreted in its original shape in the feces. Drug liberation depends solely on its solubility in GI fluids and is completely independent of pH, enzyme activity, concentration, or GI motility.

A certain amount of drug is released immediately upon administration. This is the drug that is on the surface of the dosage form and can therefore be dissolved immediately. Further release depends on the penetration of GI fluid into the pores of the skeleton. If an increased amount of the active ingredient is required for the initial phase, then the manufacture of double-layer, or sandwich, tablets is indicated. Here, one layer contains the rapidly disintegrating initial phase only, while the second layer contains the skeleton of the depot phase. Skeleton tablets can also be used as cores for compressed-coated or sugar-coated tablets, for which they contain the initial phase in the coat. Disadvantages of plastic matrix tablets are that slightly soluble or insoluble drugs cannot be released from this type of dosage form.[64,65]

8.   Repeat action

Repeat-action preparations contain two doses, one of which is released immediately upon administration, followed by a second dose, which is not a depot phase as discussed previously, but is a dose that is released after a certain time interval or in a certain environment. This is achieved by using enteric coating for the second dose. The second dose, which is a repeat dose, is a normal tablet coated by an enteric film. The initial phase is administered around the core in the form of a sugar coat or by compression coating.

9.   Hydrophilic matrix

Oral retard preparations based on the hydrophilic-matrix principle are prepared by mixing the active ingredients with nondigestible hydrophilic gums and compressing the mixture into tablets. Upon administration, a rapid dissolution of the drug from the surface of the tablet is usually observed. When hydration and gelation of the gum at the tablet/liquid interface progresses, a viscous gel barrier is formed. The drug in this gelated form is then released at a much slower rate. The release rate of the drug is markedly influenced by the percentage and type of gum used. Liberation rate also depends on the physical and chemical properties of the active ingredient. A prerequisite for this type of dosage form is high solubility of the active ingredient. The gums used are sodium carboxymethylcellulose and hydroxypropylmethylcellulose.

Drug release *in vitro* follows a constant or zero-order release. Both inter- and intrasubject variations in *in vivo*-absorption kinetics have been found in studies with prolonged-release dosage forms containing aspirin in a hydrophilic gelating agent. Following a lag time, individual absorption data were found to follow first-order kinetics in most instances. Using averaged data, a zero-order plot for absorption was obtained. Levy and Hollister[66] have warned of erroneous conclusions from average data if all or the majority of individual data can not be fitted satisfactorily to the model. Investigating the factors controlling the rate of drug release from hydrophilic matrices indicates that release is controlled more by drug diffusibility than by dissolution of polymer and water penetrability. As long as the integrity of the hydrated polymer is maintained, the release of drug is diffusion-controlled.

10.   Polymer resin beads

Using epoxy resins, drugs can be incorporated into the plastic material, either by dissolving or suspending the active ingredient in the liquid plastic monomer. The solution or suspension is then dispersed in a hydrophilic or lipophilic medium, producing an emulsion. The bead size of the plastic monomer depends on the agitation intensity, surface tension, and degree of incorporation of protective colloids. Polymerization occurs upon heating the mixture to 50 to 60°C, and the liquid plastic droplets solidify within 2 to 4 hours to form beads.

Epoxy compounds cured with primary amines dissolve in strong acidic buffers and may, therefore, liberate the drug in the stomach. Epoxy compounds cured with acids dissolve in weakly acidic or neutral mediums and therefore release the drug in the intestine only. Resins containing the active ingredients can be obtained in bulk as well as in bead form. Dissolution rate is enhanced with an increased concentration of 2-amino-2-ethyl-1,3-propandiol in the epoxy resin. Low concentrations of chloramphenicol in such polymerization resins have no effect on dissolution rate. However, dissolution rate decreases with increasing concentration of chloramphenicol core in the form of a sugar coat or by compression coating.

The *in vitro* release of chloramphenicol from different bead polymers containing methyl methacrylate and α-methacrylic acid in various buffer solutions was found to depend on the amount of α-methacrylic acid content in the polymer and the bead particle size. Plastic polymer beads may also be formed by extrusion molding. Polymers, being solid and brittle at room temperature but liquefying at higher temperatures, are suitable for extrusion molding. For preparation, a free-flowing solid mixture of drug and thermoplastic material is melted at 100 to 110°C and injected into cooled metal molds. Polymers between drug and epoxy-amine resins are soluble in an acidic environment (initial phase), whereas polymers between drug and vinyl acetate and crotonic acid are soluble in a slightly acidic and neutral environment (depot phase).[67]

11.   Passage-sponge formation

A new method to obtain depot preparations has been described. Soft gelatin capsules can be prepared by dissolving or suspending the active ingredients in a polyethylene glycol solution of shellac or polyvinyl acetate. Additional vehicle substances, such as stearates, acids, bases, or phosphates, may be added. The filling material is then incorporated into a gelatin solution for the manufacture of soft gelatin capsules by the usual method. The gelatin goes into solution in the aqueous gastrointestinal fluids. The interior of the capsule becomes spongelike due to the penetration of the aqueous media into the capsule from the surface. Finally, the whole interior is converted into a spongelike skeleton as the aqueous medium penetrates deeper into the capsule. The active ingredient is released from this microporous sponge by diffusion. Since the sponge-like wall is quite thin at the beginning, a large amount of drug is liberated during the initial phase. Usually, about 30 to 40% of the drug content is released within the first hour. Further drug release follows continuously and is complete after approximately six hours.

Another new method of preparing depot dosage forms based on the passage-sponge formation uses a soluble alginate (sodium alginate) and a calcium ion donator ($CaHPO_3$) with other vehicles. The dry mixture of these substances and a solid drug are compressed into tablets. Upon administration, a spongelike matrix is formed under the influence of the GI fluids, from which the drug is released by dissolution and diffusion. The sponge is formed progressively from the outside to the inside of the tablet. The GI fluid dissolves the alginate and the calcium compound. The alginate and calcium ions react immediately with each other, forming a spongelike layer of calcium alginate.[68]

12.   Drug complex formation

Depot preparations can be made with drugs having an amine group in the molecule. Examples of these are alkaloids, antihistamines, and amphetamine, which can be complexed with tannic acid. An alcoholic solution of the amine and the tannic acid is combined, and the precipitated complex is washed, dried, and mixed with additional vehicles and either compressed into tablets or granulated and filled into capsules. A preparation of methylcellulose salts of basic amines is also possible for this type of formulation. Usually, the solubility of the complex is greatest at acidic pH. Therefore, other vehicle substances, such as buffers or hydrophilic gums, are added to prevent too rapid dissolution. The different groups of oral prolonged-action dosage forms, their manufacturing characteristics, and drug release characteristics are listed by Cavallito et al. and Ritschel.[69,70]

13.   Bioadhesives

One of the simplest concepts for prolonging the duration of drug presence in the GI tract and localizing it in a specific region involves binding the product to the mucin/epithelial surface of the GI tract. This is the premise of bioadhesion. Although the concept is old, it is receiving renewed attention because of a better understanding of polymers and the GI tract. To this end, it is now possible to attach a number of polymeric substances noncovalently to mucous tissue and keep them localized for an extended period of time. One of the early researchers in this area was Nagai et al.,[71] who used the bioadhesion principle to treat aphtha, an inflammation of the mouth. He used an anti-inflammatory drug mixed with a bioadhesive polymer that would attach to the tongue or cheek and remain in place for many hours. He has since extended the clinical application of this concept to the treatment of cervical cancer and to the nasal delivery of peptides. Extended, local release of the drug has yielded good clinical results in the treatment of both aphtha and cervical cancer.

For the past decade, work at the University of Wisconsin, School of Pharmacy, has been directed to understanding the mechanisms of bioadhesion and controlling them for drug delivery purposes. Experimental work at Wisconsin, with drugs in the eye and GI tract, has led to once-daily administration and uncovered a number of other advantages, including improved duration of blood or local drug levels, improved fraction of dose absorbed, improved local drug targeting, strategies for drug–polymer pro-drugs, platforms for enzyme inhibition (peptidases), and membrane permeability for enzyme change in a restricted area.

One of the great potential advantages of an oral bioadhesive is in its use with peptide drugs. Protein and polypeptide drugs, which are expected to increase substantially in number as a result of genetic engineering, are subject to peptidase inactivation in the GI tract and commonly have difficulty crossing the intestinal barrier because of their size.[70] To overcome these concerns, it is necessary to localize a dosage form in a specified region of the GI tract to inhibit local peptidase activity and perhaps modify intestinal membrane permeability. Bioadhesives offer the potential to partially accomplish this goal and also offer the best and most significant opportunity to improve controlled oral delivery.

14.   Local, targeted systems

An effort is being made to find specific binding sites in the GI tract to which drugs can be targeted. Knowing there is a specific sugar-binding site at a specific region of the intestine could, for example, conceivably permit attachment of a drug to that sugar and possibly achieve localization. In a similar manner, small peptides, such as fibronectin fragments, can bind to epithelial cells, and might be good platforms for drug delivery. These studies seem further from commercialization than the more physical systems described earlier, but they have considerable potential to target drugs to specific locations.[72,73]

15.   Synchron system

The Synchron system is Forest Laboratories' patented procedure based on the blending of cellulose and noncellulose material with a drug. These materials are combined into a homogeneous mixture from which tablets are made. When the Synchron system tablet comes in contact with water, the outer

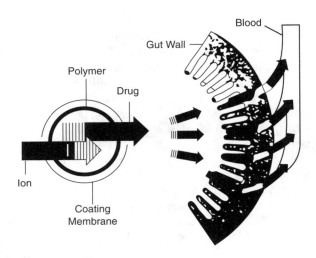

Figure 5.2 Schematic drawing of a Pennkinetic system.

layer of the matrix softens to a gel-like consistency, which allows the trapped drug to release at a controlled rate. The simplicity of this system allows the completion of a desired drug formulation within a matter of months. Forest has marketed Theochron, a controlled-release theophylline product using the Synchron system (see Figure 5.2).

16. *Pennkinetic and other liquid controlled-release systems*
The Pennkinetic system is Pennwalt's proprietary liquid system, which makes use of two controlled-release technologies: ion exchange and membrane diffusion control. The Pennkinetic system is formed by reacting a drug in its ionic state with a suitable polymer matrix. This polymer-drug complex is then subjected to polyethylene glycol 4000, which imparts plasticity and stability to the complex. A coating of ethylcellulose is applied by air to the preparation to form a water-insoluble but ionic and drug-permeable coating. To be effective, this system requires that a drug interact ionically with the ion-exchange polymer.

Since the ion concentration in the human GI tract is remarkably consistent, medication release from the Pennkinetic system is quite precise and unaffected by variations in pH, temperature, or contents in the stomach or intestine. Pennwalt has used this system in making a variety of long-lasting nonprescription drug products. Its first product was Delsym, a 12-h cough product containing dextromethorphan. Pennwalt also introduced 12-h cold preparations called Corsym and Cold Factor 12, which employ the same delivery system to supply chlorpheniramine and phenylpropanolamine, respectively.

In addition to prolonged, precise release of medication, the Pennkinetic matrix system makes the drug tasteless, which is helpful in masking the bitter taste of many drugs, especially in pediatric formulations. Elan Corpo-

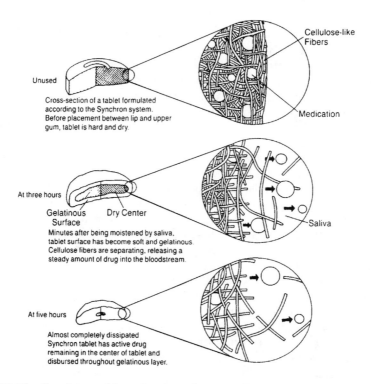

Cellulose-like Fibers

Unused

Cross-section of a tablet formulated according to the Synchron system. Before placement between lip and upper gum, tablet is hard and dry.

Medication

At three hours

Gelatinous Surface   Dry Center

Minutes after being moistened by saliva, tablet surface has become soft and gelatinous. Cellulose fibers are separating, releasing a steady amount of drug into the bloodstream.

Saliva

At five hours

Almost completely dissipated Synchron tablet has active drug remaining in the center of tablet and disbursed throughout gelatinous layer.

Figure 5.3 The Synchron tablet-release mechanism. (From *Pharm. Tech.*, The Latest Developments in Drug Delivery Systems, Conf. Proc., Oct. 1985, 31. With permission.)

ration has also developed a liquid sustained-release system called Pharmazome. While the company has not disclosed the mechanism of action of this system, it is believed to provide the same benefits of long action and taste masking offered by the Pennkinetic system (see Figure 5.3).

17. Controlled-release capsules
While drugstore shelves are full of many ethical and proprietary preparations of conventional and prolonged-release capsules, the introduction of pH-independent, controlled-release capsules has occurred only during the past few years. These capsule products use different technologies to achieve zero-order release of active ingredients.

Inderal LA, a prescription drug, has been introduced by Ayerst. It uses polymer-coated, controlled-diffusion technology to achieve 12-hour release of therapeutic levels of propranolol. Polymer coating used for preparing Inderal LA beads gives the drug higher than normal density of 1.1 to 1.3. Higher-density formulation helps keep the drug in the upper alimentary canal for a substantially longer time.

Searle's Theo-24 was the first 24-hour theophylline therapy on the market. Theo-24 uses a chemical timing complex to produce very small theophylline-coated beads that provide dependable, zero-order controlled drug release. A tiny sphere of sugar and starch forms the core of the bead. The core is first coated with theophylline and then with a timing complex. The resulting beads are put into capsules for oral administration. When the capsule dissolves in the GI tract, the timing coating on the bead, which is insoluble, slowly erodes. The drug, which is highly soluble, moves through the coating into the GI tract. In the core, the starch swells and pushes the drug out, while the dissolving sugar also helps carry the drug through the chemical timing complex. This results in a constant release.

When the Theo-24 capsule dissolves, many tiny beads are widely dispersed throughout the GI tract and there is a more even distribution of the drug than would otherwise be achieved with a tablet. Because of this dispersion, the beads are less affected than a single tablet would be by variations in stomach-emptying time and rate of movement through the intestine. The dispersion of the beads also helps to overcome the potential problem of localized high concentration of drugs that can irritate the gastric mucosa.

Burroughs Wellcome Co. introduced Lanoxicaps, a new form of digoxin in a soft elastic gelatin (SEG) sustained-release capsule formulated by R.P. Scherer Company. Scherer's sustained-release SEG capsule is a controlled-release delivery system embodying a unique matrix. The matrix allows the drug to diffuse out of the capsule, providing a constant level of drug in the blood over a period of 12 h. Digoxin therapy with Lanoxicaps allows digoxin to be much more rapidly and completely absorbed. Whereas digoxin tablet bioavailability is only in the range of 60 to 80%, bioavailability with Lanoxicaps is similar to that following IV administration (greater than 90%).

18.   Controlled-release tablets

The wax-matrix delivery system employs a tablet made up of a honeycomb-type of wax matrix. As the tablet passes through the GI tract, the active ingredient is slowly released from the matrix and is absorbed in the body. Ciba-Geigy's Slow-K (potassium chloride) tablet uses a wax matrix. Ciba-Geigy has also introduced a slow iron tablet in a wax matrix called Slow-Fe. While Slow-K is widely used and Slow-Fe is well accepted, some recent studies have shown that Slow-K matrix tablets tend to cause more gastric irritation than the microencapsulated Micro-K.

Theo-Dur tablets use Key Pharmaceutical's patented controlled-release tablet formulation to achieve zero-order drug availability. Unlike Theo-24, Theo-Dur requires 12-h dosing. However, Theo-Dur was on the market long before Theo-24 and still leads the theophylline market in sales.

Unlike conventional tablets, buccal or transmucosal tablets pass directly into the bloodstream through the oral mucosa. This avoids liver extraction, which occurs with orally administered drugs. Buccal tablets are not swallowed but are kept in the buccal pouch between the cheeks and the gum. They are dissolved rapidly in the mouth. Merrell-Dow's Susadrin tablets are buccal tablets that use Forest Lab's Synchron system to release nitroglycerine in a controlled manner over a period of 6 hours. Zetachron Co. also has a buccal delivery system for nitroglycerine.

19. Hoffmann-La Roche's Web Delivery System

Hoffmann-La Roche owns a series of patents on a high-tech drug delivery system called Web Delivery System (WDS). The Web Delivery System consists of an edible web formed by paperlike polymeric material on which a drug is deposited in suspension or powder form. The coated drug webs are then laminated to produce a multilayered structure of 6 to 20 layers. The WDS system uses a number of drug-release mechanisms, such as diffusion, disintegration, and erosion, to achieve controlled release of active ingredients at a desirable rate. Roche has used this system to prepare oral dosage forms for benzodiazepines and digoxin. However, none of these products have yet been marketed.

20. Hydrodynamic cushion system

Elan Corporation has developed an oral solid dosage form using a cushioned material. This cushioned material allows drug-bearing granules to be compressed into a unique tablet. Unlike conventional tablets, this tablet is made from cushioned material that breaks apart immediately after entering the GI tract and releases drug granules for controlled release. According to Elan, incorporation of the cushion material allows more active ingredients per dose and is cheaper to produce.

21. Floating delivery system

The 3M Company has developed an oral dosage form in which the drug-carrying matrix is covered on either side by a bubble-type barrier film. The barrier layer causes the tablet to float. The matrix layer releases the drug in zero-order fashion in the stomach. This system has been used to deliver theophylline.

22. Meter release system

This is a controlled-release drug delivery system developed by KV Pharmaceutical Company. It consists of beads or granules coated with a rate-controlling membrane system specific for each drug compound. This flexibility of rate-controlled membrane system allows precise control of drug-release rates. The meter release system has been used for preparing a long-acting capsule form of Actifed®. It has also been used for many other compounds, including antihistamines and cardiovascular agents.

23. Hydrodynamically Balanced System

Hoffmann-La Roche has developed a patented oral drug delivery system called Hydrodynamically Balanced System (HBS). It contains one or more active ingredients combined with a hydrocolloid in such a way that the entire formulation becomes hydrodynamically balanced. When the formulation enters the gastric fluid, it acquires a specific gravity of less than 1. Low specific gravity allows it to become buoyant in this fluid, and it stays in the stomach for a prolonged period until all of the active ingredients are released. This system is especially useful for drugs that are absorbed in the upper portion of the duodenum, undergoing abrupt changes in solubility in different pH media, intended to act in the stomach contents, and likely to cause gastric irritation. Roche's controlled-release form of Valium®, called Valrelease®, is a good example of this system.

24. *Other oral controlled drug delivery systems*

Avitek has an exclusive licensing agreement from Yissum for an innovative submicronized fat-emulsion drug delivery system (SES formula) for oral or parenteral administration. It is expected that stable emulsions of certain drugs will improve efficacy and reduce side effects. Preclinical studies with diazepam have been successfully performed, and work is now underway with other compounds.[74]

Destab is a broad line of more than 14 directly compressible tablet excipients prepared by Desmo Chemical (KV). The products are designed for tablet formulations in which optimal compression or flow characteristics are desired. The technology has been extended to incorporate active ingredients, including paracetamol, niacinamide, riboflavin, thiamin, and various minerals. Descote is a delivery system for encapsulating small-particle vitamins, minerals, and pharmaceutical chemicals by the same company. It provides superior taste masking, improved stability profiles, and homogeneous particles of combinations of materials. A broad line of Descote B vitamins, ferrous fumarate, potassium chloride, paracetamol, zinc gluconate, copper gluconate, ascorbic acid, magnesium oxide, ferrous lactate, and many other vitamins and minerals are currently available.

Pharmedix (IVAX) has developed a granular drug delivery system for use with certain ethical and OTC products. The drug is incorporated into granules, each of which is a microencapsulated delivery system. They can be administered either by sprinkling the granules from a premeasured capsule onto food or directly into the mouth, by swallowing a capsule containing the granules or suspending the granules in water. The delivery system results in improved therapeutic characteristics of the drug and a more convenient mode of administration.[74]

Elan has developed a new delivery system for the oral administration of highly insoluble drugs. INDAS (insoluble drug absorption system) is currently being applied to certain dihydropyridine compounds and is further being used in a range of insoluble compounds from various therapeutic classes. To date, it has enabled the development of once-daily formulations of isradipine, nicardipine, nifedipine, and a formulation of hydergine. This new tabletting technique has proven to be highly suitable in the development of long acting tablets with excellent bioavailability for highly insoluble drugs and other problem compounds.[74]

Gacell Laboratories has reported on the firm's Multipor controlled-release technology. Tablets prepared using this technology have a porous outer membrane composed of a water-insoluble polymer and a soluble pore-forming substance. When exposed to gastric fluid, the pore-forming substance dissolves, which allows the fluid to penetrate into the tablet core as the drug diffuses outward at a constant rate. According to the manufacturer, the technology allows for the controlled release of drugs independent of pH values, peristaltic movements, and intake of food and water. In addition, the outer membrane protects patients from GI irritation, masks unpleasant tastes, and makes the tablets easy to swallow. This technology can be applied to tablets of various shapes, colors, and sizes, and the outer coating can accept printed text or trademarks.[74]

Biotechnology Australia is investigating an oral delivery system for drugs, hormones, and vaccines by linking them to vitamin B-12. Vitamin B-12 is rapidly absorbed from the gut via a receptor for intrinsic factor (IF), a naturally occurring protein that complexes with vitamin B-12. Thus, substances that can be coupled to vitamin B-12 in a way that does not affect the formation of the receptor-IF-vitamin B-12 complex or its subsequent absorption are potential candidates for this method of oral delivery.[74]

Benzon is developing a multiple-unit, controlled-release tablet formulation of propranolol using its Repro-Dose technology. The formulation is unique in that it is a multiple-unit tablet using a water-based, diffusion-coating system.[74]

Elan has recently announced the production of Asprilan Retard, containing aspirin, and Elangesic Tablets, containing ibuprofen. These formulations were made using SODAS (solid oral drug absorption system).

The first potassium tablet to deliver 20 mEq of potassium (twice the amount in other potassium tablets) was developed by Key Pharmaceuticals. The product, K-Dur 20, utilizes a patented microburst release system and is indicated for prevention and treatment of hypokalemia. K-Dur 20's high-tech system is said to give the product a high safety profile, sparing patients from many of the side effects of conventional potassium medications. Like a liquid, K-Dur 20 is designed to disperse immediately, distributing minute sustained-action particles over a wide surface in the stomach. As a result of its delivery system, K-Dur 20 minimizes contact between concentrated quantities of potassium and the lining of the GI tract, thereby reducing the risk of gastric irritation.[74]

KV Pharmaceuticals has developed a drug delivery system that allows unpalatable solid drug particles to be combined with liquids and taken orally in a taste-free manner. Marketed under the trade name Liquette®, it consists of a solid dispersion of the active drug in an inert, biodegradable, particulate matrix. The delivery system allows larger volume doses of solid drugs to be administered and allows the rate of release of the active drug to be controlled in order to reduce GI irritation or to prolong drug absorption. Two or more drugs can be incorporated simultaneously in the Liquette particles, which can be coated to provide additional control of drug release, enhanced drug stability, uniform suspension of the particles in liquids, and alteration of GI transit time, thus enhancing bioavailability.[74]

Micro-Release is a long-acting delivery system developed by KV Pharmaceutical Co. The finished products are in the form of minispheres of encapsulated particles, with the active ingredient contained in a biochemically matched matrix. Sphere diameters vary from 100 to 500 µm and are suitable for use in encapsulated, tableted, or bulk form. Variation in matrix components provides a wide range of both rate and duration of release (including once-daily dosing) throughout the GI tract and protection from moisture, pH effects, and enzymatic dissolution. Micro-Release products are claimed to offer such benefits as effective utilization of the product and improved content uniformity.[74]

VI. Survey of oral controlled-release products

(Brand names are in parentheses)

Acetazoamide (Diamox Sequels)
Disopyramide (Norpace CR)
Isosorbide dinitrate (Isordil)
Nitroglycerine (Nitrospan, Nitrobid)
Papaverine HCl (Pavacen Cenules)
Pentaerythritol tetranitrate (Pentraspan SR)
Propranol (Inderal LA)
Quinidine sulfate (Quinidex Extentabs)
Quinidine gluconate (Quinaglute)
Verapamil (Isoptin SR, Calan SR)
Aspirin (Measurin)
Chlorpromazine (Thorazine Spansules)
Dextroamphetamine sulfate (Dexedrine Spansules)
Diazepam (Valrelease)
Diethylpropion HCl (Tenuate Dospan)
Fluphenazine HCl (Permitil Chronotabs)
Indomethacin (Indocin SR)
Lithium (Lithobid)
Meprobamate (Meprospan)
Methamphetamine HCl (Desoxyn Gradumets)
Methylphenidate HCl (RitalinSR)
Morphine sulfate (RoxanolSR)
Ophenadrine citrate (Norflex)
Phenylpropanolamine HCL (Acutrim, Dexatrim)
Prochlorperazine (Compazine Spansules)
Hexocyclium (Tral Gradumets)
Clinoril (Sulindac)
Aminophylline (Phyllcontin)
Antitussive combinstions (Rescap, Ornade Spansules)

Brompheniramine maleate (Bromphen, Dimtane)
Chlorpheniramine maleate (Chlor-Trimeton)
Decongestant and antihistamine (ResaidSR, NovafedSR Dristan)
Decongestant, antihistamine, and anticholinergic (Dallergy, Supres)
Pseudoephedrine HCl (SudafedSA)
Theophylline (Gyrocaps, Theo-24, Theobid, Theovent)
Trimeprazine (Temaril Spansules)
Tripelennamine (PBZ-SR)
Xanthine combinations (Isofil, TedralSA)
Ascorbic acid (Ascorbicap, Cevi-Bid)
Ferrous sulfate (Mol-Iron, Filmtabs Feosol Spansules)
Nicotinic acid (Nicobid, Nico-400)
Potassium (Micro-K, Slow-K, Klotrix)
Vitamin combinations (NeoVicaps)
Naproxen (Naprosyn)
Procainamide HCl (ProcanSR, PronestlySR)
Lanoxin (Lanoxicaps)
Iron (Slow-Fe)
Metoprolol (Lopressor)
Salbutamol (Volmax, Ventolon)
GITS-Nifedipine (Procardia)
GITS-Prazosin (Minipress)
Vitamin C (AcuSystem C)
Methyldopa (Elanpres)
Ibuprofen (Motrin)
Diltiazem (Cardizem)
Spironolactone (Aldactone, Aldactazide)
Thioridazine (Mellaril)
Diclofenac (Diffucap)
Acetaminophen (Paracetamol)
Cimetidine (Tagamet)

VII. Recent advances

- Anderson and Powell have synthesized enterically active microcapsules with controlled release in aqueous environments. These microcapsules exhibit rapid and relatively slow release of material in aqueous acid environments.[75]
- Rembaum has reported that ions that covalently bind to small, polymeric spheres can be used for binding anions and polyanions in separation, analytical, diagnostic, and clinical applications.[76]
- Waxlike materials have been used by Blichare et al.[77] to prepare controlled-release granules. Among the number of waxlike materials that can be used are the following: glyceryl monostearate, hydrogenated tallow, castor wax, myristyl alcohol, white beeswax, myristic

acid, stearyl alcohol, substituted monoglycerides, diglycerides, triglycerides, carnauba wax, acylated monoglycerides, and stearic acid.

- A carrier, depot, or bonding system for a drug that allows sustained release of a drug has been used by Baukal et al.[78] A wide variety of drugs can be used with the carrier to produce a dosage form that can be administered orally, externally, or by implantation. The carrier material consists of physiologically innocuous, inorganic, or organic materials that are totally or almost totally nonabsorbable in the body. For its properties as a carrier of active pharmaceutical substances, what is decisive is the special porous structure. It consists of "inkwell pores" (i.e., it contains cavities connected to the outer surface of the bonding substance by narrow passages (pore necks)). The drug is embedded in the cavities.

- A process for preparing tablets containing microcapsules without rupture of the microcapsules has been prepared by Estevenel et al.[79] These tablets contain a number of superposed layers, of which the medial layer is essentially constituted of microcapsules containing an active substance. The exterior layers, which may possibly also contain identical or different active substance and which have a composition usual for the formulation of tablets, constitute means of protecting the microcapsules of the medial layer, particularly against compression shock.

- Gastric-resistant gelatin capsules having two coatings have been described by Leiberich et al.[80] The capsules are characterized by a gastric juice-resistant outer layer consisting of an anionic polymerizate of methacrylic acid and acrylic acid esters. They also contain an intermediate layer consisting of a cationic polymerizate of di-lower alkylamino-lower alkylmethacrylate with other neutral methacrylic acid esters between this outer layer and the gelatin shell.

- Capsules that are completely dissolved, or slurried, within short periods of time have been developed by Controulis et al.[81] The capsule shell is apertured, and the holes are covered by a water-soluble barrier film that seals the holes and blocks any escape of the contents from the shell. The film is more water-soluble than the cap and the body parts of the shell so that when the package is contacted with water, as in the digestive tract, the film rather than the shell dissolves first, exposing the contents for dissolution or release by way of the apertures, while the shell is still intact.

- A rigid canister dispenser has been described by Higuchi and Leeper.[82] This osmotically driven fluid dispenser for use in an aqueous environment is comprised of a shape-retaining canister having controlled permeability to water; an osmotically effective solute confined in the canister, which, in solution, exhibits an osmotic pressure gradient against water in the environment; and an outlet in the canister wall. The dispenser includes a flexible bag of relatively impervious material that holds the fluid to be dispensed and is housed in the canister with its open end in sealed contact with the canister such that the canister outlet communicates with the bag interior.

- A multizone or multilayered tablet is produced by the process described by Beringer and Woltmann.[83] The process is characterized by a nonplastic tablet and a plastic chewing gum mass. One of the masses contains at least one pharmaceutically active ingredient and is compressed to form the joined tablet. The joined tablet has at least one plastic zone comprising the chewing gum mass. The chewing gum mass contains a water-soluble portion, which, although it can be kneaded in the mouth, cannot be dissolved or chewed.

- The process developed by Michaelis[84] provides a method of preparing improved controlled gastric-residence formulations that involves treating the polymeric film coating of such formulations with a volatile amine. Volatile amines include those which are volatile at ambient temperature, may be volatilized by raising the polymer-treatment temperature, or lowering the polymer-treatment pressure (e.g., vacuum treatment).

- Nitrofurantoin is an antibacterial agent for the treatment of urinary tract infections. The drug is remarkably well tolerated in humans. However, adverse reactions occur, including anorexia, nausea, and emesis. Numerous attempts have been made to alleviate these undesirable side effects while providing a dosage form requiring less frequent administration. Huber developed improved, pharmaceutically acceptable, layered tablets containing nitrofurantoin in sustained-release form.[85]

- It has been found that some of the more active polyene macrolides (e.g., candicidin, fungimycin, hamycin) are somewhat unstable under the acidic conditions in the stomach and cause GI irritation (i.e., emesis and diarrhea) in some patients. This has hindered achieving optimum effectiveness by the oral route. A method has been found by Gordon and Schaffner.[86] for increasing overall effectiveness, including stability and GI tolerability, of these drugs. Compositions containing a polyenic macrolide and a suitable absorbent material, preferably in bead form, are used in treating various conditions.

- Macrolide antibiotics are sparingly water-soluble substances. In orally administrable formulations, the use of an amorphous solid form, having better solubility, can lead to full effectiveness of these antibiotics. Attempts to obtain amorphous solids of macrolide antibiotics by ordinary techniques (e.g., lyophilization or the rapid cooling of a molten liquid) result in products containing crystals or products that are readily converted to crystals with the passage of time. Consequently, it is difficult to obtain crystal-free amorphous solids that are stable with the passage of time. Sato et al.[87] have succeeded in developing a process to overcome these problems.

- Erythromycin salts and esters, such as the alkylsulfate salts or the mono-alkyl erythromycin esters of dicarboxylic acids (e.g., the erythromycin ethyl succinate), have enjoyed excellent acceptance due to their wide spectrum of antibacterial activity. Unfortunately, some of these esters or salts have a number of physical and chemical properties that are objectionable for administration in the form of liquid suspensions. For instance, erythromycin ethyl succinate has a bitter taste which is very difficult to mask; even worse, it is known that when exposed to an acidic environment, it eventually converts to an anhydro form that is inactive. The process described by Farhadieh[88] is designed to protect particles of erythromycin derivatives from being inactivated by the pH of the stomach and simultaneously cover their objectionable taste.

- An early method for making multilayer aspirin tablets, including a timed-release layer, has been developed by Guy and Powers.[89] Hill[90] has further described improvements in connection with several other analgesic and antipyretic tablets. APAP (N-acetyl-p-aminophenol) has long been known to be useful as an analgesic or antipyretic agent and has found its way into several commercially available products. However, the speed at which its action takes effect and the amount of it which is absorbed is less than desirable. This is at least partly due to the relatively slow rate at which it is absorbed into the bloodstream from the GI tract. Weintraub et al.[107] have devised a tablet formulation that provides improved absorption.

- A new method for preparing galenic forms able to deliver a drug with a constant rate has been described by Vergnaud et al.[91] It consists of surrounding a sphere made of drug dispersed in a polymer-matrix with a layer of Gelucire. The layer of Gelucire plays the role of a membrane, while the drug-polymer mixture provides the drug. As a result, this technique provides the drug in synthetic gastric liquid without any potential danger, the drug being dispersed in the polymer.

- Self-emulsifying systems are well known to the herbicide and pesticide industries for their advantage in the transportation of lipophilic products. The system for pharmaceutical use described by Pouton et al.[92] utilizes a vegetable oil and a nonionic surfactant, which are likely to be acceptable for oral ingestion.

- Many of the undesirable side effects associated with current oral contraceptives are dose-related. If the drug is absorbed slowly over a period of time, lower doses can be effective and side effects reduced. The objective of studies by Schlameus et al.[93] was to prepare and evaluate sustained-release oral formulations of marketed contraceptive steroids (e.g., ethynyl estradiol, norethindrone, norethindrone acetate, and mestranol). Selected formulations were tested for reduction of daily peak concentrations, body burden, and contraceptive efficacy. Evaluation of the formulations was accomplished by *in vitro* release-rate testing, selected *in vivo* studies using baboons, and clinical studies using the most promising systems.

- Theophylline ethylcellulose microcapsules, prepared by using ethylene-vinyl acetate (EVA) as a coacervation-inducing agent, have exhibited a sustained-release behavior *in vitro* that correlates well with *in vivo* bioavailability in rats. In a study by Lin and Yang,[94] the effect of compression pressure, particle size, and types of excipients used on physical parameters and dissolution properties of tablets made from theophylline ethylcellulose microcapsules have been investigated.

- A report by Chattaraj et al.[95] concerns the development of a viable microencapsulated, controlled-release drug delivery system. Microcapsules containing ranitidine, which was selected as the core material, were prepared by phase-separation coacervation of ethyl cellulose in nonaqueous solvents. The effects of different concentrations of the coacervation-inducing agent polyisobutylene on drug release were studied.

- Located throughout the GI tract of man and other mammals are distinct lympho-reticular follicles (Peyer's patches) that possess IgA precursor B cells. Subsequent to antigen sensitization, these precursor B cells migrate throughout the body and repopulate the lamina propria regions of the GI and upper respiratory tracts and differentiate into mature IgA-synthesizing plasma cells. This migration pattern provides a common mucosal immune system by continually shuttling sensitized B cells to mucosal sites for responses to gut-encountered environmental antigens and potential pathogens. To take advantage of the mucosal system, Gilley et al.[96] have developed microcapsule formulations that target Peyer's patches and release antigens at controlled rates. The microcapsules protect the antigens from degradation in the GI tract and are effectively taken up by Peyer's patches. After uptake, the microcapsules release the antigen, resulting in sensitization of precursor B cells.

- Microparticles (containing propranolol or quinidine sulfate) or nanoparticles (spray-dried latex particles) have been dispersed into aqueous solutions of ionic polysaccharides (e.g., chitosan or sodium alginate) and then mixed with aqueous solutions of suitable counterions (e.g., tripolyphosphate or calcium chloride). The ionic character of the polysaccharides allows site-specific release of the microparticles in the GI tract. Chitosan beads, which dissolve below pH 6, release the microparticles in gastric juice, while sodium alginate beads stay intact in gastric juice but rapidly disintegrate in intestinal fluids. The beads could be taken as prepared or placed into capsules.[97]

- Research by Shefer and Kost[98] have focused on the application of starch from various vegetative sources for enzymatic targeted drug delivery. Starch is commonly used as food and is known to undergo enzymatic breakdown by amylase. Starch microbeads have been produced using a concentrated emulsion (loaded with a releasing agent) treated with a strong base and a calcium chloride solution. It was found that entrapment efficiency decreases as the molecular weight of the entrapped molecule increases. Microbeads prepared from different sources of starch undergo different breakdown rates. The release of high molecular weight molecules is due to matrix degradation, while small molecules are released by diffusion and degradation. Parameters affecting release kinetics are polymer source, molecular weight, and release environment (e.g., pH, enzymatic activity).

- Attributes of the ideal contraceptive drug delivery system include safety, efficacy, reversibility, absence of side effects, minimum steroid load, and high patient compliance. The objective of the work reported by Eldem et al.[99] was to formulate ultrafine lipid pellets as steroid carriers for oral contraception by using spray drying and congealing techniques. By taking into consideration the basic mechanism of fat absorption, physiologic lipid carriers, such as triglycerides and lecithin, were used to promote the lymphatic absorption of steroids, thus avoiding first-pass metabolism by the liver and increasing their bioavailability.

- Many hydrophilic polymers have been used in controlled-release tablet formulations, but modified starches have never been investigated extensively for this purpose. Herman and Remon[100] reported the use of starches containing different amounts of amylose and modified by spray drying, drum drying, or extrusion in controlled-release formulations. The influence of silicium dioxide and some lubricants on drug-release rate from tablets containing starch: theophylline (60:40 w/w) has been investigated. Most starches containing less than 30% amylose show a dramatic reduction in drug release. Silicium dioxide had no influence on release rate, while magnesium stearate and polyethylene glycol increase the release rate dramatically.

- A bioadhesive tablet of metronidazole has been developed for oral or vaginal administration. It was found that pH in the range of 2 to 7, although known to modify the swelling of the carbopol, had no significant effect on the bioadhesive power of the tablet in conditions of weak hydration. This was explained by the substantial difference between the time required for swelling and that required for a detachment test and also by the specific buffer capacity of carbopol. On the other hand, ionic strength had a clear effect on the bioadhesive power, which decreased with an increase in ionic strength.[101]

- An orally applicable pulsatile drug delivery system in dry-coated tablet form has been prepared using diltiazem as a model drug and a polyvinyl, chloride-hydrogenated, castor oil-polyethyleneglycol mixture as the outer shell of the tablet. *In vitro* drug release from the prepared tablet exhibited a typical pulsatile pattern with a 7-hour lag phase.[102]

- Ampicillin has been embedded in a chitosan matrix to develop an oral release dosage form. It appears that the drug forms a crystal structure within the chitosan beads, which slowly dissolves out to the dissolution medium through the micropores of the chitosan matrix.[103,104]

- The oral delivery of O-(N-morpholino-carbonyl-3L-phenylaspartyl-L-leucinamide or (2S,3R,4S)-2-amino-1-cyclohexyl-3,4-dihydroxy-6-methylene, a new renin inhibitor, has been studied in an *in vivo* rat model using emulsion formulations. The components of the emulsion formulations were chosen based on their proposed effects on membrane structure, fluidity, and solute transport. The results suggest that in the intestine, the particle size of the emulsion is reduced in the presence of bile fluid while the drug resides primarily in the oil phase.[105]

- Cephalosporin has been enterically coated with an absorption-promoting excipient for oral administration. The novelty claimed for this preparation resides in a two-component absorption-enhancing agent. The first component is ethoxylated n-dodecanol, while the second component is a salt of caprylic acid.[106]

- Delayed-release osmotic devices for delivery of verapamil have been described. This involves a tablet formulation that is intended to be taken at bedtime, but that releases verapamil only in the early morning hours. A drug-containing layer was prepared with verapamil, Polynox N-750 (EO polymer), polyvinylpyrrolidone K29–32, sodium chloride, and magnesium stearate. Drug and osmotic pump layers were co-tableted and then coated with a wall-forming composition. Exit orifices were drilled on the drug-containing side of the tablet.[107]

- Nicotine has been delivered osmotically to the oral mucosa using a coated tablet that provides a readily absorbable form of nicotine *in situ*. The bitartrate salt of nicotine was tableted with sodium carbonate, PEO, HPMC, sodium saccharin, and flavorants. Nicotine tartrate exhibits good stability during storage and is readily converted to the absorbable base form in the mouth.[108]

- A Scherer dosage form, the Pulsincap, provides a dose of drug at either a predetermined time or a predetermined place in the GI tract. The system, which resembles a capsule, has a water-insoluble body that contains the active agent: either a powder or liquid. A water-soluble "cap" protects a hydrogel plug that is seated in the neck of the main compartment. Another type of Pulsincap has an enteric film coating over the water-soluble cap. This modification allows drugs to get past the stomach and into the colon — a good direct-deposit way of delivering treatment for inflammatory bowel disease.[109]

- Dispersing a drug into Gelucire, with the addition of a small amount of a polymer called Sumikagel®, has been described. Gelucire plays the role of an erodible polymer matrix with a low rate of erosion. Sumikagel swells to various extents, depending on pH. This new dosage form disintegrates completely in an aqueous solution of pH 8 in less than 1 hour, while the rate of drug delivery remains constant.

Delivery of drug occurs by transient diffusion when the pH is between 1 and 2.[110]

- The transmucosal absorption of various peptides, such as insulin, calcitonin, tetragastrin, and thyrotropin-releasing hormone (TRH), could be improved by using additives, such as absorption enhancers and protease inhibitors.[125]
- Lectins have been used as specific bioadhesives, with many suitable properties for targeting of cells in the GI tract.[126]
- Oral absorption of parathyroid hormone in rats and monkeys as models of osteoporosis was facilitated by N-8(2hydroxy-4-methoxy)benzoylaminocaprylic acid as a novel delivery agent.[127]
- The introduction of biotin moiety in certain nonapeptides can alter its intestinal transport pathway, resulting in a significant improvement in the absorptive permeability by enhancing nonspecific passive and carrier-mediated uptake by means of a sodium-dependent multivitamin transporter.[128]
- A possible method to enhance oral absorption is to exploit the phenomenon of lipophilic modification and mono- and oligosaccharide conjugation. The delivery system can be conjugated to the drug in such a way as to release the active compound after it has been absorbed (i.e., the drug is converted to a pro-drug), or to form a biologically stable and active molecule (i.e., the conjugate becomes a new drug moiety). The use of lipid, sugar, and lipid–sugar conjugates has resulted in enhanced drug delivery.[129]
- "Lipid" formulations for oral administration of drugs generally consist of a drug involved in a blend of two or more excipients, which may be triglyceride oils, partial glycerides, surfactants, or co-surfactants. The primary mechanism of action that leads to improved bioavailability is usually avoidance or partial avoidance of the slow dissolution process, which limits the bioavailability of hydrophobic drug from solid dosage forms. Ideally, the formulation allows the drug to remain in a dissolved state throughout its transit through the GI tract. The availability of the drug for absorption can be enhanced by presentation of the drug as a solubilizate within a colloidal dispersion. This objective can be achieved by formulation of the drug in a self-emulsifying or self-microemulsifying system or, alternatively, by taking advantage of the natural process of triglyceride digestion. In practice, "lipid" formulations range from pure oils, at one extreme, to blends that contain a substantial proportion of hydrophilic surfactants or cosolvents, at the other extreme.[130]
- As a new oral drug delivery system for colon targeting, enteric-coated, timed-release, press-coated tablets (ETP tablets) have been developed by coating enteric polymer on timed-release, press-coated tablets composed of an outer shell of hydroxypropylcellulose and a core tablet containing diltiazem hydrochloride as a model drug. The re-

sults indicated that the tablets showed both acid resistance and timed release and they reached the colon after gastric emptying.[131]

- pH-sensitive interpolymer interactions between high molecular weight polyoxyethylene and poly(methacrylic acid co-methyl methacrylate) (EudragitEUD L100 of S100) were demonstrated and exploited to prepare coevaporates, or physical mixtures, of compressed matrix tablets containing prednisolone in order to deliver them to sites in the GI tract. Matrices based on plain EUD were found to exhibit a comparatively low release rate, more suited to an extended delivery to the colon than to a specific delivery to the ileum.[132]

- In order to develop an enzymatically controlled, pulsatile drug-release system based on an impermeable capsule body that contains the drug, an erodible pectin/pectinase plug was prepared by direct compression of pectin and pectinase in different ratios. It was found that drug release was controlled by the enzymatic degradation and dissolution of pectin.[133]

- The ability of glycostenoid (TC002) was investigated to increase the oral bioavailability of gentamicin. TC002 was found to be significantly more efficacious than sodium taurocholate, but similar in cutotoxicity. TC002 remained primarily in the GI tract following oral or intestinal administration and cleared rapidly from the body. It was only partly metabolized in the GI tract, but was rapidly and completely converted to its metabolite in plasma and urine.[134]

- Lectin-mediated mucosal delivery of drugs and vaccines, mucoadhesive DL-lactide/glycolide copolymer nanospheres coated with chitosan to improve oral delivery of elactonin, microspheres containing dexamethasone, synthetic peptides encapsulated in PLG microparticles, nanoparticles linked to vitamin B-12, and chitosan-cellulose multicore microparticles for controlled drug delivery were prepared.

- Cardinal Health, Inc. has developed controlled-release, oral, sustained-action technology (OSAT). This is a multiparticulate, HPMC-based, coating bead system that allows the active drug to diffuse out of pores in the bead. This system utilizes multiple beads that eliminate the concerns of dose dumping and has taste-masking properties.

VIII. Current development of oral drug delivery systems[74]

Developer	Product under Development
Cortecs & Rhone-Poulenc Rorer	Calcitonin and the diuretic peptide DDAVP
Cortecs	Insulin using macromol delivery system, Indomethacin formulation
Ethical Pharmaceuticals	Amiophylline formulation, Rhotard Delivery System, morphine and verapamil formulations

Developer	Product under Development
Gacell Laboratories and Pan	Multipore drug delivery system using diltiazem
Medica	Metoclopramide formulation
Hafslund, Nycomed	Furosemide in multiple unit, controlled-release capsule, Naproxen enteric-coated, Indomethacin and morphine using Repro-dose control-release system
Siegfried	Nifedipine capsule formulation
SmithKline Beecham	Mesalazine formulation
Erbamont, Proctor & Gamble	Mesalazine formulation
Lab Phoenix	Ranitidine sustained-release system
Taiyo Pharmaceutical	Sodium picosulfate
Kabi Pharm	Silfasalazine enteric-coated
Vuman	For treatment of hyperglycemia
Pharma Logic	Dantrolene, microCRYSTAL formulation for malignant hyperthermia
Biovail	Verapamil once-daily formulation
Orion	Verapamil formulation
Forest Laboratories	Cognine Synapton, physostigmine Synchron delivery system
Forest Labs, Sandoz	Thioridazine (Synchron)
Pharmed:Ferring	Vasopressin, Insulin
Pharmaceutical Development Associates	Insulin
R.P. Sherer:Johnson& Johnson	Loperamide, Polysol Sheresol system
Glenfair Pharmaceuticals	Magnesium chloride enteric-coated
Pharmos: Yissum	Submicron emulsion (SME) delivery system, lipophilic drugs in uniform minute droplets, physostigmine
TheraTech	STDC for site-specific targeted delivery in the colon
Recordati	Control-release suspension system (CRSS)
Faulding Glaxo Dainippon	Morphine sustained-release system Theophylline formulation
Nikken Chemical	Valproate sodium once-daily granule formulation
Elf Sanofi:Kyowa Hakko	Valproate sodium
Gebro Broschek	Theophylline long-acting
Pierre Fabre	Theophylline slow-release
Schering-Plough:Recordati	Theophylline once-daily
Verex	Indomethacin SR Formulation
Verex:Biovail	Naproxen Formulation OLipHEX (Osmotic lipid hydrogel complex) system, Zidovudin once daily for AIDS
Hisamatsu:Nissan Chemical Solvay	Ketoprofen formulation
Pharmatec International	Ketoprofen SURECAPS capsule delivery system
Alfa Schiapparelli	Naproxen formulation

Developer	Product under Development
Wassermann Monsanto Research Triangle Pharmaceuticals	Carbamazepine, microCRYSTAL
CytRX	Emulsion technology
Fisons	Pennkinetic delivery system dextromethorpham
Sparta	Spartaject,microcrystal/micro-droplet delivery system for Busulfan doxorubicin and aphidicolin
KV Pharmaceutical	Caltrate D, FerroSequels, nutritionals Liquette, solid drug delivery system for antacids. Meter-release containing beads or granules with the active drug coated with a rate-controlling system, e.g., antihistamines, nitroglycerine, theophylline, Vitamin C long-acting capsule
KV Pharmaceutical, Taisho Warner-Lambert	KV/24 drug delivery system
Alza	MOSTS (mucosal oral therapeutic system) Chronset Controlled-release Osmotic dosage formulation system
Alza:Monsanto	Verapamil, OROS
Alza:Pfizer	Glipizide, OROS
Alza:Pfizer:Bayer	Adalat, OROS; Procardia, OROS
Alza:Ciba-Geigy	Lopressor, OROS
Alza:Pfizer	Alpress. Prazosin, GITS, Minipress, OROS
Eurand	Isosorbide 5'-mononitrate using Diffutab control-release system Theophylline-Liquitard, Prazosin Diffutab, Diclofenac, Diffucaps, Ibuprofen, Diffutab system, Minitabs, multiparticulate dosing formulation Liquitard, drugs are microencapsulated by MICROCAP system and then are in the suspension form, MICROCAP for taste masking
Eurand:E.Merck	Pancreatin, lipase capsules
Elan	Sulindac-capsule, SODAS (Solid Oral Drug Absorption System), Cough-cold product, EL-715 for osteoporosis Verapamil, Trimethoprim/sulfamethoxazole using PharmaZome
Elan	INDAS (Insoluble Drug Absorption System) for dihydropyridine compounds, e.g., nifedipine, isradipine, nicardipine Formulations for propranolol, indomethacin, prazozin, Capsules, Carbamazepine taste masking.
Elan:Syntex:Roche	Naproxen formulation
Elan:Pasteur Merieux	Trimethoprim/silfamethoxazole using PharmaZome technology
Elan:Roussel-Uclaf	Theophylline using PharmaZome system

Extensive studies with inhaled insulin, nasal insulin, and oral insulin have produced interesting findings with pulmonary delivery for coverage, with short-acting insulin having the brightest prospects. Encapsulated islets and biohybrid systems that place liver islets into an implanted device are in stages of development. Closing the loop with a continuous glucose sensor will be the only way to achieve truly normal blood glucose homeostasis by directing insulin delivery automatically on demand. Alternately, insulin has been delivered by a variety of routes (e.g., transdermal, buccal, ocular, rectal, vaginal, uterine, and subcutaneous).[135,143]

Successful oral delivery of insulin involves overcoming the barriers of enzymatic degradation, achieving epithelial permeability, and taking steps to conserve bioactivity during formulation processing. The use of enzyme (protease) inhibitors, permeation enhancers, calcium chelators, and polymer systems (with absorption modifiers) has been attempted to overcome these barriers. A synergistic approach, however, works best. The development of dosage forms with dual controlled-release characteristics using chicken or duck ovomucoids were investigated for enzymatic stability, permeability, and dissolution stability experiments. Biodegradable and nondegradable microspheres or nanospheres were studied for oral insulin delivery.[139,140–142,144,145]

Ovasome technology (Endorex Corp., Chicago, IL) is developing encapsulation of insulin/protein in liposomes, while Enisphere technology (New York) works with non-acylated alpha-amino acids as carriers for oral delivery of macromolecules and insulin. The M2 system (Nobex Corp., Research Triangle Park, NC) is based on the attachment of low molecular weight polymers to specific sites in the protein. These polymer conjugates have been reported to improve stability and absorption when compared with the performance of native protein.

In oral drug delivery, R.P. Scherer, Jenssen Pharmaceutica, and Pharmalyoc use lyophilization process and Zydis, Qucksolv, and Lyoc technologies, respectively,[149] while Cima Labs, Yamanouchi Pharma, Elan, Ethypharm, and Eurand use the tabletting process and Orasolv/Durasolv, WOWTABS, FEDAS, Flashtab, and Ziplets technologies, respectively. Biovail (Fuisz) uses the cotton-candy process and the Flashdose technology. Alza initially worked on the "Ringcap" technology, which was acquired by Alkermes. This system is based on a tablet preferentially film-coated, which is subsequently partially coated with a series of "rings" using an adaptation of the capsule-banding process. In this technology, the number of "rings" applied, and their respective thicknesses, provide the primary means for moderating the rate at which the drug is released from the final dosage form. In the matrix technology, two approaches were used in Contramid (Lactopharm) and Geomatrix (Skyepharma). Further developments include introduction of Smartrix and GlaxoSmithKline's Procise system. Combining conventional HPMC matrix technology with an upper and lower layer comprised mainly of the matrix polymer, this device purports to moderate drug release by matching an increase in surface area with the concomitant reduction in drug concentration within the device. The core matrix, in combination with an upper and lower compressed coating layer that erodes at a specific rate, is intended to provide a greater degree of precision over the manner in which the drug is released.

In the processing technologies,[146,147] BASF Pharma (now Abbott), Therics Sarnoff, Delsys, and Phoqus have developed new processes. In the Theriform (Therics) process, the technique uses an adaption of inkjet printing to fabricate tablets with precise architectures capable of providing a broad range of drug delivery possibilities. Delsys uses the Accudep process to apply electrostatically charged particles of a drug to a polymeric substratum held by an electrostatic module. Subsequently, the drug-loaded substratum is laminated with a second layer of polymeric film, and discs containing the drug are punched out from the laminate to create the final dosage form.[150-152] The technology employed by Phoqus represents an adaption of the electrophotography process employed in all common photocopying machines. Electrostatically applied coatings can be used to create unique appearance attributes, and an inherent ability to apply different coating formulations to different parts of the same tablet, or only to partially coat a tablet surface, provide a broad space in facilitating the design of highly specialized drug delivery systems (see Figure 5.4).[148]

Reo and Fredrickson[153] have discussed the latest developments in taste-masking science. Agents like sodium chloride, phosphatidic acid, and peppermint flavor are known to inhibit bitterness of select active pharmaceutical ingredients (API) molecules via a mechanism that takes place at the bitterness receptor in the taste buds. API crystallization techniques, such as crystal size distribution (CSD), spherical crystal agglomeration (SCA), and quasi-emulsion solvent diffusion (QESD), developed by solid-state scientists, chemical processing engineers, and formulation chemists can save time and resources for producing suitable API particles for taste and masking processing.[154-156]

Parenteral low molecular weight heparin (LMWH) has replaced warfarin as the standard of care for the prevention of deep-vein thrombosis and pulmonary embolism in high-risk hospitalized patients undergoing joint replacement or abdominal surgery. Compared with warfarin, LMWH has a significantly lower incidence of drug–drug interaction. The major disadvantage of LMWH therapy has been that it must be parenterally administered because it is ineffective when given orally. Several recent attempts to develop effective oral LMWH formulations have been reviewed by Sastry et al.[152] For example, complexes with tertiary amines, lipid-matrix-containing phosphatidylcholine from soy protein and medium-chain monoacyl glycerol and the use of glycerol esters of fatty acids and non-ionic surfactants. These authors also report the use of 8-[N2-hydroxybenzoyl)amino] caprylate (SNAC) and sodium 10-[N-(2-hydroxybenzoyl)amino]decanoate (SNAD) as delivery agents. They found that SNAC and SNAD facilitate the transport of LMWH across Caco-2-epithelial cells without opening the tight junctions or adversely affecting the structural integrity of the cell monolayer. Their studies also demonstrate that SNAC and SNAD facilitate oral LMWH absorption in rats and monkeys, and their combinations are not cytotoxic in a Caco-2 cell culture model.[136-138]

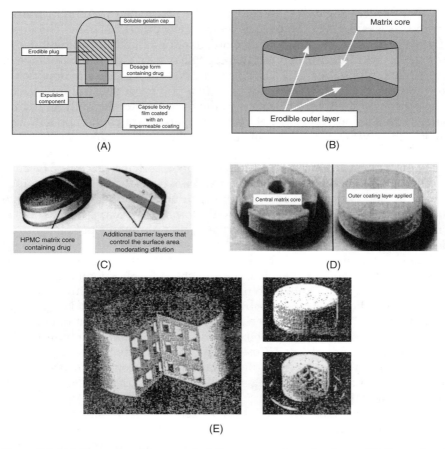

Figure 5.4 (A) Example of temporal delivery capsule technology. (B) Example of Smartrix technology. (C) Example of Geomatrix tablet. (D) Example of Procise technology. (E) Example of Therisys technology. (With permission, Russell Publ., *Am. Pharm. Rev.*, 4, 3, 28, 2001.)

In other experiments, it was reported that polymeric nanoparticles (NPs) prepared with biodegradable poly-epsilon-caprolactone and poly(lactic-co-glycolic)acid and nonbiodegradable positively charged polymers (Eudragit RS & RL), used alone or in combination, were evaluated *in vitro* and *in vivo* after a single oral administration of heparin-loaded NPs in rabbits. The authors concluded that the significant increases in anti-factor Xa activity and (aPTT)activated partial thromboplastin time confirmed the oral absorption in rabbits of heparin released from polymeric NPs.[157–160]

IX. Conclusion

The potential value of therapeutic drug delivery systems lies in a continuous controlled-release process that can proceed unattended for relatively long periods. Ideally, these systems will eliminate the need for frequent dosing and control fluctuating blood levels.

Oral sustained-release dosage forms are, to a large extent, elementary in their design and often imprecise in their ability to release a drug at a constant rate. However, because GI transit time limits these drug delivery systems to 8 to 12 hours, and because of our lack of knowledge of fundamental processes in the GI tract at the molecular and cellular levels, design must be either self-contained systems (i.e., independent of the environment) or systems that are elementary. Presumably, the next generation of controlled-release oral dosage forms will be based in part on a strategy developed from a mechanistic understanding of GI physiology.[111]

Traditionally, an important element of oral controlled-release dosage forms has been the need for strict adherence to zero-order kinetics. Given that many drugs enjoy a reasonably wide therapeutic range and that 10 to 30% differences in blood-drug levels will usually not show a change in biological response, perhaps too much has been made of this requirement. Within experimental error, a number of release-rate kinetic orders cannot be distinguished on the basis of the resulting blood levels.[112–118]

It is apparent that controlled drug delivery is a strategy that will remain popular for the foreseeable future and that the oral route will be a dominant approach. To date, the majority of new products claiming to be controlled-release systems are really extensions of old technologies with no great improvement in clinical performance. Nonetheless, given the current efforts being made in oral controlled delivery and our increasing knowledge base in GI physiology, it is likely that a substantial number of new products will emerge in this decade.[119–124]

References

1. Banker, G.S., Pharmaceutical applications of controlled release: an overview of the past, present, and future. In *Medical Applications of Controlled Release*, Vol. 2, Langer, R.S. and Wise, D.L., Eds., CRC Press, Inc., Boca Raton, FL, 1–34, 1984.
2. Blythe, R.H., U.S. Patent 2,738,303, 1956.
3. Anon., Oral sustained products — pro's and con's, *Drug and Therapeutics Bulletin*, 22, 57–60, 1984.
4. Shaw, J.E., Drug delivery systems. In *Annual Reports in Medicinal Chemistry*, Vol. 15, Academic Press, Inc., New York, 302–315, 1980.
5. Zaffaroni, A., *Proc. Sixth Int. Congress of Pharmacology*, Vol. 5, Tuomisto, J. and Paasonen, M.K., Eds., Forsan Kirjapaino Oy Helsinki, 53, 1975.
6. Heilmann, K., Therapeutic systems-pattern-specific drug delivery: concept and development, *G. Thieme*, Stuttgart, 1978.
7. Yates, F.E., Benson, H., Buckles, J., Urquhart, J., and Zaffaroni, A., *Advances in Biomedical Engineering*, Vol. 5, Brown, J.H.U. and Dickson, J.F. III, Eds., Academic Press, New York, 1, 1975.

8. Urquhart, J., *Proc. Sixth Int. Congress of Pharmacology*, Vol. 5, Tuomisto, J. and Paasonen, M.K., Eds., Forsaan Kirjapaino Oy Helsinki, 63, 1975.

9. Zaffaroni, A., In *Drug Metabolism Review*, Vol. 8, DiCarlo, F., Ed., Marcel Dekker, New York, 191, 1978.

10. Davis, S.S., *Evaluation of the Gastrointestinal Transit and Release Characteristics of Drugs*, Johnson, P. and Lloyd-Jones, J.G., Eds., VCH Publishers, Chichester, 164–179, 1987; also see Ganderton, D., Technological advances in oral drug delivery, 150–163.

11. Ho, N.F.H., Merkle, H.P., and Higuchi, W.I., Quantitative, mechanistic and physiological realistic approach to the biopharmaceutical design of oral drug delivery systems, *Drug Development and Industrial Pharmacy*, 9, 1111–1184, 1983.

12. Antonin, H.K.H., Bieck, P., Scheurlen, M., Jedrychowski, M., and Malchow, H., Oxprenolol absorption in man after single bolus dosing into two segments of the colon compared with that after oral dosing, *Br. J. Clin. Pharmac.*, 19, 137S-142S, 1985.

13. Bruck, S.D., Pharmacological basis of controlled drug delivery. In *Controlled Drug Delivery*, Vol. 1, Basic Concepts, Bruck, S.D., Ed., CRC Press, Inc., Boca Raton, FL, 1–13, 1983.

14. John, V.A., Shotton, P.A., Moppert, J., and Theobald, W., Gastrointestinal transit of Oros drug delivery systems in healthy volunteers: a short report. *Br. J. Clin. Pharmac.*, 19, 203S-206S, 1985.

15. Davis, S.S., The use of scinigraphic methods for the evaluation of novel delivery systems. In *Directed Drug Delivery: A Multidisciplinery Problem*, Borchardt, R.T., Repta, A.J., and Stella, V.J., Eds., Humana Press, Totowa, NJ, 319–340, 1985.

16. Peppas, N.A., Mathematical models for controlled release kinetics. In *Medical Applications of Controlled Release*, Vol. 2, Langer, R.S. and Wise, D.L., Eds., CRC Press, Inc., Boca Raton, FL, 169–187, 1984.

17. Hopfenberg, H.B., Controlled release from edible slabs, cylinders and spheres. In *Controlled Release Polymeric Formulations*, Paul, D.R. and Harris, F.W., Eds., American Chemical Society Symposium Series, Washington, D.C., 33, 26, 1976.

18. Lee, P.I., Diffusional release of a solute from a polymeric matrix: approximate analytical solutions, *J. Membr. Sci.*, 7, 255, 1980.

19. Anderson, J.A. and Olanoff, L.S., Pharmacokinetic modeling and bioavailability. In *Medical Applications of Controlled Release*, Vol. 2, Langer, R.S. and Wise, D.L., Eds., CRC Press, Inc., Boca Raton, FL, 189–219, 1984.

20. Baker, R.W. and Lonsdale, H.K., Controlled release: Mechanisms and rates. In *Controlled Release of Biologically Active Agents*, Tanquary, A.C. and Lacey, R.E., Eds., Plenum Press, Inc., NY, 15, 1974.

21. Notari, R.E., *Biopharmaceutics and Pharmacokinetics*, 2nd ed., Marcel Dekker, New York, 1975.

22. Schneider, H., Nightingale, C.H., Quintrilliani, R., and Fanagan, D.R., Evaluation of an oral prolonged-release antibiotic formulation, *J. Pharm. Sci.*, 67, 1620, 1978.

23. Beckett, A.H. and Slipper, J.A., The importance of dissolution test media in *in vitro* and *in vivo* correlations of formulations of disopyramide. In *FIB 81 Abstracts, Programme of Short Communications*, 41st Int. Cong. Pharm. Sci., Vienna, Austria, 1981, 133.

24. Turi, P., Dauvois, M., and Michaeles, A.S., Continuous dissolution rate determination as a function of the pH of the medium, *J. Pharm. Sci.*, 65, 806, 1976.

25. Good, W.R. and Lee, P.I., Membrane-controlled reservoir drug delivery systems. In *Medical Applications of Controlled Release*, Vol. 1, Langer, R.S. and Wise, D.L., Eds., CRC Press, Inc., Boca Raton, FL, 1–39, 1984; also see Wagner, J.G., Biopharmaceutics and relevant pharmacokinetics, *Drug Intelligence Publications*, Hamilton, IL, 1971.
26. Harris, M.S., Preparation and release kinetics of potassium chloride microcapsules, *J. Pharm. Sci.*, 70, 391, 1981.
27. Bakan, J.A., Microcapsule drug delivery systems. In *Polymers in Medicine and Surgery*, Kronenthal, R.L., Oser, Z., and Martin, E., Eds., Plenum Press, New York, 1975.
28. Sears, B.D., U.S. Patent 4,145,410, 1979.
29. Shank, J.L., U.S. Patent 4,001,480, 1977.
30. Kawashima, Y., Ohno, H., and Takenaka, H., Preparation of spherical matrixes of prolonged-release drugs from liquid suspension, *J. Pharm. Sci.*, 70, 913, 1981.
31. Heller, J. and Trescony, P.V., Controlled drug release by polymer dissolution, II. Enzyme-mediated delivery device, *J. Pharm. Sci.*, 68, 919, 1979.
32. Theeuwes, F. and Higuchi, T., U.S. Patent 3,916,899, 1975.
33. Theeuwes, F., Elementary osmotic pumps, *J. Pharm. Sci.*, 64, 1987, 1975.
34. Johnson, J.C., *Sustained Release Medications*, Noyes Data Corp., Park Ridge, NJ, 1980.
35. Chandrasekaran, S.K., Theeuwes, F., and Yum, S.I., The design of controlled drug delivery systems. In *Drug Design*, Vol. 8, Academic Press, New York, 133–167, 1979.
36. Hendeles, L., Bighley, L., Richardson, R., Heples, C.D., and Carmichael, J., *Drug. Intell. Clin. Pharm.*, 11, 12–18, 1977.
37. Park, K., Wood, R.W., and Robinson, J.R., Oral controlled-release systems. In *Medical Applications of Controlled Release*, Vol. 1, Langer, R.S. and Wise, D.L., Eds., CRC Press, Inc., Boca Raton, FL, 159–201, 1984.
38. Michaels, A.S., Wong, P.S.L., Prather, R., and Gale, R.M., *AIChE J.*, 21, 1073, 1975.
39. Good, W.R. and Mueller, K.F., *Controlled Release of Bioactive Materials*, Baker, R., Ed., Academic Press, New York, 155, 1980.
40. Good, W.R., *Polymeric Delivery Systems*, Vol. 5, Kastelnick, R., Ed., Midland Macromolecular Monograph, Gordon & Breach, New York, 139, 1978.
41. Mueller, K.F. and Heiber, S.J., *J. Appl. Polym. Sci.*, 27, 1982.
42. Lee, P.I., *Controlled Release of Bioactive Materials*, Baker, R., Ed., Academic Press, New York, 135, 1980.
43. Lee, P.I., *Proc. Ninth Int. Symp. Controlled Release of Bioactive Materials*, Controlled Release Society, 54, 1982.
44. Yasuda, H., Lamaze, C.E., and Peterlim, A.J., *Polymer Sci.*, Part A, 9, 1117, 1971.
45. Zentner, G.M., Cardinal, J.R., and Gregonis, D.E., Progestrin permeative through polymer membranes, III. Polymerization solvent effect on progesterone permeation through hydrated membranes, *J. Pharm. Sci.*, 68, 794, 1979.
46. Chen, R.Y.S., Polymer preparation, Am. Chem. Soc., *Div. Polym. Chem.*, 15(2), 387, 1974.
47. Wisniewski, S.J., Gregonis, D.E., Kim, S.W., and Andrade, J.D., *Hydrogels for Medical and Related Applications*, Andrade, J.D., Ed., American Chemical Society, Washington, D.C., 1976.

48. Higuchi, T., Rate of release of medicaments from ointment bases containing drugs in suspension, *J. Pharm. Sci.*, 50, 874, 1961.
49. Higuchi, T. Mechanism of sustained action medication: theoretical analysis of rate of release of solid drugs dispersed in solid matrices, *J. Pharm. Sci.*, 52, 1145, 1963.
50. Ginzburg, B.Z. and Katchalsky, A., *J. Gen. Physiol.*, 47, 403, 1963.
51. Helfferich, F., *Ion Exchange*, McGraw-Hill, New York, 339, 1962.
52. Lightfoot, E.N., *Transport Phenomena and Living Systems*, John Wiley & Sons, New York, 1974.
53. Flynn, G.L., Yalkowski, S.H., and Roseman, T.J., Mass transport phenomena and models: theoretical concepts, *J. Pharm. Sci.*, 63, 479, 1974.
54. Watanabe, S., Kayano, M., Ishino, Y., and Miyao, K., U.S. Patent 3,976,764, 1976.
55. Sheth, P.R. and Tossounian, J.F., U.S. Patent, 4,126,672, 1978.
56. Timko, R.J. and Lordi, N.G. *In vitro* evaluation of three commercial sustained-release papaverine hydrochloride products, *J. Pharm. Sci.*, 67, 496, 1978.
57. Amidon, G.L., Leesman, G.D., and Elliott, R.L. Improving intestinal absorption of water-insoluble compounds: a membrane metabolism strategy, *J. Pharm. Sci.*, 69, 1363, 1980.
58. Luzzi, C.A. and Gerraughty, R.J., Effect of additions and formulation techniques on controlled release of drugs from microcapsules, *J. Pharm. Sci.*, 56, 1174, 1967.
59. Luzzi, C.A., Zoglio, M.A., and Maulding, H.V., Preparation and evaluation of the prolonged release properties of nylon microcapsules, *J. Pharm. Sci.*, 59, 338, 1970.
60. Lehmann, K., *Pharm. Int.*, 3, 34, 1971.
61. Kakemi, K., Arita, T., Sezaki, H., and Sugimoto, I., *Arch. Pract. Pharm.*, 25, 19, 1965.
62. Ponomareff-Bauumann, M., Soliva, M., and Speiser, P., *Pharm. Acta Helv.*, 43, 158, 1968.
63. Ritschel, W.A. and Clotten, R., Entwicklung einer peroralen Nitroglycerin-Proxyphyllin-Retard-Form, *Arzneim-Forsch*, 20, 1180, 1970.
64. Determann, H. and Lotz, R., *Pharm. Ind.*, 32, 469, 1970.
65. Huber, H.E. and Christenson, G.L., Utilization of hydrophilic gums for the control of drug substance release from tablet formulations, II. Influence of tablet hardness and density on dissolution behavior, *J. Pharm. Sci.*, 57, 164, 1968.
66. Levy, G. and Hollister, L.E., Dissolution rate limited absorption in man: Factors influencing drug absorption from prolonged release dosage form, *J. Pharm. Sci.*, 54, 1121, 1965.
67. Khanna, S.C., Jecklin, T., and Speiser, P., Bead polymerization technique for sustained-release dosage form, *J. Pharm. Sci.*, 59, 614, 1970.
68. Widmann, A., Eiden, F., and Tenczer, J., Die Wirkstoff-Freigabe aus Depot-Weichgalatinekapseln, *Arzneim-Forsch*, 20, 283, 1970.
69. Cavallito, C.J., Califez, L., and Miller, L.D., Some studies of sustained release principle, *J. Pharm. Sci.*, 52, 259, 1963.
70. Ritschel, W.A., Peroral solid dosage forms with prolonged action. In *Drug Design*, Vol. 4, Academic Press, New York, 37–73, 1973.
71. Nagai, T., Yi, Q.D., Akitoshi, Y., and Takayama, K., Effect of cyclohexanone derivatives on percutaneous absorption of ketoprofen and indomethacin, *Program and Abstracts of the 15th Int. Symp. Control. Rel. Bioact. Mater.*, 87, August 1988.

72. Robinson, J.R., Recent developments in controlled oral drug delivery. In *The Latest Developments in Drug Delivery Systems, Conf. Proc. Pharm. Tech.*, 48–52, 1985.

73. DeCoursin, J.W., The controlled-release oral drug delivery opportunity. In *The Latest Developments in Drug Delivery Systems, Conf. Proc. Pharm. Tech.*, 29–32, 1985.

74. Pharmaprojects, 1993.

75. Anderson, J.L. and Powell, T.C., U.S. Patent 3,909,444, 1975.

76. Rembaum, A., U.S. Patent 4,046,750, 1977.

77. Blichare, M.S. and Jackson, G.L. Jr., U.S. Patent 4,132,753, 1979.

78. Baukal, W., Kinkel, H.J., Robens, E., and Walter, G., U.S. Patent 3,923,969, 1975.

79. Estevenel, Y.F.M.J., Thely, M.H., and Coulon, W.A., U.S. Patent 3,922,338, 1975.

80. Leiberich, R. and Gabler, W., U.S. Patent 3,959,540, 1976.

81. Controulis, J., Larsen, K.N., and Wheeler, L.M., U.S. Patent 3,823,816, 1974.

82. Higuchi, T. and Leeper, H.M., U.S. Patent 4,034,756, 1977.

83. Beringer, M. and Woltmann, S., U.S. Patent 4,139,589, 1979.

84. Michaelis, A.F., U.S. Patent 4,088798, 1978.

85. Huber, H.E., U.S. Patent 4,122157, 1978.

86. Gordon, H.W. and Schaffner, C.P., U.S. Patent 4,064,230, 1977.

87. Sato, T., Kobashi, T., Mayama, T., and Okada, A., U.S. Patent 4,127,647, 1978.

88. Farhadieh, A., U.S. Patent 3,922,379, 1975; also see Amann, A.H., U.S. Patent 3,865,935, 1975.

89. Guy, M.G. and Powers, R.G., U.S. Patent 4,025,613, 1977.

90. Hill, W.H., U.S. Patent 3,946,110, 1976.

91. Vergnaud, J.M., Magron, P., Rollet, J., and Taverdet, J.L., Modeling of composite polymers-drug compounds for controlled release of drug in stomach, *Proc. Int. Symp. Control. Rel. Bioactive Mater.*, 14, 73, Controlled Release Society, Inc., 1987.

92. Pouton, C.W., Wakerly, M.G., and Meakin, B.J., Self-emulsifying systems for oral delivery of drugs, *Proc. Int. Symp. Control. Rel. Bioactive Mater.*, 14, 113, Controlled Release Society, Inc., 1987.

93. Schlameus, H.W., Swynnerton, N.F., Mangold, D.J., Gayton Jr., J.H., et al., Development of orally-active sustained-release dosage forms for steroids, *Proc. Int. Symp. Control. Rel. Bioactive Mater.*, 14, 119, Controlled Release Society, Inc., 1987.

94. Lin, S.Y. and Yang, J.C., Tablet properties and dissolution behaviour of compressed theophylline ethylcellulose microcapsules, *Proc. Int. Symp. Control. Rel. Bioactive Mater.*, 14, 154, Controlled Release Society, Inc., 1987.

95. Chattaraj, S.C., Das, S.K., and Gupta, B.K., *In vivo–in vitro* correlation of drug release from ethyl cellulose microcapsules containing ranitidine hydrochloride, *Proc. Int. Symp. Control Rel. Bioactive Mater.*, 14, 308, Controlled Release Society, Inc., 1987.

96. Gilley, R.M., Eldridge, J.H., Opitz, J.L., Hanna, L.K., et al., Development of secretory immunity following oral administration of microencapsulated antigens, *15th Int. Symp. Control. Rel. Bioactive Mater.*, Abstract No. 72, Controlled Release Society, Inc., 1988.

97. Oh, K.H. and Bodmeier, R. A., novel approach to the oral delivery of micro- and nanoparticles, *15th Int. Symp. Control. Rel. Bioactive Mater.*, Abstract No. 194, Controlled Release Society, Inc., 1988.

98. Shefer, S. and Kost, J., Starch microbeads for enzymatic controlled oral drug delivery, *15th Int. Symp. Control. Rel. Bioactive Mater.*, Abstract No. 198, Controlled Release Society, Inc., 1988.

99. Eldem, T., Speiser, P., and Hincal, A., Formulation studies on lipid pellets as steroid carriers for oral contraception, *15th Int. Symp. Control. Rel. Bioactive Mater.*, Abstract No. 247, Controlled Release Society, Inc., 1988.

100. Herman, J. and Remon, J.P., Modified starches as hydrophilic matrices for controlled oral delivery systems, *Program and Abstracts, 15th Int. Symp. Control. Rel. Bioact. Mater.*, 126, August 1988.

101. Lejoyeux, F., Ponchel, G., Wouessidjewe, D., Peppas, N.A., and Duchene, D., Influence of the composition of the testing medium on the adhesion of a bioadhesive tablet to a biological fabric, *15th Int. Symp. Control. Rel. Bioactive Mater.* Abstract No. 261, Controlled Release Society, Inc., 1988.

102. Ishino, R., Yoshino, H., Hirakawa, Y., and Noda, K., Design and preparation of pulsatile release tablet as a new oral drug delivery system, *Chem. Pharm. Bull.*, 40, 3036–3041, 1992.

103. Ishikawa, M., Matsuna, Y., Noguchi, A., and Kuzuya, M., A new drug delivery system (DDS) development using plasma-irradiated pharmaceutical aids, *Chem. Pharm. Bull.*, 41, 1626–1631, 1993.

104. Chandy, T. and Sharma, C.P., Chitosan matrix for oral sustained delivery of ampicillin, *Biomaterials*, 14, 939–944, 1993.

105. Kararli, T.T., Needham, T.E., Griffin, M., Schoenhard, G., Ferro, L.J., and Alcorn, L., Oral delivery of a renin inhibitor compound using emulsion formulations, *Pharm. Res.*, 9, 888–893, 1992.

106. Bachynsky, M. et al., U.S. Patent 5,190,748, March 2, 1993.

107. Weintraub, H. and Gibaldi, M., Rotating-flask method for dissolution-rate determinations of aspirin from various dosage forms, *J. Pharm. Sci.*, 59, 1792, 1970.

108. Place, V. et al., PCT Application (WO), 92 01,445.

109. Starr, C., Word of mouth: a review of new oral delivery systems, *Drug Topics*, March 23, 1992, 29–30.

110. Bidah, D. and Vergnaud, J.M., New oral dosage form with two polymers: Gelucire and Sumikagel, *Int. J. Pharm.*, 72, 35–41, 1991.

111. Eckenhoff, B., Theeuwes, F., and Urquhart, J., Osmotically actuated dosage forms for rate-controlled drug delivery, *Pharm. Tech.*, 11, 96–105, 1987.

112. Smith, P.L., Wall, D.A., Gochoco, C.H., and Wilson, G., Oral absorption of peptides and proteins, *Adv. Drug Del. Rev.*, 8, 253–290, 1992.

113. Friend, D.R. in *Oral Colon-Specific Drug Delivery*, CRC Press, Inc., Boca Raton, FL, 268, 1982.

114. Chang, R., *Pharm. Tech.*, March 1992, 134.

115. Lee, V.H.L., Oral route of peptide and protein drug delivery, *Bio. Pharm.*, July–August 1992, 39–42.

116. Ichikawa, M., Kato, T., Kawahara, M., Watanabe, S., and Kayano, M., A new multiple-unit oral floating dosage system, II., *J. Pharm. Sci.*, 80, 1153–1156, 1991.

117. Ichikawa, M., Watanabe, S., and Miyake, Y., A new multiple-unit oral floating dosage system, I., *J. Pharm. Sci.*, 80, 1062–1066, 1991.

118. Harris, D. and Robinson, J.R., Drug delivery via the mucous membranes of the oral cavity, *J. Pharm. Sci.*, 81, 1–10, 1992.

119. Yacobi, A. and Halperin-Walega, E., In *Oral Sustained Release Formulations: Design and Evaluation*, A. Wheaton & Co., Exeter, U.K., 1988.

120. Robinson, J.R. and Lee, V.H.L., *Controlled Drug Delivery, Fundamentals and Applications*, 2nd ed., Marcel Dekker, New York, 1987.
121. Baker, R., *Controlled Release of Biologically Active Agents*, John Wiley & Sons, New York, 1987.
122. Morley, J.S., *Drug Design and Delivery*, Harwood Academic Publications, New York, 1986.
123. Hsieh, D.S.T., *Controlled Release Systems: Fabrication Technology*, CRC Press, Boca Raton, FL, 1988.
124. Hoffman, A., Babay, D., and Benita, S., The design of controlled release indomethacin microspheres for oral use, *Proc. 14th Int. Symp. Control. Rel. Bioact. Mater.*, 115, August 1987.
125. Yamamoto, A., Improvement of transmucosal absorption of biologically active peptide drugs, *Yakugaku Zasshi.*, 121, 929–948, 2001.
126. Lavelle, E.C., Targeted delivery of drugs to the gastrointestinal tract, *Crit. Rev. Ther. Drug Carrier Syst.*, 18, 341–386, 2001.
127. Leone-Bay, A. et al., Oral delivery of biologically active parathyroid hormone, *Pharm. Res.*, 18, 964–970, 2001.
128. Ramnathan, S. et al., Targeting the sodium-dependent multivitamin transporter (SMVT) for improving the oral absorption properties of a retro-inverseo Tat nonapeptide, *Pharm. Res.*, 18, 950–956, 2001.
129. Wong, A. and Toth, I., Lipid, sugar and liposaccharide based delivery systems, *Curr. Med. Chem.*, 8, 1123–1136, 2001.
130. Pouton, C.W., Lipid formulations for oral administration of drugs, non-emulsifying self-emulsifying and self-microemulsifying drug delivery system, *Eur. J. Pharm. Sci.*, 11 Suppl 2, S93–S98, 2000.
131. Fukui, E. and Miyamura, N., Preparation of enteric coated timed-release press-coated tablets and evaluation of their function by *in vitro* and *in vivo* tests for colon targeting, *Int. J. Pharm.*, 204, (1–2) 7–15, 2000.
132. Carelli, V. and Di Colo, G., Polyoxyethylene-poly(methacrylic acid-co-methyl methacrylate) compounds for site-specific peroral delivery, *Int. J. Pharm.*, 202, (1–2), 103–112, 2000.
133. Krogel, I. and Bodmeier, R., Evaluation of an enzyme-containing capsular shaped pulsatile drug delivery system, *Pharm. Res.*, 16, 1424–1429, 1999.
134. Axelrod, H.R. and Kim, J.S., Intestinal transport of gentamicin with a novel glycosteroid drug transport agent, *Pharm. Res.*, 15, 1876–1881, 1998.
135. Leone-Bay, T., O'Shaughnessy, C., et al., Oral low molecular weight heparin absorption, *Pharm. Tech.*, 26, 38–46, 2002.
136. Herr, D., Increasing the enteral absorption of heparin or heparinoids, U.S. Patent 4,656,161, 1987.
137. Gonze, M.D. et al., Orally administered unfractionated heparin with carrier is therapeutic for deep vein thrombosis, *Circulation*, 2638–2661, 2000.
138. Quan, Y.S. et al., Effectiveness and toxicity screening of various absorption enhancers using Caco-2 cell monolayers, *Biol. Pharm. Bull.*, 21, 615–620, 1998.
139. Agarwal, V. and Khan, M.A., Current status of the oral delivery of insulin, *Pharm. Tech.*, 25, 76–90, 2001.
140. Johnson, O., Formulations of proteins for incorporation into drug delivery systems. In *Protein Formulation and Delivery*, McNally, E.I., Ed., Marcel Dekker, New York, 2000.

141. Forbes, R.T. et al., Water vapor sorption studies on the physical stability of a series of spray-dried protein/sugar powders for inhalation, *J. Pharm. Sci.*, 87, 1316–1321, 1998.

142. Tozaki, H. et al., Degradation of insulin and calcitonin and their production by various protease inhibitors in rat caecal contents: implications in peptide delivery to the colon, *J. Pharm. Pharmacol.*, 49, 164–168, 1997.

143. Agarwal, V. et al., Polymethylacrylate microcapsules of insulin for oral delivery, Preparation and *in vitro* dissolution stability in the presence of enzyme inhibitors, *Int. J. Pharm.*, 225, 31–39, 2001.

144. Marschutz, M.K. and Bernkop-Schnurch, A., Oral peptide drug delivery: polymer inhibitor conjugates protecting insulin from enzymatic degradation *in vitro*, *Biomaterials*, 21, 1499–1507, 2000.

145. Damge, C. et al., New approach for oral administration of insulin with polyalkylcyanoacrylate nanocapsules as drug carrier, *Diabetes*, 37, 246–251, 1988.

146. Milstein, S.J. et al., Partially unfolded proteins efficiently penetrate cell membranes: implications for oral drug delivery, *J. Controlled Release*, 53, 259–267, 1998.

147. McPhillips, A. et al., Evaluation of fluid-bed applied acrylic polymers for the targeted peroral delivery of insulin, *STP Pharma. Sciences*, 7, 476–482, 1997.

148. Porter, S.C., Novel drug delivery: review of recent trends with oral solid dosage forms, *Am. Pharm. Rev.*, 4, 28–35, 2001.

149. Seager, H., Drug delivery products and the Zydis fast dissolving dosage form, *J. Pharm. Pharmacol.*, 50, 375–382, 1998.

150. McConville, J.T. et al., Processing induced variability of time-delayed delivery from a pulsatile capsule device, *Proc. AAPS Annual Meeting*, Indianapolis, 2000.

151. Zerbe, H.G. and Ktrumme, M., Design characteristics and release properties of a novel, erosion controlled oral delivery system. In *Modified Release Drug Delivery Technology*, Rathbone, Hadgraft, and Roberts, Eds., Marcel Dekker, in press.

152. Sastry, S.V. et al., Recent technological advances in oral drug delivery: a review, *PSST*, 3(4) 138–145, 2000.

153. Reo, J.P. and Fredrickson, J.K., Taste masking science and technology applied to compacted oral solid dosage, Part I, *Am. Pharm. Rev.*, 5, 8–14, 2002.

154. Desijan, S., Anderson, S.R., et al., Crystallization challenges in drug development: scale-up from laboratory to pilot plant and beyond, *Cur. Opin. Drug Dis. Dev.*, 3, 723–733, 2000.

155. Rapaport, H. et al., From nucleatuin to engineering of crystalline architectures at air-liquid interfaces, *J. Phy. Chem. Part B.*, 104, 1399–1428, 2000.

156. Shekunov, Y. and York, P., Crystallization processes in pharmaceutical technology and drug delivery design, *J. Crystl. Growth*, 211, 122–136, 2000.

157. Kawashima, Y. et al., Preparation of spherically granulated crystals of waxy drug(tocopherol nicotinate) for direct tableting by spherical crystallization technique, *World Cong., Part. Technol.*, 3, 1121–1130, 1998.

158. Espitalier, F. et al., Modelling of the mechanism of formation of spherical grains obtained by the quasi-emulsion crystallization process, *TransIChemE*, 75(A2), 257–267, 1997.

159. Reo, J.P. and Fredrickson, J.K., Taste masking science and technology applied to compacted oral dosage forms, Part 3, *Am. Pharm. Rev.*, 5, 8–14, 2002.

160. Hauss, D.J., Liquid-based systems for oral drug delivery: enhancing the bioavailability of poorly water soluble drugs, *Am. Pharm. Rev.*, 5, 22–28, 2002.

section four

Transdermal, intranasal, ocular, and miscellaneous drug delivery

chapter six

Transdermal drug delivery*

Contents

I.   Introduction

Although some drugs have inherent side effects that cannot be eliminated in any dosage form, many drugs exhibit undesirable behavior that is specifically related to a particular route of administration. One recent effort at eliminating some of the problems of traditional dosage forms is the development of transdermal delivery systems.

Oral administration of drugs has been practiced for centuries and, most recently, through tablets and capsules. Injectables came into being approxi-

* Adapted from Ranade, V.V., Drug delivery systems. 6. Transdermal drug delivery, *J. Clin. Pharmacol.*, 31, 401, 1991. With permission of *J. Clin. Pharmacol.* and J.B. Lippincott Publishing Company, Philadelphia, PA.

mately 130 years ago, but have only become acceptable since the development of a better understanding of sterilization. Topical application has also been used for centuries, predominantly in the treatment of localized skin diseases. Local treatment requires only that the drug permeate the outer layers of the skin to treat the diseased state, with the hope that this occurs with little or no systemic accumulation.[1]

Transdermal delivery systems, on the other hand, are specifically designed to obtain systemic blood levels and have been used in the U.S. since the 1950s. Transdermal permeation, or percutaneous absorption, can be defined as the passage of a substance, such as a drug, from the outside of the skin through its various layers into the bloodstream. Any time there is systemic access of a drug, unwanted side effects or toxic effects can occur. Certainly, each dosage form has its unique place in medicine, but some attributes of the transdermal delivery system provide distinct advantages over traditional methods. Cleary[1] has listed important advantages and disadvantages of transdermal delivery systems. The advantages are: the system avoids the chemically hostile gastrointestinal (GI) environment; no GI distress or other physiological contraindications of the oral route exist; the system can provide adequate absorption of certain drugs; there is increased patient compliance; the system avoids the first-pass effect; the system allows for the effective use of drugs with short biological half-lives; the system allows for the administration of drugs with narrow therapeutic windows; the system provides controlled plasma levels of highly potent drugs; drug input can be promptly interrupted should toxicity occur. Disadvantages of this system include: drugs that require high blood levels cannot be administered; the adhesive used may not adhere well to all types of skin; drug or drug formulation may cause skin irritation or sensitization; the patches can be uncomfortable to wear; and this system may not be economical for some patients.[1,2]

In the development of transdermal delivery systems, a series of interrelated elements must be taken into consideration. These elements can be classified into five basic areas: bioactivity of the drug, skin characteristics, formulation, adhesion, and system design. The transport of drugs through the skin is complex since many factors influence their permeation. To simplify the situation somewhat, one should consider the following: skin structure and its properties, the penetrating molecule and its physical–chemical relationship to the skin and the delivery platform, the platform or delivery system carrying the penetrant, and the combination of skin, penetrant, and delivery system as a whole. The major emphasis of this chapter is on discussing each of these factors, their complexities, and their interdependencies in the development of transdermal delivery systems.[3,4]

II.   Structure of human skin

As has been discussed by Barry et al.,[5] human skin consists of two distinct layers: the stratified avascular cellular epidermis and an underlying dermis of connective tissue. A fatty subcutaneous layer resides beneath the dermis.

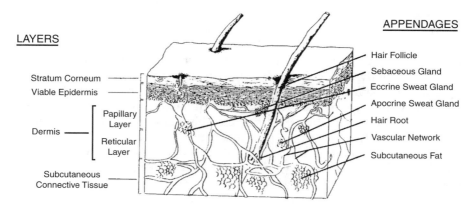

LAYERS

Stratum Corneum
Viable Epidermis

Papillary Layer
Dermis
Reticular Layer

Subcutaneous Connective Tissue

APPENDAGES

Hair Follicle
Sebaceous Gland
Eccrine Sweat Gland
Apocrine Sweat Gland
Hair Root
Vascular Network
Subcutaneous Fat

Figure 6.1 Basic diagram of skin structure. (From Langer and Wise, Eds., *Medical Applications of Controlled Release*, CRC Press, Boca Raton, FL, 1984, 207.)

Hairy skin develops hair follicles and sebaceous glands, and the highly vascularized dermis supports the apocrine and eccrine sweat glands, which pass through pores in the epidermis to reach the skin surface. With respect to drug permeation, the most important component in this complex membrane is the stratum corneum, or horny layer, which usually provides the rate-limiting or slowest step in the penetration process.

The transport mechanisms by which drugs cross the intact skin have not yet been completely elucidated. However, possible macro-routes may comprise the transepidermal pathway (across the horny layer either intra- or intercellularly) or via the hair follicles and sweat glands (the appendageal route). The appendageal route may be of significance for short diffusional times and for polar molecules. Until recently, it was believed that, for polar molecules, the probable route was via the hydrated keratin of the corneocyte. However, it now seems more probable that the dominant pathway is via the polar region of intercellular lipid, with the lipid chains providing the non-polar routes[6–10] (see Figure 6.1).

The relative importance of these routes depends upon numerous factors, such as the time-scale of permeation (steady-state vs. transient diffusion), the physicochemical properties of the penetrant (e.g., pKa, molecular size, stability, binding affinity, solubility, and partition coefficient), integrity and thickness of the stratum corneum, density of sweat glands and follicles, skin hydration, metabolism, and vehicle effects.

In order to develop a topical system, there is a definite need for a stable preparation of the drug with a correct partition coefficient relative to the drug reservoir, device membrane, and skin layers. For the type of transdermal delivery device that incorporates a rate-controlling membrane, the flux across this barrier should be low enough so that the underlying skin acts as a sink. This could be a severe restriction because of the general impermeability of the stratum corneum. If the horny layer cannot be utilized as a sink, then the individual patient's skin will control drug input, and variable consequences can ensue due to the significant biological variability existing between people and from different skin sites.

Many pharmacologically active drugs have inappropriate physiochemical properties to partition into the skin. An important effort in the future will undoubtedly be devoted to synthesizing suitable pro-drugs to optimize the partition coefficient, stratum corneum penetration, and vehicle. In developing new drug entities, more attention will have to be paid to producing chemicals with low melting points (preferably liquids at biological temperatures) and to include penetration-enhancing substances.

In traversing the skin, the drug must partition into the stratum corneum and diffuse through this nearly impermeable barrier. Following this pathway, the molecules will have to interact with many potential binding sites, possibly forming a reservoir operating for days or even weeks. Free drug will eventually reach the interface between the stratum corneum and the epidermis, where the drug will have to partition into this water-rich tissue. There is a potential problem here in that a drug or pro-drug designed to partition from a vehicle into the horny layer may then have difficulty leaving the stratum corneum to enter the epidermis. For drugs that are lipid-soluble, clearance from the living tissue may replace diffusion through the stratum corneum, and this could be the rate-limiting step.[11-15]

Light, oxygen, and bacteria can influence the microenvironment of the skin surface. For example, skin microflora can destroy nitroglycerin and steroid esters. Occlusive systems, such as transdermal devices, when applied for several days, may cause problems with changes in skin flora, as well as with maceration and irritation of the skin, since prolonged application can make sweat glands ineffective.[16] In addition, the skin is a storehouse of enzymes which can have activities 80 to 90% as efficient as those present in the liver. Hydrolytic, oxidative, reductive, and conjugative reactions can all take place in the skin. One possible reason why activities approach those in the liver is the extreme dilution at which molecules cross the epidermis. As a result, the process renders them subject to attack. However, this is counterbalanced by the much greater permeation rates compared with those operating within the stratum corneum. Metabolism can alter permeation pharmacokinetics, activating pro-drugs and destroying active drugs, while generating active and inactive metabolites.

A future possibility may be to incorporate enzyme inhibitors into the devices to protect the drugs. In the epidermis, the drug comes in contact with pharmacological receptors as it approaches the epidermal/dermal boundary, where it then partitions into the dermis. Since both tissues consist mainly of water, it is preferable that the partition coefficient be approximately 1, provided that no different binding sites are in close proximity on either side of the interface. It is possible that, over time, sensitization reactions can occur in a small percentage of the patient population when any chemical is delivered via an unusual route (i.e., one to which the body is not accustomed). This phenomenon of sensitization has been observed with clonidine, and it may occur with other drugs, enhancers, enzyme inhibitors, adhesives, and vehicle components.[17,18]

After the penetrating drug partitions into the dermis, metabolic and depot sites may intervene as the drug gradually moves to a blood capillary, partitions into the wall, and then exits into the blood. The lymph system can also aid in drug removal. A portion of the drug may also partition into subcutaneous fat and underlying muscle to form further depots, even though this finding would appear insignificant based on theoretical considerations.[19,20]

III.   Theoretical advantages of the transdermal route

It is customary to compare the percutaneous route with oral delivery since the latter provides the most popular way for delivering drugs. Transdermal delivery of a drug may eliminate several variables associated with oral intake since it bypasses GI absorption. In the GI tract, changes occur in pH as a molecule moves from gastric acid, with a pH as low as 1, to the intestine, with a pH of up to 8. Other variables that may be obviated include gastric emptying, intestinal motility and transit times, the activity of human and bacterial enzymes, and the influence of food.

In transdermal delivery, the drug enters the systemic circulation without first passing into the hepatic portal system and traversing the liver. This route, therefore, avoids the first-pass phenomenon by which the liver can significantly reduce the amount of intact drug. Additionally, the drug avoids the enzymes present in the gut wall. However, as has been emphasized earlier, the skin itself possesses some metabolic capability for biotransformation.

Percutaneous administration of a drug can control administration and limit pharmacological action, while the corresponding oral or injectable formulation may well elicit several effects, including toxic reactions. Patient compliance may be achieved by the continuity of delivery of drugs with short half-lives (see Figure 6.2).

Transdermal administration, under suitable rate control, may minimize pulse entry of a drug into the bloodstream. However, it is difficult to deliberately provide a controlled on/off action because intact skin membranes are intrinsically slow-response systems with prolonged lag times, at least when shunt diffusion via the appendageal route is negligible.

IV.   Optimization of percutaneous absorption

Two main strategies for the formulation of dermatological preparations have been described.[5] In the first strategy, a vehicle or device is utilized in order to maximize drug partition into the skin without significantly affecting the physicochemical properties of the stratum corneum. Thus, the vehicle in this instance promotes drug release by optimizing the absorption potential of the drug. However, if hydration occurs, even the most innocuous of vehicles tends to change the nature of the stratum corneum.

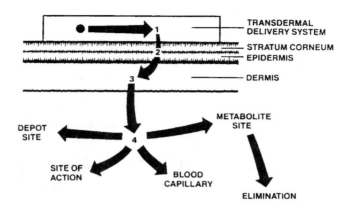

Figure 6.2 Process of transdermal permeation. (From Higuchi, T., *Curr. Prob. Dermatol.*, 7, 121, 1978. With permission of S. Karger, AG Basel, Switzerland.)

The alternate strategy incorporates materials such as penetration enhancers into the formulation. These enhancers are chemicals that enter the skin and reversibly alter it to promote the penetration of a drug. The desirable attributes of enhancers include: they should be pharmacologically inert, preferably not interacting with receptors in the skin or elsewhere in the body; the enhancer should not be toxic, irritating, or allergenic; the onset of enhancer activity and the duration of effect should be predictable and controllable; the skin should show an immediate and full recovery of its normal properties when the enhancer leaves the tissue; the accelerant should promote penetration into the skin without developing significant problems of loss of body fluids, electrolytes, or other endogenous materials; the chemical should be compatible with a wide range of drugs and pharmaceutical adjuvants; where appropriate, the substance should be a suitable solvent for the drug; for traditional formulations, the material should spread well on the skin, and it should have a suitable skin "feel;" the chemical should formulate into creams, ointments, gels, lotions, suspensions, aerosols, skin adhesives, and delivery devices; and it should be odorless, tasteless, colorless, and relatively inexpensive.[21]

V.   The theory for penetration-enhancer activity

Penetration enhancers can interact with the polar head groups of lipid via hydrogen and ionic bonding. The subsequent change in hydration spheres of the lipids, and alterations in head group interactions, will affect the packing at the head region. This change can decrease the retarding action, which then can affect the diffusion of polar penetrants. A second response may be to increase the volume of the aqueous layer so that more water enters the tissue. Subsequently, the swelling that occurs provides a greater cross-sectional area for polar diffusion and a larger fractional volume that is distinct from the structured water at the lipid interface.

This modification may also happen with simple hydration. The change in interfacial structure can alter the packing of the lipid tails such that the lipid hydrophobic route becomes more disordered and more easily traversed by a lipid-like penetrant.

In addition to any effect a penetration enhancer has on the aqueous region by increasing its water content, there can be a direct action whereby temporal changes can occur in its chemical constitution. With high concentrations of solvents, such as dimethylsulfoxide, propylene glycol or ethanol, in a vehicle or device, a large quantity may penetrate into the aqueous region of the tissue, thereby becoming a better solvent for steroidal molecules, such as hydrocortisone and estradiol. The partition coefficient in this instance favors elevated drug concentration in the skin. The solvent then diffuses out into the dermis, followed by the drug diffusing down its concentration gradient.[22]

An important feature of the activity of certain penetration enhancers is the correct choice of a cosolvent for materials such as Azone (1-dodecylaza-cycloheptane-2-one) and cis-unsaturated oleic acid. For these enhancers to reach the polar surface of the lipid bilayer in relatively large amounts, they may need an additive, such as propylene glycol. This addition can alter the polarity of the aqueous region and therefore increase its solubilizing ability for lipid-like materials.

The polar heads of oleic acid and Azone can place themselves between the head groups of the lipid and the enhancer tails and flip over to insert between the hydrophobic groups of the membrane lipids, thus increasing the fluidity of the lipid domain. Azone is not readily soluble in water, and under extreme conditions it may move fully into the internal region of the lipid to provide maximum disordering. This relationship between the elements of cosolvent systems operates particularly with Azone/propylene glycol mixtures. Not only does propylene glycol help the penetration of Azone into the stratum corneum, but Azone also increases the flux of propylene glycol through the skin, which subsequently increases the amount of Azone in the tissue.

When the resistance of the horny layer is reduced to that of an equivalent thickness of viable tissue, even more drastic disorder in the intercellular domain may result.[5] This situation can permit drug penetration at rates that are several orders of magnitude greater than those operating in the unaffected horny layer. The final stage in this process would be the dissolution of the lipid to form a homogeneous phase with little resistance to molecular diffusion. This disruption would occur only in the presence of high concentrations of molecules with good solvent properties for lipid components. If, for a particular penetrant, the intracellular route supplies a significant permeation pathway, the enhancer could interact with whatever lipid remains within the corneocyte.

Regarding the keratin fibrils, it is important to be cognizant of typical interactions, which materials such as the aprotic solvents (e.g., dimethylsulfoxide) and surfactants undergo with proteins. These mechanisms include interactions with polar groups, relaxation of binding forces, and alterations in helix conformations. Pore routes may form through this tissue. Most investigators now largely reject the fact that the transcellular route presents a significant pathway for molecular diffusion through the stratum corneum. Nonetheless, the corneocyte may sequester and retain certain molecules within its structure.

VI.   *Development of the transdermal therapeutic system*

A.   *Transdermal penetration of drugs*

In the past 50 years, many terms have been used to describe one of the objectives of a transdermal delivery system (i.e., penetration of a substance from the outside of the skin through the skin and into the bloodstream), such as percutaneous absorption. Other terms, such as persorption, permeation, and penetration, have been used also. All these processes relate to passively driven mass transfer; some terms, such as sorption, have other conflicting meanings. No matter how it is referred to, absorption through the skin involves passive diffusion through the outer and middle structures of the skin until the systemic circulation is attained.[23–25]

As described previously, the skin is stratified histologically into the stratum corneum, epidermis, dermis, and subcutaneous tissue, and as such it can be considered a laminate of barriers. This laminate consists of the stratum corneum, the viable epidermis, and a portion of the dermis. For most purposes, subcutaneous tissue is not considered to be involved in percutaneous absorption, although it may act as a potential depot. To review, permeation can occur by diffusion via transcellular penetration through the stratum corneum, intercellular penetration through the stratum corneum, and transappendageal penetration, especially including the sebaceous pathway of the pilosebaceous apparatus and the aqueous pathway of the salty sweat glands. The first two mechanisms require further diffusion through the rest of the epidermis and dermis. The third mechanism allows diffusional leakage into the epidermis and direct permeation into the dermis.[26–30]

B.   *Formulation*

The formulation of transdermal systems is essential for providing suitable delivery rates of drugs. The components of the system impact on the rate the drug is released to the skin and on the adherence of the device to the skin, and thus on the design of the final product.

The drug must be incorporated into some type of physical structure that both serves as a reservoir and provides for diffusive "communication" of the drug with the surface of the skin. This physical structure, or laminar construction, serves as a "platform" for the drug. The platform could consist of a liquid, a semisolid, a nonflowing (three-dimensionally stable) material, or a combination of any of these. A liquid by itself is rather impractical for any extended wearing. However, if well contained, it could be made useful.

The semisolid platform, exemplified by the traditional ointment or semisolid gel material, with containment, is truly acceptable for wearing on the skin. Even without containment, such materials are ideal for spreading over irregular surfaces. A three-dimensionally stable material (such as a polymeric film or rubbery gel) has a discrete size and shape and can be easily contained. This type can be called a "solid-state" platform. The solid-state delivery system is more amenable for wearing and removing from the skin. On the other hand, it may not as easily conform to the application area, and complete system-to-skin contact is less certain.

Platforms thus consist of materials that are liquid, semisolid, or solid. Some investigators have referred to these platforms as monoliths, slabs, reservoirs, vehicles, films, polymer matrices, or just matrices. A matrix can be totally morphous and of varying viscosities, crystalline, or a combination of both. If a barrier or some material is placed in the path of the diffusing molecule so that it controls the rate of flux, it will be referred to as a membrane or film. Hwang and Kammermeyer[31] have classified membranes in terms of their nature, structure, application, or mechanism of action. The nature of a membrane can be said to be either natural (such as skin or intestinal walls) or synthetic (such as polymeric films). Defining membranes structurally, they can be either porous (such as microporous polymeric films, filters, etc.) or nonporous (such as films of polyethylene, vinyl, or other polymers commonly used in packaging).

The analysis of data on matrix or film diffusion can be presented in several formats. The most common methods are to observe either the cumulative amount of a drug that permeates or by the rate that it diffuses out of or through a matrix or membrane. Depending on the system selected, the drug will have a particular release-rate profile curve. Mathematical diffusion models have been reviewed extensively and are useful references.[32-38]

C. Adhesion

The modern transdermal product is a unique delivery system in that it is worn on the skin. This requires good skin contact over the total area of application and ease of applying and removing the transdermal patch. Also, if the transdermal delivery system is made of two or more laminating structures, good bonding between these layers must take place. Other parts of the system must not adhere well, such as the release liner (peel-away strip that is removed). If the drug is to be formulated into the adhesive itself, care must be taken that the drug or any adhesives do not influence the adhesiveness of the adhesive.

Along with an understanding of the effect of the formulation on drug release, one has to consider trade-offs with optimized adhesive properties. A good understanding of adhesion, adhesive properties, and adhesive materials, particularly in relation to pressure-sensitive adhesives, is helpful when dealing with these materials. Although the literature provides little specific information on pressure-sensitive adhesives, there are some reviews on the practical and theoretical aspects of adhesives. Generally, the adhesive–cohesive properties, peel-strength, tack, and creep qualities of adhesives are basic properties used in formulating suitable pressure-sensitive adhesives. The basic construction of pressure-sensitive tapes has been reviewed in the literature. The facestock, or backing, can be a material that is occlusive (serves as a barrier, such as vinyl, polyethylene, polyester films, etc.) or nonocclusive (allows water and gases to readily flow through, such as nonwoven or porous films). The backing serves as a platform or carrier for the adhesive and is essential for application to and removal from the skin.[39,40]

The adhesive layer is pressure-sensitive and the anchor of the system. The American Society for Testing and Materials (ASTM) definition of a pressure-sensitive adhesive is a viscoelastic material which in solvent-free form remains permanently tacky.[41] Such material will adhere instantaneously to most solid surfaces with the application of slight pressure. The adhesive can then be removed from a surface, such as the skin or release liner, without leaving a residue. The pressure-sensitive adhesives (called adhesive mass) commonly used in medical applications are based on natural or synthetic rubbers, polyacrylates, or silicone. The release liner (also called release paper or peel-away strip) is a sheet that serves as a protectant or carrier for an adhesive film or mass, which is easily removed from the adhesive mass prior to use. The release liner consists of paper, polystyrene, polyethylene, polyester, or other polymeric films with a light coating of such compounds as silicones, long-chain branched polymers, chromium complexes, fluorochemicals, or various hard polymers.[42,43]

In a transdermal delivery system (TDD), the choice or design of adhesive is critical because it will have a strong effect on a patch's drug release, stability, and wear properties. The most common pressure-sensitive adhesives used for TDD systems are acrylates. Silicones tend to contain fairly limited properties, whereas acrylates can be tailored to achieve a wide range of performance in regards to various drugs, excipients, and particular product requirements. Cantor and Wirtanen[189] described novel acrylates adhesives — hydroxyethyl acrylate or pyrrolidoneethyl acrylate — as polar monomers to control drug stability and a graft macromer to control adhesive performance in 3M's latitude transdermal systems. These investigators studied solubility of drugs such as buprenophine, cyproheptadine, phenobarbital, testosterone, captopril, haloperidol, morphine, and atenolol.

D.   Bioactivity

Other dosage forms intended to deliver drugs to the systemic circulation often provide highly fluctuating levels in the blood and tissues, especially after repeated dosing. The transdermal method offers an alternative whereby this problem is minimized. To determine if the transdermal route is indeed a workable alternative, one must ask what problems exist with the current dosage forms of a particular drug. In most cases, the therapeutic effect of a drug is related to drug concentration. There is an upper and lower limit of a drug that will establish a "therapeutic window." In this range, the diseased state can be treated with minimal side effects. Some drugs may have nominal inherent side effects in this window but reach toxic proportions when higher levels are achieved. When levels go below the therapeutic threshold, the drug essentially becomes ineffective (e.g., a subtherapeutic level). Ideally, a drug delivery system should provide drug levels within the limits of the therapeutic window.[44]

In order to achieve systemic levels from a transdermal delivery system, the drug must first dissolve in the matrix and then migrate from the matrix through the skin and into the capillary plexus. Pharmacokinetic treatment of percutaneous absorption in the literature concentrates largely on drugs permeating into rather than through the skin. However, Beckett et al.[45] compared the transdermal route against the oral route of four ephedrine derivatives. They showed that metabolites were formed in smaller amounts and that the combination of unchanged drug and its metabolites was less using the percutaneous route. Riegelman[46] also showed the skin is rate-limiting and indicated that by adjusting drug loading, vehicle components, and surface area, prolonged steady-state blood levels can be sustained.

The use of pharmacokinetic parameters provides a useful tool for the development of transdermal systems. It can allow one to establish what steady-state fluxes of the drug are needed to reach a therapeutic level systemically. Pharmacokinetic parameters are also important from the biopharmaceutics point of view as part of the U.S. Food and Drug Administration review for market approval in order to support drug labeling. Furthermore, the system must show reproducibility of plasma levels and that these levels are within the therapeutic limits of a standard dosage form.

E.   Polymers in transdermal delivery systems

Polymers are the backbone of transdermal delivery systems. These systems are fabricated as multilayered, polymeric laminates in which a drug reservoir or a drug–polymer matrix is sandwiched between two polymeric layers: an outer, impervious backing layer that prevents the loss of drug through the backing surface and an inner polymeric layer that functions as an adhesive or rate-controlling membrane. The physicochemical and mechanical properties of various polymers that are currently used in commercially available transdermal drug delivery systems are summarized in the following tables. This summary is intended as a guide for the selection of polymers for developing such systems.

VII. Examples of transdermal applications

Transdermal systems, such as Nitrodur and Nitrodisc, are referred to as monolithic systems because they contain the drug as a semisolid solution or dispersion. With these systems, the drug reservoir is manufactured by dissolution of all components, including the polymer that serves as the matrix, with subsequent casting and drying. In some cases, the solvent may form the continuous phase of the matrix, and processing may involve mixing high-viscosity fluid at an elevated temperature before forming the gelled matrix, either in sheet form or as a solid cylinder. The individual units must then be punched from the sheet or sliced cylinder.[47]

Once the drug reservoir, having the specified surface area, is obtained, it must be assembled with the system backing, peripheral adhesive, and protective liner. This process is the most labor-intensive and, consequently, the most expensive part of the manufacturing process. In the future, monolithic systems will undoubtedly be manufactured by more continuous processes, such as extrusion, injection molding, and laminating lines.[48–51]

Transderm-Nitro and Transderm-Scop are examples of membrane-controlled transdermal systems. Their methods of manufacture are somewhat different, however, in that the former is a product of technologies originating in the packaging industry, referred to as form-fill-seal, while the latter system derives purely from lamination processes. The technologies for both processes are well established, having been applied for some time in the food and cosmetics industries. Hence, these processes make it possible to produce pharmaceutical products under good manufacturing practices (GMP) regulations (see Figure 6.3).

In the case of form-fill-seal systems, the formulation of the drug reservoir can be accomplished by techniques utilized in the pharmaceutical industry. With the processes of lamination, however, dosing of the drug

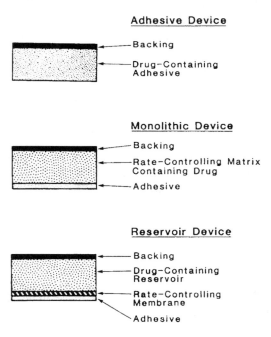

Figure 6.3 Types of transdermal delivery devices. (From *Pharm. Tech.*, The Latest Developments in Drug Delivery Systems, Conf. Proc., 1987, 27. With permission.)

reservoir and heat sealing must be refined and adapted somewhat before the overall manufacturing process becomes general and routine. Nevertheless, it seems this technology may be closer to finding a place in pharmaceutical production than those technologies needed for efficient production of monolithic systems.

The female reproductive hormones estradiol and progesterone are obvious choices for transdermal delivery. Estradiol is particularly promising because its oral administration causes a large fraction of the dose to be converted in the liver to the less-active metabolite estrone. Transdermal administration avoids most hepatic metabolism and results in therapeutic blood levels of estradiol at total doses much lower than those required by oral administration.

Diseases of the cardiovascular system lend themselves quite readily to transdermal administration of drugs because of the nature of the diseases. Drug treatment of hypertension and angina is generally a protracted process, often requiring continuous use for many years. As such, compliance with the established regimen is important and can be a problem — particularly with hypertension, because the disease is often asymptomatic, giving the patient no incentive to take his or her medication on time. Two beta blockers, timolol and propranolol, have been studied in their free-base form in skin-permeation models and have been shown to provide sufficient skin permeability to obtain significant blood levels. Both of these compounds are used in oral form to treat hypertension and angina. Neither of these is cardioselective, and several of the hepatic metabolites of propranolol are active beta-adrenergic antagonists. Timolol has been introduced in an ocular formulation for the treatment of ocular hypertension (glaucoma). It seems likely that both timolol and propranolol, administered transdermally, would have some efficacy in reducing blood pressure.[52,53]

Compounds used to control pain continue to be of general interest in the medical and pharmaceutical communities. It is important, however, to understand when a transdermal delivery system, or any controlled delivery system for that matter, is an advantage in the control of pain. Clearly, the amelioration of acute pain requires fast onset of action and probably is not an appropriate use of transdermal therapy. Still, control of chronic pain may well lend itself to transdermal therapy. At least one group has studied transdermal delivery of salicylates. It appears, however, that dosing requirements may prove too great for common nonnarcotic analgesics. At the same time, many fundamental questions regarding the development of tolerance during continuous dosing must be answered before any transdermal analgesics can become a reality.[54]

There may be a need for continuous delivery of both over-the-counter (OTC) and prescription antihistamines, particularly in the treatment of certain allergies. At least one pharmaceutical company is developing a transdermal delivery system for chlorpheniramine. The primary advantage of continuous transdermal delivery of antihistamines is the possibility of maintaining histamine-receptor antagonism while reducing the occurrence of central nervous system (CNS) side effects, such as drowsiness. Because chlorpheniramine has a relatively long half-life, it is believed that its transdermal administration may not provide major advantages in a dosing interval, unless the system can be designed to last more than one day. Substantial benefit in minimizing side effects, however, may well overcome modest benefits in duration of effect. The primary drawback to transdermal administration of antihistamines, particularly the tertiary amines, is the possibility of skin irritation or hypersensitization.

In a paper describing skin permeability[55] of physostigmine, a cholinesterase inhibitor, the authors studied a transdermal system that delivered the drug at a sufficient rate through pig skin *in vivo* to inhibit the breakdown of acetylcholine by 30 to 40% over 4 days. This mode of treatment could have far-reaching effects for certain dementias involving a deficit in CNS acetylcholine, including Alzheimer's disease. One must, however, be cautious, because physostigmine is not specific to the CNS, and peripheral side effects must be carefully controlled. Nonetheless, this system provides a convenient means of delivering physostigmine at a controlled rate to the systemic circulation — bypassing hepatic metabolism — over a long period of time. It should prove useful in studying the treatment of these diseases and their responses to cholinesterase inhibition.

Tables 6.1 and 6.2 contain partial lists of transdermal controlled-release products and devices.

The following drugs are also under development using a transdermal therapeutic system: ketoprofen, 5-fluorouracil, metoprolol, terodiline, primaquine, ibuprofen piconol, nitrendipine, diclofenac, corticosteroids, sandimune (cyclosporine A), fluazifopbutyl, glyceryl trinitrate, azido-profen esters, methotrexate, medroxyprogesterone acetate, levonorgestrel, mepindolol, oxycodone, prostaglandins, and 9-β-D-arabinofuranosyladenine (Ara-A).

A.   Iontophoresis

An alternate strategy to drive drugs through the skin that seems to be enjoying a revival of interest is iontophoresis. In this method, a battery is connected to two electrodes on the skin. If an ionized drug is placed in contact with one electrode, it will migrate under the influence of the voltage gradient through the skin and enter the systemic circulation. Substantial delivery can be obtained in this way (see Figure 6.4).

The earliest patents describing the essential features of iontophoresis date back to the 1890s, although apparently their objective was to shock their subjects rather than drug them. The first modern device appeared in 1972, and advances since then have enabled smaller and smaller devices to be built. The newest devices, from Drug Delivery Systems, have a built-in battery layer and are comparable in size to a normal transdermal patch. The patents in this area so far deal with device design and do not specify particular drugs. There is considerable potential for innovative work in this specialized area.

Table 6.1 Transdermal controlled-release products and devices

Drug	Trade name	Type of device	Indication
Scopolamine (Hyoscine)	Transderm-Scop Kimite Patch	Reservoir	Motion sickness
Nitroglycerine[a]	Transderm-Nitro	Reservoir	Angina
	Deponit	Mixed monolithic reservoir	Angina
	Nitro-Dur	Monolithic	Angina
	Nitrodisc	Monolithic	Angina
	NTS	Monolithic	Angina
Isosorbide-dinitrate	Frandol Tape	Monolithic	Angina
Clonidine	Catapress-TTS	Reservoir	Hypertension
Estradiol	Estraderm	Reservoir and ethanol enhancer	Hormone treatment
Estradiol esters	—	**	Hormone treatment
Testosterone	TheraDerm-LRS	**	Hormone treatment
Timolol	—	**	Cardiovascular
Propranolol	—	**	Cardiovascular
Fentanyl	Duragesic	—	Opioid analgesic
Glycol salicylate	—	**	Analgesic
Methyl salicylate	—	—	—
Chlorpheniramine	—	**	Antihistamine
Diphenhydramine	Zenol	—	Antihistamine
Physostigmine	—	**	Cholinergic
Insulin	—	**	Diabetes
Albuterol	—	**	Bronchodilator
Piroxicam	—	**	Arthritis
Ketorolac (Toradol)	—	**	Nonnarcotic analgesic
Flurbiprofen	Zepolas	—	Anti-inflammatory
Indomethacin	Indomethin	—	Anti-inflammatory
Bufuralol	—	**	Angina, hypertension
Bupranolol	—	**	Angina, hypertension, antiglaucoma agent
Nicotine	Habitrol, Nicoderm, Nicotrol, PROSTEP	—	Aid to smoking cessation, Tourette's syndrome

[a] Other trade names are Diafusor, Minitran, Nitriderm, Nitrol Patch, Nitrocine, Deponit, Millistrol Tape, and Herzer.

** In research and development.

Table 6.2 Transdermal products under development

Drug	Trade name	Producer/marketer
Minocycline	(Topical) Sunstar	American Cyanamid, Takeda
Eperisone	E-2000	Eisai
Estradiol+ Norethisterone	Estracombi TIS	Ciba-Geigy, Alza, Ethical Pharmaceuticals
Estradiol+Progestin	—	Cygnus Research, Elf Sanofi
Estradiol	Menorest	Noven Pharmaceuticals, Cygnus Research, Ciba-Geigy, Elf Sanofi, Pierre Fabre, Rhone-Poulenc, Johnson & Johnson, Warner-Lambert, Rotta Research Fournier, Forest Labs, Hercon, Ethical Pharm., Nikko Denko, Pharmed, Pharmetrix Recordati, Teikoku Hormone
Estrogen+ Progestogen	—	Noven Pharm., Rhone-Poulenc-Rorer, Fournier, 3M Pharm., Pharmetrix Biosearch
DHEA (Androgen)	—	Pharmedic
Eptazocine	—	TheraTech, Nichiiko
Fentanyl	—	Anaquest, CygnusResearch
Pain-Drug	—	Syntex-Roche, TheraTech
Progesterone	—	TheraTech, Solvay
Analgesic	—	Ethical Pharm., TheraTech, Syntex-Roche
Lipophilic iron Chelators	—	Yissum
Buprenorphine	—	Pierre Fabre, Cygnus Research, Whitby Pharmaceuticals
Triamcinolone acetonide	—	Whitby Pharmaceuticals
Antoproliferative compound	Topical formulation	Yissum
Anthralin	Percutaneous delivery	Vuman

The iontophoretic system currently marketed (Phoresor, Motion Control, Inc.) uses a continuous, waveless, unidirectional current of low voltage (DC). All ions are either positive or negative. For a drug to be phoresed, it must be ionizable and its polarity determined. The drug is then injected into a reservoir in the active pole (electrode). This electrode is smaller than the inactive or indifferent electrode in order to concentrate the drug's effects. When the pads are placed, they should be as directly opposite each other as possible (e.g., on either side of the elbow). When the system is activated, the drug is driven out of the active pole toward the inactive pole. The inactive pole, being the opposite polarity of the drug will, therefore, theoretically attract the drug, allowing it to be distributed to the tissues between the two electrodes.

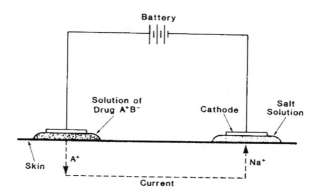

Figure 6.4 Schematic diagram illustrating the principles of iontophoresis. (From *Pharm. Tech.*, The Latest Developments in Drug Delivery Systems, Conf. Proc., 1987, 31. With permission.)

Human skin has a limited tolerance for flow of electric current, however. Therefore, the unit must be turned on and off slowly to avoid muscle stimulation. Turning the unit on or off suddenly, changing the electrode placement, or changing the polarity while the unit is running may cause the patient to receive a shock. When lower voltages are used, the patient will have less sensation of penetration, but the level of drug penetration will also be lower. The amount of drug delivered is equal to the current applied multiplied by the duration of treatment. The recommended treatment time is 20 minutes, and the recommended maximum current is 4 mA. Therefore, the amount of drug delivered would be 80 mA/min. Iontophoresis is currently used for the treatment of acute musculoskeletal and neuromuscular inflammatory problems using a mixture of lidocaine and dexamethasone or dexamethasone alone. Lidocaine alone is also used for local anesthesia. Many drugs are being studied for the feasibility of their delivery via iontophoresis. They are listed in Table 6.3.

VIII. Transdermal controlled-release products and devices

Lectec Corporation has developed a solid-state, hydrophilic reservoir system that uses body heat and humidity to hydrate the skin and allows the diffusion of drug through the skin for systemic absorption.

Health-Chem Corporation has developed a transdermal laminar system that releases a drug by using different polymers in the reservoir and protective layers. The Zetachron Company has developed its own transdermal system that can slow down skin permeation of drugs that are highly permeable. This is useful in transdermally delivering low-dose, potent drugs, such as antihypertensive and antianginal agents. Its transdermal systems are believed to be easier to manufacture than conventional transdermal patches.[56]

Table 6.3 Transdermal iontophoretic delivery

Drug	Use
Lidocaine	Local anesthesia
Dexamethasone	Arthritis
Hydrocortisone	Arthritis
Acetic acid	Calcified tendonitis
Iodine	Scar tissue removal
Penicillin	Burns
Salicylates	Arthritis, myalgias
Histamine	Peripheral vascular disease
Hyaluronidase	Edema
Lithium	Gouty arthritis
Magnesium	Arthritis
Calcium	Myospasm
Copper	Fungal infections
Zinc	Scars, adhesions
Acetate	Calcifications
Isopropamide	Anticholinergic
Piroxicam	NSAID
Sufentanil	Analgesic, anesthetic
Insulin	Diabetes
Sotalol	Antianginal, antiarrhythmic
Leuprolide	Antineoplastic
ACE inhibitors	Hypertension
Amino acid derivatives	—
Alanine tripeptides	—
Melatonin, melanin	Mediator of photic-induced antigonadotrophic activity
Verapamil	Antianginal, antiarrhythmic

The Elan Company has developed two transdermal systems: Dermaflex and Panoderm. Both of these systems are to be worn like bracelets. The active ingredients are absorbed from the bracelet by electrical impulses.

The Moleculon Biotech Company has developed a poroplastic membrane system. This system is a molecular sponge that can hold within its pores a large quantity of solid, solubilized compounds. This membrane system is quite flexible. It can alter release rate by adding various compounds to deliver drugs from a few hours to months (see Figures 6.5 and 6.6).[56]

Finally, some examples of skin applications are pressure-sensitive adhesive compositions containing chlorhexidine or PVP-1 and iodine as antimicrobial agents and for administering tretinoin for acne; topical treatments for dermatological conditions (e.g., tricyclic antidepressants, such as imipramine, amitryptyline, and doxepin, for pruritis and anthracenone derivatives for psoriasis)[57] and antiphlogistic analgesic adhesive containing indomethacin for arthritis.[58] Electrically assisted delivery by iontophoresis or electroporation was used *in vitro* to deliver the calcium-regulating hormones salmon calcitonin (sCT) and parathyroid hormone (PTH) through

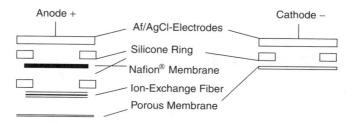

Figure 6.5 Transdermal iontophoresis of tacrine. The structure of the ion-exchange fiber device. (With permission, Kluwer Publishers, *Pharm. Res.*, 19, 5, 704, 2002.)

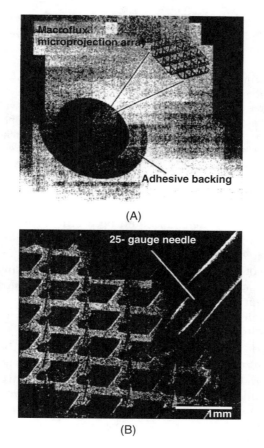

Figure 6.6 (A) Schematic representation of the Macroflux® microprojection array integrated with an adhesive patch. (B) Scanning electron photomicrograph of an array of microprojections (330 μm length). For scale, a 25-gauge needle is shown adjacent to the array. (With permission, Kluwer Publishers, *Pharm. Res.*, 19, 1, 64, 2002.)

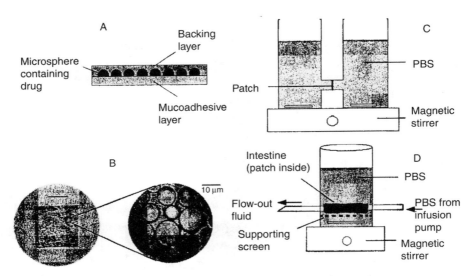

Figure 6.7 (A) Schematic representation of the patch design. The patch consists of a film of a mucoadhesive polymer. A monolayer of cross-linked bovine serum albumin (BDA) microspheres (10–30 µm) is dispersed on the mucoadhesive film. The drug to be delivered is encapsulated in the microspheres. The microsphere monolayer is covered by a film of poorly permeable polymer. (B) Intestinal patches (4 mm²). (Right figure indicates the microstructure of the patch.) (C) Schematic representation of the diffusion cell used to measure release of model drugs from the patch. (D) Schematic representation of flow-through setup for measurement of transport across the intestinal wall. (With permission, Kluwer Publishers, *Pharm. Res.*, 19, 4, 391, 2002.)

human epidermis. Such delivery could be useful for chronic treatment of postmenopausal osteoporosis and other clinical indications as a superior alternative to parenteral delivery.[128–130] Transdermal and topical delivery of macromolecules of at least 40 kDa was also achieved by skin electroporation. Spatially constrained skin electroporation with sodium thiosulfate and urea was found to create transdermal microconduits.[131–135]

Gelatin-containing, microemulsion-based organogels (MBGs) (see Figures 6.7 and 6.8) have been formulated using pharmaceutically acceptable surfactants and oils, such as Tween 85 and isopropyl myristate. MBGs provide a convenient means of immobilizing a drug such as sodium salicylate and are rheologically similar to their hydrogel counterparts at comparable gelatin concentrations. MBGs also offer improved microbial resistance in comparison to aqueous solution or hydrogels.[141–147] Bhatia and Singh[158] investigated the effects of 5% terpenes (e.g., limonene, carvone, thymol, and cineole) and iontophoresis on the *in vitro* permeability of leutinizing hormone (LH-RH) through the porcine epidermis and biophysical changes in the stratum corneum (SC) lipids by Fourier transform infrared (FT-IR). They found that terpenes/EtOH increased permeability by enhancing the extraction of the SC lipids. Iontophoresis synergistically enhanced the permeabil-

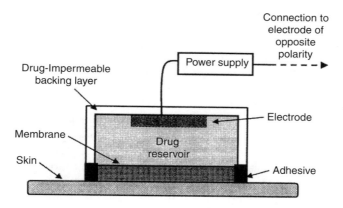

Figure 6.8 Schematic drawing of a transdermal drug delivery patch in contact with the skin. For iontophoretic delivery, an electrode of the same polarity as the charge of the drug is placed in the drug reservoir. The electrical circuit is completed by the application of a second electrode of the opposite polarity at a different skin site. (With permission, Elsevier, *J. Control Rel.*, 81, 335–345, 2002.)

ity of LHRH through terpenes/EtOH-treated epidermis. Other researchers have also investigated transdermal iontophoresis of oligonuclide drugs, the electrotransport of representative bases (uracil and adenine), and nucleosides (uridine and adenosine) and nucleotides (AMP, ATP, GTP, and imido-GTP) across mammalian skin *in vitro*. Vanbever et al.[179] found that skin electroporation could be a good way to improve the transdermal diffusion of fentanyl. Langer[38] found that application of therapeutic ultrasound (frequency 1 to 3 KHz and intensity 0 to $2W/cm^2$) enhances transdermal drug transport, although typically by a factor of less than 10. They studied permeants such as estradiol, salicylic acid, corticosterone, sucrose, aldosterone, water, and butanol across human cadaver skin. They concluded that low-frequency ultrasound enhances transdermal transport of drugs more effectively than that induced by therapeutic ultrasound. Cevc[182] described transferosomes, which are supramolecular aggregates better than liposomes or niosomes. These are found to increase the agents' diffusivity or partitioning in the organ.

IX.   Recent advances

Transdermal drug absorption can be enhanced to a degree by various chemical and physical methods. Chemical enhancers exert their influence on lipids in the stratum corneum as well as on lower dermal layers, and possibly capillary beds. Physical enhancers seem to promote the penetration of the stratum corneum, while diffusional permeation seems to be important in the lower layers of the skin. In addition, the effect that the chemical enhancers might have on the activity of the drug in the delivery device must always be considered. A means of enhancement that can provide reproducible transdermal delivery through a variety of skins under various conditions is needed. Iontophoresis has an advantage over chemical methods because it apparently offers better control of transdermal drug delivery. However, it requires a device separate from, and in addition to, the drug delivery reservoir and therefore often is considered cumbersome to use and uncertain from a regulatory standpoint. This is an important consideration for companies attempting to commercialize such a product. Rolf[59] has described some examples of amphoteric enhancers, such as sodium lauryl sulfate, lauryl amine oxide, azone decylmethyl sulfoxide, lauryl ethoxylate, and octanol.

Using the cell or the cylinder method, Aiche et al.[60] have evaluated the rate of release and dissolution of trinitrine from a membrane-reservoir transdermic delivery system. Both methods yielded the same results in terms of the quantity of drug released per unit area per hour and thus ensure a satisfactory quality control of the system. Regardless of the method used, the drug release is zero-order at 1 hour after diffusion and thereafter. The authors conclude that the method proposed by the supplier (the cylinder method) is validated against that described by the pharmacopoeia.

Despite the great need for effective transdermal permeation enhancers, the search is still largely empirical. Very few studies have involved systematic evaluation of enhancer congeners. The enhancer congeners that have been evaluated by Chow and Hseih[61] include surfactants of alkyl sulfates, saturated fatty acids, fatty alcohols with different numbers of double bonds, unsaturated fatty acids with equal numbers of double bonds at different positions or with different configurations, and cyclic compounds with various carbon numbers and sizes.

Pressure-sensitive adhesives (PSAs) are necessary components in transdermal systems because they ensure intimate contact of the device with the skin. PSAs are used in many system designs that can be configured using an adhesive overlay face adhesive, adhesive matrix, and multilaminated PSA matrix. The science and engineering involved in the selection, formulation, and optimization of PSA properties is critical to the successful development of transdermal systems. Adverse interactions between the drug, excipients, cosolvents, and permeation enhancers in reservoir or matrix-type systems can compromise the performance of the adhesive, resulting in system failure.[62]

The skin is a vital metabolic and immunocompetent organ that serves as the body's first line of defense against environmental attack. Certain chemicals, however, are capable of producing immediate and delayed hypersensitivity reactions within the skin by interacting directly or indirectly with certain cells in the epidermis and dermis. For this reason, the delivery of drugs through the skin might produce adverse reactions by affecting responsive cells. Dunn[63] has discussed work regarding the biological response of whole skin and isolated epidermal keratinocytes to phorbol esters, potent drugs, irritants, and mitogens.

The article by Pfister[64] illustrates how silicone pressure-sensitive adhesives can be customized to accommodate specific drug, material, and coating requirements of transdermal delivery systems. Physiochemical properties of silicone PSAs and their end-use properties, such as tack, adhesion, and cohesive strength, are characterized. The article also describes how these properties can be varied either chemically — by altering silanol functionality, resin-to-polymer ratio, or choice of solvent — or physically — by adjusting coating thickness. Finally, relationships between silicone PSAs and drug-release kinetics are addressed, and methods of developing formulations to optimize system performance are suggested.

Because of the side effects associated with the oral administration of tetra-hydrocannabinol (THC), Touitou et al.[65] tested the use of the skin as a noninvasive portal for the sustained delivery of the drug. Rat skin was found to be approximately 13 times more permeable than human skin. Autoradiographs showed that after 24 hours, the drug was concentrated in the stratum corneum, in the upper epidermis, and around the hair follicles, which suggests that THC penetrates through the lipophilic pathways.

Touitou[66] have also investigated the permeation-enhancement properties of n-decyl methyl sulfoxide (decylMSO) in the presence of water and propylene glycol *in vitro* through hairless mouse skin. 5-Fluorouracil and idoxuridine were used as test drugs because of their respective hydrophilic and hydrophobic properties. Results showed that the enhancement of permeation by decylMSO occurred only in an aqueous medium and only at concentrations greater than the critical micelle concentrations.

Ashton et al.[67] have investigated the influence of sodium lauryl sulfate (SLS) and Brij 36T on the thermodynamic activity of methyl nicotinate in aqueous gels. The permeability of skin *in vivo* was assessed by measuring the time required for nicotine esters and hexyl nicotinate in aqueous gels. The time required for SLS gels to cause erythema correlates with *in vitro* release rates. Because SLS is considered to be a powerful penetration enhancer, the results of this study indicate that these two surfactants exert their influences in different ways.

Key Pharmaceuticals has received approval to market Nitro-Dur II (nitroglycerine) transdermal infusion system for prevention of severe angina pectoris. Applied once a day to the chest or upper arm, it delivers nitroglycerine for a full 24 hours.[56]

Cygnus Research, in collaboration with Family Health International, is developing a weekly contraceptive patch. Patches would be replaced weekly for three weeks, and a drug-free patch worn on the fourth week.[56]

Forest Laboratories has formulated nitroglycerine in a transdermal polymer gel. The gel, which Forest will market, is applied in liquid form to the skin, where it quickly dries and is absorbed.[56]

A transdermal formulation of ketoprofen for orthopedic use is being developed for the treatment of osteoarthritis, tenditis, and bursitis. The formulation comprises a flexible pad and adhesive layer containing the water-based drug.[56]

MacroChem has filed a patent application for enhancing the transdermal delivery of minoxidil. This technology will be employed in the company's

Dermelec product, a transdermal device to be worn and adjusted by patients to control the rate and amount of dosage.[56]

Transdermal delivery of glibenclamide from polymeric matrices of eudragits, ethylcellulose, hydroxypropylmethyl cellulose, polyvinyl pyrrolidone carboxymethyl cellulose, and polyvinyl acetate with plasticizers has been studied. It was reported that the permeation rate was enhanced, depending on the type and the concentration of the enhancers. The advantage of using an enhancer combination was also observed.[68]

Occlusion of skin under a transdermal patch may facilitate the occurrence of adverse dermal reactions. In order to minimize such reactions, a novel system has been developed which is ultrathin, breathable (oxygen- and moisture-permeable), and has excellent conformability to the skin. This system is ideally suited for topical application of medications such as antibiotics, anti-inflammatory, and antifungal agents and for transdermal delivery of relatively nontoxic and nonvolatile drugs.[69]

During the course of work on the development of a transdermal levonorgestrel (LN) delivery system, a number of permeation enhancers have been investigated that can be used in conjunction with ethanol to achieve therapeutically effective fluxes of LN through the intact stratum corneum. The effectiveness of this enhancer for 5-fluorouracil, estradiol, and hydrocortisone was also studied.[70]

The article by Bodde et al.[71] focuses on two aspects of transdermal peptide delivery: transepidermal penetration and intra(epi)dermal biotransformation using the example of desenkephalin endorphin, a highly potent neuropeptide. *In vitro* studies with this peptide, using both intact human skin samples and cultured human skin cells, showed transdermal fluxes (without enhancers). From these results, it is anticipated that the transdermal delivery of small peptides, even hydrophilic ones, is a distinct possibility.

Based on long-term physical and chemical stability results, a transdermal contraceptive (TCS) formulation has been developed. Extensive effort was then devoted to the development of procedures and technology for scale-up manufacturing of TCS patches. A continuous operation-type fabrication machine (SFM) was designed. The patches fabricated were evaluated by measuring their weight variation and content uniformity, as well as the release and skin-permeation rates of levonorgestrel and estradiol against the patches prepared by the hand-operated, compression-coated (HCC) process.[72]

A transdermal delivery system for verapamil was developed and applied for a 24-hour period on the chest skin of eight healthy male volunteers. Plasma concentration was monitored during 48 hours after application. Verapamil and its active metabolite (norverapamil) were detected in plasma. Plasma concentration reached steady state within approximately 10 hours after application. Clinical data was found to be comparable to *in vitro* penetration of hairless mouse skin with the help of a computer simulation technique.[73]

A transdermal polymeric delivery system for hydromorphone has been developed. Various penetration enhancers, such as isopropylmyristate, azone, hexamethylene palmitamide, hexamethy lauramide, aliphatic acids, alcohols, and esters, were incorporated in the polymer matrix. The rate of drug penetration across hairless mouse skin increased and lag time decreased as enhancer concentration increased. Among the enhancers investigated, hexamethyl lauramide most significantly improved penetration of hydromorphone.[74]

The transdermal route offers several advantages over other routes of administration. However, a key problem is the low permeability of skin to most drugs. Low skin permeability often requires impractically large devices if useful drug delivery rates are to be achieved. Highly potent drugs that are effective at low dosage rates, and hence do not demand large devices, are promising candidates for the transdermal delivery route. LN is one such drug and is capable of suppressing ovulation.[75]

A multilaminate-type transdermal drug delivery (mTDD) system was recently developed for controlled administration of various drugs. The skin-permeation rates of progestins and other drugs were found to be substantially enhanced, to varying degrees, by releasing different types of skin-permeation enhancers from the surface adhesive layers to modify skin permeability.[76]

BIOTEK has developed a Universal Transdermal Delivery System, which is highly versatile and adaptable to a wide variety of drugs and dosing requirements. Its unique features include a macroporous non-rate-controlling membrane, a viscous liquid base as a solvent for the drug, and suspended drug microparticles as reservoirs. After application, the system maintains a thin film of drug solution in direct contact with the skin, providing for skin occlusion. The system is compatible with enhancers and additives, and its delivery rate and duration are controllable by formulation variables. The system has been evaluated *in vitro* and *in vivo* for the simultaneous delivery of estradiol and levonorgestrel.[77]

Polydimethylsiloxane (PDMS) PSAs are used in transdermal drug delivery systems, in part because of excellent biocompatibillity and high permeability of this class of materials. BIO-PSA® 355 silicone pressure-sensitive adhesive is well-suited as a contact adhesive in reservoir-type delivery systems. Its properties are somewhat compromised, however, when co-formulated with amine-functional agents. BIO-PSA® Q7-2920 was developed to exhibit amine resistance. PSA either functions as a contact adhesive or may potentially act as a drug-loaded adhesive matrix, a conceptually simple, yet technologically complex, drug delivery system. Preliminary suitability of BIO-PSA® Q7-2920 as a drug-loaded matrix was determined by characterizing the release kinetics of nitroglycerine, indomethacin, estradiol, progesterone, propranolol, and testosterone from the PSA and testing the adhesive-tape properties (release, adhesion, and tack) of the drug-loaded matrices as a function of time.[78]

Actibase (Schering Corp., Kenilworth, NJ) is an optimized vehicle of propylene glycol, propylene glycol stearate, white wax, and white petrolatum used in the formulation of topical betamethasone dipropionate.[79] Erythromycin formulated with a hydroalcoholic solution composed of ethanol and propylene glycol seems to be effective, as does tetracycline (e.g., Topicycline, Proctor & Gamble, Cincinnati, OH) formulated with the enhancer decyl methyl sulfoxide.[79]

Actiderm (Bristol Myers Squibb, Princeton, NJ), a patch that does not contain any drug, was introduced in 1988 for use as an occlusive dressing. The patch is placed over topically applied corticosteroids to enhance their efficacy by promoting hydration of the stratum corneum. This treatment leads to enhanced percutaneous absorption and prolonged activity, thus minimizing the need for high-potency steroids.[80]

Hercon has developed a laminated reservoir system for the controlled transdermal delivery of agents to the systemic circulation, achieving steady-state blood levels for extended periods while minimizing side effects. The system is thin and flexible and consists of two to four layers, including a backing membrane, the drug reservoir, a rate-controlling membrane, and an adhesive that holds the system to the skin. The system is suited to compounds that require either a one-day or seven-day frequency of delivery. Hercon has signed agreements with several pharmaceutical companies to develop or market its polymeric transdermal system for selected products, which include antiarthritics, antiemetics, antihistamines, beta-blockers, antihypertensives, antiasthmatics, antiaddictives, calcium antagonists, tranquilizers, and hormonal agents.[81]

The penetration of azidoprofen through excised hairless mouse skin has been investigated. Formulation factors influencing skin permeation, such as pH and solute and cosolvent concentrations, were studied and found related to physicochemical parameters such as pka and partition coefficient. In addition, the effect of a range of penetration enhancers on the transport of azidoprofen was also assessed. Pretreatment with azone in propylene glycol resulted in an increased flux with increasing pH, and thus appeared to facilitate penetration of the ionized species.[82]

The feasibility of achieving transdermal delivery of the opioid analgesic ketobemidone in human skin penetration studies *in vitro*, using both ketobemidone and three carbonate ester pro-drugs, has been studied. Whereas ketobemidone had only limited ability to permeate the skin from either polar or apolar vehicles, the ester pro-drugs readily penetrated the skin when present in certain solvents, such as isopropyl myristate, ethanol, and ethanol-water. This study demonstrated the feasibility of achieving transdermal delivery of ketobemidone based on enzymatic conversion and favorable skin-penetration properties of the ester pro-drugs, which, in turn, is attributed to their high solubilities in both polar and apolar solvents.[83]

Pro-drug fatty acid esters of N-(2-hydroxyethyl)-2-pyrrolidone have also been synthesized in order to test the previously mentioned approach. It was found that a twofold order of magnitude increase in permeability for hydrocortisone through mouse skin could be achieved *in vitro* with these enhancers. The ester linkage was readily cleaved by hydrolytic enzymes in plasma and skin homogenates, while having relatively good solution stability at neutral and slightly acidic pH. These agents appear to have much less irritation potential than traditional penetration enhancers.[84]

The effect of simultaneous use of 1-menthol and ethanol on skin permeation of six potent cardiovascular agents — nicardipine, atenolol, captopril, nifedipine, vinpocetine, and nilvadipine — has been investigated to evaluate the feasibility of their use in a transdermal therapeutic system. *In vitro* diffusion experiments were carried out using excised hairless rat and human skin. The application area of the transdermal system required for the minimum effect was estimated by pharmacokinetic calculation. Marked enhancement of penetration by the 1-menthol-ethanol system was found independent of drug lipophilicity, while the mode of drug action was dependent on lipophilicity.[85]

The synthesis of ε-aminocaproic acid esters has been described. Two representative members from a group of five analogues of 1-alkylazacycloheptanone derivatives were evaluated *in vitro* for their effectiveness on transport of theophylline through excised human cadaver skin in comparison with azone. The 1-octyl and 10-dodecyl-ε-aminocaproic acid esters (OCEAC and DDEAC) showed excellent penetration enhancement. OCEAC and DDEAC did not exhibit acute dermal irritation *in vivo* on rabbits at a 5% concentration in white petrolatum.[86]

Hisetal contains properties of melanotropin, an endogenous pituitary peptide hormone. The permeability coefficient of hisetal is on the same order of magnitude as that of amino acids (5.58×10^{-5} cm · hr^{-1}). Oleic acid enhanced the permeation of hisetal by a factor of 28. Dodecyl N,N-dimethylamino acetate (3%) enhanced the permeation of hisetal 1.5 times more than azone at the same concentration. The effects of the penetration enhancers were irreversible within 12 hours. For the treatment of multiple sclerosis, assuming the same permeation rate as in hairless mouse skin, this would not achieve desired delivery of hisetal.[87]

A technique to deliver drugs through the skin by means of a millisecond, high-voltage pulse has been described by scientists from the Massachusetts Institute of Technology. The method, which the investigators call electroporation, temporarily alters the permeability of the skin. Millisecond pulses of 100 volts applied to human skin preparations or to anesthetized small animals every five seconds delivered approximately 1 microgram of test compound per square centimeter of skin per hour. Test compounds were calcein, lucifer yellow, and a derivative of erythrosine, all chosen for their detectability by fluorescence.[88]

An attempt has been made to establish a predictive method for determining the steady-state permeation rate of drugs through human skin. The method is based on the assumption that the stratum corneum is the main barrier in the skin and that it can be considered a membrane with two permeation pathways: lipid and pore. The authors derived an equation for predicting the steady-state permeation rate. Results showed that the skin-permeation potential of each drug in humans was different than that occurring in the hairless rat. The permeability of lipophilic drugs was slightly higher in humans than in the hairless rat, however, that of hydrophilic drugs was lower than in the hairless rat. Factors accounting for other species differences in skin permeability were discussed.[89]

Recently, patches containing polyisobutylene, azone, liquid paraffin, and 50 mg of nitrendipine (a calcium channel blocker) have been studied. *In vitro* release rates revealed that the cumulative release of nitrendipine was 31.5% of the initial loading dose in 34 hours and 40% in 72 hours. The results showed that this form of drug delivery not only decreases blood pressure effectively, but also reduces the adverse side effects induced by high plasma concentrations of the drug. Clinical trials involving 150 hypertensive patients showed that the patches reduced both systolic and diastolic blood pressure to within normal limits in 86% of the patients. The patches, applied to different skin locations, caused no skin irritation in either rabbits or human subjects during a 3-day period.[90]

The transfer of 13 drugs from transdermal patches to intact and stripped rat skin has been carried out to correlate transfer with the physicochemical properties of the drug. The drugs tested had melting points up to 234°C, lipophilic indexes of 0.475 to 5.336, and molecular weights of 122 to 392. The percentage of drug transferred to intact skin was lower when the melting point, lipophilic index, and molecular weight were high. Using stripped skin, the authors obtained similar results, although the percentage of drug transferred was markedly higher. The impact of the stratum corneum against drug transference tended to be greatest when the melting point and lipophilic index were low.[91]

The authors investigated the effects of various additives on the crystallization of ketoprofen in polyisobutylene adhesive matrix. The addition of Tween 80, Labrasol, or PVP K 30 significantly reduced the decrease in the flux of ketoprofen within this matrix during a storage time of 3 weeks.[148,149]

Terpenes, menthol, terpineol, cineole, and menthone were found to be effective permeation enhancers for imipramine HCl. Results of this study were explained with the help of H-bond breaking potential and self-association of terpenes. In order to elucidate the effect of terpenes on stratum corneum, FT-IR was used.[154,155]

Oral administration of tripolidine and antihistamines may cause many adverse side effects, such as dry mouth, sedation, and dizziness, and transdermal drug delivery was therefore considered. The transdermal controlled-release of the tripolidine system could be developed using the poly(4-methyl-1-pentene [TPX]) polymer, including the plasticizer. Among the plasticizers used, such as alkyl citrates, phthalates, and sebacate, tetra ethyl citrate showed the best enhancing effects.[151,152]

To formulate a transdermal drug delivery system of captopril, monolithic, adhesive-matrix-type patches containing 20% captopril, different pressure-sensitive adhesives, and various permeation enhancers were prepared using a labcoater. Fatty alcohols resulted in a pronounced enhancing effect on the skin permeation of captopril, while dimethyl sulfoxide, N-methyl-2-pyrrolidone, oleic acid, transcutol, and polysorbate 20 showed no significant enhancing effect.

Transdermal enhancement effects of electroporation applied only on the stratum corneum by two electrode types, the stamp-type electrode and the frog-type electrode, were investigated *in vitro* using excised rat skin. Carboxyfluorescein was selected as a model compound and used successfully in this work.

Ketotifen fumarate is effective in low doses in the treatment of bronchial asthma, particularly types of allergic origin. It is substantially metabolized when given orally. Isopropyl myristate and a linoleic acid combination and isopropyl myristate alone produced promising results in drug-release kinetics and skin-permeation profiles.

The influence of an erbium, Nd:YAG laser on the transdermal delivery of drugs across skin, was studied *in vitro*. Indomethacin and nalbuphine were selected for these studies. The authors found that the use of this technique for enhancing transdermal absorption of both lipophilic and hydrophilic drugs was acceptable since it allowed precise control of stratum corneum removal, and this ablation of SC can be reversible to the original normal status.[156,157]

Takahashi and Rytting[136] reported a novel approach to improve permeation of ondansetron, an antagonist of the 5-HT3 receptor used for the treatment of chemotherapy-induced emesis, across shed snakeskin as a model membrane. Oleic acid enhanced the permeation of ondansetron, probably in two ways: by a direct effect on the stratum corneum or via counter-ion formation of an ion-pair.

Venter et al.[137] reported on a comparative study of an *in situ* adapted diffusion cell and an *in vitro* Franz diffusion cell method for transdermal absorption of doxylamine. They found that excised skin might undergo sublethal injury (necrosis) during *in vitro* experiments.

Ilic et al.[138] described the microfabrication of individual 200-micron-diameter transdermal microconduits using high-voltage pulsing in salicylic acid and benzoic acid. They hypothesized that spatially localized electroporation of the multilamellar lipid bilayer membranes provides rapid delivery of salicylic acid to the keratin within corneocytes, leading to localized keratin disruption and then to a microconduit.

Recently, the FDA approved Ortho-McNeill's (J & J Co.) Ortho-EVRA as a transdermal patch containing ethinyl estradiol/norgestromin for contraception.

Lake and Pinnock[139] reported on a transdermal drug-in-adhesive estradiol patch system that is more acceptable to patients than the reservoir system for the treatment of postmenopausal estrogen deficiency. Characteristics of this patch system include ease of remembering once-weekly patch application, improved cosmetic appearance, and better adhesion.

The Cygnus transdermal fentanyl device showed great variability in the rate of fentanyl absorption, resulting in highly variable plasma fentanyl concentrations, but sometimes leading to toxicity. The currently available Duragesic transdermal fentanyl device has been contraindicated for postoperative analgesia. Vanbever et al.[179] used skin-electroporation techniques to improve the transdermal diffusion of fentanyl. According to Lehmann et al.,[173] however, the transdermal fentanyl patch, if properly used, could be effective in providing a background of analgesia in various pain states.

Ramachandran and Fleisher[140] discuss the feasibility of delivering drugs such as biphosphonates across the skin for the treatment of bone diseases. According to Zitzmann and Nieschlag,[143] transdermal systems provide the pharmacokinetic modality closest to natural diurnal variations in testosterone levels. Verma and Iyer[145] reported on controlled transdermal delivery of propranol using hydoxypropylmethylcelluslose matrices. In another study, estradiol transdermal system (OESCLIM) was developed for hormone replacement therapy (HRT), and it was shown that this system was as effective as Estraderm TTS at reducing vasomotor symptoms, even in highly symptomatic women.

Foldvari[150] investigated delivery of interferon (IFN) alpha, an antiviral agent used in the treatment of condylomata acuminata (genital warts), using lipid-based delivery systems (LBDS). They investigated the use of liposomes and fatty acylation as ways to increase IFN alpha delivery into human skin.

Chang et al.[144] used delta sleep-inducing peptide (DSIP), a peptide of nine amino acid residues, as a model drug to investigate the effects of pH, electric current, and enzyme inhibitors on the transdermal iontophoretic delivery of peptide drugs.

The polarities of four elastomers made of silicon oligomers of different viscosities were investigated by measuring the uptake of swelled solvent in different polarity solvents after 24, 48, and 72 hours of treatment. The solvent uptake provided a good characterization for the polarity of the inside of the matrix.

A proniosome-based transdermal system of LN was developed and extensively characterized, both *in vivo* and *in vitro*. The proniosomal structure was a liquid crystalline-compact niosomes hybrid, which could be converted into niosomes upon hydration. The system was evaluated *in vitro* for drug loading, rate of hydration (spontaneity), vesicle size, polydispersity, entrapment efficiency, and drug diffusion across rat skin. This study demonstrated the utility of proniosomal, transdermal-patch-bearing LN for effective contraception.[159,160]

Use of electroporation pulses as a physical penetration enhancer enabled delivery of a significant amount of cyclosporine-A (CSA) for the treatment of psoriasis. Transdermally delivered CSA was mostly bound to the skin, and only a small amount was seen to cross the full skin into the receiver compartment.[161,163]

According to Hippius et al.,[171] although topical drugs are usually applied at a convenient site, the target for the drug interaction may be systemic. Phonophoresis is the use of ultrasound to enhance the delivery of topically applied drugs. The purpose of their study was to investigate the *in vitro* penetration and the *in vivo* transport of flufenamic acid in dependence of ultrasound. Percutaneous absorption studies were performed in various *in vitro* models to determine the rate of drug absorption via the skin. These investigators designed a phonophoretic drug delivery system to study the influence of ultrasound on transmembrane transport of different drugs.

Dinslage et al.[174] reported on a new transdermal delivery system for pilocarpine in glaucoma treatment. They studied the intraocular pressure

(IOP)-lowering effects and the side effects of the new system (known as TDS). A substantial amount of pilocarpine was released from the TDS to the dermis, causing detectable plasma levels of pilocarpine at 12 and 20 hours after administration.

According to Thacharodi and Rao,[176] and Rao and Diwan,[162] membrane permeation-controlled transdermal delivery devices for the controlled delivery of nifedipine were developed using collagen and chitosan membranes as a rate-controlling membrane. To increase the stability of nifedipine in the systems, alginate gel was used as a drug reservoir. Drug release was found to depend on the type of membrane used to control the drug delivery, suggesting that drug delivery is efficiently controlled in this system by the rate-controlling membranes.

According to Pillai et al.,[153] epidermal enzymes play an important role in the process of differentiation of keratinocytes. Their preliminary study was undertaken to observe if topical enzyme treatment influenced permeation of compounds across the skin. Their study showed that phospholipase A2 significantly enhanced permeation of benzoic acid and mannitol, while it did not have any effect of the penetration of testosterone.

A homologous series of N-acetic acid esters of 2-pyrrolidone and 2-piperidinone were prepared and evaluated for their ability to enhance the skin content and flux of hydrocortisone 21-acetate in hairless mouse skin *in vitro*. Enhancement ratios (ER) were determined for flux (J), 24-hour diffusion cell receptor cell concentrations (Q24), and 24-hour full-thickness mouse skin steroid content (SC) and compared to control values. In this study, 2-oxopyrrolidine-alpha-acetic acid decyl ester showed the highest enhancement ratio of (SC).[166,167]

Transdermal systems bearing captopril were developed using a low-temperature casting method and aqueous-based polymers (e.g., Eudragit RL-100 and polyvinylpyrrolidone).[164,165]

Finally, developments continue for the transdermal delivery of old compounds, such as nitroglycerine, nicotine, isosorbide dinitrate, and insulin. Other developments have also been reported for drugs and therapeutic agents such as albuterol, chlorpheniramine maleate, nadolol, terbutaline sulfate, selegiline, ethylcellulose-polyvinyl pyrrolidone films containing diltiazem HCl and indomethacin, diclofenac diethyl ammonium in a pressure-sensitive adhesive system, Clonidine (M-5041T system), Zidovudine (AZT), pro-drug of gestodene, physostigmine (for organophosphate poisoning), propranolol (chitosan-based), tacrine for treating symptoms of Alzheimer's disease, and dideoxynucleoside-type anti-HIV drugs.[170–188]

X. Conclusion

Many factors must be considered in designing a delivery system for a drug to be applied via the skin. Certain aspects, such as drug stability, physical stability of the formulation, irritation and sensitization properties, preservation, and aesthetic acceptability, are all critical parameters. None of these considerations can be neglected in developing a new drug for transdermal delivery. There is little doubt that the vehicle can grossly affect drug bio-availability and, thus, influence the clinical efficacy of the drug. Unfortunately, there is no blueprint that can be followed to ensure development of an optimal product. Much depends on the specific pharmacologic properties of the drug, its physicochemical properties, and its clinical function. In addition, there can be no assurance that maximizing drug penetration into the skin is, in every case, synonymous with optimizing drug delivery. Topical products can be applied to skin that has been completely stripped of its barrier properties, as well as to skin that is anatomically intact and enormously resistant to drug diffusion. These two situations only define the extremes as far as the diffusional resistance of skin is concerned. It should be recognized that the same topical product cannot be ideal, in terms of drug bioavailability, for every type of skin disease or for every patient.[92-95]

There is no doubt that the physicochemical properties of the drug determine the ease or difficulty with which it passes through the skin barrier. However, in view of recent evidence, it now seems clear that the vehicle must be regarded as something more than a solvent in which the drug is placed to ensure uniform contact with the skin surface. If one's intent is to manipulate the diffusion rate of a drug across the skin, there are two general mechanisms by which this might be accomplished. One is to change the degree of interaction between drug and vehicle (i.e., affect the drug's thermodynamic activity). The other is to produce changes in the stratum corneum that will affect its diffusional resistance. In general terms, one can describe these two approaches as involving either drug-vehicle interactions or vehicle-barrier interactions. Both effects are generally involved, and distinction of the specific mechanism may be difficult. Careful characterization of the physical properties of a delivery system and the solubility and partitioning properties of the drug in this system will aid considerably in analyzing subsequent *in vitro* and *in vivo* penetration data involving human skin.[96-106]

For the great majority of substances, it is diffusion through the stratum corneum that represents the rate-limiting step in percutaneous absorption. Almost all substances used as drugs can be expected to penetrate even intact skin to some degree. Even particles of considerable size appear to pass through skin, although the rates are infinitesimally small. Characteristically, the penetration rate of most drugs will be small, and only a fraction of the total applied to the skin will reach the systemic circulation and be excreted. Obviously, if a finite rate of absorption occurs, the drug will ultimately be completely absorbed if it remains on the skin surface. In practice, much of the drug, along with the debris of the vehicle in which it is applied, will be removed by contact with dressings, clothing, and other objects, or simply be washed off by the patient. Because the skin is a complex, biological barrier that is not yet fully understood, generalizations about its relative permeability to different types of compounds must be made with considerable caution.[56,107-117]

Transdermal therapy appears to be ready for a rapid expansion of rate-controlled administration of potent, nonallergenic agents with suitable physicochemical properties where current methods of administration pose problems. By the mid-1990s, approximately 70% or more of all drugs potentially might have been delivered by transdermal delivery systems. However, because of the constraints imposed by drug potency, skin permeability, or topical reactions, transdermal administration may not become the preferred dosage route for a high percentage of drugs. Problems exist, such as cutaneous metabolism and the fact that a small volume of the skin has to deliver the entire load of a drug. Possibilities for future transdermal systems include making more use of pro-drugs, penetration enhancers, and specific nontoxic enzyme inhibitors. Certainly, a need exists for significant expansion in research on the fundamental understanding of skin metabolism as it affects drug transformation as well as pro-drug activation/inactivation.[118–121]

A specific challenge for future drug therapy is to efficiently deliver peptide drugs developed by the biotechnology industry. At present, it would not seem probable that simple application to the skin of a peptide would produce desirable clinical results. One possible approach may be to develop delivery devices that will synchronize the introduction of a suitable penetration enhancer into the stratum corneum together with the peptide. Another possibility would be to use iontophoresis, a technique that has been employed for a number of ionic drugs, and possibly use it in conjunction with penetration enhancers.[122–125]

Drug molecules may also be redesigned to achieve higher skin penetration. Most drugs in today's market are not only structured to elicit a particular pharmacological response, but also designed to have suitable solubilities, particularly with respect to oral and parenteral dosage forms. Perhaps more lipid-soluble molecules (pro-drugs) could be made from currently approved drugs to provide a more favorable prognosis for the transdermal approach in cases where drugs do not have the requisite physiochemical attributes.[81,126,127,168]

References

1. Cleary, G.W., Transdermal controlled-release systems. In *Medical Applications of Controlled Release*, Vol. 1, Langer, R.S. and Wise, D.L., Eds., CRC Press, Inc., Boca Raton FL, 203–251, 1984.
2. Kydonieus, A.F., *Controlled-Release Technologies: Methods, Theory, and Applications*, CRC Press, Inc., Boca Raton, FL, 213, 1987.
3. Juliano, R.L., Ed., Biological approaches to the controlled delivery of drugs, *Ann. NY Acad. Sci.*, 507, 364, 1987.
4. Chien, Y.W., Ed., Transdermal Controlled Medications, Marcel Dekker, New York, 440, 1987.
5. Barry, B.W., Johnson, P., and Lloyd-Jones, J.G., Eds., *Transdermal Drug Delivery Systems Fundamentals and Techniques*, Ellis Horwood Publishers, Chichester, 200–223, 1987.
6. Idson, B., Percutaneous absorption in topics in medicinal chemistry. In *Absorption Phenomena*, Rabinowitz Myerson, R.M., Ed., Wiley-Interscience, New York, 4, 181, 1976.

7. Katz, M., Design of topical drug product: pharmaceutics. In *Drug Design*, Ariens, E.J., Ed., Academic Press, New York, 4, 93–148, 1973.

8. Katz, M. and Poulsen, B.J., Absorption of drugs through the skin. In *Handbook of Experimental Pharmacology*, Brodie, B.B. and Gillette, J., Eds., Springer-Verlag, New York, 28, 103, 1971.

9. Poulsen, B.J., Design of topical drug products: biopharmaceutics. In *Drug Design*, Ariens, E.J., Ed., Academic Press, New York, 4, 149–192, 1973.

10. Higuchi, T., Pro-drug, molecular structure and percutaneous delivery. In *Design of Biopharmaceutical Properties through Pro-drugs and Analogs*, Roche, B., Ed., American Pharmaceutical Association, Washington, D.C., 409–421, 1977.

11. Scheuplein, R.J., The skin as a barrier, skin permeation, site variation in diffusion and permeability. In *The Physiology and Pathophysiology of the Skin*, Jarret, A., Ed., Academic Press, New York, 1693–1731, 1978.

12. Flynn, G.L., Topical drug absorption and topical pharmaceutical systems. In *Modern Pharmaceutics*, Banker, G.S. and Rhodes, C.T., Eds., Dekker, New York and Basel, 263, 1979.

13. Chien, Y.W., *Novel Drug Systems*, Dekker, New York and Basel, 149, 1982.

14. Schafer, H., Zesch, A., and Stuttgen, G., *Permeability*, Springer-Verlag, New York, 1982.

15. Bronaugh, R.L. and Maibach, H.I., Eds., *Percutaneous Absorption*, Marcel Dekker, New York and Basel, 1985.

16. Denyer, S.P., Guy, R.H., Hadgraft, J., and Hugo, W.B., The microbial degradation of topically applied drugs, *J. Pharm. Pharmacol.*, 37, 89, 1985.

17. Wester, R.C. and Noonan, P.K., Relevance of animal models for percutaneous absorption, *Int. J. Pharm.*, 7, 99, 1980.

18. Noonan, P.K. and Wester, R.K., Cutaneous metabolism of xenobiotics. In *Percutaneous Absorption*, Bronaugh, R.L. and Maibach, H.I., Eds., Marcel Dekker, New York and Basel, 65, 1985.

19. Guy, R.H. and Hadgraft, J., Pharmacokinetics of percutaneous absorption and concurrent metabolism, *Int. J. Pharm*, 20, 43, 1984.

20. Marty, J.P., Guy, R.H., and Maibach, H.I., Percutaneous penetration as a method of delivery to muscle and other tissues. In *Percutaneous Absorption*, Bronaugh, R.L. and Maibach, H.I., Eds., Marcel Dekker, New York and Basel, 1985.

21. Woodford, R. and Barry, B.W., Penetration enhancers and the percutaneous absorption of drugs: an update, *J. Toxicol. Cut. Ocular Toxicol.*, 5, 165, 1986.

22. Southwell, D., Barry, B.W., and Woodford, R., Variations in permeability in human skin within and between specimens, *Int. J. Pharm.*, 18, 19, 1984.

23. Schuplein, R.J., and Blank, I.H., Permeability of the skin, *Physiol. Rev.*, 51, 702, 1971.

24. Schuplein, R.J., Molecular structure and diffusional processes across intact epidermis, Report No. 7, *Edgewood Arsenal*, Maryland, 1966.

25. Ebling, F.J., *Dermatotoxicology and Pharmacology*, Marzulli, F.N. and Maibach, H.I., Eds., John Wiley & Sons, New York, 56, 1977.

26. Barr, M., Percutaneous absorption, *J. Pharm. Sci.*, 51, 395, 1962.

27. Katz, M. and Poulsen, B.J., Corticoid, vehicle and skin interaction in percutaneous absorption, *J. Cosmet. Chem.*, 23, 565, 1972.

28. Shaw, J.E., Taskovich, L., and Chandrasekaran, S.K., Properties of skin in relation to drug absorption *in vitro* and *in vivo*. In *Current Concepts in Cutaneous Toxicity*, Drill, V.A., Ed., Academic Press, New York, 127, 1980.

29. Elias, P.M., Epidermal lipids, membranes, and keratization, *Int. J. Dermatol.*, 20, 1, 1981.

30. Wepierre, J. and Martz, J.P., Percutaneous absorption of drugs, *Trends Pharm. Sci.*, 1, 23, 1979.

31. Hwang, S. and Kammermeyer, K., Membranes in separations. In *Techniques of Chemistry*, Vol. 7, Weissberger, A., Ed., Wiley-Interscience, New York, 3, 1975.

32. Crank, J., *The Mathematics of Diffusion*, Oxford University Press, London, 1956.

33. Higuchi, W.I., Diffusional models useful in biopharmaceutics, *J. Pharm. Sci.*, 56, 315, 1967.

34. Baker, R.W. and Lonsdale, H.K., Controlled-release mechanism and rates. In *Controlled Release of Biologically Active Agents*, Tanquary, T.C. and Lacy, R.E., Eds., Plenum Press, Inc., New York, 15, 1974.

35. Crank, J. and Park, G.S., Eds., *Diffusion in Polymers*, Academic Press, London, 1968.

36. Flynn, G.L., Yalkowski, S.H., and Roseman, T.J., Mass-transport phenomena and models: Theoretical concepts, *J. Pharm. Sci.*, 63, 479, 1974.

37. Flynn, G.L., Influence of physicochemical properties of drug and system on release of drugs from inert matrices. In *Controlled Release of Biologically Active Agents*, Tanquary, T.C. and Lacy, R.E., Eds., Plenum Press, New York, 72, 1974.

38. Langer, R., Polymer delivery systems for controlled drug release, *Chem. Eng. Commun.*, 6, 1980.

39. Kaeble, D.H., *Physical Chemistry of Adhesion*, John Wiley & Sons, New York, 1971.

40. Wake, W.C., Theories of adhesion and uses of adhesives: a review, *Polymer*, 19, 219, 1978.

41. ASTM Designation D 907–74 Stanford Definitions of Terms Relating to Adhesives, American Society for Testing and Materials, Philadelphia, 1974.

42. Fukuzawa, K. and Satas, D., Packaging tapes. In *Handbook of Pressure-Sensitive Adhesive Technology*, Satas, D., Ed., Von Nostrand Reinhold, New York, 426, 1982.

43. Adair, W.H., Pressure-sensitive fastening systems, *Adhes. Age*, 18, 31, 1975.

44. Higuchi, T., Design of chemical structure for optimal dermal delivery, *Curr. Probl. Dermatol.*, 7, 121, 1978.

45. Beckett, A.H., Gorrod, J.W., and Taylor, D.C., Comparison of oral and percutaneous routes in man for the systemic administration of ephedrines, *Pharm. Pharmacol.*, 24, 65P, 1972.

46. Riegelman, S., Pharmacokinetic factors affecting epidermal penetration and percutaneous absorption, *Clin. Pharmacol. Therap.*, 16, 873, 1974.

47. Good, W.R., Transdermal drug delivery systems. In The Latest Developments in Drug Delivery Systems Conference Proceedings, *Pharma. Tech.*, 40-48, 1985.

48. Schwenkenbecker, A., Studies on skin absorption, *Arch. Anal. Physiol.*, 28, 121, 1904.

49. Blank, I.H., Factors which influence the water content of the stratum corneum, *J. Invest. Derm.*, 18, 433, 1952.

50. Hadgraft, J. and Somers, G.E., Percutaneous absorption, *J. Pharm. Pharmacol.*, 8, 625, 1956.

51. Scheuplein, R.J., Mechanism of percutaneous absorption, routes of penetration and influence of solubility, *J. Invest. Derm.*, 45, 334, 1965.

52. Vlasses, P.H., Ribeiro, L., Rotmensch, H., et al., Initial evaluation of transdermal timolol, serum concentrations and beta blockade, *J. Cardiovas. Pharmacol.*, 7(2), 245, 1985.

53. Nagai, T., Yoshiaki, S., Nambu, N., and Machida, Y., Percutaneous absorption of propranolol from gel ointment in rabbits, *J. Control Rel.*, 1(3), 239, 1985.

54. Rabinowitz, J.L., Absorption of labeled triethanolamine salicylate. In *Proc. 12th Int. Symp. on Control. Rel. of Bioact. Mater.*, July 8–12, 1985, *Control. Rel. Soc.*, 347, 1985.

55. Baker, R.W. and Farrant, J., Patents in transdermal drug delivery. In The Latest Developments in Drug Delivery Systems, *Pharm. Tech.*, 26–31, 1987.

56. Pharmaprojects, 1993.

57. Bernstein, J.E., U.S. Patent 4,395,420, 1983.

58. Nagai, H., Wada, Y., Kobayashi, I., Tamada, M., et al., U.S. Patent 4,390,520, 1983.

59. Rolf, D., Chemical and physical methods of enhancing transdermal drug delivery, *Pharm. Tech.*, 12, 130–140, 1988.

60. Aiche, J.M., Cardot, J.M., and Aiche, S., *Int. J. Pharm.*, 55, 2, 3147–3155, 1989.

61. Chow, D.S.L. and Hsieh, D., Structure-activity relationship of permeation enhancers and their possible mechanisms, *Pharm. Tech.*, 13, 37, 1989.

62. Pfister, B. Compatibility of permeation enhancers with pressure-sensitive adhesives used in transdermal systems, *Pharm. Tech.*, 13, 37, 1989.

63. Dunn, J.A., Safety and toxicity considerations in the design of topical drug delivery systems, *Pharm. Tech.*, 11, 47, 1987.

64. Pfister, W.R., Customizing silicone adhesives for transdermal drug delivery systems, *Pharm. Tech.*, 13, 126–138, 1989.

65. Touitou, E., Fabin, B., Dany, S., and Almog, S., Transdermal delivery of tetrahydrocannabinol, *Int. J. Pharm.*, 43, 9–15, 1988.

66. Touitou, E., Skin-permeation enhancement by n-decyl methyl sulfoxide: Effect of solvent systems and insights on mechanism of action, *Int. J. Pharm.*, 43, 1–7, 1988.

67. Ashton, P., Hadgraft, J., Brain, K.R., Miller, T.A., and Walter, K.A., Surfactant effects in topical drug delivery, *Int. J. Pharm.*, 41, 189–195, 1988.

68. Das, S.K., Chattraj, S.C., and Gupta, B.K., Transdermal delivery of glibenclamide for blood-glucose control in diabetic rabbits, Program and Abstracts of the 15th Int. Symp. on Control Rel. Bioact. Mater., Basel, August 15–19, 1988, Paper No. 51.

69. Shah, K.R., Apostolopoulos, D.V., Franz, T.J., Sochan, T., and Kydonieus, A.F., Novel transdermal drug delivery system, *Program and Abstracts of the 15th Int. Symp. on Control Rel. Bioact. Mater.*, Basel, August 15–19, 1988, Paper No. 53.

70. Friend, D.R., Catz, P., Heller, J., and Baker, R., Transdermal permeation enhancers for levonorgestrel and other drugs, *Program and Abstracts of the 15th Int. Symp. on Control Rel. Bioact. Mater.*, Basel, August 15–19, 1988, Paper No. 92.

71. Bodde, H.E., Verhoff, J., and Ponec, M., Transdermal peptide delivery, *Program and Abstracts of the 15th Int. Symp. on Control Rel. Bioact. Mater.*, Basel, August 15–19, 1988, Paper No. 163.

72. Chien, Y.W., Chien, T., and Huang, Y.C., Transdermal fertility regulation in females, II. Scale-up process development and *in vivo* clinical evaluation, *Program and Abstracts of the 15th Int. Symp. on Control Rel. Bioact. Mater.*, Basel, August 15–19, 1988, Paper No. 168.

73. Tojo, K., Shah, H.S., Chien, Y.W., and Huang, Y.C., *In vivo/in vitro* correlation for transdermal verapamil delivery, *Program and Abstracts of the 15th Int. Symp. on Control Rel. Bioact. Mater.*, Basel, August 15–19, 1988, Paper No. 169.

74. Tojo, K., Chiang, C.C., Chien, Y.W., and Huang, Y.C., Development of transdermal delivery system for hydromorphone: Effect of enhancers, *Program and Abstracts of the 15th Int. Symp. on Control Rel. Bioact. Mater.,* Basel, August 15–19, 1988, Paper No. 234.

75. Friend, D.R., Catz, P., Heller, J., Reid, J., and Baker, R.W., Transdermal delivery of levonorgestrel, *Proc. Intern. Symp. Control. Rel. Bioact. Mater.,* 14, 135, 1987.

76. Lee, C.S. and Chien, Y.W., Transdermal-controlled delivery of progesterone: Enhancement in skin-permeation rate by alkanoic acids and their derivatives, *Proc. Intern. Symp. Control. Rel. Bioact. Mater.,* 219–220, 1987.

77. Tsuk, A.G., Nuwayser, E.S., and Gay, M.H., A new system for transdermal drug delivery, *Proc. Intern. Symp. Control. Rel. Bioact. Mater.,* 227–228, 1987.

78. Marinan, D.S., Noel, R.A., Pfister, W.R., Swarthout, D.E., et al., Evaluation of release kinetics of selected therapeutic agents and physical properties of silicone adhesive transdermal matrices, *Proc. Intern. Symp. Control. Rel. Bioact. Mater.,* 265–266, 1987.

79. Pfister, W.R. and Hsieh, D.S.T., Permeation enhancers compatible with transdermal drug delivery systems, Part I, Selection and formulation considerations, *Pharm. Tech.,* 14, 132–140, 1990.

80. Queen, D. et al., Assessment of the potential of a new hydrocolloid dermatological (Actiderm) in the treatment of steroid-responsive dermatoses, *Int. J. Pharm.,* 44, 25–30, 1988.

81. Pfister, W.R. and Hsieh, D.S.T., Permeation enhancers compatible with transdermal drug delivery systems, Part II. System design considerations, *Pharm. Tech.,* 14, 54–60, 1990.

82. Naik, A., Irwin, W.J., and Griffin, R.J., Percutaneous absorption of azidoprofen, *Int. J. Pharm.* (Amst), 90, 129–140, 1993.

83. Hansen, L.B., Fullerton, A., Christrup, L.L., and Bundgaard, H., Enhanced transdermal delivery of ketobemidone with pro-drugs, *Int. J. Pharm.* (Amst), 84, 253–260, 1992.

84. Lambert, W.J., Kudla, R.J., Holland, J.M., and Curry, J.T., A biodegradable-transdermal penetration enhancer based on N-2-hydroxyethyl-2-pyrrolidone I, *Int. J. Pharm.* (Amst), 95, 181–192, 1993.

85. Kobayashi, D. et al., Feasibility of use of several cardiovascular agents in transdermal therapeutic systems with 1-menthol-ethanol system on hairless rat and human skin, *Biol. Pharm. Bull.,* 16, 254–258, 1993.

86. Dolezal, P., Hrabalek, A., and Semecky, V., Epsilon-aminocaproic acid esters as transdermal penetration-enhancing agents, *Pharm. Res.,* 10, 1015–1019, 1993.

87. Ruland, A., Kreutert, J., and Rytting, J.H., Transdermal delivery of the tetra-peptide hisetal (melanotropin 6–9), *Int. J. Pharm.,* 101, 57–61, 1994.

88. *Chem. and Eng. News,* August 3, 1992, p. 24.

89. Morimoto, Y., Hatanaka, T., Sugibayashi, K., and Omiya, H., Prediction of skin permeability of drugs, *J. Pharm. Pharmacol,* 44, 634–639, 1992.

90. Ruan, L., Liang, B., Tao, J., and Yin, C., Transdermal absorption of nitrendipine from adhesive parches, *J. Control Rel.,* 20, 231–236, 1992.

91. Izumoto, T., Aioi, A., Uenoyama, S., Kuriyama, K., and Azuma, M., Relationship between the transference of a drug from a transdermal patch and the physicochemical properties, *Chem. Pharm. Bull.,* 40, 456–458, 1992.

92. Wolter, K.M.E,, A transdermal delivery system containing textile fabrics, *Chem. Pharm. Bull.,* 273–274, 1987.

93. van Ham, G.S. and Herzog, W.P., The design of sunscreen preparations. In *Drug Design*, Vol. 4, Eriens, E.J., Ed., 193–235, 1973.

94. Baker, R., *Controlled Release of Biologically Active Agents*, John Wiley & Sons, New York, 1987.

95. Shaw, J.E. and Chandrasekaran, S.K., Controlled topical delivery of drugs for systemic action, *Drug Metab. Rev.*, 8, 223, 1978.

96. Kasting, G.B., Theoretical models for iontophoretic delivery, *Adv. Drug Del. Rev.*, 9, 177–199, 1992.

97. Pikal, M.J., The role of electroosmotic flow in transdermal iontophoresis, *Adv. Drug Del. Rev.*, 9, 201–237, 1992.

98. Yoshida, N.H. and Roberts, M.S., Structure-transport relationship in transdermal iontophoresis, *Adv. Drug Del. Rev.*, 9, 239–264, 1992.

99. Sage, B.H. Jr. and Riviere, J.E., Model systems in iontophoresis transport efficacy, *Adv. Drug Del. Rev.*, 9, 265–287, 1992.

100. Ledger, P.W., Skin biological issues in electrically enhanced transdermal delivery, *Adv. Drug Del. Rev.*, 9, 289–307, 1992.

101. Phipps, J.B. and Gyory, J.R., Transdermal ion migration, *Adv. Drug Del. Rev.*, 9, 137–176, 1992.

102. Cullander, C., What are the pathways of iontophoretic current flow through mammalian skin? *Adv. Drug Del. Rev.*, 9, 119–135, 1992.

103. Santus, G.C. and Baker, R.W., Transdermal-enhancer patent literature, *J. Control Rel.*, 25, 1–20, 1993.

104. Knutson, K., Harrison, D.J., Pershing, L.K., and Goates, C.Y., Transdermal absorption of steroids, *J. Control Rel.*, 24, 95–108, 1993.

105. Leveque, J.L., de Rigal, J., Saint-Leger, D., and Billy, D., How does sodium lauryl sulfate alter the skin-barrier function in man? *Skin Pharmacol.*, 6, 111–115, 1993.

106. Singh, J. and Maibach, H.I., Topical iontophoretic drug delivery *in vivo*, *Dermatology*, 187, 235–238, 1993.

107. Cullander, C. and Guy, R.H., Routes of delivery case studies: transdermal delivery of peptides and proteins, *Adv. Drug Del. Rev.*, 8, 291–329, 1992.

108. Ghosh, T.K. and Banga, A.K., Methods of enhancement of transdermal drug delivery, *Pharm. Tech.*, April 1993, 62.

109. Ghosh, T.K. and Banga, A.K., Part I. Physical and biochemical approaches, *Pharm. Tech.*, March 1993, 72.

110. Ghosh, T.K. and Banga, A.K., Part II. Chemical permeation enhancers, *Pharm. Tech.*, May 1993, 68.

111. Kydonieus, A.F. and Berner, B., *Transdermal Delivery of Drugs*, Vols. 1–3, CRC Press, Boca Raton, FL, 1987, 560.

112. Shah, U.P., Behl, C.R., Flynn, G.L., Higuchi, W.I., and Schefer, H., Principles and criteria in the development and optimization of topical therapeutic products, *Skin Pharmacol.*, 6, 72–80, 1993.

113. Walters, K.A. and Hadgraft, J., Eds., *Pharmaceutical Skin-Penetration Enhancement*, Marcel Dekker, New York, 1993, 448.

114. Theiss, U., Kuhn, I., and Lucker, P.W., Iontophoresis — Is there a future for clinical application? *Methods Find Exp. Clin. Pharmacol.*, 13, 353–359, 1991.

115. Asmussen, B., Transdermal therapeutic systems — actual state and future, *Methods Find Exp. Clin. Pharmacol.*, 13, 343–351, 1991.

116. Gurny, R. and Junginger, H.E., *Bioadhesion Possibilities and Future Trends*, CRC Press, Boca Raton, FL, 1989, 206.

117. Gurny, R. and Teubner, A., *Dermal and Transdermal Drug Delivery*, CRC Press, Boca Raton, FL, 1993, 200.

118. Hymes, A.C., Transdermal drug delivery from a solid state hydrophilic reservoir system. In *Recent Advances in Drug Delivery Systems*, Anderson, J.M. and Kim, S.W., Eds., Plenum Press, New York and London, 1984, 309–313.

119. Karim, A., Transdermal delivery systems. In *Drug Delivery Systems*, McCloskey, J., Ed., Aster, Springfield, OR, 1983, 28.

120. Lenaerts, V.M. and Gurny, R., Eds., *Bioadhesive Drug Delivery Systems*, CRC Press, Boca Raton, FL, 1989, 200.

121. Nimmo, W.S., The promise of transdermal drug delivery, *Brit. J. Anesth.*, 64(1), 7, 1989.

122. Lelawongs, P., Liu, J.C., Siddiqui, O., and Chien, Y.W., Transdermal iontophoretic delivery of arginine-vasopressin, 1. Physicochemical considerations, *Int. J. Pharm.*, 56(1), 13, 1989.

123. Williams, A.C. and Barry, B.W., Urea analogs in propylene glycol as penetration enhancers in human skin, *Int. J. Pharm.*, 56(1), 43, 1989.

124. Jones, D.A., *Transdermal and Related Drug Delivery Systems*, Noyes Data Corporation, NJ, 1984.

125. Hoelgaard, A. and Mollgaard, B., Dermal drug delivery — improvement by choice of vehicle or drug derivative. In *Advances in Drug Delivery Systems*, Anderson, J.M. and Kim, S.W., Eds., Elsevier, Amsterdam, 111, 1986.

126. Rosoff, M., Ed., *Controlled Release of Drugs, Polymers and Aggregate Systems*, VCH, New York, 1989, 315.

127. Buyukyaylaci, S., Joshi, Y.M., Peck, G.E., and Banker, G.S., Polymeric pseudolatex dispersions as a new topical drug delivery system. In *Recent Advances in Drug Delivery Systems*, Anderson, J.M. and Kim, S.W., Eds., Plenum Press, NY and London, 1984, 291–307.

128. Kim, J.H. and Choi, H.K., Effect of additives in the crystallization and the permeation of ketoprofen from adhesive matrix, *Int. J. Pharm.*, 236(1–2), 81–85, 2002.

129. Jain, A.K. et al., Transdermal drug delivery of imiprimine hydrochloride, I. Effect of terpenes, *J. Control Release*, 79(1–3), 93–101, 2002.

130. Shun, S.C. and Yoon, M.K., Application of TPX polymer membranes for the controlled release of tripolidine, *Int. J. Pharm.*, 232 (1–2), 131–137, 2002.

131. Park, E.S. et al., Effects of adhesives and permeation enhancers on the skin permeation of captopril, *Drug Dev. Ind. Pharm.*, 27, 975–980, 2001.

132. Fukushima, S. et al., Transdermal drug delivery by electroporation applied on the stratum corneum of rats using stamp-type electrode and frog-type electrode *in vitro*, *Biol. Pharm. Bull.*, 24, 1027–1031, 2001.

133. Bhattacharya, A. and Ghosal, S.K., Effect of hydrophobic permeation enhancers on the release and skin-permeation kinetics from matrix-type transdermal drug delivery system of ketotifen fumrate, *Acta. Pol. Pharm.*, 58, 101–105, 2001.

134. Riviere, J.E. and Papich, M.G., Potential and problems of developing patches for veterinary applications, *Adv. Drug Deliv. Rev.*, 50, 175–203, 2001.

135. Lee, W.R. and Shen, S.C., Transdermal drug delivery enhanced and controlled by erbium:YAG laser: a comparative study of lipohilic and hydrophilic drugs, *J. Control Release*, 75(1–2), 155–166, 2001.

136. Takahashi, K. and Rytting, J.H., Novel approach to improve permeation of ondansetron across shed snake skin as a model membrane, *J. Pharm. Pharmacol.*, 53, 789–794, 2001.

137. Venter, J.P. et al., A comparative study of an *in situ*-adapted diffusion cell and an *in vitro* Franz diffusion cell method for transdermal absorption of doxylamine, *Eur. J. Pharm. Sci.*, 13, 169–177, 2001.

138. Ilic, L. et al., Microfabrication of individual 200-micron-diameter transdermal microconduits using high-voltage pulsing in salicylic acid and benzoic acid, *J. Invest. Dermatol.*, 116, 40–49, 2001.

139. Lake, Y. and Pinnock, S., Improved patient acceptability with a transdermal drug-in-adhesive estradiol patch, *Aust. NZ J. Obstet. Gynaecol.*, 40, 313–316, 2000.

140. Ramachandran, C. and Fleisher, D., Transdermal delivery of drugs for the treatment of bone diseases, *Adv. Drug Deliv. Rev.*, 42, 197–223, 2000.

141. Mitragotri, S. and Kost, J., Low-frequency sonophoresis: A noninvasive method of drug delivery and diagnostics, *Biotechnol. Prog.*, 16, 488–492, 2000.

142. Manna, A. et al., Statistical optimization of transdermal drug delivery system of terbutaline sulfate by factorial analysis, *Boll. Chim. Farm.*, 139, 34–40, 2000.

143. Zitzmann, M. and Nieschlag, E., Hormone substitution in male hypogonadism, *Mol. Cell. Endocrinol.*, 161, 73–88, 2000.

144. Chang, S.L. et al., The effect of electroporation on iontophoretic transdermal delivery of calcium regulating hormones, *J. Control Release*, 66, 127–133, 2000.

145. Verma, P.R. and Iyer, S.S., Controlled transdermal delivery of propranolol using HPMC matrices: design and *in vitro* and *in vivo* evaluation, *J. Pharm. Pharmacol.*, 52, 151–156, 2000.

146. Lombry, C. et al., Transdermal delivery of macromoleculess using skin electroporation, *Pharm. Res.*, 17, 32–37, 2000.

147. Kim, J., Cho, Y., et al., Effect of vehicles and pressure-sensitive adhesives on the permeation of tacrine across hairless mouse skin, *Int. J. Pharm.*, 196, 105–113, 2000.

148. Monoz, A., OESCLIM: an advanced delivery system for HRT, *Maturitas*, 33 Suppl, S39–S47, 1999.

149. Groning, R. and Kuhland, U., Pulsed release of nitroglycerine from transdermal drug delivery systems, *Int. J. Pharm.*, 193, 57–61, 1999.

150. Foldvari, M. et al., Dermal and transdermal delivery of protein pharmaceuticals: lipid-based delivery systems for interferon alpha, *Biotechnol. Appl. Biochem.*, 30(pt. 2), 129–137, 1999.

151. Ilic, L. and Gowrishankar, T.R., Spatially constrained skin electroporation with sodium thiosulfate and urea creates transdermal microconduits, *J. Control Release*, 61, 185–202, 1999.

152. Kantaria, S. and Rees, G.D., Gelatin-stabilized microemulsion-based organogels: Rheology and application in iontophoretic transdermal drug delivery, *J. Control Release*, 60, 355–365, 1999.

153. Pillai, O. et al., Transdermal iontophoresis, Part II: peptide and protein delivery, *Methods Find Exp. Clin. Pharmacol.*, 21, 229–240, 1999.

154. Ocak, F. and Agabeyoglu, I., Development of a membrane-controlled transdermal therapeutic system containing isosorbide dinitrate, *Int. J. Pharm.*, 180, 177–183, 1999.

155. Gowrishankar, T.R. et al., Spatially constrained localized transport regions due to skin electroporation, *J. Control Release*, 60, 101–110, 1999.

156. Fang, J.Y. et al., *In vitro* study of transdermal nicotine delivery: Influence of rate-controlling membranes and adhesives, *Drug Dev. Ind. Pharm.*, 25, 789–794, 1999.

157. Devi, K. and Paranjothy, K.L., Pharmacokinetic profile of a new matrix-type transdermal delivery system: diclofenac diethyl ammonium patch, *Drug Dev. Ind. Pharm.*, 25, 695–700, 1999.

158. Bhatia, K.S. and Singh, J., Mechanism of transport enhancement of LHRH through porcine epidermis by terpenes and iontophoresis: permeability and lipid extraction studies, *Pharm. Res.*, 15, 1857–1862, 1998.

159. Chetty, D.J. and Chien, Y.W., Novel methods of insulin delivery: an update, *Crit. Rev. Ther. Drug Carrier Syst.*, 15, 629–670, 1998.

160. Arra, G.S. et al., Transdermal delivery of isosorbide 5-mononitrate from a new membrane reservoir and matrix-type patches, *Drug Dev. Ind. Pharm.*, 24, 489–492, 1998.

161. Chiang, C.H. et al., Effects of pH, electric current, and enzyme inhibitors on iontophoresis of delta sleep-inducing peptide, *Drug Dev. Ind. Pharm.*, 24, 431–438, 1998.

162. Rao, P.R. and Diwan, P.V., Formulation and *in vitro* evaluation of polymeric films of diltiazem hydrochloride and indomethacin for transdermal administration, *Drug Dev. Ind. Pharm.*, 24, 327–336, 1998.

163. Wagner, O., Development of a new silicon-based transdermal system, I. Study of silicone elastomers and effect of liquid ingredients, *Drug Dev. Ind. Pharm.*, 24, 243–252, 1998.

164. Benech, H. et al., Development and *in vivo* assessment of a transdermal system for physostigmine, *Methods Find Exp. Clin. Pharmacol.*, 20, 489–498, 1998.

165. Lipp, R. et al., Pro-drugs of gestidene for matrix-type transdermal drug delivery systems, *Pharm. Res.*, 15, 1419–1424, 1998.

166. Vora, B. et al., Proniosome-based transdermal delivery of levonorgestrel for effective contraception, *J. Control Release*, 54, 149–165, 1998.

167. Oh, Sy. et al., Enhanced transdermal delivery of AZT(Zidovudine) using iontophoresis and penetration enhancer, *J. Control Release*, 51(2–3), 161–168, 1998.

168. Wang, D.M. and Lin, F.C., Application of asymmetric TPX membranes to transdermal delivery of nitroglycerine, *J. Control Release*, 50, 187–195, 1998.

169. Wang, S. et al., Transdermal delivery of cyclosporine-A using electroporation, *J. Control Release*, 50, 61–70, 1998.

170. Mikulak, S.A. et al., Transdermal delivery and accumulation on indomethacin in subcutaneous tissues in rats, *J. Pharm. Pharmacol.*, 50, 153–158, 1998.

171. Hippius, M. et al., *In vitro* investigations of drug release and penetration-enhancing effect of ultrasound on transmembrane transport of flufenamic acid, *Int. J. Clin. Pharmacol. Ther.*, 36, 107–111, 1998.

172. Barrett, J.S. and DiSanto, A.R., Toxicokinetic evaluation of a selegiline transdermal system in the dog, *Biopharm. Drug Dispos.*, 18, 165–184, 1997.

173. Lehmann, L.J. et al., Transdermalfentanyl in postoperative pain, *Reg. Anesth.*, 22, 24–28, 1997.

174. Dinslage, S. et al., A new transdermal delivery system for pilocarpine in glaucoma treatment, *Ger. J. Ophthalmol.*, 5, 275–280, 1996.

175. Kalish, R. and Wood, J.A., Sensitization of mice to topically applied drugs: Albuterol, chlorpheniramine, clonidine, and nadolol, *Contact Dermatitis*, 35, 76–82, 1996.

176. Thacharodi, D. and Rao, K.P., Rate-controlling biopolymer membranes as transdermal delivery systems for nifedipine, development and *in vitro* evaluations, *Biomaterials*, 17, 1307–1311, 1996.

177. Van der Geest, R. et al., Iontophoresis of bases, nucleosides, and nucleotides, *Pharm. Res.*, 13, 553–558, 1996.
178. Krishna, R. and Pandit, J.K., Carboxymethylcellulose sodium-based transdermal drug delivery system for propranolol, *J. Pharm. Pharmacol.*, 48, 367–370, 1996.
179. Vanbever, R. et al., Transdermal delivery of fentanyl by electroporation, I. Influence of electrical factors, *Pharm. Res.*, 13, 559–565, 1996.
180. Mitragotri, S. et al., Transdermal drug delivery using low-frequency sonophoresis, *Pharm. Res.*, 13, 411–420, 1996.
181. Michniak, B.B. et al., Synthesis and *in vitro* transdermal penetration enhancing activity of lactam N-acetic acid esters, *J. Pharm. Sci.*, 85, 150–154, 1996.
182. Cevc, G., Transfersomes, liposomes, and other lipid suspensions on the skin: Permeation enhancement, vesicle penetration, and transdermal drug delivery, *Crit. Rev. Ther. Drug Carrier Syst.*, 13, 257–388, 1996.
183. Kimira, K. et al., Effects of a newly developed transdermal clonidine delivery system (M-5041T) on EEG sleep–wake cycle in relation to plasma concentration in rabbits, *Gen. Pharmacol.*, 27, 73–77, 1996.
184. Andronis, V., Mesiha, M.S., et al., Design and evaluation of transdermal chlorpheniramine maleate drug delivery system, *Pharm. Acta. Helv.*, 70, 301–306, 1995.
185. Fiset, P. et al., Biopharmaceutics of a new transdermal fentanyl device, *Anesthesiology*, 83, 459–469, 1995.
186. Jenner, J. and Saleem, A., Transdermal delivery of physostigamine: A pretreatment against organophosphate poisoning, *J. Pharm. Pharmacol.*, 47, 206–212, 1995.
187. Thacharodi, D., Rao, K.P., Development and *in vitro* evaluation of chitosan-based transdermal drug delivery systems for the controlled delivery of propranolol hydrochloride, *Biomaterials*, 16, 145–148, 1995.
188. Kandavilli, S. et al., Polymers in transdermal drug delivery systems, *Pharm. Tech.*, 26, 62–80, 2002.
189. Cantor, A.S. and Wirtanen, D.J., Novel acrylate adhesives for transdermal drug delivery, *Pharm. Tech.*, 26, 28–38, 2002.

chapter seven

Intranasal and ocular drug delivery

Contents

I.   Intranasal drug delivery

A.   Introduction

In view of the vascularity of the nasal mucosa, the possibility of bypassing hepato-gastrointestinal (GI) first-pass elimination, and the ease of administration, the nasal route would seem to be an ideal alternative for daily administration of some drugs. The use of the nasal route for the administration of drugs has, in fact, engaged the attention of mankind since ancient times. Nasal therapy, for example, is a recognized form of treatment in the Ayurvedic system of East Indian medicine. Psychotropic drugs and hallucinogens have been used as snuffs by the natives in South America for centuries.

Over the last decade, the possibility that intranasal administration might be useful for many compounds that are not absorbed orally has received increasing attention. In particular, with the availability of proteins and peptides from advanced biotechnology (e.g., insulin, growth hormone, etc.), the research and development of intranasal drug delivery systems has become even more vital.[1]

Not all drugs can be administered nasally. For example, some drugs cannot be absorbed through the nasal mucosa because of their chemical characteristics. Others are absorbed only with great difficulty and require added permeation enhancers — pharmaceutical ingredients that often produce their own side effects. For drugs that can be delivered nasally, however, there are potential advantages: lower doses, more rapid attainment of therapeutic blood levels, quicker onset of pharmacological activity, and fewer side effects.

Not all of these benefits accrue to every drug that can be delivered nasally. In rare instances, a drug that is absorbed nasally will show none of these benefits. In such cases, the only advantage of nasal delivery may be convenience or compliance of administration — reason enough to continue to evaluate the nasal route of administration. For drugs that can be delivered orally, nasal delivery might not offer the advantages of increased efficacy, absorption rate, compliance, and convenience.

Nudelman[2] has reported that a drug should be considered for development as a nasal product if it fulfills one of the following conditions: it is administered parenterally; it is in an inconvenient dosage form, such as a suppository; it is absorbed poorly; or it is absorbed slowly and produces undesirable side effects when administered orally.

Many drugs absorbed through the rich blood supply of the nasal mucosa enter the systemic circulation more rapidly than when they are administered orally. For example, properly formulated into a nasal dosage form, the beta blocker propranolol can abort a migraine attack even after the symptoms have started. Similarly, nasally administered meclizine (an antihistamine) can reduce or eliminate dizziness and nausea associated with motion sickness.

B. Nasal physiology and intranasal drug administration

Even with a cursory examination of nasal morphology and physiology, it becomes obvious that the nasal passage is quite different from the remainder of the airway. Figure 7.1 illustrates the upper airway as seen from the midline. The dashed line just beyond the nostrils marks the beginning of the nasal valve, while the dotted line shows approximately the beginning of the ciliated epithelium region. Large aerosol particles deposit largely in the zone between the dashed and dotted lines. The dashed line near the nasopharynx indicates the posterior termination of the nasal septum. Materials applied topically to the nasal conjunctiva will enter the nose through the nasolacrimal duct, just beneath the anterior end of the inferior turbinate. The other conducting airways provide conduits permitting the passage of respired air with a minimum resistance to airflow.

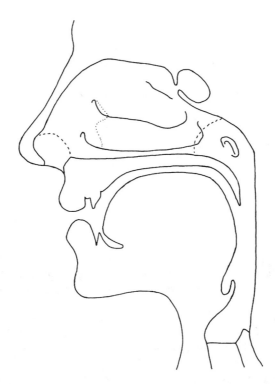

Figure 7.1 The upper airways as seen from the midline. (From Chien, Y.W., Ed., *Transnasal Systemic Medications, Fundamentals, Developmental Concepts and Biomedical Assessments*, Elsevier Science Publishers, Amsterdam, 1985, 102. With permission.)

The nasal airway accounts for as much resistance as all the remainder of the respiratory tract. This results from the bifurcation of the nose into two halves by the nasal septum. Each half, in turn, is convoluted by the folds of the turbinates, an arrangement which, at the cost of added resistance to airflow, permits an intimate contact between the air stream and the mucosal surfaces.[3]

Figure 7.2 illustrates a section through the main nasal passage showing the nasal septum, folds of the turbinates, and airway. The stippled area indicates the olfactory region, which is generally free of inspiratory airflow. Horizontal lines mark the metal spaces, through which there is very little airflow, but in which there exists communications with the paranasal sinuses and naso-lacrimal duct. The clear areas mark the zone of inspiratory airflow and the region lined with richly vascular erectile tissue. This is the site primarily reached by medications applied intranasally (e.g., nose drops or fine aerosol sprays).

Modification of inspired air within the nose includes stabilization of temperature and water vapor content. These adjustments become possible because of the close contact between the narrow airstreams and mucosal

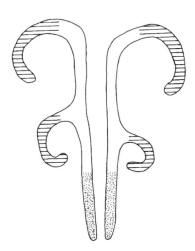

Figure 7.2 Section through the main nasal passage. (From Chien, Y.W., Ed., *Transnasal Systemic Medications, Fundamentals, Developmental Concepts and Biomedical Assessments,* Elsevier Science Publishers, Amsterdam, 1985, 103. With permission.)

surfaces and because of the nature of the circulatory and mucociliary systems. Therefore, the nasal vascular system presents a substantial surface area to inspired materials (e.g., gases or aerosols) that is extremely rich and highly adjustable.[4,5]

The mucociliary system consists of a great number of submucosal glands and goblet cells that provide the mucus and cilia that transport fluids to the nasopharynx, where they can be swallowed or expectorated. Of special importance is the fact that both circulatory and secretory mechanisms are susceptible to a variety of influences. For example, if a factor produces significant vasoconstriction, the capability of the nose to transmit surface materials to the systemic circulation can be significantly reduced.

Since a drug may be introduced into the nose in liquid or nasal spray form (e.g., aerosol or powder), it is necessary to understand the factors that influence these delivery forms. In the anterior area of the nose, there is a constriction known as the nasal valve. To pass this point, air must flow at a high-linear velocity and change direction. These two characteristics result in deposition of most aerosols or dusts in the anterior region of the nose. The larger particles lodge far enough anteriorly to be in front of the exchange region of the nose and, therefore, are not subject to nasal absorption into the body. Insoluble particles, even if they pass this point and deposit in the main passage, are likely to be carried backward by the mucociliary system and dispatched to the stomach. If a drug is introduced as a vapor or in soluble form, it may readily pass through the surface secretions and into the systemic circulation.

The presence of existing nasal pathology is also important. Nasal obstruction as a result of extensive nasal polyposis, for example, would reduce the capacity of nasal absorption. In addition, atrophic rhinitis or severe vasomotor rhinitis can also reduce the usefulness of the nose to absorb a drug. In some individuals, excessive response of the mucous cells to some irritants may drain away whatever is introduced prior to absorption. Such a tendency may exist in persons with severe nasal allergies.[6,7]

Of all of the parenteral routes, intravenous administration serves as the reference standard for establishing the basis of bioavailability. Not only does it bypass the absorption process, but it results in no presystemic metabolism. Intramuscular injection, unlike intravenous, does not always ensure rapid or complete absorption. Like intramuscular and intranasal, subcutaneous administration also depends upon the vascularity and blood supply at the administration site, and these factors can influence the rate or extent of absorption.[8]

Although surfactants and other absorption promoters may stimulate the absorption of macromolecular drugs by other routes, intranasal administration offers a much more favorable opportunity for the absorption of such large bioactive molecules.[9,10]

In comparison with the more traditional nonoral routes of administration, the intranasal route is experiencing increasing interest, especially for hormones, peptides, vaccines, and other drugs. This is a clear advantage for drugs that undergo extensive hepatic first-pass elimination, gut wall metabolism, or destruction in GI fluids. In some cases, such as with an influenza vaccine, a large population of individuals will be more willing to accept intranasal rather than parenteral administration, and this could have significant public health implications.[11]

C. Nasal drug delivery devices

In the development of nasal drug delivery devices, two principal systems will be discussed: the mechanical pump system and the pressurized aerosol system. Because both systems are capable of delivering drugs accurately, they are widely used. The selection of either the mechanical pump system or the pressurized aerosol system depends upon the nature of the drug to be developed. In general, the mechanical pump system is simpler than the pressurized aerosol system. Once the final formulation has been assured to be stable — both chemically and physically — and compatible with all the components of the delivery device, the use of a pump system should be straightforward. However, the pressurized aerosol system can be more complicated because of the presence of propellants in the formulation.

If an ingredient in the formulation is required to be dissolved or dispersed, the physicochemical compatibility of the drug with the propellant, co-solvents, or dispersing agents will require evaluation. An aqueous system should certainly be the first choice, and then its use with a mechanical system should be straightforward. However, if an active ingredient has solubility and stability problems in an aqueous system, a nonaqueous solvent system should be considered. Once a specific formulation is determined, three basic vehicle systems can be considered (i.e., solution, suspension, and emulsion).

When a formulation is finalized, it is essential to evaluate how the product will maintain its stability under the variable conditions of time, temperature, and pressure. Accelerated stability testings, in which the final formulation is subjected to the stability evaluation under more extreme conditions, will provide some preliminary information. Stability studies, in addition to assessing the active ingredient, should include testing for weight loss, delivery rate, tail-off, pressure, and pH. The studies must be conducted with the formulation in a glass container to permit the observation of any physical changes if the final product is to be in metal. During storage, the adsorption of a drug by plastic components could occur, leading to a reduction in drug concentration delivered to the patient. Although aerosol products, like oral dosage forms, need not be sterile, they should be free from any bacterial contamination.

With regard to evaluation of the physical stability of an aerosol system, the pertinent parameters include polymorphism, crystal growth, phase separation, dispersability, and dose distribution. Products are subjected to stability testing at temperatures of $-8°C$, $4°C$, room temperature, and a cycling temperature ranging from $-8°C$ to $40°C$ to mimic shipping conditions. A wrong choice of polymorph can result in some physical instability. Furthermore, the presence of a less stable crystal form may cause crystal growth at a later stage, which may subsequently affect aerosol performance. It should be kept in mind that since the propellant content in the formulation can vary once the product is in use, the dose distribution from the first dose could be significantly different from the last dose. Therefore, dose distribution must be fully studied.

The aerosol release valve plays perhaps the most important role in any aerosol product. It must mechanically function each time and must repeatedly deliver the drug in a specified quantity. Therefore, the valve components need to be compatible with the formulation. Plastic parts used in the valve may be subject to swelling, softening, and cracking. The metal parts of the valve may also be corroded, depending upon the formula involved. Dip tube growth, for instance, is a common problem in aerosols. Therefore, separate testing for each valve part by the total immersion technique should be conducted to detect any incompatibility problems.

The plasticizers and lubricants required in the molding of the plastics may be extracted by various solvents used in the formulation. These materials should not have any adverse effects on the physiological properties of the drug and its efficacy. For example, pumps or aerosol systems employ at least one rubber gasket, which comes in contact with the contents of the product. These gaskets almost always contain plasticizers, antioxidants, lubricants, and other substances. Compatibility of these gaskets with the formula must be evaluated. The gaskets fabricated from rubber products such as buna and neoprene are commonly utilized in the aerosol industry because of their acceptable compatibility with most products.

No matter how well a valve is designed, variation in the volume dispensed will occur from one valve to another and from one actuation to another, even with the same valve. The limits of acceptable variation depend entirely on the formulation to be dispensed and the safety of the medication to be administered.

There is no doubt that drug distribution within the nasal cavity is an important factor for nasal uptake. Because the mode of administration will affect drug distribution, it will, in turn, affect the efficacy of a medication. Mygind et al.[12] have demonstrated that a significant variation in drug distribution occurs in a model cast of the human nose following intranasal drug administration by different drug delivery devices.

The drug, and its final dosage form, must be subjected to both acute and chronic toxicity evaluations. Most of the ingredients used in aerosol formulations are generally regarded as safe, so that no major toxicity issues should be of concern. With regard to the active compound, acute toxicity is fairly easy to evaluate, since toxic manifestations show up within a relatively short period of time during preclinical testing. This data should be available in time for starting preformulation and designing dosage forms. Chronic toxicity presents a greater problem because of the long waiting time required for determination of toxicity under normal conditions of exposure and use. Nevertheless, like other dosage-form products, a 30-day toxicity program on the finished product should be sufficient for single-dose clinical trials and a 90-day toxicity program for multiple-dose clinical trials.[1]

Phasing out of chlorofluorocarbon (CFC) propellants in pressurized inhalers under the terms of the Montreal Protocol, together with the desire to use the lungs as a portal to the systemic circulation, has resulted in the development of many innovative techniques. Since the introduction of the first generation of passive unit dry-powder inhalers (DPIs), Fison's Spinhaler and GSK Rotahaler powder inhalers, many advances with respect to both complexity and performance have been made (see Table 7.1). Inhance Pulmonary Delivery system utilizes compressed air to pre-aerosolize the formulation, independent of the patients' inspiratory effort, into a transparent holding chamber, thereby enabling patients to view the aerosol before inhalation. This device has been designed for the systemic delivery of insulin and other proteins. Marketed multiunit dose devices include GSK Diskhaler and Accuhaler. Other innovative multiunit device systems include Spiros S2, the technology of which involves the use of electro-mechanical energy (breath-actuated, battery-operated propeller) to aerosolize and disperse powdered medication, rather than depending upon the patients' inspiratory effort or propellants. The development of multidose reservoir powder inhalers was pioneered by AstraZeneca with the Turbohaler. The design of this delivery system enables the efficient aerosolization and dispersion of pure aggregated drug material without excipients.

Optimization and control of particle–particle and particle–inhaler interactions is of critical importance in the development of efficient drug-powder inhaler systems. Drug particles should be less than 5 mm aerodynamic

Table 7.1 Dry-powder inhalers at various stages of development

Passive powder inhalers	Classification	Dispersion mechanism
Spinhaler (Fisons)	Unit dose	Pierced capsule rotates on impeller — vibratory dispersion
Rotahaler (GSK)	Unit dose	Capsule separates with dispersion via plastic grid
Inhalator (Boehringer-Ingelheim)	Unit dose	Stationary capsule pierced — dispersion via capillary fluidization
Aerosolizer (Novartis)	Unit dose	Pierced capsule rotates in chamber — dispersion aided by grid
Solo (Inhale Therapeutic Systems)	Unit dose	Dispersion via turbulent airflow pathway
Orbital (BrinTech International)	Unit dose	Dispersion via centrifugal acceleration mechanism
U.S. Patent 6,092,522 (RPR)	Unit dose	Pierced capsule rotates rapidly within a chamber
U.S. Patent 6,102,035 (Astra)	Unit dose	Disposable inhaler — airflow pathway entrainment and dispersion
Diskhaler (GSK)	Multiunit dose	Pierced blister — dispersion via turbulent airflow pathway and grid
Accuhaler (GSK)	Multiunit dose	Pierced blister — dispersion via turbulent airflow pathway
Inhalator M (Boehringer-Ingelheim)	Multiunit dose	Stationary capsule pierced — dispersion via capillary fluidization
Flowcaps (Hovione)	Multiunit dose	Capsule-based device — dispersion via turbulent airflow pathway
Spiros S2 (Elan Corporation)	Multiunit dose	Dispersion via free-floating beads and a dosing chamber
Technohaler (Innovata Biomed)	Multiunit dose	Dispersion via turbulent airflow pathway
U.S. Patent 5,469,843 (3M)	Multiunit dose	Pierced capsule rotates rapidly within a chamber
U.S. Patent 5,724,959 (AEA Technology)	Multiunit dose	Dispersion via impaction and turbulent flow
U.S. Patent 6,182,655 (Jago Research)	Multiunit dose	Dispersion via turbulent airflow pathway
U.S. Patent 6,209,538 (Innova Devices)	Multiunit dose	Airflow diversion around powder until optimal flow rate achieved
U.S. Patent 6,237,591 (Dura)	Multiunit dose	Turbine-powdered inhaler with impeller
Turbuhaler (AstraZeneca)	Multidose reservoir	Dispersion via turbulent airflow pathway
Easyhaler (Orion)	Multidose reservoir	Dispersion via turbulent airflow pathway
Clickhaler (Innovata Biomed)	Multidose reservoir	Dispersion via turbulent airflow pathway

Table 7.1 Dry-powder inhalers at various stages of development (Continued)

Passive powder inhalers	Classification	Dispersion mechanism
Pulvinal (Chiesi)	Multidose reservoir	Dispersion via turbulent airflow pathway
Twisthaler (Schering-Plough)	Multidose reservoir	Dispersion via turbulent airflow pathway
SkyePharma DPI (SkyePharma)	Multidose reservoir	Dispersion via turbulent airflow pathway
Taifun (Leiras)	Multidose reservoir	Dispersion via turbulent airflow pathway
Novolizer (Sofotec GmbH)	Multidose reservoir	Dispersion via turbulent airflow pathway
MAGhaler (Mundipharma)	Multidose tablet	Dispersion via turbulent airflow; formulation present as tablet
U.S. Patent 5,505,196 (Bayer)	Multidose reservoir	Dispersion via turbulent airflow in a "swirl chamber"
U.S. Patent 5,699,789	Multidose reservoir	Dispersion via turbulent airflow pathway
U.S. Patent 5,975,076 (Kings College)	Multidose reservoir	Dispersion via turbulent airflow pathway

Active powder inhalers	Classification	Dispersion mechanism
Inhance PDS (Inhale)	Unit dose	Gas-assisted — compressed air disperses powder formulation
Spiros (Elan Corporation)	Multiunit dose	Electromechanical energy — battery-operated impeller
Prohaler (Valois)	Multiunit dose	Gas-assisted — built-in pump provides compressed air
U.S. Patent 5,349,947	Multiunit dose	Explosive blister is crushed between piston and anvil
U.S. Patent 5,388,572 (Tenax)	Multiunit dose	Gas-assisted — inhalation-activated piston
U.S. Patent 5,875,776 (Vivorx)	Multiunit dose	Gas-assisted — electrostatic charge discharges on spacer
U.S. Patent 6,142,146 (Microdose)	Multiunit dose	Electronic circuitry with dispersion via vibration
U.S. Patent 6,237,590 (Delsys)	Multiunit dose	Electrostatic powder dosing coupled with electronic release

Source: Russell Publishing, *Am. Pharm. Rev.,* Fall 2001, 38. With permission.

diameter to produce efficient lung deposition, but should also exhibit acceptable flow properties required for accurate dose metering. Therefore, micronized powders are often blended with "coarse" inert carriers (e.g., lactose or glucose), or alternatively pelletized as loose agglomerates to improve powder flow. In recent years, the industry has focused on two types of alternative particle-generation technologies (e.g., spray drying and supercritical fluid condensation). Generally, spray-drying particles are spherical and often hollow, resulting in a powder with a low bulk density in comparison to the starting material. The major drawback of the spray-drying process is that metastable, high-energy amorphous forms that may crystallize over time and influence product performance are created. Improved aerosol efficiency can be achieved by spray drying with excipients such as sodium chloride, human serum albumin, or carbohydrates (e.g., lactose, mannitol, trehalose, or combinations thereof). Particles of insulin, delta-1-amitrypsin and beta-interferon have been successfully prepared by spray drying with excipients. Proteins are spray dried with "glass forming" sugars to form an amorphous glass state in which the liquid has a high viscosity. The glass state will remain stable for long periods of time when stored well below the glass-transition temperature.

In another approach, large porous particles (comprising poly[lactic acid-co-glycolic acid] or DL-a-phosphatidylcholine) have been prepared with geometric diameters in the order of 5 to 20 μm. Because of the reduced number of surface contacts, interparticle interactions are minimized, and thus particles are claimed to be less cohesive and demonstrate improved flow and dispersability. Also, these large particles are less likely to be phagocytosed than small particles and can reside in the lungs for relatively long periods of time and offer sustained release characteristics. Spray freeze drying produces large protein particles with light and porous particles, demonstrating improved aerosol performance compared to spray-dried particles. Hollow and porous particles are prepared by a two-stage process. Initially, a drug is dissolved in the continuous phase of a fluorocarbon in water emulsion. The resulting emulsion is spray dried, with the dispersed fluorocarbon serving as a blowing agent, keeping the particles inflated and creating pores in the drying aerosol droplets.

The inhalation particles can also be prepared by using supercritical fluid condensation (SCF) methods. SCFs are fluids at or above their critical temperature and pressure. In this region, SCFs exist as a single phase and possess the solvent power of liquids (also used in high-pressure liquid chromatographic separation of chemicals) together with the mass-transfer properties of gases. Carbon dioxide is the most commonly used SCF because it is nontoxic, noninflammable, inexpensive, and has a critical temperature of 31°C, which allows for easy operation under ambient conditions.

During the past few years, advances relating to formulation-related pMDIs include: incorporation of HFA-miscible co-solvents into the formulation, inclusion of various surfactant systems, encapsulation of drug particles, use of perforated microparticles, and use of other nontoxic stabilizing excipients. Device-related pMDI advances include incorporation of actuation mechanism (e.g., Smartmist, Aradigm, Hayward, CA) and use of spacers and plume modifiers (e.g., Azmacort, Rhone-Poulenc Rorer Co., Collegeville, PA; Aerohaler, Bespak, UK; and Spacehaler, Evans Medical, UK).

Nebulizers are drug delivery systems that can be used to generate solutions or suspensions for inhalation. These are suitable for deep-lung delivery.

Two types of nebulizers are currently marketed: jet and ultrasonic. Jet nebulizers use the Venture Effect to draw solution through a capillary tube and disperse droplets in air at high velocity. Ultrasonic nebulizers use oscillating ultrasonic vibration, which is conveyed by means of piezoelectric transducer to a solution that creates droplets suitable for inhalation. A portable, battery-operated aerosol generator has been developed (AeroGen, Sunnyvale, CA). This device has been used for delivery of liposomes and can be used to store freeze-dried compounds, which can be dissolved in a solution (also stored in a device) immediately before being aerosolized. This is particularly useful in the case of proteins and peptides, which are more stable in the solid state. The AERx (Aradigm) system has been shown to be useful in the delivery of peptide drugs, narcotics, and insulin. A portable, piezoelectric aqueous delivery system has been developed for the delivery of drugs in solution. A portable, breath-activated delivery system, the Halolite (Medic-Aid, UK) has also been developed. This device is capable of producing a precise dose and prevents the waste of drugs during exhalation. A device that uses an electric field to form an aerosol of fine droplets from a liquid has been developed (Battelle Pulmonary Therapeutics, Columbus, OH). The aerosol formed from this system in monodisperse, and the total delivered dose, dose reproducibility, and particle-size distributions generated can be controlled by changes in the drug formulations or electric field.

DPIs can be divided into two classes: passive and active devices. Passive devices rely solely upon the patients' inhalatory flow through the DPI to provide the energy needed for dispersion. Active devices have been under investigation for several years, but no active device has been on the market yet. These devices use an external energy source for powder dispersion. However, complexity of these active devices probably has contributed to their inability to achieve regulatory approval, which could increase their cost. Besides Allen & Hanbury's Rotahaler and Fison's Spinhaler, several passive devices are available (e.g., AstraZeneca's Turbuhaler, Schering-Plough's Twisthaler, and Spiro's inhalers).

The addition of five ternary components has increased fine-particle fraction (FPF) of various drug particles. Ternary components so far examined include magnesium stearate, lactose, L-leucine, PEG-6000, and lecithin. Possible mechanism for improved FPF by ternary components could be the saturation of active sites on the carrier, electrostatic interactions, and drug redistribution on the ternary component.

Current commercial DPI formulations are based on drug agglomerates or carrier-based interactive mixtures. Excipients act as diluents and stability enhancers and improve flowability and aerosol dispersability. Surfactants, such as dipalmitoylphosphatidylcholine, can be incorporated to further improve powder flow, aerosol dispersion, and lung deposition. Large-sized particles have been found to enhance mouth deposition and reduce lung deposition. Commercial formulations predominantly deliver bronchodilators, anticholinergics, and corticosteroids for the local treatment of asthma and chronic airway obstruction. New formulations contain multiple drug components, such as fluticasone and salmeterol. Several therapeutic agents, such as analgesics (fentanyl and morphine), antibiotics, peptides (insulin, vasopressin, growth hormone, calcitonin, and parathyroid hormone), RNA/DNA fragments for gene therapy, and vaccines, are under investigation for inhalation. A new therapy using DPI formulations is zamamivir (Relenza, GSK, Research Triangle Park, NC), and it is mainly targeted at the upper respiratory tract for the treatment of influenza.

Nanosystems, PDC, and BioSante have technologies dealing with particulates containing drugs and formulation additives and absorption enhancers, such as bile acids and surfactants. The potential advantage of all of the particulate or molecular-transport promoters is that they may improve the bioavailability of the drug, thereby maximizing the proportion of the dose that reaches the site of action. According to one report, self-reported asthma prevalence in the U.S. increased 75% between 1980 and 1994 and to 17.3 million cases in 1998. In children between the ages of 5 and 14, asthma was prevalent in 74.4 children for every 1000 in 1994. Chronic obstructive pulmonary disease (COPD) was the fourth leading cause of death in 1998, with incidence rates of 6.9 per 1000 for all ages and 32.4 per 1000 for age 65 and over. Therapeutic drugs that potentially could be used for lung delivery include antimicrobial agents, such as antitubercular compounds; vaccines; proteins, such as insulin for diabetes therapy; and nucleic acids or oligonuclides for cystic fibrosis gene therapy.

The market for compounds to treat respiratory diseases (e.g., asthma and COPD) was approximately $12 billion worldwide in 2001 and is projected to grow to $20 billion in the next 5 years. In 2001, the DPI share of this market was around 20%, and this percentage is likely to grow as pMDIs are slowly phased out and new products with better therapeutic profiles are phased in. Compounds intended for systemic delivery represent an even larger potential market. The overall systemic market is projected to be nearly $40 billion during the first decade of this millennium.

D.   Examples of intranasal drug delivery systems

1. Su et al.[11] have reported nasal absorption studies with compounds such as clofilium tosylate, enkephalin analogs, and dobutamine hydrochloride. In particular, they demonstrated that a compound with a short biological half-life can be designed for mimicking intravenous infusion by applying an intranasal sustained-release formulation approach.

2. Kumar et al.[13] reported that intranasal administration of progesterone and norethisterone can prevent ovulation in rhesus monkeys. These steroids were given to 15 animals to determine their systemic absorption through the nasal mucosa and conjunctival sac and to evaluate the existence of a specific pathway from the eye and nose to the cerebrospinal fluid.

3. Lindsay[14] has reported his observations with 93 patients having nasal surgery whose bleeding was controlled by diathermy and postoperative application of a nasal aerosol called Tobispray. Tobispray is a dry, metered-dose nasal aerosol containing a vasoconstrictor (tramazoline), a steroid (dexamethasone isonicotinate), and an antibiotic (neomycin sulfate). This treatment achieved a success rate of 94.6%.

4. Xylometazoline is a long-acting topical nasal decongestant used for the relief of congestion due to coryza or allergic rhinitis. Hamilton[15] evaluated the ability of xylometazoline nasal spray in the reduction of nasal congestion in normal subjects with coryza as a result of upper respiratory infection.

5. Hyde et al.[16] have reported that sublingual administration of scopolamine is definitely inferior to both the intranasal and subcutaneous routes of administration.

6. Atropine sulfate has been administered intranasally, using an atomizer, to patients with rhinorrhea caused by allergic rhinitis and viral rhinitis. All but one of the 31 patients studied demonstrated a visible reduction in secretions. None of the patients reported the occurrence of common side effects, such as dry mouth or visual disturbance.[17]

7. Ipratropium is a parasympatholytic drug with topical activity and, when supplied in aerosol, has been used as a bronchodilator for the treatment of broncho-constructive diseases. Borum and Mygind[18] developed a simple test for the measurement of nasal reactivity in healthy subjects and patients with perennial rhinitis.

8. Dyke et al.[19] have made a comparative study on the efficacy of cocaine by oral and intranasal administrations. Their results indicated that following intranasal administration, cocaine was detected in the plasma by 15 min, reached peak concentrations at 60 to 120 min, and then decreased gradually over the next 2 to 3 h. On the other hand, by oral administration, cocaine was not detected in the plasma until 30 min, and it then increased rapidly for the next 30 min.

9. Angard[20] topically administered PGE_1, PGE_2, and $PGF_{1\alpha}$ to subjects and reported the observation of increased pharmacological potency in some subjects taking PGE_1 and PGE_2. The most likely mechanism of action for the increase of nasal potency results from the vasodilating effect of prostaglandins on nasal blood vessels.

10. Sulbenicillin, cephacetrile, and cefazoline are poorly absorbed from the GI tract because of their high water solubility and lack of lipophilic properties. Hirai et al.[21] carried out an *in vivo* absorption study in rats to compare the bioavailability of these antibiotics following intranasal, oral, and intramuscular administrations. After oral administration, poor absorption was confirmed for all three drugs. After intranasal administration, the percentage excreted in the urine was one-half of that following intramuscular injection.

11. Absorption of aminoglycosides from the GI tract can be enhanced by coadministration with a nonionic surfactant. Rubinstein et al.[22] have reported the observation of increased absorption of gentamicin from the nasal passages in healthy human subjects. Apparently, the presence of a surfactant, such as glycocholate, is required to obtain a significant concentration of gentamicin in the circulation.

12. When antiviral drugs are administered as nasal drops to animals infected with viruses in the upper respiratory tract, antiviral activity is always found to be much less than expected. Bucknall[23] studied the factors that may be responsible for the reduction of the effectiveness of antiviral drugs taken intranasally.

13. Enviroxime, a substituted benzimidazole derivative, is virustatic for rhinoviruses. Delong and Reed[24] have studied the clinical prophylactic and therapeutic effects of enviroxime given as a nasal spray in a placebo-controlled, double-blind study in volunteers infected with rhinovirus Type 4 (RV4). A metered-dose nasal spray was used to deliver either the enviroxime or a placebo in an alcohol solution with a freon propellant. No abnormalities were observed in the total or differential leukocyte count, hemoglobin concentration, or renal and hepatic function tests that were attributable to the intranasal administration of enviroxime by nasal spray.

14. The potential of intranasal administration of two antihistamines, prophen-pyridamine maleate and chlorphenpyridamine maleate, was evaluated in patients with allergic rhinitis. The combination was significantly more effective than chlorpheniramine maleate alone. The observations suggest the equal importance of H_1 and H_2 receptors in nasal blood vessels and an additive effect of H_1 and H_2 antihistamines.[25]

15. The efficacy of sodium cromoglycate in powder or solution form has been compared with placebo in a group of patients with allergic rhinitis over a period of 4 weeks. A crossover trial was further carried out in some patients to compare the efficacy of sodium cromoglycate in powder and solution in individuals whose main symptoms were nasal obstruction.[26]

16. The absorptive ability of the sinus membrane for phenol red was studied over 50 years ago by Childrey and Essex in dogs. They found that the dye appeared in the urine 1 hour and 50 minutes after the injection and only faint traces were present at 6 hours and 45 minutes later.[27]

17. Nasal absorption of CsCl, $SrCl_2$, $BaCl_2$ and $CeCl_3$ has been studied in Syrian hamsters and compared with GI absorption. Results indicated that more than 50% of the radioactive Cs, Sr, and Ba deposited on the nasal membrane is absorbed directly into the general circulation, but less than 4% of the Ce is absorbed. For all the isotopes studied, nasal bioavailability was approximately equal to or greater than oral bioavailability in the first four hours postadministration.

The data suggested that the nasopharynx may be the most important site of absorption for aerosols with a median mass aerodynamic diameter greater than 5 microns, where nasal deposition greatly exceeds deposition in all other areas of the respiratory tract.[28]

18. Czeniawska[29] investigated the possibility of penetration of radioactive colloidal gold (Au) from the mucous membrane of the olfactory region into the cerebrospinal fluid of the subarachnoid space in the anterior part of the brain. The results demonstrated that the radioactive isotope Au penetrates from the mucous membrane of the nasal olfactory region directly into the cerebrospinal fluid of the anterior cranial fossa.

19. Nebulized aqueous solutions are similar in efficiency to metered-dose inhalers (MDIs). Nevertheless, penetration of the lung's periphery — as opposed to tracheobronchial deposition — appears to be more effective with nebulized aqueous solutions than with MDIs. DPIs are much less efficient than either MDIs or nebulizers. Byron[30] has discussed pulmonary targeting, especially with aerosols.

20. The invention reported by Mahl et al.[31] is directed toward reducing the transmission of viral infections, such as respiratory, without significantly changing normal behavioral patterns. A substantially dry, flexible, impregnated wipe having virucidal properties against common cold viruses is the basis of this technology.

21. The Food and Drug Administration (FDA) has approved a nasal spray formulation of desmopressin acetate (DDAVP) for the control of nocturnal enuresis. Marketed by Rorer Pharmaceuticals, DDAVP Nasal Spray stimulates production of arginine vasopressin, an antidiuretic hormone that regulates urine production. The absence of a normal nighttime rise in levels of arginine vasopressin is thought to be responsible for many cases of nocturnal enuresis. DDAVP has a biphasic half-life consisting of a 7.8-minute fast phase and 75.5-minute slow phase. Its use results in decreased urinary output, increased urine osmolality, and decreased plasma osmolality.[32]

22. Researchers at the University of Nottingham, UK, and Novo-Nordisk A/S, Gentofte, Denmark, found that administering an insulin solution intranasally in combination with an enhancer produced a 65% decrease in blood glucose levels. They also found that the palmitoyl and stearyl components of lysophosphatidylcholine, in 0.5% concentration, produced effects similar to those produced by the parent compound, indicating that these lysophospholipids are equally potent absorption enhancers when used in nasal delivery.[33]

23. Researchers at the University of Nottingham, UK, have administered a gelling bioadhesive microsphere delivery system containing gentamicin to rats and sheep using the nasal route. The uptake of the drug across the nasal membrane was increased using the microsphere delivery system described. Lysolecithin was incorporated into the delivery system as an absorption enhancer, and the bioavailability of

gentamicin was increased by a factor of 50%, compared with an increase of less than 1% for a simple nasal gentamicin solution.[34]

24. Nasally delivered medications can be effective in treating migraine headaches. As mentioned previously, nasal administration of propranolol is more effective than oral administration, acting faster and avoiding a developing migraine.[35]

25. Sodium taurodihydrofusidate (STDHF) is a novel protein absorption enhancer whose parent compound, sodium fusidate, is isolated from the fermentation products of *Fusidium coccineum*. Interest in this molecule as an absorption enhancer was stimulated by its similarity to the bile salts, which are known enhancers of protein absorption.[36]

26. Other compounds under development for intranasal administration are: flunisolide (Aerobid); narcotic antagonists, such as naloxone and naltrexone; nitroglycerine; LHRH analog-buserelin; hydralazine; interferon; adrenocorticotropin; HOE 471, a synthetic LHRH analog for cryptorchism; oxytocin; nafarelin acetate, an LHRL antagonist for contraception; lypressin; vasopressin; secretin; dye T-1824; pentagastrin; potassium ferrocyanide; dopamine; bradykinin receptor antagonist; insulin using dimethyl-beta-cyclodextrin; physostigmine; arecoline; flurazepam; midazolam; triazolam; amphotericin B; budesonide; benzalkonium chloride; vaccines; epinephrine; thiophene; azelastine; chlorhexidine acetate; acyclovir; nicotine; dextromethorphan HCl; and isosorbide dinitrate.[37]

27. Since it was first described in 1981, nasal continuous positive airway pressure (CPAP) has gained widespread use and is generally accepted as first-line therapy of obstructive sleep apnea. Several types of nasal CPAP devices are currently available at about the same cost as nocturnal nasal oxygen systems. Nasal CPAP is thought to act as a "pneumatic splint," forcing the posterior nasopharynx open to prevent its collapse during sleep. In addition to abolishing apneas, nasal CPAP eliminates snoring. Side effects of nasal CPAP are few, but include conjunctivitis, nasal stuffiness, and ear pain. A minority of patients, however, do not tolerate nasal CPAP. Nasal oxygen is also a logical therapy for sleep apnea, since many of the sequelae, such as arrhythmias and impaired cognition, are thought to result from oxygen deprivation during sleep. Several studies have demonstrated the safety of nasal oxygen and its efficacy in improving oxygenation during sleep.[38–40]

28. The results of a 1-year, controlled, randomized trial of intranasal salmon calcitonin in 79 healthy women have shown that the agent can counteract early postmenopausal bone loss by inhibiting bone resorption and, perhaps temporarily, uncoupling the mechanisms of resorption and formation, according to researchers from the University of Liege, Belgium.[41]

A partial list of transnasal drugs is given in Table 7.2.

Table 7.2 A partial list of transnasal drugs

Drug	Trade name	Use	Producer-marketer
Amiloride	—	Cystic fibrosis	Glaxo
Salmeterol	—	Asthma	Glaxo
Fluticasone	Flixonase	Perennial rhinitis	Glaxo
Pentigetide	Pentyde	Allergic rhinitis	Dura Pharmaceuticals
Vitamin B-12	—	Pernicious anemia	Nastech
Meclizine	—	Antiemetic	Nastech
Cimetidine, ranitidine	—	Antihistaminic	Nastech
Doxylamine, azatidine	—	Antihistaminic	Nastech
Butorphanol tartrate	Stadol NS	Analgesic	Bristol Myers Squibb
Triamcinolone	Nasacort	Allergic rhinitis	Rhone-Poulenc Rorer

E.   Recent advances

Ketorolac tromethamine is a potent nonnarcotic analgesic with moderate anti-inflammatory activity. A series of spray and lyophilized powder formulations of ketorolac was administered into the nasal cavity of rabbits, and their pharmacokinetics profiles were assessed. Nasal spray formulations were significantly better absorbed than powder formulations. A nasal spray formulation of ketorolac tromethamine showed the highest absorption, with an absolute bioavailability of 91%. Interestingly, the absolute bioavailability of ketorolac tromethamine from a powder formulation is only 38%, indicating that the drug may not be totally released from the polymer matrix before it is removed from nasal epithelium by mucociliary clearance.[79]

Nasal glucagon delivery using microcrystalline cellulose in healthy volunteers was reported by Teshima et al.[80] The spray solution caused strong irritation, but the powder form did not. Their results suggested usefulness of the powder form of glucagon for the treatment of pancreatectomized patients.

Biodegradable microparticles containing gentamicin were prepared using chitosan hydroglutamate (CH), hyaluronic acid (HA), and a combination of both polymers by a solvent evaporation method. The bioavailability of gentamicin was poor when administered as a nasal solution (1.1%) and dry powder (2.1%) when compared with IV. However, the microparticulate systems composed of CH and HA/CH considerably enhanced the bioavailability of gentamicin (31.4 and 42.9%, respectively).[81]

Carboxymethyl cellulose (CMC) powder formulation of apomorphine was prepared by lyophyilization and characterized with respect to the *in vitro* and intranasal *in vivo* release of apomorphine in rabbits. This was compared to apomorphine release from degradable starch microspheres (DSM) and lactose. *In vitro* apomorphine release from CMC was sustained, unlike that of DSM and lactose. The sustained plasma level of apomorphine by CMC was achieved, with relative bioavailabilities equivalent to subcutaneous injection.[82]

Emulsion formulations of testosterone for nasal administration were reported by Ko et al.[83] Three differently charged testosterone submicron-size emulsion formulations with various zeta potentials were prepared as nasal spray formulations. Both the positively and negatively charged emulsion formulations provided a better bioavailability than the neutrally charged emulsion, probably indicating that the charged particle interactions between emulsion globules and the mucus layer prolong the contact of the drug with nasal membrane, thus enhancing drug absorption.

Lizio et al.[84] reported on the pulmonary absorption and tolerability of various formulations of the decapeptide cetrorelix acetate in rats by aerosol delivery system (ASTA-ADS) for intratracheal application. The histologic examination of the lungs revealed different tolerability of the various tested formulations, ranging from locally intolerable to well tolerated. The measurement of the lung-function parameters did not reveal any compound or formulation-related changes.

The purpose of investigation reported by Moore and Pham[85] was to assess hydraulic high-pressure nebulization as a means for respiratory drug delivery. A hydraulic high-pressure nebulizer was designed and constructed. The efficiency of the hydraulic high-pressure nebulizer appears to be correlated with the calculated properties of the liquid jet. For respiratory drug delivery, the hydraulic high-pressure nebulizer provides reasonably high outputs of respirable particles, independent of time, from a single pass of liquid through the nebulizer.

The effect of mixing of fine carrier particles on dry powder inhalation property of salbutamol sulfate was investigated by Iida et al.[86] They concluded that this could be a suitable method for improving the dry powder inhalation properties of therapeutic agents.

Direct delivery of medication to the sinuses with standard nebulizers is sometimes difficult to achieve. The nasal inhalation of aerosolized medications is dependent on the size of the particles and the pressure with which they are delivered. The ability of topical medications to treat sinus disorders can be improved if the medication could be delivered directly to the sinuses. The authors tested the ability of the RinoFlow nasal aerosol delivery device to deposit aerosol directly to the paranasal sinuses. Tc99m was used nasally, and nuclear scanning was used to detect deposition in the frontal and maxillary sinuses. The results of this study were promising.[87]

Particle-size distribution of the sodium cromoglycate preparations, CROPOZ PLUS and CROMOGEN EB, generated with MDI and for underpressure releasing methods were measured. Results of measurements indicate a significant repeatability of each sample properties. An average contribution of mass of the respirable fraction for both aerosolized pharmaceuticals is in the range of 40% of the generated dose. High contribution of submicron particles of CROMOGEN EB with optimizer gives efficient penetration and deposition of these particles in the lungs.[88]

In one study reported by Musoh et al.,[89] the bronchoconstriction induced by histamine inhalation was significantly inhibited by tulobuterol tape in comparison with its placebo tape. Twenty-four hours after binding, the inhibitory effect of tulobuterol tape gradually diminished. These results suggest that tulobuterol tape has a long-lasting bronchodilatory action.

Pulmonary vasodilation with a 100-ppm concentration of Nomin (NO), given as a short burst of a few milliliters at the beginning of each breath was compared with conventionally inhaled NO, in which a full breath of 40 ppm of NO was inhaled (NOCD). A small volume of NO inhaled at the beginning of the breath was equally effective as NOCD, but reduced the dose of NO per breath by 40-fold.[90]

The incidence of invasive pulmonary aspergillosis has increased in patients receiving immunosuppressive therapy or organ transplantation. For prophylaxis against aspergillus infections, amphotericin B may be a useful drug when inhaled as aerosol. In this reported study, the aerosolization of amphotericin B was investigated using eight different medical nebulizers under various operating conditions and with different amphotericin B concentrations in the solution. Three out of eight devices proved suitable for amphotericin treatment via inhalation.[91]

Kraemer[92] reported on Babyhaler, a new pediatric aerosol device. Nebulizers have, until recently, been the mainstay of drug delivery by inhalation in babies and young children. The willingness of a young child to cooperate, however, is limited, and the 10 to 12 minutes needed to deliver a drug using a nebulizer often limits the compliance with this mode of administration in infants. Therefore, drug delivery systems using the MDI as the aerosol generator attached to valves holding chambers were developed. In brief, the Babyhaler consists of a tubular chamber 230 mm long, with a volume of 350 ml and low-resistance inspiratory and expiratory valves, among other things.

Fuller[93] reported on the Diskus, a new multi-dose powder device. The mass of drug substance (mass median aerodynamic diameter [MMAD]), less than 6 microns, delivered from the Diskus remains relatively constant at different flow rates, unlike the reservoir powder inhaler, in which the fine particle mass is more dependent on flow rate. The doses of drug in the Diskus are protected from moisture. In clinical studies, salmeterol, 50 micrograms twice daily, and fluticasosne propionate, 50 to 500 micrograms twice daily, have been shown to be equally effective and well tolerated when delivered by Diskus as compared with Diskhaler.[94–96]

II   Ocular drug delivery

A.   Introduction

Ophthalmic preparations, including solutions, suspensions, and ointments, can be applied topically to the cornea or instilled in the space between the eyeball and lower eyelid (the cul-de-sac or conjunctival sac of the lower lid). When drops of an aqueous solution are applied onto the cornea, through which the drug must penetrate to reach the interior part of the eye, the solution in the drops is immediately diluted with tears and washes away rapidly through the lachrymal apparatus. Consequently, eye drops do not remain in contact with the eye for a long time, and they must be administered at relatively frequent intervals. Suspensions have the advantage of longer contact time in the eye, but also the disadvantage of an irritation potential, due to the particle size of the suspended drugs. Irritation may produce excessive tearing and, consequently, rapid drainage of the instilled dose. Ointments have the advantages of longer contact time and greater storage stability, but also the disadvantage of producing a film over the eye, thereby blurring vision. In addition, ointments can interfere with the attachment of new corneal epithelial cells to their normal base. The disadvantages of various types of ophthalmic preparations can be overcome by controlled delivery systems that release a drug at a constant rate for a relatively long time.

The typical administration of an ocular drug delivery system has been pulse entry of the drug, followed by a rapid, first-order decline of drug concentration. Adequate therapy from eyedrops may be achieved either by providing a sufficient magnitude of the pulse, so that its effect is extended for a useful period of time, or by giving more frequent applications of a less-concentrated pulse.[42]

Some of the new ophthalmic drug delivery systems have been reported to have enhanced corneal absorption. While these systems prolong the desired effect with less frequent applications than eyedrops require, side effects are also enhanced. Thus, these systems are limited to use with drugs with dose-related side effects that are not serious or that can be tolerated by the patient. Representative examples of these delivery systems are described in this section.

B.   Relevant anatomy and physiology of the eye

The human eye (see Figure 7.3) has a spherical shape with a diameter of 23 mm. The structural components of the eyeball are divided into three layers: the outermost coat comprises the clear, transparent cornea and the white, opaque sclera; the middle layer comprises the iris anteriorly, the choroid posteriorly, and the ciliary body; and the inner layer is the retina, which is an extension of the central nervous system.[43]

The cornea (see Figure 7.4) is often the tissue through which drugs in ophthalmic preparations reach the inside of the eye. Because the structure of the cornea consists of epithelium–stroma–epithelium, which is equivalent to a fat–water–fat structure, the penetration of nonpolar compounds through the cornea depends on their oil/water partition coefficients. The fluid systems in the eye — the aqueous humor and the vitreous humor — also play an important role in ocular pharmacokinetics. The aqueous humor fills the anterior and posterior chambers of the eye and is secreted continuously from the blood through the epithelium of the ciliary body. This fluid is transported from the posterior to the anterior chamber, and hence escapes through Schlemm's canal. The vitreous humor has the same origin as the aqueous

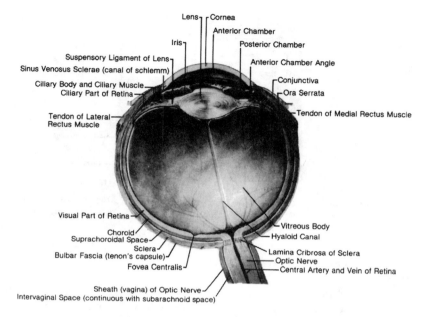

Figure 7.3 Cross-sectional view of the eye. (From Robinson, J.R., Ed., Ophthalmic drug delivery systems, *J. Pharm. Sci.*, 1, 1980. With permission of the American Pharmaceutical Association.)

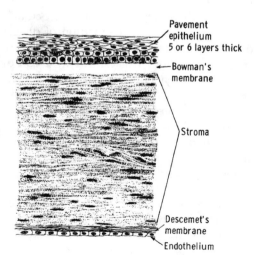

Figure 7.4 Corneal cross-section. (From Robinson, J.R., Ed., Ophthalmic drug delivery systems, *J. Pharm. Sci.*, 10, 1980. With permission of the American Pharmaceutical Association.)

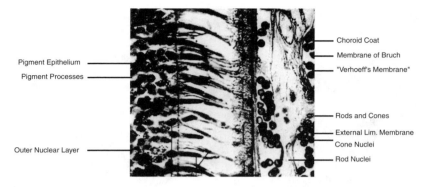

Choroid Coat

Membrane of Bruch

"Verhoeff's Membrane"

Pigment Epithelium

Pigment Processes

Rods and Cones

External Lim. Membrane

Cone Nuclei

Outer Nuclear Layer

Rod Nuclei

Figure 7.5 Structural detail of the retina. (From Robinson, J.R., Ed., Ophthalmic drug delivery systems, *J. Pharm. Sci.*, 94, 1980. With permission of the American Pharmaceutical Association.)

humor, but diffuses through the vitreous body and escapes from the eye through the uveo-scleral route.

From the perspective of ocular pharmacokinetics, the dynamics of the aqueous humor are more important than those of the vitreous humor because ocular drugs are usually applied to the cornea and the aqueous humor has a relatively fast turnover rate. The structural details of the retina, which belongs to the inner coat of the eye, are illustrated in Figure 7.5.

Drug disposition in the eye following topical application is a complex phenomenon resulting from both drug-dependent and independent parameters. In order to describe the pharmacokinetics of ocular drugs, it is necessary to consider the distribution and disposition of drugs in three areas of the eye: the precorneal area, the cornea, and the interior of the eye.

The internal ocular structures are critical to a comprehensive understanding of ocular drug pharmacokinetics. Binding to both aqueous humor and tissues, aqueous flow and turnover, partitioning into and binding within tissues, and various distribution equilibria are all determinants in drug-disposition kinetics in the eye.[43]

When a drug is instilled into the eye, there exist a large number of factors that can influence its distribution and movement into various parts of the eye or the body as a whole. Topically applied ocular drugs may be intended to exert a local effect, or to penetrate into the anterior chamber, to be distributed to various eye tissues. The events that take place in the precorneal area of the eye are critical factors in determining how much of any instilled or applied dose is available to exert its pharmacologic effect. These precorneal factors include the effects of tear production and instilled fluid drainage, protein binding, metabolism, tear evaporation, and nonproductive absorption/adsorption.

The role of the cornea in ocular drug disposition is important. The cornea comprises the anterior one-sixth of the globe and is the membrane through which drugs must pass if they are to reach the inner areas of the eye, such as the anterior chamber and the iris. As such, the cornea is critical to an overall understanding of ocular drug disposition after topical dosing. It is generally conceded that there are three main factors contributing to the efficiency of corneal penetration of topically applied ophthalmic drugs: the corneal structure and its integrity, the physical–chemical properties of the applied drug, and the formulation in which the drug is prepared.[43]

Once a drug has penetrated the cornea, there are several factors that need to be considered in the ultimate pharmacokinetic description of that drug's fate: the volume or spaces (tissues) into which the drug distributes; binding of drug in both aqueous humor and tissues; partitioning behavior of drug between aqueous humor and the various ocular tissues, such as iris, lens, and vitreous humor; possible differences in equilibration time between aqueous humor and the various ocular tissues; possibility of drug metabolism in eye fluid or tissues; and drug effects to either stimulate or inhibit aqueous humor production and turnover.

The traditional ophthalmic dosage forms have been solutions, suspensions, and ointments, although there have been several other forms tried. Relatively few new efforts have seen any real success, and the newest, the ocular insert, is still uncertain as to its real place in drug delivery. The characteristic parts of an ophthalmic dosage form — the drug, the vehicle, the preservative, and the other additives — occupy the same general relationship to each other as they do in other drug solution, suspension, and ointment products. However, the eye itself has several specific characteristics that affect the expected performance of each of these parts.

In order of economic importance, the topical dosage forms used to treat diseases fall into three specific and one rather broad category: solutions, suspensions, ointments, and a rather amorphous group. Solutions are without question the most generally used and accepted forms. They are relatively straightforward to make, filter, and sterilize, and they all use the standard formulation parameters. Suspensions, while not as common as solutions, are widely used for formulations involving ocular steroids and came into broad, general use with the post-World War II availability of these drugs for the treatment of inflammatory diseases. Ointments have traditionally been the cheapest form of ocular therapy, but for years presented significant problems. They could not, for example, be effectively filtered to free them from particles; they could not be made truly sterile; and no adequate test had been devised to indicate the suitability of added preservatives.

In 1970, with the advent of oil-stable microbial filters, most of these problems were solved. Shortly thereafter, sterile, filtered ophthalmic ointments appeared on the U.S. market, although they are certainly still a distant third in economic importance. Inserts have been described in the pharmaceutical literature for more than 50 years, but a resurgence of interest has been stimulated by the fundamental improvement over the original gelatin leaflet offered by the Ocusert®.[44]

Unlike most systemic drug therapy, the major portion of a topically instilled drug leaves the potential absorption site (the cornea) unused, unabsorbed, and lost to therapy. This occurs, in part, because some drug forms do not penetrate the corneal epithelium well and, more important, because tear dilution and subsequent washout eliminate the drug rapidly. This produces, in some cases, an undesired drug load for the systemic circulation when adequate concentrations are used to provide the desired ophthalmic effects. Physiologic factors prevent some areas of the optical globe from being treated with topical products. For example, the posterior parts of the eye are protected from externally applied drugs by the intrinsic flow patterns within the globe. Efforts to treat posterior-chamber inflammation and retinal disease, where the aqueous flow opposes the diffusion path from cornea to the ciliary body, require large systemic doses, and topical therapy is largely ineffective.

While normal saline is an acceptable vehicle for ophthalmic drugs, slightly more viscous solutions are generally recognized by physicians and patients as more satisfying to use. However, this satisfaction results only over a relatively narrow range of viscosity. This narrow band of acceptable viscosity is dictated by the fact that these products must have negligible visual effects if they are to be used during waking hours, as well as be comfortable, filterable, and sterilizable.

Ophthalmic products, with their application methods and multiple-use characteristics, are, unfortunately, highly susceptible to "suck-back" contamination. Preservation, as opposed to single-use containers, has answered the problem satisfactorily, but the limited number of preservatives available has presented problems of compatibility and pH stability for the formulator. For the most part, only three preservatives are in common use — benzalkonium chloride, thimerosal, and chlorobutanol, although mixtures and enhancers, such as EDTA, have increased the spectrum of possibilities.[44]

C.   *Examples of ocular drug delivery systems*

1. The Ocusert, introduced commercially by Alza, is a membrane-controlled reservoir system used in the treatment of glaucoma. The active agent in Ocusert is pilocarpine, a parasympathomimetic agent that acts directly on target organs in the iris, ciliary body, and trabecular meshwork, increasing the outflow of aqueous humor and decreasing the intraocular pressure. The copolymer used in the Ocusert is ethylene-vinyl acetate. Pilocarpine is surrounded on both sides with two polymer membranes (see Figure 7.6). Alginic acid, a carbohydrate extracted from seaweed, is also placed in the core of the Ocusert to act as a carrier for pilocarpine. There is also a white annular border around the device consisting of the ethylene-vinyl acetate copolymer impregnated with titanium dioxide, a powdered pigment. The border makes the Ocusert easier for the patient to visualize. To use the Ocusert, the patient places the device in the eye's cul-de-sac where it floats on the tear film. No major complications occur with the

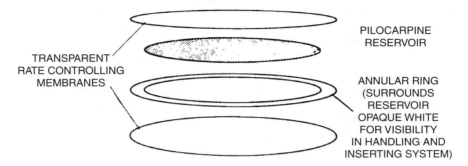

PILOCARPINE
RESERVOIR

TRANSPARENT
RATE CONTROLLING
MEMBRANES

ANNULAR RING
(SURROUNDS
RESERVOIR
OPAQUE WHITE
FOR VISIBILITY
IN HANDLING AND
INSERTING SYSTEM)

Figure 7.6 Schematic diagram of Ocusert. (From Langer, R.S. and Wise, D.L., Eds., *Medical Applications of Controlled Release*, Vol. II, CRC Press, Boca Raton, FL, 1984, 67.)

Ocusert. The patients who are candidates for Ocuserts are those in whom drugs such as beta blockers do not produce adequate pressure control and who respond well to pilocarpine eyedrops, but are too young to tolerate the marked variation in visual acuity that occurs with pulsed-drop medication.

2. Patients with dry eyes (keratitis sicca) are one of the most common and difficult management problems in ophthalmology. These patients generally demonstrate a wide range of abnormalities of tear production and lid function. In an effort to augment tear function, liquid tear substitutes have been designed to replace the aqueous component of tears and to stabilize the tear film in much the same way that mucous does. The Lacrisert, a substitute for artificial tears, has been developed by Merck. The Lacrisert is inserted into the eye with a special reusable applicator. The system is placed in the conjunctival sac, where it softens within 1 hour and completely dissolves within 14 to 18 hours. The Lacrisert acts to stabilize and thicken the precorneal tear film and prolong the tear film break-up time, which is usually accelerated in patients with dry-eye states.

At least 25 products have been marketed for dry-eye syndrome since 1955. Currently, product formulators and clinical research groups are examining the influence of immunological factors on dry-eye syndrome. It is anticipated that these factors may offer considerable additional insight into establishing more precise rational approaches to dry-eye syndrome.

3. An ophthalmic gel used for the delivery of pilocarpine is poloxamer 407. This vehicle was chosen because of its low viscosity, optical clarity, and mucomimetic properties and for its previous acceptability in ophthalmic preparations. This formulation enhances pilocarpine activity, as indicated by miosis measurements in rabbits, compared to an aqueous pilocarpine solution of equal drug concentration. A pilocarpine emulsion in eyedrop form (Piloplex) reportedly[45] pro-

longs therapeutic effectiveness compared with pilocarpine hydro-chloride eyedrops. In this formulation, pilocarpine is bound to a polymeric material, and this complex makes up the internal, dispersed phase of the emulsion system. Facilitated transport in animals has been used successfully to enhance the movement of the mast cell stabilizer sodium chromoglycate (the dianion) across the cornea.[46]

4. The first ophthalmic pro-drug, dipivalylepinephrine (Dipivefrin, Propine), was recently described in 1980. By diesterification, the compound was made more lipophilic, resulting in a tenfold increase in its corneal absorption. Upon absorption, esterases within both the cornea and the aqueous humor act rapidly to liberate the epinephrine.[47]

A number of soluble, solid-state drug carriers have been utilized for ophthalmic medication. "Lamellae," described as early as 1948 in the British Pharmacopoeia, were atropine-containing gelatin wafers intended for placement beneath the eyelid. Delivery of an antibiotic by an ocular insert made of succinylated, enzyme-solubilized collagen has also been described, and this approach appears promising for the treatment of ocular infection. One study compared ^{14}C-gentamicin levels in rabbit tear film and in ocular tissue when the drug was administered by eyedrops, ointments, subconjunctival injection, or by solid wafers. The inserts gave superior levels of drug in the tears, sclera, and cornea. Prolongation of the pulse entry, as compared to ointment delivery or periocular injection, are evident.[48]

Experimental continuous-delivery systems based upon the osmotic properties of an incorporated drug have been developed and have undergone early clinical testing. Several sizes and shapes have been developed. They range from a thin, flat layer of different shapes to a contoured, three-dimensional unit designed to conform to the supratarsal space of the upper cul-de-sac. The latter system has been utilized in the delivery of diethylcarbamazine in ocular onchocerciasis. The nonhydrophilic polymer matrix contains the incorporated drug, which is dispersed in the solid state as numerous, extremely small domains, each as a discrete compartment separated by polymer material. Drug delivery proceeds at a fairly constant rate for the life of the system, at which time the device is removed and replaced. The useful life of these systems is limited to a large extent by drug-volume constraints; there being an upper limit to the size of the device the eye will tolerate and retain. Systems have been developed that deliver therapeutic drugs levels for 2 weeks.[49–51]

5. Topically applied peptides can also be absorbed into the bloodstream via the blood vessels in the conjunctival mucosa. Indeed, in one study, the conjunctival mucosa played a more significant role than did the nasal mucosa in the systemic absorption of [D-ala^2] met-enkephalinamide. This is demonstrated by the small change in the area under the curve of concentration plotted against time when the drainage apparatus was blocked to deny the peptide access to the nasal mu-

cosa. When contact between the peptide and the conjunctiva was prolonged by increasing the viscosity of the aqueous solution, the percentage of [D-ala^2] metenkephalinamide systemically absorbed was doubled, but absorption was still far from complete. To achieve systemic delivery of peptides using the ocular route, absorption of the peptide must be enhanced by ensuring that peptidase-mediated degradation of the peptide in the corneal epithelium is prevented.[52]

6. Transport of drugs across the corneal barrier can sometimes be facilitated by formation of a chemical derivative. A distinction is made between temporary derivatives (pro-drugs), from which the active parent compound is regenerated following absorption and derivatives that are made to improve some useful property, such as their bioavailability. A recently reported success with the latter approach involves removing one alkyl group from the quaternary nitrogen of carbachol and converting it into a tertiary nitrogen. The new derivative, N-demethylated carbachol, possesses an enhanced ability to penetrate the cornea with retention of miotic activity.[53]

7. Clinical studies have been conducted on 466 patients waiting for senile cataract surgery and receiving chloromycetin, gentamycin, or carbenicillin subconjunctively or through New Sauflon 70 and New Sauflon 85 lenses. Soft contact lenses provided significantly higher drug penetration than subconjunctival therapy. Both modes of treatment provided therapeutically effective levels against most common ocular pathogens for intervals of 2 to 12 h.[54]

8. Development of an extended-duration ocular drug delivery system is particularly challenging, due to extensive precorneal-loss parameters, as evidenced by the fact that very few ocular products are available for once-daily/weekly therapy. Patient comfort, compliance, and dosing are additional constraints of the product profile. Researchers at the University of Wisconsin have developed an ocular device, the Minidisc, that resolves patient compliance issues with design features that are based on eye anatomy and pharmacokinetic aspects of ocular drug disposition. The disc can be hydrophilic or hydrophobic to permit use of both water-soluble and water-insoluble drugs. For developmental purposes, the researchers selected sulfisoxazole and gentamicin as model drugs. It was found that the Minidisc is an effective and versatile prolonged-release ocular drug delivery system.[55]

9. Corneal penetration and bioconversion of ocular pro-drugs for an anticataract drug, catalin, has been investigated using freshly excised rabbit cornea. A horizontal-type *in vitro* apparatus was developed for studying long-term transcorneal drug penetration/bioconversion kinetics. The appearance rate of the drug after the bioconversion of methyl, ethyl, propyl, and butyl esters was much higher than the penetration rate of the parent drug. The appearance rate of catalin after pro-drug bioconversion improves with increasing alkyl chain length of the esters.[56]

10. Investigation of the impact of the dosage form, whether suspension or ophthalmic film, and formulation variables in the film delivery system on dexa-methasone pharmacokinetics in ocular tissue has been carried out. The results reveal some characteristic features for the disposition of the drug in ocular tissues when the drug is applied in suspension form.[57]

11. An objective in the development of an ophthalmic formulation is the close resemblance of *in vitro* or animal models with the clinical situation. For this reason, experiments with pilocarpine nitrate in conventional eyedrops or adsorbed to poly-(butyl cyanoacrylate) nanoparticles has been carried out.[58]

12. Extensive drug loss due to the highly efficient precorneal elimination process occurs upon eyedrop instillation. The addition of viscosity-enhancing polymers increases precorneal retention and hence bioavailability. A mucoadhesive polymeric solution (Carbopol 934 P) has been compared with an equiviscous (60 cps) nonmucoadhesive solution (PVA), measuring pilocarpine bioavailability and polymer-retention times in the rabbit eye. The polymers were labeled with radioactivity in and their deposition and clearance studied by lachrymal scintigraphy. Different clearance kinetics were observed for the Carbopol 934 P and the PVA, with the former exhibiting extended corneal retention.[59]

13. An ocular therapeutic system for releasing a drug to the eye at a controlled and continuous rate for a prolonged period of time has been described. The system is shaped, sized, and adapted for insertion and retention in the eye. The system contains an ophthalmically acceptable drug, such as hydrocortisone, and it is formed of a polymeric material permeable to the passage of drug by diffusion.[60]

14. 6-Hydroxy-2-benzothiazolesulfonamide is useful for the topical treatment of elevated intraocular pressure. Ophthalmic compositions, including drops and inserts, have been described.[49]

15. Polymers and hydrogels of polymers have been described. The hydrogels are preferably used for the formation of contact lenses. The hydrogels can be impregnated with a solution containing a drug. A material (e.g., drug for ocular therapy) can then be administered to a patient, and the material will gradually be released to the patient. As the drug is removed from the surface of the hydrogel, it will be replaced with a fresh supply of drug migrating to the surface from its interior.[42]

16. A treatment for glaucoma or ocular hypertension by ophthalmically applying an effective amount of 2-(3-tert-butylamino-2-hydroxy-propylthio)-4-(5-carbamoyl-2-thienyl)-thiazole has been described.[61]

17. Waltman and Kaufman[62] have used hydrophilic contact lenses (Bionite, Griffin Labs, and Soflens, Bausch & Lomb) as devices for maintaining high drug concentration in the anterior chamber of the eye. They used fluorescein as a model drug. A Bionite lens presoaked

with the drug yielded a fluorescein concentration in rabbit aqueous humor four times greater than that from drops. In human studies, a Bionite lens could maintain the fluorescein concentration in ocular tissues for 24 h, despite the known rapid exit of the drug.

18. Kaufman et al.[63] have shown the usefulness of soft contact lenses for drug delivery to the eye in several experiments: antiviral idoxuridine (IDU) drops plus a soft contact lens significantly improved the therapeutic index for eyes infected with McKrae herpes virus; polymyxin B 0.25% and a lens soaked in polymyxin solution were administered to rabbit corneas infected with *Pseudomonas aeruginosa* (the presence of the lens in the eye had neither a beneficial nor a harmful effect); and the advantage of a soft contact lens on the effect of pilocarpine on the eye was investigated.

19. Praus et al.[64] have studied the release of antibiotics from presoaked (0.1% chlor-amphenicol or tetracycline) hydrogel contact lenses. In an *in vitro* experiment, the amount of released antibiotics was determined spectrometrically. During the first 3 hours, lenses of 0.3- and 0.9-mm thickness released 50% and 40% of tetracycline and 75% and 60% of chloramphenicol, respectively. The duration of release was up to eight hours for the thinner lens and more than 4 hours for the thicker one.

20. Corticosteroids are useful for the treatment of ocular inflammation. Hull et al.[65] studied the ocular penetration of prednisolone in the rabbit eye and the effect of a hydrophilic contact lens on penetration. The contact lenses made from PHP (hefilcon-A) copolymer (80% 2-hydroxyethyl methacrylate and 20% N-vinyl-2-pyrrolidone) were 16 mm in diameter and 0.3 mm thick, and their hydration was 40% to 45%. Lenses presoaked in prednisolone for 2 min were able to maintain the aqueous and corneal levels two to three times higher, at 4 h, than the levels after topical administration without the lens.

21. Other polymeric devices for drug delivery are soluble ocular inserts, such as the poly(vinyl alcohol) insert (PVAI); the soluble ophthalmic drug insert (SODI); and polypeptide devices.[66] Seven different combinations of SODI and drugs including pilocarpine, atropine, neomycin, kanamycin, sulfapyridazine, tetracaine, and idoxuridine have been studied. These studies established that SODIs are well tolerated by eye tissue and that when an SODI is inserted into the conjunctival sac, it absorbs tears rapidly, swells, and dissolves in about 30 to 90 minutes, releasing the active substance. The dissolution property of the SODIs frees the patient from the task of removing the device after the drug has been released completely.

22. An interesting enzymatically degradable pharmaceutical carrier has been produced by Capozza,[67] and it is made of poly(N-acetyl-D-glucosamine)(chitin), an important structural polysaccharide of invertebrates. Chitin is converted enzymatically to a decomposed form, which serves as a matrix for the ocular inserts. Pilocarpine, which is

released from the eroding surface of the insert, produces pupillary miosis for 6 h.

23. Ueno and Refojo[68] have investigated the sustained release of chloramphenicol and lincomycin from closed-cell, silicone-rubber, scleral-buckling material (sponge) (Dow Corning Silastic sponge, Lincoff design). The sponge was immersed in a saturated solution of lincomycin in propylene oxide for three days at room temperature and then dried. The antibiotic was released into seeded agar plates at a nearly constant rate for about 3 weeks from the cylindrical sponge and for more than one month from the oval-shaped sponge. The cylindrical sponge also released chloramphenicol at a nearly constant rate for about 2 weeks, but then the release rate slowly declined.

The uptake mechanism was thought due to propylene oxide swelling the silicone rubber of the sponge, converting it to a gel; and the antibiotics dissolved in propylene oxide diffuse through the network of the swollen rubber into the cells of the sponge. After the propylene oxide evaporates, the swollen sponge shrinks and returns to its original shape, but the antibiotics remain in the cells of the sponge. These antibiotic-impregnated materials, used in conjunction with standard pre- and postoperative therapy, can reduce even further the rate of infection in scleral-buckling procedures.

24. Ueno and Refojo[68] also have developed a device for the delivery of hydrophobic drugs consisting of a silicone-rubber system. The methodology is especially useful for the treatment of intraocular malignancies with 1,3-bis(2-chloroethyl)-1-nitrosourea (BCNU). BCNU is a useful chemotherapeutic agent for the treatment of a variety of human cancers. It has also been found effective against Brown–Pearce epithelioma and Greene melanoma implanted in the anterior chamber of the rabbit eye, which are useful animal models for ocular cancer research. BCNU is a liposoluble drug that decomposes rapidly to yield alkylating and carbamoylating intermediates at physiologic pH. BCNU produces various adverse effects, particularly when administered in therapeutic doses to the whole body. Ueno and Refojo have worked on the basis that ideally one should minimize the amount of drug given to the whole body while maximizing drug level at the tumor site. The silicone-rubber drug delivery device fulfilled these goals for the administration of BCNU to eye tumors in the rabbit.

25. The double-stranded complex of polyriboinosonic acid and polyribocytidylic acid (poly I:C) has been successfully used to induce resistance to systemic, as well as localized, viral infections through production of endogenous interferons. Of particular interest, poly I:C has been applied topically for clinical treatment of herpetic infections of the cornea and conjunctiva of the eye. However, a disadvantage associated with topical ophthalmic application of poly I:C has been the apparent need for frequently repeated applications to ensure

adequate exposure of the infected tissue. Major improvements in ophthalmic medication systems can be realized either by providing for the controlled release of drug subsequent to instillation in the medication of the eye or by increasing the contact time for the drug with eye tissues.[69]

D. Recent advances

The objectives of the study were to prepare a biodegradable polyisobutyl-cyanoaacrylate (PIBCA) colloidal particulate system of pilocarpine to incorporate it into a Pluronic F127 (PF 127)-based gel delivery system and to evaluate its ability to prolong the release of pilocarpine. PIBCA nanocapsules of pilocarpine were prepared by interfacial polymerization. This system can also be used for other, more hydrophobic drugs.[97]

The purpose of the study reported by Kim and Gao[98] was to prepare a chemically and physically stable rhEGF/HP-bta-CD poloxamer complex gel to investigate its possibility of ophthalmic delivery. The poloxamer gel containing the complex increased the area under the concentration-time curve, or area under the curve (AUC), rhEGF in tear fluid compared with gel containing rhEGF solution. This also indicated that rhEGF may be retained in the precorneal area for prolonged periods.

The objective of the study reported by Kawakami et al.[99] was to examine the ocular absorption behavior of an amphiphilic pro-drug after instillation onto the cornea of rabbits. A micellar solution of O-palmitoyl tilisolol (PalTL) an amphiphilic pro-drug, was prepared. After instillation of tilisolol (TL) and PalTL, the drug concentrations in the tear fluid, cornea, aqueous humor, iris-ciliary body, vitreous body, and blood were measured. PalTL exhibited increased retention in the precorneal area compared with the parent drug, TL, resulting in improved ocular absorption of the parent drug.

Poly(ortho esters) (POE) are hydrophobic and biodegradable polymers that have been investigated for pharmaceutical use since the early 1970s. Among the four described generations of POE, the third (POEIII) and fourth (POEIV) are promising viscous and injectable materials that have been investigated in numerous biomedical applications. POEIII has been extensively studied for ophthalmic drug delivery since it presents an excellent biocompatibility, and is currently under investigation as a vehicle for sustained drug delivery to treat diseases of the posterior segment of the eye.[100]

The report by Ghelardi and Tavanti[101] describes the efficacy of a novel mucoadhesive polymer, the tamarind seed polysaccharide, as a delivery system for the ocular administration of hydrophilic and hydrophobic antibiotics. The increased drug (e.g., gentamicin or ofloxacin absorption) and the prolonged drug-elimination phase obtained with the viscosified formulations indicate the usefulness of the tamarind seed polysaccharide as an ophthalmic delivery system for topical administration of antibiotics.

Systemic absorption of insulin from a Gelfoam ocular device was reported by Lee and Yalkowski[102] Gelfoam ocular devices containing 0.2 mg of sodium insulin prepared with either water or 10% acetic acid were evaluated in rabbits. The results suggest that a change in the Gelfoam upon treatment with acid is responsible for the efficient systemic absorption of insulin from these enhancer-free devices.

The overall objective of the study was to develop pluronic F127 (PF127)-containing formulations of pilocarpine HCl suitable for controlled-release ocular delivery of PHCl. On the basis of the *in vitro* results, the PF127 formulations pf PHCl containing methylcellulose or hydroxypropyl methylcellulose as an additive showed potential for use as controlled-release ocular delivery systems for PHCl.[103]

Sodium insulin and zinc insulin ocular devices are developed for the systemic delivery of insulin. Commercially available Humulin R was selected as another source of zinc insulin and was used as an eyedrop, as well as one device preparation. Only 10% acetic acid solution-treated insulin devices produce significant blood glucose reduction. The dose of insulin used in this study is less than 50% of that used in the reported insulin devices.[104]

Mitomycin C was studied in the rabbit eye. The mitomycin C concentrations in the target tissues were dose-dependent and decreased rapidly over 24 hours. Both the initial mitomycin C concentrations, as well as AUCs in these eyes treated with mitomycin C, dissolved in a reversible thermosetting gel, were higher than those in eyes treated similarly in a study in which the gel was not used. Therefore, applied subconjunctively in the rabbit eye, mitomycin C dissolved in the reversible thermosetting gel-enhanced transfer of the agent to the sclera and the conjunctiva.[105]

Rafferty and Elfaki[106] reported on the preparation and characterization of a biodegradable microparticle antigen/cytokine ocular delivery system. They found that the inclusion of cytokines in the antigen-containing biodegradable microparticles enhanced teat IgA antibody levels following ocular optical delivery P2o, while elevated VW IgA responses occurred following intraperitoneal delivery of P2o and P3o. These data demonstrate that antigen/cytokine-loaded microparticles can potentiate long-term mucosal antibody responses at both target and distal effector sites, as well as elicit circulating antibodies.

E.   Conclusion and future outlook

Experimental and clinical studies have confirmed that nasal and ocular routes of administration are practical approaches to therapy with many drugs, with the advantages of rapid absorption in some cases, along with ease of administration and good local tolerance. Nasal spray formulations, especially, have facilitated the diagnostic applications of peptides and biotechnology products by reducing side effects commonly observed in IV testing and treatment of infants and children in which repeated injections are a disadvantage[70,71] (see Figure 7.7).

The potential therapeutic advantages offered by ophthalmic and nasal drug delivery systems are numerous and significant. Despite this, the avail-

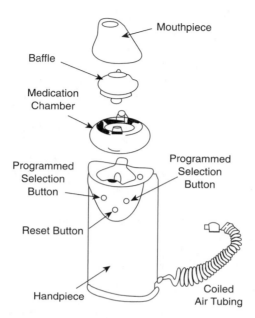

Mouthpiece

Baffle

Medication
Chamber

Programmed
Selection
Button

Programmed
Selection
Button

Reset Button

Handpiece

Coiled
Air Tubing

Figure 7.7 Halolite delivery system (Medic-Aid, Profile Therap. Subsidiary, U.K.).

able systems have not yet gained widespread acceptance. This situation may change as improved delivery systems are developed and as continuous administration systems are mandated by the emergence of important new drugs that have short half-lives.

When drugs are given in eyedrop form, 80% or more of the volume of an administered eyedrop, which is known to drain rapidly through the nasolacrimal canal, avoids the first-pass effect and is totally available for systemic absorption through the highly vascularized mucosa. Thus, an eyedrop is more like an intravenous dose.

Until recently, the side effects of frequently used and relatively safe ophthalmic drugs have been of little consequence, or at least have not been serious enough to alter prescribing habits in favor of new drug delivery systems. The development and rational use of more potent drugs, however, which may have serious side effects, may require concomitant development and use of improved methods for their controlled (i.e., non-pulsed) delivery.

Another feature of some ophthalmic and nasal delivery systems that may encourage their eventual acceptance is their freedom from the need for preservatives and other vehicle ingredients. The deleterious effects of these agents are not widely appreciated, but they are certainly real. Systems that provide continuous, controlled drug release to the eye may in time find important uses in the treatment of ophthalmic diseases, which, due to special circumstances, are otherwise difficult to treat effectively. The most important example is trachoma, an infectious ocular disease that is the leading cause of blindness worldwide.[72]

Finally, controlled-release systems could prove beneficial in a number of other ocular indications. These have been summarized by Jones[73] as follows: short, topical, ocular half-life (e.g., heparin for ligneous disease); small, topical, ocular therapeutic index (e.g., pilocarpine for chronic open-angle glaucoma, possibly nucleoside, or antiviral); systemic side effects (e.g., timolol for glaucoma and cyclosporin A for graft rejection); need for combination therapy (e.g., cromoglycate and corticosteroid for asthma and allergies, corticosteroid and indomethacin, or possibly corticosteroid, cyclosporin A, and indomethacin for prevention of corneal graft rejection; combination of antibiotics for septic keratitis (e.g., gentamicin or other aminoglycosides with methicilin or a cephalosporin); the need for a predetermined profile of drug delivery over a prolonged period of days, weeks, or months (e.g., acute corneal infections, acute-becoming chronic inflammation, and corneal graft rejection episodes); and long-continued low dosage for therapy or prophylaxis (e.g., for prevention of corneal graft rejection, prevention of recrudescence of inflammation, and prevention of or recurrence of herpetic disease).

In forecasting the future of rate-controlled topical delivery of nasal and ophthalmic drugs based on the examples cited, it is important to note that certain arbitrary choices about design were made early in this field. Much subsequent work needs to be done regarding reassessment of these early design features in the search for greater ease of system insertion, placement, and removal.[74,75]

References

1. Chien, Y.W., In *Transnasal Systemic Medications, Fundamentals, Developmental Concepts and Biomedical Assessments*, Elsevier, New York, 226, 1985.
2. Nudelman, I., Nasal delivery: a revolution in drug administration. In The Latest Developments in Drug Delivery Systems, Conf. Proc., *Pharma. Tech.*, 43–48, 1987.
3. Proctor, D.F., Nasal physiology in intranasal drug administration. In *Transnasal Systemic Medications, Fundamentals, Developmental Concepts and Biomedical Assessments*, Elsevier, New York, 101–119, 1985.
4. Batson, O.V., The venous networks of the nasal mucosa, *Ann. Otol. Rhinol. Laryngol.*, 63, 571–580, 1954.
5. Cauna, N., Blood and nerve supply of the nasal lining. In *The Nose, Upper Airway Physiology and the Atmospheric Environment*, Proctor, D.F. and Anderson, I., Eds., Elsevier, Amsterdam, 45–70, 1982.
6. Dawes, J.D.K. and Prichard, M.N.L., Studies of the vascular arrangements of the nose, *J. Anat.*, 87, 311–322, 1953.
7. Hall, L.J. and Jackson, R.T., Effects of alpha and beta adrenergic agonists on nasal blood flow, *Ann. Otol. Rhinol. Laryngol.*, 77, 1120–1130, 1968.
8. Jackson, R.T. and Burson, J.H., Effect of inflammatory mediators on nasal mucosa, *Arch. Otolaryngol.*, 103, 441–444, 1977.
9. Tovall, R. and Jackson, R.T., Prostaglandins and nasal blood flow, *Ann. Otol. Rhinol. Laryngol.*, 76, 1051–1060, 1967.
10. Watanabe, K., Saito, Y., Watanabe, I., and Mizuhriva, V., Characteristics of capillary permeability in nasal mucosa, *Ann. Otol. Rhinol. Laryngol.*, 89, 377–382, 1980.

11. Su, K.S.E., Wilson, H.C., and Campanale, K.M., Recent advances in intranasal drug delivery systems. In *Drug Delivery Systems, Fundamentals and Techniques,* Johnson, P. and Lloyd-Jones, J.G., Eds., VCH Publishers, London, 224–242, 1987.

12. Mygind, N., Rasmussen, F.V., and Molgaard, F., Cellular and neurogenic mechanisms in nose and bronchi, *Eur. J. Respir. Dis.*, 64(Suppl. 128), 483–554, 1983.

13. Kumar, A.T.C., David, G.F.X., and Puri, V., Nasal sprays for controlling ovulation in rhesus monkeys. In *Recent Advances in Primatology*, Vol. 4, Chivers, D.J. and Ford, E.H.R., Eds., Academic Press, New York, 1978.

14. Lindsay, W.W., Tobispray in nasal surgery, *Med. J. Aust.*, 1, 751, 1977.

15. Hamilton, L.H., Effect of xylometazoline nasal spray on nasal conductance in subjects with coryza, *J. Otolaryngol.*, 10(2), 109, 1981.

16. Hyde, R.W., Tonndorf, J., and Chinn, H.E., Absorption from the nasal mucous membrane, *Ann. Otol. Rhinol. Laryngol.*, 62, 957, 1953.

17. Tonndorf, J., Chinn, H.I., and Lett, J.E., Absorption from the nasal mucous membrane: systemic effect of hyoscine following intranasal administration, *Ann. Otol. Rhinol. Laryngol.*, 62, 630, 1953.

18. Borum, P. and Mygind, N., Nasal methacholine challenge and ipratropium therapy: Laboratory studies and a clinical trial in perennial rhinitis, *Acta. Otol-Rhinol-Laryngologica Belgica*, 33(4), 528, 1979.

19. Dyke, C.V., Jatlow, P., Ungerer, P., Barash, P.G., and Byck, R., Oral cocaine: plasma concentrations and central effects, *Science*, 24, 271, 1978.

20. Angard, A., The effect of prostaglandins on nasal airway resistance in man, *Ann. Otol. Rhinol. Laryngol.*, 78, 657, 1969.

21. Hirai, S., Yashiki, T., Matswzawa, T., and Mima, H., Absorption of drugs from the nasal mucosa of rat, *Int. J. Pharm.*, 7, 317, 1981.

22. Rubinstein, A., Rubinstein, E., Toitum, E., and Donbrow, M., Increase of intestinal absorption of gentamicin and amitracin by nonionic surfactant, *Antimicrob. Agents Chemother.*, 19, 696, 1981.

23. Bucknall, R.A., Why aren't antivirals effective when administered intranasally? In *Chemotherapy and Control of Influenza*, Oxford, J.S. and Williams, J.D., Eds., Academic Press, New York, 77–80, 1976.

24. Delong, D.C. and Reed, S.E., Inhibition of rhinovirus replication in organ cultures by a potential antiviral drug, *J. Infect. Dis.*, 141, 87, 1980.

25. Schaffer, N. and Seidman, E.E., The intranasal use of prophenopyridamine maleate and chlorprophenpyridamine maleate in allergic rhinitis, *Ann. Allergy*, 10, 194, 1952.

26. Resta, O., Barbars, M.P.F., and Carnimea, N., A comparison of sodium cromo-glycate nasal solution and powder in the treatment of allergic rhinitis, *Br. J. Clin. Pract*, 36, 94, 1982.

27. Childrey, J.H. and Essex, H.E., Absorption from the mucosa of the frontal sinus, *Arch. Otolaryngology*, 14, 564, 1931.

28. Cuddihy, R.G. and Ozog, J.A., Nasal absorption of CsCl, SrCl, BaCl, and CeCl in Syrian hamsters, *Health Physics*, 25, 219, 1973.

29. Czerniawska, A., Experimental investigations on the preparation of Au from nasal mucous membrane into cerebrospinal fluid, *Acta. Otolaryng.*, 70, 58, 1970.

30. Byron, P.R., Pulmonary targeting with aerosols, *Pharm. Tech.*, 11, 42–56, 1987.

31. Mahl, M.C., Dick, E.C., and Walter, G.R. Jr., U.S. Patent 4,355,021, 1982.

32. *Drug Therapy*, CORE Medical Journals, Lawrenceville, NJ, 96, 1990.
33. Illum, L., Farraj, N.F., Critchley, H., Johansen ,B.R., and Davis, S.S., Enhanced nasal absorption of insulin in rats using lysophosphatidylcholine, *Int. J. Pharm.*, 57, 49–54, 1989.
34. Illum, L., Farraj, N., Critchley, H., and Davis, S.S., Nasal administration of gentamicin using a novel microsphere delivery system, *Int. J. Pharm.*, 46, 261–265, 1988.
35. Kornhauser, D.M., Wood, A.J.J., Wood, R.E., Vestal, G.R., et al., Biological determinants of propranolol distribution in man, *Clin. Pharmacol. Ther.*, 23, 165–174, 1978.
36. Lee, V.H.L., Gallardo, D., and Longnecker, J.P., Protease inhibition as an additional mechanism for the nasal absorption enhancement effect of sodium taurodihydrofusidate, *Proc. Intl. Symp. Control Rel. Bioact. Mater.*, 14, 55–56, 1987.
37. Chien, Y.W., Su, K.S.E., and Chang, S.F., *Nasal Systemic Drug Delivery*, Marcel Dekker, New York, 320, 1989.
38. Gold, A.R., Bleeker, E.R., and Smith, P.L., The effect of chronic nocturnal oxygen administration upon sleep apnea, *Am. Rev. Respir. Dis.*, 134, 925–969, 1986.
39. Phillips, B.A., Schmitt, F.A., Berry, D.T., Lamb, D.G., et al., Treatment of obstructive sleep apnea, *Chest*, 98, 325–330, 1990.
40. Phillips, B.A. and Berry, D., Sleep apnea in the elderly, *Drug Therapy*, 20, 65–74, 1990.
41. Lee, W.A., Ennis, R.D., Longenecker, J.P., and Bengtsson, P., The bioavailability of intranasal salmon calcitonin in healthy volunteers with and without a permeation enhancer, *Pharm. Res.*, 11, 747–750, 1994.
42. Robinson, J.R., In *Ophthalmic Drug Delivery Systems*, APhA Academy of Pharmaceutical Sciences, 137, 1980.
43. Cumming, J.S., Relevant anatomy and physiology of the eye. In *Ophthalmic Drug Delivery Systems*, Robinson, J.R., Ed., APhA Academy of Pharmaceutical Sciences, 1–27, 1980.
44. Langer, R. and Conn, H., Ocular applications of controlled release. In *Medical Applications of Controlled Release*, Vol. 2, CRC Press, Inc., Boca Raton, FL, 65–76, 1984.
45. Ticho, U., Blumenthal, M., Zonis, S., Gal, A., et al., A clinical trial with Piloplex — a new long-acting pilocarpine compound, preliminary report, *Ann. Ophthalmol.*, 11, 555–561, 1979.
46. Wilson, C.G., Tomlinson, E., Davis, S.S., and Olejnik, O., Altered ocular absorption and disposition of sodium chromoglycate upon ion-pair and complex coacervate formation with dodecylbenzyldimethylammonium chloride, *J. Phar., Pharmacol.*, 31, 749–753, 1981.
47. Krause, P.D., Dipivefrin (DPE): preclinical and clinical aspects of its development for use in the eye. In *Ophthalmic Drug Delivery Systems*, Robinson, J.R., Ed., APhA Academy of Pharmaceutical Sciences, 91–104, 1980.
48. Bloomfield, S.E., Miyata, T., Dunn, M.W., Bueser, N., et al., Soluble gentamicin ophthalmic inserts as drug delivery systems, *Arch. Ophthalmol.*, 96, 885–887, 1978.
49. Shell, J.W., New systems for the ocular delivery of drugs. In *Drug Delivery Systems, Fundamentals and Techniques*, Johnson, P. and Lloyd-Jones, H., Eds., VCH Publishers, London, 243–265, 1987.

50. Lee, V.H.L., Ophthalmic delivery of peptides and proteins, *Pharm. Tech.*, 11, 26–38, 1987.

51. Sieg, J.W. and Robinson, J.R., Vehicle effects on ocular drug bioavailability, I. Evaluation of fluorometholone, *J. Pharm. Sci.*, 64, 931–936, 1975.

52. Stratford Jr., R.E., Carson, L.W., Dodda-Kashi, S., and Lee, V.H.L., Systemic absorption of ocularly administered enkephalinamide and insulin in the albino rabbit: extent, pathways and vehicle effects, *J. Pharm. Sci.*, 77, 838–842, 1988.

53. Trzeciakowski, J. and Chiou, G.C., Effects of demethylated carbachol on iris and ciliary muscles, *J. Pharm. Sci.*, 69, 332–334, 1980.

54. Jain, M.R., Drug delivery through soft contact lenses, *Brit. J. Ophthal.*, 72, 150–154, 1988.

55. Bawa, R., Dais, M., Nandu, M., and Robinson, J.R., New extended-release ocular drug delivery system-design: characterization and performance of minidisc inserts, Paper No. 63, *Program and Abstracts of the 15th Int. Symp. Cont. Rel. Bioact. Mater.*, August 15–19, 1988, Basel, Switzerland.

56. Desai, D.S., Chien, Y.W., and Tojo, K., Bioconversion of ocular pro-drugs across rabbit cornea *in vitro*, Paper No. 80, *Program and Abstracts of the 15th Intl. Symp. Cont. Rel. Bioact. Mater.*, August 15–19, 1988, Basel, Switzerland.

57. Attia, M.A., Impact of formulation factors on the pharmacokinetics of dexamethasone in ocular tissues, Paper No. 118, *Program and Abstracts of the 15th Intl. Symp. Cont. Rel. Bioact. Mater.*, August 15–19, 1988, Basel, Switzerland.

58. Kreuter, J., Diepold, R., Andermann, G., Gurny, R., et al., Comparison of different *in vitro* and *in vivo* test-models for pilocarpine using conventional and depot eyedrops (nanoparticles), Paper No. 120, *Program and Abstracts of the 15th Intl. Symp. Cont. Rel. Bioact. Mater.*, August 15–19, 1988, Basel, Switzerland.

59. Davies, N.M., Farr, S.J., Hadgraft, J., and Kellaway, I.W., The effect of a mucoadhesive polymer on the bioavailability of pilocarpine, Paper No. 222, *Program and Abstracts of the 15th Intl. Symp. Cont. Rel. Bioact. Mater.*, August 15–19, 1988, Basel, Switzerland.

60. Lerman, S., Davis, P., and Jackson, W.B., Prolonged-release hydrocortisone therapy, *Can. J. Ophthalmol.*, 8, 114–118, 1973.

61. Gurny, R., Preliminary study of prolonged-acting drug delivery systems for the treatment of glaucoma, *Pharm. Acta. Helv.*, 56, 130–132, 1981.

62. Waltman, S.R. and Kaufman, H.E., Use of hydrophilic contact lenses to increase ocular penetration of topical drugs, *Invest. Ophthalmol.*, 9, 250, 1970.

63. Kaufman, H.E., Uotila, M.H., Gasset, A.R., Wood, R.O., and Ellison, E.D., The medical uses of soft contact lenses, *Trans. Am. Acad. Ophthalmol. Otolaryngol.*, 75, 361, 1971.

64. Praus, R., Brettschneider, H.F., Krejci, L., and Kalvodova, D., Hydrophilic contact lenses as a new therapeutic approach for the topical use of chloramphenicol and tetracycline, *Ophthalmologica*, 165, 62, 1972.

65. Hull, D.S., Edelhauser, H.F., and Hyndiuk, R.A., Ocular penetration of prednisolone and the hydrophilic contact lens, *Arch. Opthalmol.*, 14, 413, 1974.

66. Maichuk, Y.F., Polymeric drug delivery systems in ophthalmology. In *Symp. Ocular Therapy*, Vol. 9, Leopold, I.H. and Burns, R.P., Eds., John Wiley & Sons, New York, 1976.

67. Capozza, R.C., Enzymically decomposable bioerodible pharmaceutical carrier, German Patent 2,505,305, (Chem. Abstr. 84, 35314s, 1976), 1976.

68. Ueno, N. and Refojo, M.F., Ocular pharmacology of drug release devices. In *Controlled Drug Delivery.* Vol. 2, Clinical Applications, Bruck, S.D., Ed., CRC Press, Boca Raton, FL, 89–109, 1983.

69. Harwood, R.J., Perry, H.C.B., and Field, K.A., Antiviral activity of an interferon inducer in a biosoluble ophthalmic system. In *Controlled Release Delivery Systems*, Roseman, T.J. and Mansdorf, S.Z., Eds., Marcel Dekker and Basel, New York, 187–197.

70. Byron, P.R., *Respiratory Drug Delivery*, CRC Press, Boca Raton, FL, 304, 1989.

71. Ganderton, D. and Jones, T., Eds., *Drug Delivery to the Respiratory Tract*, VCH Publishers, New York, 141, 1987.

72. Shaw, J.E., Drug delivery systems, *Ann. Rep. Med. Chem.*, 15, 302–315, 1980.

73. Jones, B.R., Role of new delivery systems in ophthalmic delivery. In *Better Therapy with Existing Drugs: New Uses and Delivery Systems*, Bearn, A., Ed., Merck Sharp & Dohme, 163, 1981.

74. Niven, R.W., Delivery of biotherapeutics by inhalation aerosols, *Pharm. Tech.*, July 1993, 72.

75. Hickey, A.J., in *Pharmaceutical Inhalation Aerosol Technology*, Marcel Dekker, New York, 384, 1992.

76. Edman, P., *Biopharmaceutics of Ocular Drug Delivery*, CRC Press, Boca Raton, FL, 224, 1993.

77. Maurice, D.M., In *Ophthalmic Drug Delivery, Biopharmaceutical, Technological and Clinical Aspects*, Fidia Research Series, Vol. 11, Saettone, M.S., Ed., Padova, Italy, 19–26, 1987.

78. Harris, D., Liaw, J.H., and Robinson, J.R., Ocular delivery of peptide and protein drugs, In *Ophthalmic Drug Delivery, Biopharmaceutical, Technological and Clinical Aspects*, Fidia Research Series, Vol. 11, Saettone, M.S., Ed., Padova, Italy, 8/2–3, 331–339, 1992.

79. Quadir, M. et al., Development and evaluation of nasal formulations of ketorolac, *Drug Deliv.*, 7, 223–229, 2000.

80. Teshima, D. et al., Nasal glucagon delivery using microcrystalline cellulose in healthy volunteers, *Int. J. Pharm.*, 233, 61–66, 2002.

81. Lim, S.T. et al., *In vivo* evaluation of novel hyaluron/chitosan microparticulate delivery systems for the nasal delivery of gentamicin in rabbits, *Int. J. Pharm.*, 231, 73–82, 2002.

82. Ikechukwu-Ugwoke, M. et al., Intranasal bioavailability of apomorphine from carboxymethylcellulose-based drug delivery system, *Int. J. Pharm.*, 202, 125–131, 2000.

83. Ko, K.T. et al., Emulsion formulations of testosterone for nasal administration, *L. Microencapsul.*, 15, 197–205, 1998.

84. Lizio, R. et al., Systemic delivery of cetrorelix to rats by a new aerosol delivery system, *Pharm. Res.*, 18, 771–779, 2001.

85. Moore, J.M. and Pham, S., Hydraulic high-pressure nebulization of solution and dispersions for respiratory drug delivery, *Pharm. Dev. Technol.*, 5, 105–113, 2000.

86. Iida, K. et al., Effect of mixing of fine carrier particles on dry powder inhalation property of salbutamol sulfate (SS), *Yakugaku Zasshi*, 120, 113–119, 2000.

87. Negley, J.E. et al., RinoFlow nasal wash and sinus system as a mechanism for deliver medications to the paranasal sinuses: results of a radiolabeled pilot study, *Ear Nose Throat J.*, 78, 550–552, 1999.

88. Gradon, L. and Sosnowski, T.R., Comparative studies of particle distribution range of aerosol cromolyn sodium generated by MDI systems, *Pol. Merkuriusz. Lek.*, 6, 253–255, 1999.

89. Musoh, K. et al., The effect of tulobuterol tape on histamine-induced bronchoconstriction in conscious guinea pigs: long duration of action, *Jpn. J. Pharmacol.*, 79,401–79,402, 1999.

90. Katayama, Y. et al., Minimizing the inhaled dose of NO with breath-by-breath delivery of spikes of concentrated gas, *Circulation*, 98, 2429–2432, 1998.

91. Roth, C. et al., Characterization of amphotericin B aerosols for inhalation treatment of pulmonary aspergillosis, *Infection*, 24, 354–360, 1996.

92. Kraemer, R., Babyhaler — a new pediatric aerosol device, *J. Aerosol Med.*, 8(Suppl 2:S), 19–26, 1995.

93. Fuller, R., The Diskus: A new multi-dose powder device — efficacy and comparison with Turbuhaler, *J. Aerosol Med.*, 8 (Suppl. 2:S), 11–17, 1995.

94. Peart, J. and Clarke, M.J., New developments in dry powder inhaler technology, *Am. Pharm. Rev.*, 4, 37–45, 2001.

95. Jones, L.D. et al., Analysis and physical stability of pharmaceutical aerosols, *Pharm. Tech.*, 24, 40–54, 2000.

96. Crowder, T.M. et al., 2001: An odyssey in inhaler formulation and design, *Pharm. Tech.*, 25, 99–113, 2001.

97. Desai, S.D. and Blanchard, J., Pluronic F127-based ocular delivery system containing biodegradable polyisobutylcyanoacrylate nanocapsules of pilocarpine, *Drug Deliv.*, 7, 201–207, 2000.

98. Kim, E.Y. and Gao, Z.G., rhEGF/HP-beta-CD complex in poloxamer gel for ophthalmic delivery, *Int. J. Pharm.*, 233, 159–167, 2002.

99. Kawakami, S. et al., Ocular absorption behavior of palmitoyl tilisolol: an amphiphilic pro-drug of tilisolol for ocular drug delivery, *J. Pharm. Sci.*, 90, 2113–2120, 2001.

100. Einmahl, S. et al., Therapeutic applications of viscous and injectable poly(ortho esters), *Adv. Drug Deliv. Rev.*, 53, 45–73, 2001.

101. Ghelardi, F. and Tavanti, A., Effect of a novel mucoadhesive polysaccharide obtained from tamarind seeds on the intraocular penetration of gentamicin and ofloxacin in rabbits, *J. Antimicrob. Chemother.*, 46, 831–834, 2000.

102. Lee, Y.C. and Yalkowski, S.H., Systemic absorption of insulin from a Gelfoam ocular device, *Int. J. Pharm.*, 190, 35–40, 1999.

103. Desai, S.D. and Blanchard, J., *In vitro* evaluation of pluronic F-127-based controlled-release ocular delivery systems for pilocarpine, *J. Pharm. Sci.*, 87, 226–230, 1998.

104. Lee, Y.C. et al., Systemic delivery of insulin via an enhancer-free ocular device, *J. Pharm. Sci.*, 86, 1361–1364, 1997.

105. Ichien, K. et al., Mitomicin C dissolved in a reversible thermosetting gel: target tissue concentrations in the rabbit eye, *Br. J. Ophthalmol.*, 81, 72–75, 1997.

106. Rafferty, D.E. and Elfaki, M.G., Preparation and characterization of a biodegradable microparticle antigen/cytokine delivery system, *Vaccine*, 14, 532–538, 1996.

chapter eight

Miscellaneous forms of drug delivery

I. Introduction

Three basic approaches are used to address the problem of improving drug absorption: the formulation approach, the pro-drug (reversible-derivative) approach, and the analog (irreversible-derivative) approach. Each of these approaches should be contemplated whenever there is a problem with drug efficacy.

Since it involves no synthesis and only minimal investigational new drug (IND) amending, the formulation approach is the quickest, easiest, and least expensive of the three; it should, therefore, be considered first. By altering the formulation, it is usually possible to increase or decrease a drug's aqueous solubility or dissolution rate. However, the formulation approach is of almost no value for increasing membrane transport, and it cannot always be used to alter drug stability. In general, the formulation approach, when applied to drugs that are insoluble (or too soluble) or that are degraded in the stomach, offers a high probability of success for a comparatively small investment.

Analogs are generally defined as molecular modifications consisting of a skeletal transformation or a substituent group synthesis. These irreversible derivatives are synthesized with the intent of altering or improving intrinsic activity. Because they often interact differently with receptors, analogs frequently have a different spectrum of activity and side effects than the parent drug. For these reasons, the analog approach is not normally used to improve absorption, although, in cases of metabolism-limited bioavailability, this approach is worthy of consideration. While the formulation and analog approaches have been classical strategies to increase drug efficacy, the development of pro-drugs is of a more recent vintage.

II. Pro-drugs

The term pro-drug is employed for that class of drug derivatives that is converted *in vivo* to the desired compound. The important distinction between analogs and pro-drugs is that the former are biologically active, whereas the latter require *in vivo* conversion in order to elicit biological activity. The primary utility of analogs is to improve potency and to achieve specificity of action, whereas the pro-drug is used to improve pharmaceutical properties. Because it does not alter the primary structure of the parent drug, pro-drug synthesis is usually much less difficult than analog synthesis, and the probability of a pro-drug being active may be greater than for an analog.

In the case of the most common pro-drugs (i.e., simple esters and amides) it might be possible to accelerate the development and registration process by using an abbreviated preclinical testing program. One of the important applications of pro-drugs is in improving oral absorption. The unique feature of the pro-drug is that the physicochemical properties of the resulting deriv-

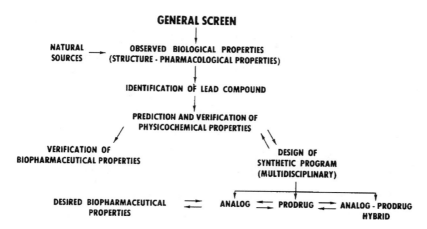

Figure 8.1 Perspective in drug design. (Copyright 1977 by the American Pharmaceutical Association, *Design of Biopharmaceutical Properties through Pro-Drugs and Analogs.* Reprinted with permission of the American Pharmaceutical Association.)

ative can be carefully tailored by means of structural modification of the pro-moiety. The intrinsic activity of the parent drug is assured through *in vivo* cleavage of the pro-drug.

The pro-drug approach has been successfully applied to a wide variety of drugs. It is most effective when an undesirable characteristic of the parent drug needs to be eliminated, especially if that characteristic can be related to a physicochemical property, such as melting point, boiling point, solubility, or partition coefficient. In these instances, the characteristic to be altered is related as much as possible to a physicochemical property (see Figures 8.1 and 8.2).

The economics of synthesizing a pro-drug should be such that the cost is not significantly higher than that of the parent drug. Single-step pro-drug synthesis using inexpensive pro-moieties is preferred. The pro-moiety selected should yield a fragment, upon cleavage of the pro-drug, that is free of toxicity or side effects and preferably free of biological activity. The choice of the pro-moiety is also dependent upon the nature of the parent drug. For example, the pro-moiety chosen for a parent drug with an effective dose of 1 mg may not be acceptable with another parent drug given at a high dosage (e.g., 500 mg) because of either the unacceptably high weight of an equivalent dose of the pro-drug or the toxicity or other side effects of the pro-moiety at this high dosage level.

The pro-moiety should be rapidly cleaved once the pro-drug is absorbed in order to elicit a pharmacokinetic profile similar to that of the parent drug. A pro-drug with both improved absorption and prolonged action through sustained release requires that the pro-moiety be carefully tailored with respect to lability. Finally, the intact drug should not produce drug distribution patterns that could lead to unfavorable tissue distribution.

The rational design of pro-drugs having oral activity can be divided into three basic steps: the determination of physical properties required for max-

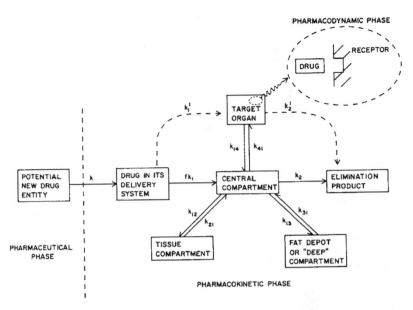

Figure 8.2 Drug in different phases. (From Stella, V.J. et al. in *Drug Delivery Systems*, Juliano, R.L., Ed., Oxford University Press, NY, 1980, 115. With permission.)

imum efficacy, the selection of a chemical linkage between the parent drug and the pro-moiety that will be cleaved in the desired biological compartment, and the design and synthesis of pro-drugs that have the proper physiochemical properties as well as the proper chemical lability. The selection of optimum physicochemical parameters is accomplished through the aid of *in vitro* and *in vivo* experimentation and modeling. If the biological system is clearly understood, it is usually possible to devise models that give reliable estimates of what physicochemical parameters are important and of their optimal values.[1]

For a drug, most often an organic chemical, to elicit a pharmacologic response, it must reach a "site of action." The term "site of action" refers to the fact that a chemical must reach and interact with a receptor in some host target site in order elicit an effect. There are barriers that can limit the ability of a drug to reach its site of action. Two examples are: a barrier may be as simple as low aqueous solubility, such that when a drug is administered to an animal for evaluation of a particular pharmacologic effect, it may be absorbed very poorly or not at all; and even though the agent may interact strongly with a receptor, in an *in vitro* test, it may not reach the receptor site in the *in vivo* test, due to its impermeability to the outer membrane of the cells containing the particular receptor.

The term "pro-drug," or "pro-agent," was first used to describe compounds that undergo biotransformation prior to eliciting a pharmacologic effect. It was suggested that this approach could be used to alter the properties of certain drugs, in a temporary manner, to increase their usefulness or to alter or decrease their toxicity.[2]

Local drug delivery involves the administration of a drug contained in a dosage form to a local surface or tissue of the body. The therapeutic success achieved is a matter of the efficiency of the release of the drug from the dosage form and the absorption or transport of the drug across the biological membranes to which the delivery system is applied. The efficiency is a net result of drug-dosage form and drug-biological interactions. These interactions are a function of the physicochemical properties of the drug, dosage-form factors, and biological structures and characteristics.

Approaches other than the pro-drug approach in local drug delivery manipulate the drug-dosage form by maximizing or optimizing thermodynamic activity of the drug at the absorbing membrane surface. Since the flux of a drug across a membrane is a function of the product of the permeability of the membrane and the concentration of the drug at the absorbing interface, such approaches can optimize the flux or absorption of a drug to a certain extent. However, the absorption of the drug and, consequently, the therapeutic success obtained by the delivery method can be unacceptably poor because of intrinsically poor permeability of the limiting membrane to the drug. Since the permeability of a membrane is a function of drug properties, in addition to the properties of the membrane, the pro-drug approach offers possible solutions to problems in absorption and drug transport across biological membranes.

The chemical structural changes made in the pro-drug approach, which are changes made by design to be either chemically or enzymatically reversible, result in changes in drug properties, such as solubility and partition coefficient. By design, the result is improved membrane permeability. The pro-drug approach in this regard represents an alteration in drug-membrane interactions such that membrane permeability is enhanced.

The structural features of a therapeutic agent that make it selective for various target tissues or cells has been an area of scientific interest and research for a number of years. In the case of pharmacologically important alkaloids and other natural products, the important structural features have been incorporated into the drug by nature. Others are fortitous accidents of drug synthesis. Some synthetic modifications in the early years, however, were actually products of design intended to improve or otherwise change a biological property.[3]

A strategy may be divided into three general areas wherein chemical modification can be employed to alter pharmacokinetics. These are the input function, which includes both rate and amount; elimination by excretion metabolism; and distribution to active and inactive binding sites. The input function is the most commonly altered pharmacokinetic property. The two most common goals in controlling drug input are to increase bioavailability or to program the drug time course. The bioavailability of orally administered drugs has been successfully increased by increasing gastric stability, decreasing binding to foods, optimizing the partition coefficient, increasing solubility, and decreasing intestinal metabolism or first-pass effect. The most common goal in attempting to improve drug input is to increase duration of action. The control of drug input may also be used to decrease toxicity.

Elimination may limit the success of a drug if it results in a short duration. Molecular modification could be designed to reduce excretion or metabolism in order to increase duration. Reduced metabolism may also be necessitated to avoid formation of a toxic metabolite. Conversely, a specific metabolic route may be enhanced if an active metabolite is formed. Distribution is probably the least understood of the three areas. Few generalities can be made with confidence regarding structural effects on distribution. Isolated examples of success can be found, but these do not provide sufficient basis for prediction. The goals, if less attainable, are perhaps more significant. Specificity is undoubtedly the single most important desirable trait. Thus, increased distribution to a specific site is considered a prime goal in effecting specificity and decreasing toxicity. Increasing tissue distribution can also be a means of increasing duration. This would be achieved by increasing the deposition of drugs in sites that are not available to either metabolism or excretion.[4]

There are many examples of widely used drugs that have a well-recognized pharmacokinetic limitation. Such agents are candidates for irreversible derivatives (analogs) or bioreversible derivatives (pro-drugs). In both cases, optimization of the pharmacokinetic profile is aimed at the specific limitation of the original drug. Thus, derivatization has been employed to increase oral absorption, control drug delivery rate, decrease metabolism (or first-pass effect), increase duration, increase site specificity, or reduce side effects. All of the improvements result from an alteration of the physical chemistry of the molecule. It is unlikely that such an alteration would affect only one aspect of the pharmacokinetic profile since these kinetic processes are influenced by the physicochemical properties of the agent. The exception to this is a rapidly reversible pro-drug designed to increase absorption. Although the rationale for developing analogs and pro-drugs is often identical, their pharmacokinetic evaluation and optimization presents dissimilar problems. This is due to the fact that the active drug remains the same in the case of a pro-drug, whereas an analog is, in fact, a new drug. Plasma time course for a pro-drug may be compared directly to that obtained by administration of the original drug product. Conversely, the pharmacokinetics of an analog must be completely defined, and its plasma data cannot be directly compared to the original drug. Pro-drugs pose an additional kinetic problem in that the site for bioreversal influences the results. The ideal site for bioreversal depends upon the goal. This, in turn, determines the relative desirability of circulating pro-drug. Thus, a lack of assay specificity may sometimes result in misinterpretation of pharmacokinetic profiles.

Antibiotics represent the compounds most widely modified for pharmacokinetic reasons. Improved oral absorption is the most frequent goal. The modification of penicillins, tetracyclines, lincomycin, erythromycin, and cephalosporins are typical examples. Structural effects on the kinetics of first-pass metabolism are not presently well defined. Pro-drugs, which survive first-pass reversal, may also lack the required rate of bioreversal. The prediction of structural effects on pharmacokinetic behavior has not yet been adequately developed, and satisfactory interpretation of kinetic data has not always been achieved. Both of these areas represent significant areas for future research.

A physical-model approach to drug design to improve intestinal absorption is a quantitative and mechanistic approach that utilizes the basic principles of thermodynamics and mass transport. The mathematics are rigorously applied to describe the processes in terms of physically and chemically meaningful thermodynamic and kinetic parameters. Within the framework of these parameters, one has access to the relevant physicochemical descriptors of the drug molecule itself (such as pKa, molecular size, solubility, diffusivity in water, etc.) and of the drug-biomembrane relationship (such as membrane-water partition coefficient, diffusivity in the membrane, molecular size relative to the effective pore size, etc.). The physical model predicts a sigmoidal relationship between the absorption-rate constant and lipophilicity.

The physical-model approach has been applied to evaluating different formulation systems (suspensions and carrier-mediated systems). Formulation factors influence absorption by affecting thermodynamic drug activity in the intestinal lumen, and this is clearly delineated from the optimal penetrability of the biomembrane by the molecularly modified drug. By increasing the permeability of the membrane for the drug molecule, the total rate of intestinal absorption is enhanced. One of the important avenues for future research is the detailed investigation of the structure-absorptivity correlations with the rat intestinal system for the various drugs not yet investigated by the physical-model approach. Intestinal absorption of antibiotics in man has always appeared to have been a problem from the drug-design standpoint. The present approach should allow the determination of metabolism (both cavital and gut wall) and absorption factors on a quantitative basis for the penicillins and the tetracyclines. Nucleosides and nucleotides are generally highly polar compounds and represent another class of drugs with bioavailability problems because they often permeate the lipoidal barriers with only great difficulty.

The effective design of pro-drugs through the consideration of enzyme-substrate specificities requires considerable knowledge of the particular enzyme or enzyme systems. In addition to the enzyme's specificity (both kinetic and binding), the type of reaction catalyzed, the enzyme distribution and level, and the functional role of the enzyme in cellular biochemistry should be known. The advantages of designing drugs based on this knowledge of cellular biochemistry are clearly recognized. A review of the specificities of several enzymes in the hydrolase class suggests potential use as general sites for pro-drug reconversion.[5]

Metabolic studies are an integral part of the testing procedures applied to evaluate the safety and efficacy of all new drugs, as well as other environmental chemicals, such as food additives, pesticides, and industrial chemicals. Such studies generally lead to a better understanding of a drug's mode of action, toxicity, interactions with other drugs and chemicals, and possibly provide some insight into the biochemical reaction mechanisms involved in its biotransformation. Hopefully, this insight can be used to increase the efficacy of the drug. In general terms, this can be brought about by decreasing undesirable toxic reactions of the drug, increasing its potency, selectivity, or duration of action, or a suitable combination of any of these.

Needless to say, modifying any one physicochemical or biological property of a drug to improve its efficacy may inherently increase an undesirable feature and thereby alter the overall pharmacodynamic situation *in vivo.* Several biotransformation pathways have been explored in an attempt to show the major metabolic reactions that drugs undergo. These include oxidation, reduction, hydrolysis, acylation, glucuronidation, sulfation, and mercapturic acid formation. Specific examples have been explored in each category to illustrate the basic structural requirements for a particular reaction and how modifying the structure can alter metabolism. The judicial use of deuterium and fluorine to "switch" pathways of metabolism has been particularly emphasized.[6]

The utility of pro-drugs has been illustrated in numerous review articles, and a number of pro-drugs are currently marketed with superior patient acceptance or effectiveness over the parent drug. Two approaches are used in pro-drug synthesis: random synthesis followed by screening to identify the pro-drug with the preferred properties, or prediction of the physiochemical properties required to produce the desired biopharmaceutical properties and translation of this into structural requirements. The latter approach is more appealing due to the numerous relationships established between structural and biopharmaceutical properties. In practice, however, the carefully designed pro-drug often does not yield a biologically active compound. It has been shown that the use of activated substituents in the pro-moiety is a means of ensuring *in vivo* activity of a pro-drug, and it has also become evident that a pro-drug may be inactive even though quantitatively converted to the parent drug *in vivo*, and activation of pro-moieties through substituent effects can often lead to a biologically active pro-drug[7] (see Figures 8.3 and 8.4).

The data presented on the influence of substituent effects on the pro-moiety shows that the biological activity of the pro-drug is often dictated by charge and steric effects. Pro-drugs that are biologically inactive may be improved through the incorporation of activating substituents in the pro-moiety. Control of the rate of pro-drug cleavage is necessary for special applications, such as improved absorption, prolonged action, decreased metabolism, and altered tissue distribution. The chemical modification employed to improve potency and specificity of drugs is analog, whereas modification to improve biopharmaceutical properties can consist of derivative pro-drugs, analog pro-drugs, or derivatives of the non-*in vivo* reversible

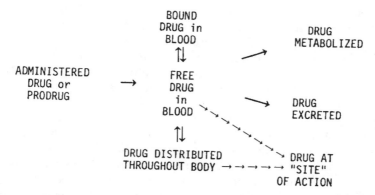

Figure 8.3 Drug undergoing biotransformation. (Copyright 1977 by the American Pharmaceutical Association, *Design of Biopharmaceutical Properties through Pro-Drugs and Analogs*. Reprinted with permission of the American Pharmaceutical Association.)

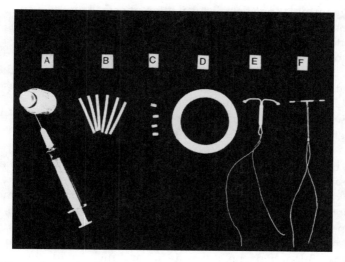

Figure 8.4 Several sustained-release forms for contraception: (A) injectable, (B) subdermal implants, (C) steroid pellets, (D) vaginal ring, (E) steroid-releasing IUD, (F) copper-releasing IUD. (From Langer, R.S. and Wise, D.L., Eds., *Medical Applications of Controlled Release*, Vol. 2, CRC Press, Boca Raton, FL, 1991. With permission.)

type. The transition between pro-drug and derivative is not clear-cut, since it is a matter of rate.

The use of pro-drug derivatives for improvement of taste properties of astringent, bitter, and tart drugs has been successful. Elimination of undesirable taste is usually accomplished by decreasing drug solubility below taste-threshold values. The most common derivative utilized is the ester since virtually all offensive-tasting drugs contain hydroxyl or carboxyl groups. Care must be taken to choose esters that decrease solubility below the taste-perception threshold in the formulated state. Tasting a drug ester as a powder is often misleading due to the inability of the drug to establish solubility equilibrium in saliva. Furthermore, limited solubility in the finished formulation is important since it is in this system that the drug will be administered, usually as a suspension. If the suspension is tasteless, the ester derivative meets taste-threshold criterion: resistance to hydrolysis in the oral cavity.

Saliva contains an abundance of hydrolytic enzymes capable of displacing a variety of ester groups from the pro-drug derivative. Once the derivative is swallowed, hydrolysis should occur within the gastrointestinal (GI) tract or systemic circulation. Most pro-drugs are bioinactive. Therefore, hydrolysis is mandatory. Amide pro-drug derivatives are not often used as taste modifiers due to their resistance to hydrolysis after absorption. Pro-drug covalent derivatives containing saccharin or cyclamate or other synthetic sweeteners may also be employed to counteract the objectionable taste of the parent drug. In some cases, absolute tastelessness will be an impossibility. The dosage formulation specialist can often physically mask a small amount of objectionable taste with a variety of flavoring agents. The chemist, for his part, should be cognizant of the physicochemical properties that result from his best modification efforts. Oils or gums are difficult to formulate as acceptable drug delivery systems, and polymorphs can have a profound effect on the taste qualities of a drug molecule. Caution must therefore be used in the final crystallization procedures of the taste substrates.

Following is a partial list of examples of therapeutic agents that have been structurally modified to yield pro-drugs.[8,9]

Antiviral/anticancer agents: Alkylaminocarboxyl derivatives of 5-fluorouracil, ancitabine, ftorafur, 5-fluorpdeoxyuridine, acyclovir (Zovirax), valacyclovir, cycladarine, trifluorothymidine, methotrexate, diethylstilbestrol, psoralen, propranolol (nitrogen mustard), mitomycin-C, hydroxy-CCNU, ara-C, adriamycin, butyric acid derivatives, N-phosphoryl derivatives of bisantrene, gamma-L-glutaminyl-4-hydroxy-3-iodobenzene, doxorubicin, and melphalan

Central Nervous System (CNS) agents: Lopiazepate, oxazepam, lorazepam, nipecotic acid, L-Dopa, phenytoin, carbamate esters of dopaminergic drugs, and benzoylphenylureas

Ophthalmic drugs: Pilocarpine, adrenalone, and propranolol (Ketoxime)

Anti-infectives: Mecillinam, cycloserine, alfonsfalin, mebendazole, polyoxins, ara-A, and Spectrobid (becampicillin)

Cardiovascular agents: Pivopril, captopril, pindolol, and amino acid derivatives of prazosin

Anti-inflammatory agents: Salicylamide, aspirin, niflumic acid, loxoprofen, diclofenac, sulindac, N-alkyllactame esters of indomethacin, and piroxicam

Antiallergy agents: Terbutaline, bambuterol, and albuterol

Miscellaneous agents: Aryloxy acetic acid diuretics, amiloride, l-cysteine nitorsourea, tornalate (bitolterol mesylate), trigonelline, epinephrine, azidothymidine (AZT), peptides, isothiazolone biocides, benzyl carbonate esters of dextran, 2,three-dimensionalidexyinosine (DDI), desmopressin (dDAVP), acyclic nucleoside phosphonates, 2,6-disubstituted 4-(2-arylethenyl)phenol (5-lipoxygenase inhibitor), benzimidazole-7-carboxylic acids (nonpeptide angiotensin II receptor antagonist), leucovorin, procysteine, phosphonoformate, 2,three-dimensionalideoxythymidine (ddT), 2-acylderivatives of BVAraU (uracil derivative), furosemide, phosphate pro-drug of peptidomimetic HIV protease inhibitors, isoniazide, anti-HIV(D4T 5-monophosphate 3,5-dioctanoyl-5-bromodeoxyuridine (BrdU-C8), phosphate ester of orally active platelet-activating factor (PAF), pro-drug NM441 (antibacterial NM394, a quinolone derivative), N-acetyl-L-gamma-glutamyl pro-drugs, cytotoxins (HPDCs), testosteronyl-4-dimethylaminobutyrate HCl, C-3 cyclic ether of cephalosporins, deoxyguanine analogs (antiviral), 9-beta-D-arabinofuranosyladenine, and antiarthritic, 3-carboxy-5-methyl-N-[(4-trifluoromethoxy)phenyl)]-4-isoxazolecarboxamide

III. Infusion devices

Controlled-release drug infusion systems allow regulated flow of drug solutions into the circulation over long periods of time. Therapeutic benefits of many intravenous drugs can be increased and side effects effectively reduced by controlled-release infusions. In addition, controlled-release infusions are definitely preferred over intermittent hypodermic injections for drugs with short half-lives or drugs that irritate the skin at injection sites.

A. Pumps

Mechanical pumps: A number of controlled-release pharmaceutical applications use mechanical pumps. For example, most patients who receive continuous intravenous infusion of drugs are connected by means of a cumbersome system of catheters to an infusing drip bottle. Several companies have devised miniaturized pumps that can be strapped to the patient with a harness, allowing the patient to be ambulatory. In addition, the patient or the physician controls the delivery rate of many devices. The simplest of these pumps has clockwork or battery motor-driven syringe or peristaltic pumps. Portable infusion pumps can be divided into several groups, depending on their functions: closed- or open-loop systems, programmable or manually controlled systems, and implantable or external systems. In addition, they may be categorized by their mechanical systems.

Closed- and open-loop systems: A closed-loop system senses the need for the drug, and then delivers the exact dose needed at the correct time. An example would be a device that monitors blood glucose levels, and then delivers the correct amount of insulin. To date, there are no truly closed-loop systems due to our inability to develop accurate and stable sensors. One system under investigation uses the drug lisuride, a dopamine agonist, in an infusion pump for patients with Parkinson's disease. The sensor in this system detects electrical signals (tremors) rather than a chemical. Currently, most infusion systems are open-loop systems, which need additional monitoring outside the system to determine the correct dosage of drug.

Programmable and manual systems: Infusion systems may be completely programmable, and the patient need not be involved with the functioning of the pump at all. Some pumps have been designed so that the rate of infusion may be changed with a computer terminal and a telephone modem. More commonly used are systems that deliver a continuous basal rate of infusion and allow the patients to deliver boli when necessary. For example, a patient with terminal cancer would use this system to deliver morphine for pain control. Alternatively, systems that deliver only bolus drugs are also available.

Implantable and external systems: Infusion pumps are available as either implantable devices or externally worn systems. Implantable pumps are placed subcutanelously, with a catheter entering a vein or the peritoneal cavity. Advantages of these devices include convenience and sterility. External pumps are more commonly used and are small enough to be worn on a belt or under clothing. Their advantages over implantable pumps are their larger volume of infusate and ease of refilling. Several external and implantable infusion pumps are available commercially.

Syringe pumps: This pump consists of a syringe with the plunger driven by a slowly advancing electromotor screw. The drug is usually delivered in pulses created by the motor turning on and off or by increasing the motor speed at periodic intervals. These pumps are normally designed for subcutaneous delivery only, as the change in hydrostatic pressure within the syringe can allow venous blood to backflow into the catheter. Syringe infusion pumps are quite accurate. However, one of the drawbacks of this type of device is that the volume of drug solution is limited by the size of the syringe.

Piston pumps: The protype in this category is an electromagnetically operated, double-acting piston pump. The system uses an electrical activator that runs off a battery. When the first piston is activated, it creates a magnetic field, driving the drug out of the system. Simultaneously, the second cylinder is recharged. In this cycle, the drug is infused. This system's unique design allows for a truly miniaturized pump.

Peristaltic pumps: These pumps deliver drug solutions by pushing them through the system with either rollers or a series of stepping motors. These pumps are popular in outpatient drug delivery and can deliver drugs intravenously, intraperitoneally, intramuscularly, and subcutaneously.

Balloon pumps: This system consists of a small cylindrical tube containing a balloon reservoir that is injected with a drug solution. As the balloon deflates, medication is delivered through an orifice, which regulates the rate of infusion. Changes in the time and rate of administration are achieved by changing the concentration and volume of the drug solution. This pump system is also available with a patient-control module (designed like a wristwatch) that allows the patient to deliver boli. This system is particularly designed for patient-controlled analgesia with drugs such as morphine and hydromorphone.

Gas-pressure pumps: In this system, the vapor pressure provided by a fluorocarbon vapor–liquid mixture forces against a collapsible bellows containing the infusate. The infusate is then moved through flow-regulating tubing and delivered into the body. The system is refilled by percutaneous injection. The pressure of the injection simultaneously refills the drug chamber and condenses the volatile vapor power source, effectively refilling and recharging the pump in one operation.

Portable infusion pumps: These pumps are miniaturized so that they are not too heavy to be worn by patients externally. Primary application of this type of pump is insulin delivery. Autosyringe brand (Baxter) portable pump provides insulin at a constant rate by driving the syringe barrel at a constant velocity; the rate is adjusted to the patient's need by adjusting the insulin concentration or barrel velocity. These methods of delivery enhancement are simple, reliable, and easily learned by patients. Another similar portable pump is Mill Hill Infuser pump. An advanced version of this type of pump is cardiac pacemaker's syringe pump. It has a more sophisticated control mechanism and microcomputer, which allows for programming in insulin units and includes the means to determine dose level and time. It also has alarms to indicate when the syringe is empty and if the motor has failed. Other portable insulin pumps are made by Cormed, Pacesetter Systems, and Brad. In recent years, similar pumps have been developed for chemotherapy and heparin.[10] Ferring Laboratories has recently introduced a portable, pulsatile delivery device called Pulsamat for dispensing luteinizing hormone-releasing hormone (LHRH). Pulsatile delivery of LHRH has helped in inducing ovulation in infertile women. The Pulsamat unit is a lightweight unit (3.7 oz) and can be worn by the patient with complete freedom of movement. The primary limitation of portable pumps is patient acceptance. Some of the commercially available pumps are still bulky and uncomfortable to wear. Another limitation is the problem of bacterial infiltration and infection associated with this type of drug delivery by the patient. In some cases, development of kinking in the pump or the catheter controllers falling out has caused problems.

Controllers: Unlike pumps, controllers regulate the rate of drug solution delivery under the force of gravity. In controllers, unlike the pumps, if inflitration occurs, an alarm is set off and the nurse can be alerted. While current controllers are primarily used for intravenous (IV) fluids, like electronic pumps, they can be used to deliver various drug solutions, such as nitroprusside, dopamine, lidocaine, and epinephrine.

B.   Other external infusion systems

There are many external infusion systems currently on the market, or are in advanced development stages, which do not fit either in pump or controller categories. One such system is Abbott's ADD-Vantage System. This system has two parts: a plastic IV bag filled with solution and a separate glass vial of powdered or liquid drug (e.g., antibiotic). A nurse locks the vial holding the prescribed dose of drug into a chamber at the top of the plastic bag and mixes the drug and the solution by removing the vial's stopper. This reconstituted drug can be infused using either pumps or controllers.

Another external system of considerable potential is a computerized feedback control system. Ideally, this type of system will measure the blood level of drug in the body and regulate the infusion rate to achieve desirable blood concentration. Pharmacontrol Co. is currently developing a feedback system called SAFCAD. This system dispenses an anesthetic agent according to the individual patient's need as shown by the patient's electroencephalogram (EEG) reading.

Finally, other research and development projects include several new delivery systems for injectable drugs based on osmotic technology. One of these, IVOS, utilizes a solid osmotic dosage form of a drug for controlled release into an infusion system. Another, Infuset, is a small, disposable, portable controlled-release system for drug infusion worn by the patient. The Baxter-Travenol Flor-Gard family of volumetric infusion pumps are good examples of peristaltic pumps that are controlled by microprocessors. Pfizer's Valley Lab also has its line of volumetric infusion pumps called Infutrol.

1.   Percutaneous catheters

A variety of devices and methods to allow simple, safe, and effective infusion-site access are either in current use or under development. These include the commonly used hypodermic needle, acute peripheral venous catheters, percutaneous central venous catheters, cerebrospinal fluid (CSF) percutaneous catheters, implantable access ports and catheters, and implantable pumps and reservoirs. A choice of systems usually can be made from the various alternatives based on infusion-site location, anticipated duration of use, patient mobility needs, and infusion protocol requirements.

The simplest and least costly infusion site-access system is the hypodermic needle. This method is preferred for many indications because it offers direct access to subcutaneous infusion sites with low risk and little discomfort to the patient. The percutaneous injection wound heals quickly and allows safe periodic reaccess. Likewise, the peripheral venous catheter is a frequently used alternative as a low-cost, acute access system for systemic vascular infusion. Typically, the system is a short, small-bore catheter that can be easily placed in the small peripheral blood vessels for a few hours or a few days. However, when access to the infusion site is frequent or prolonged or lies deep within the body, other methods of access must be considered.

Percutaneous central venous catheters were developed in an effort to target the infusion site more precisely and to reduce peripheral vessel damage by the drug or catheter. Central venous catheters usually are fabricated from a small-bore radio-opaque silicone tube, open at the infusion site and equipped with a luer-lock fitting at the external end. When used with modern imaging techniques to confirm catheter tip position, the catheter can be maneuvered from outside the body to place its tip at a predetermined infusion site deep inside the body. For systemic infusion, the catheter frequently is placed through the cephalic vein or, in some cases, the jugular vein to maneuver the catheter tip into the superior vena cava. Central venous catheters usually are externalized on the chest wall and require continuous protection by an external bandage.

To avoid blood clotting around the catheter or in the catheter lumen, percutaneous catheters terminating in the bloodstream must be flushed carefully after each use and left filled with a heparinized saline solution. To maintain patency when not in use, the catheter must be flushed daily with heparinized saline. The catheter exit site is a common source of wound infection. Externalized central venous catheters have been left in place successfully for more than a year, but generally, they are considered to be most useful for patients requiring access for a few days to a few months.

Percutaneous catheters also are utilized frequently for targeted-site drug delivery outside the blood system. The Tenckhoff catheter has long been used for direct access to the peritoneal cavity for peritoneal dialysis of patients suffering from chronic renal failure. The large-diameter Tenckhoff catheter accommodates the rapid exchange of large volumes of fluids required for peritoneal dialysis. Percutaneous fine-bore epidural or intrathecal catheters have been used for many years for targeted drug delivery to the CSF for acute or chronic pain control. These percutaneous catheters enable the targered infusion of very small doses of opiates and other analgesics into the CSF for direct action with pain receptors. This technique offers good control of pain without some of the physical or emotional side effects of intravascular or intramuscular injections of analgesics.

2. Totally implantable pump and reservoir systems

Chronic percutaneous access to an infusion site — such as the venous blood supply for nutritional support or chemotherapy, the peritoneal cavity for dialysis or chemotherapy, the hepatic artery supply for direct liver tumor infusions, or the CSF for analgesia — demonstrates the feasibility of long-term infusion-site access. With the therapeutic success of percutaneous catheters, further research and development was begun on totally implantable systems with features designed to overcome significant limitations, such as exit-site infection, catheter damage, restriction of patient activities and mobility, and patient resistance to the image of the exposed tubes and dressings. Some of the earliest implantable infusion systems were totally implantable infusion pumps. These devices are capable of storing the drug to be delivered in an implanted, refillable reservoir while continually delivering the drug from the reservoir to the infusion site through a flexible delivery catheter.

First developed in the mid-1970s, these systems soon were utilized for a variety of infusion protocols, such as the delivery of heparin for chronic anticoagulation, cytostatic drug infusion for cancer chemotherapy, morphine delivery for pain control, insulin infusion for diabetes, and numerous other special-purpose infusion protocols. Although these early systems demonstrated great potential for chronic or long-term intermittent-infusion therapy, they were too expensive for large-scale use and were limited in their capacity to accommodate changing drug delivery protocols or drug types. They did, however, improve patients' quality of life by making possible relatively safe, long-term, outpatient infusion therapy and by overcoming many of the risks and complications associated with chronic percutaneous catheter systems.

3.   Totally implantable portal and catheter systems

After several years of using totally implantable pumps and long-term percutaneous indwelling catheters, it became clear that a need existed for a system that incorporated the best features of each while achieving a low patient cost for the system and its maintenance. A totally implantable access system consisting of a subcutaneous access portal attached to a subcutaneous catheter was developed to meet this need. This device is rapidly becoming the system of choice for long-term (more than a few weeks), frequent, or chronic access to an infusion site.[11]

The subcutaneous portal is a small, hollow, plastic or metal cylinder, the top of which contains a self-sealing elastomeric septum designed to withstand several thousand needle punctures without external leakage. One end of a catheter is attached to an outlet tube on the side of the portal; the outlet end of the catheter is located at the target infusion site. The implanted system is used as follows: A low-coring hypodermic needle is passed through the skin and the self-sealing portal septum into the portal reservoir; the drug is discharged into the reservoir and through the delivery catheter to the infusion site.

The infusion may last from a few minutes to more than a week, depending on the drug therapy protocol. When the infusion is complete, the system is flushed and the percutaneous needle extracted. After the needle puncture site in the skin heals, no further dressings are required during the dormant period. During this period, blood-contacting systems usually are flushed on a monthly basis with a heparinized saline solution. Many totally implantable portal systems also are designed to allow aspiration of body fluids for blood sampling, peritoneal fluid withdrawal, and CSF sampling, as well as infusion therapy.

The demonstrated feasibility of safety and economically achieving and maintaining long-term access to deep-body, targeted infusion sites for drug therapy creates immediate and growing opportunities for services and products. Indications for long-term drug therapy that might be accommodated by a totally implantable port and catheter, or the implantable pump and reservoir, include the following: hematologic disorders, glycemia control in diabetes, cancer chemotherapy, hypertension control, intractable pain control, drug and alcohol antagonist delivery, chronic hormone supplement, and anti-arrhythmia control, to name a few. In the past, chemotherapeutic drugs requiring long-term infusion were administered in the hospital using pole-mounted infusion pumps delivering the drug through an acute peripheral venous catheter. It is now clear that, if the preferred delivery plan for an anticancer drug involves protracted, low-dose infusion or repeated bolus dosing, these catheters offer clear advantages.[12]

IV.   Insulin delivery

With the discovery and isolation of insulin in 1921, the diabetic was offered a new lifesaving therapy through subcutaneous insulin injections. Following that important development, it was observed that, although life span might be extended, long-term complications of diabetes, such as blindness, kidney failure, and neuropathy, became apparent. In an effort to reduce or eliminate these complications, many theories have been offered and tested. Central to these ideas is the need to control the blood glucose levels of the diabetic so that it closely simulates that observed in the nondiabetic.

The use of oral hypoglycemic drugs to stimulate endogenous insulin release is utilized in noninsulin-dependent diabetics, who require small increases in amounts of available insulin to maintain control. Those patients with little or no insulin production capacity resort to one or more subcutaneous insulin injections per day. However, even with frequent subcutaneous injections, the insulin-dependent diabetic finds it difficult, if not impossible, to maintain long-term glycemic control equivalent to that of the nondiabetic. Research in animals and man suggests that controlled intravenous insulin infusion may be a more appropriate method for normalizing blood glucose levels for the insulin-dependent diabetic.

The goal of therapy in insulin-dependent diabetes is to normalize blood glucose. This can be accomplished with intensive therapy consisting of either multiple injections of insulin or the continual subcutaneous infusion of insulin by pump. Although few data are available on the long-term use of either method, findings to date suggest that pump therapy results in better long-term compliance and long-term control of diabetes than conventional insulin therapy. The acute complications of pump therapy — infection at the infusion site, hypoglycemia, and diabetic acidosis — can be minimized by strict adherence to proper procedures. Thus, insulin pump treatment is a safe and effective method for achieving tight long-term control of Type I diabetes (insulin-dependent).[13]

Insulin infusion pumps, therefore, are one of several methods now available to normalize blood glucose levels to prevent the long-term complications of diabetes. These pumps permit the patient to mimic the response that a nondiabetic patient has to glucose-level loads. Open-loop infusion pumps provide a basal level of insulin throughout the day and a bolus of insulin before meals. Insulin infusion pumps have proven to be safe, effective, and convenient, and to improve the lifestyle of patients. A partial list of insulin infusion pumps on the market includes Model 2000 (Becton-Dickinson), Betatron II (Cardiac Pacemakers, Inc.), Eugly (Travenol/Autosyringe), and MiniMed504 (Pacesetters, Inc.). Surprisingly, the advantages of pump therapy, in terms of increasing the lifestyle flexibility of the patient, have not been promoted adequately. It is also surprising that with the advantage of pump therapy, so few insulin-dependent patients are using this method of treatment. It appears that in those patients who are highly motivated, properly educated, and desire to normalize blood glucose levels, the advantages of insulin pump therapy greatly outweigh the disadvantages.[14]

The concept of developing a totally artificial pancreas as a therapeutic alternative for diabetics became popular in the 1970s. In its simplest form, actually more appropriately called an artificial β-cell, it consists of a glucose sensor, computer, insulin reservoir, and pump (see Chapter 4). The device can respond to increases in the recipient's plasma glucose by administering appropriate quantities of insulin, thereby maintaining the subject's plasma glucose in the normal range.[15]

Pioneers in the development of the enzyme electrode glucose sensor were Clark and Lyons.[16] Their sensor used a glucose oxidase solution sandwiched between semipermeable polymeric membranes to catalyze the reaction between glucose and oxygen. Updike and Hicks[17] decreased the response time in a similar sensor of their own design by binding the glucose oxidase to a thin acrylamide gel layer. Their sensor used a polarographic rather than a potentiometric oxygen electrode, thus measuring electrical current instead of voltage differences.

In an attempt to refine the enzyme electrode design to make it suitable for use in an implantable artificial beta cell, Bessman and Schultz[18] modified the original design by immobilizing and stabilizing the glucose oxidase by intra- and intermolecular cross-linkages in a cloth matrix. The most advanced version of enzyme electrode glucose sensor is that developed by Miles Laboratories for their Biostator Glucose Controlled Insulin Infusion System.

One way to avoid the problem of rapid degradation of enzyme electrodes is to design a sensor that can operate without enzymes. Noble metals, such as platinum can be substituted for glucose oxidase to catalyze the oxidation of glucose. Several modes of operation are possible using this approach, including fuel cell, polarographic, potentiometric, and potentiodynamic systems. Both the enzyme electrode and electrochemical sensors have yet to solve the problem of how to prevent the sensor from encapsulation once it is implanted. This buildup of fibrotic connective tissue eventually prevents access of the reactants to the sensor.

As an alternative to these sensors, March et al.[19] designed an optical glucose sensor which they envision as incorporated into a contact lens. Their sensor would consist of a miniature laser light source, detector, power supply, and telemetry transmitter, designed to measure the optical rotation of the polarized light beam produced by the glucose in the aqueous humor of the eye. This method assumes equilibrium between glucose concentration in the aqueous humor and the blood. While it cannot be connected directly with an implanted artificial β-cell, the developers believe that a telemetric connection can be maintained, or the signal can be transmitted to an extra-corpreal receiver/display, allowing the patient or physician to manipulate the implanted unit appropriately.

One of the earliest attempts to achieve and maintain normoglycemia by means of an artificial insulin infusion device was described by Kadish.[20] His device used a Technicon Autoanalyzer to monitor glucose concentrations of blood continuously through a double-lumen catheter. Significant advances in this technique were made by Pfeiffer et al.[21] and Albisser et al.[22] More sophisticated minicomputers and control algorithms permitted adjustment of insulin infusion rates according to rates of change in glycemia, as well as static plasma glucose levels.

Clemens et al.[23] have developed an artificial endocrine pancreas. This device, called Biostator Glucose Controlled Insulin Infusion System (GCIIS), has a new glucose oxidase sensor. Bechard et al.[24] have used porous poly(ε-caprolactone) matrices to release insulin when implanted subcutaneously in rats. Heller et al.[25] used bioerodible polymers in a self-regulating insulin delivery system. These systems are based on an enzyme-substrate reaction that leads to a pH change and a pH-sensitive polymer that changes erosion rate and concomitant insulin release in response to that change.

Iontophoresis, or ion-transfer, is a process that enhances the transport of ions across the skin with a flux of electric current. Research done in this area has recently demonstrated that it is possible to control blood glucose levels in hairless rats by transdermal, iontophoretic delivery of insulin.[26] Watler and Sefton[27] have developed a piezoelectric micropump for insulin delivery.

A novel and mechanically simple implantable controlled-release system (Piezoelectric Controlled Release Micropump) capable of delivering insulin at a constant basal rate and at variable augmented rates has been developed and tested *in vitro* by Sefton et al.[28] They found that the intrinsic safety and weight of the device could be expected to make the peizoelectric micropump a desirable alternative for the treatment of insulin-dependent diabetes.

Viable mammalian cells have been encapsulated in two different water-insoluble polyacrylates: a commercially available cationic polymer (EUDRAGIT RL) and a potentially biocompatible HEMA/MMA copolymer.

Studies by Sefton et al.[28] have shown that the cells can withstand the rigors of encapsulation.

In a study by Choay and Choay,[29] water-soluble macromolecules were successfully employed in the manufacture of parenteral depot preparations, such as polyvinylpyrrolidone (PVP) for insulin. Langer and his colleagues at Massachusetts Institute of Technology, as well as Siegel et al., have done extensive work on the controlled release of insulin and other macromolecules. They used magnetically modulated systems and sintered polymers in their studies, respectively.[30, 31]

A design for a self-regulating insulin delivery system based upon the competitive binding nature of blood glucose and glycosylated insulin to lectin has been proposed. The glycosylated insulin-bound lectin is encapsulated using biodegradable or nondegradable polymers. The polymer membranes control glucose influx and insulin efflux, which depends upon the glucose concentration present: a natural biofeedback.

The chemical approach reported by Kim et al.[32] was to design a self-regulating insulin delivery system based on a combination of biological modulation and controlled release. The design of this delivery system utilized the concept of the competitive and complementary binding behavior of Concanavalin A (Con A) with glucose and glycosylated insulin. The derivatized insulin is bound to Con A, which in turn is complementary to glucose. The glycosylated insulin is then displaced from the Con A by glucose, and insulin is released in response to, and proportional to, the amount of glucose present in the blood.

The release rate of insulin also depends upon the binding affinity of a derivative to the Con A and can be influenced by the choice of the saccharide group in glycosylated insulin. By encapsulating the glycosylated insulin-bound Con A with a suitable polymer that is permeable to both glucose and insulin, the glucose influx and the insulin efflux would be controlled by the encapsulation membrane. Proper choice of the membrane criteria would provide optimal insulin release rates necessary for the maintenance of normal blood glucose levels.

A bioresponsive membrane that changes its size and ethylene glycol permeability in response to changes in glucose concentration has been reported by Horbett et al.[33] The usefulness of this system for glucose detection or controlled delivery of insulin depends on the stability of the polymeric system and the entrapped enzyme activity, the biocompatibility of the system, the response time to rapid changes in glucose concentration, the effect of physiological buffering, and the permeability of the membranes to insulin.

Related to the development of insulin infusion systems is the controversy over where the insulin should be delivered. From *a priori* physiological considerations, infusion into the portal vein is the infusion site of choice since that is where the native pancreas delivers it. Goriya et al.[34] has reported that hyperinsulinemia accompanies glycemic normalization with peripheral, but not portal, infusion. This phenomenon may be related to hepatic insulin extraction, which is reported to be 50% at first pass. Nevertheless, the potential risks of initiating portal thrombosis due to inadequate blood compatibility of cannulas have, to date, prevented the use of the portal site in the absence of documentation of adverse side effects from hyperinsulinemia.

The peritoneal cavity has been proposed as a less risky alternative to portal cannulation. While entry of the insulin may depend to some extent upon cannula tip location, this method simplifies cannula placement and, intuitively, seems to offer more safety. For the implantable pump, the intravenous, intraportal, or intraperitoneal routes can be used with little difficulty. The subcutaneous route, however, offers substantially less difficulty for portable pump infusion than does any other approach. It seems clear that good control of glycemia can be achieved by using any of the preceding infusion routes.

At the present time, there is no compelling evidence for choosing one route of administration over another, aside from appropriateness to the device and convenience to the patient and physician. Insulin infusion development is a burgeoning industrial and academic research activity still in its infancy. The dominant devices in the field at this time are portable syringe pumps and extracorporeal feedback-control devices. It seems likely that dominance will shift to implantable devices and perhaps to feedback-control devices should the glucose sensor problems be resolved. Such a device could then truly be called an artificial β-cell.[35]

V. Parenteral prolonged-action dosage forms

Parenteral dosage forms with prolonged action are of medical and economic importance. On the medical side, the physician is interested in maintaining therapeutic concentrations over a longer period of time and reducing the number of injections for a patient. Economically, only well-trained personnel can administer injections, and if frequency of administration is reduced, the costs of therapy are decreased and time is saved.

In principle, there are three ways to approach prolongation of parenteral administration, namely, by pharmacological, chemical, and physical methods. Pharmacological methods include intramuscular or subcutaneous administration instead of intravenous; the simultaneous administration of vasoconstrictors (adrenalin in local anesthetics; ephedrine in heparin solutions); and blocking the elimination of drugs through the kidneys by simultaneous administration of a blocking agent, such as probenecid with penicillin or p-aminosalicylic acid. Chemical methods include the use of salts, esters, and complexes of the active ingredient with low solubility. Physical methods include the selection of the proper vehicle, thereby giving prolonged release (use of oleaginous solutions instead of aqueous solutions); the addition of macromolecules that increase viscosity (CMC, NaCMC, PVP, tragacanth, etc.); the use of swelling materials to increase viscosity in oleaginous solutions (aluminum monostearate); the additions of adsorbents; the use of solutions from which, upon administration, the drug is precipitated when it contacts body fluids; the use of aqueous and oleaginous suspensions; and the use of implants.[36]

Complex formation and addition of macromolecules: Vaccines by depot expose the body to the antigen for a longer period of time and result in an increased formation of antibodies. Depot vaccines can be prepared by adsorption of the antigen, such as diphtheria toxoid or tetanus toxoid on the surface of aluminum hydroxide or aluminum phosphate. Another example is the complex formation between insulin and protein or metals, such as protamine insulin or zinc insulin. For vitamin B_{12} a zinc-tannate complex has been prescribed, yielding prolonged action. Water-soluble macromolecules are successfully employed in the manufacture of parenteral depot preparations, such as chorionic-gonadotropin, gelatin, or corticotropin (ACTH). In the latter case, the macromolecule does not exhibit retardant effect due to an increase of viscosity, but, rather, by inhibition of decomposition of ACTH by proteolytic enzymes in the tissue. In other cases, macromolecules form complexes. Carboxymethylcellulose is used to retard preparations of heparin, for example.

Salts of low solubility and slowly hydrolyzable esters: Drugs of high solubility can be converted to those with prolonged action by formation of salts or esters of low solubility, which are slowly hydrolyzed. The highly soluble penicillin-G forms salts of low solubility with several bases, such as procaine, dibenzylethylenediamine, and hydrabamine. Ester formation is used to prolong the action of steroid hormones by esterification of their hydroxyl groups with organic acids. In contact with body fluids of the tissue, the esters slowly hydrolyze, under the influence of esterases, to pharmacologically active steroids. By forming different esters with different rates of hydrolysis and combining these different esters into one drug product, high initial blood levels with prolonged action can be obtained upon intramuscular (IM) administration.

Aqueous suspensions: The use of aqueous suspensions results in parenteral drug products with prolonged action. The manufacture of sterile suspension products is one of the most difficult areas in pharmaceutical technology. Many methods for obtaining suitable hormone crystals and antibiotics have been described. Drug action is prolonged by increasing the crystal size (up to 100 μm) of the particle, as has been shown with testosterone isobutyrate.[36]

Oleaginous suspensions and emulsions: Dissolution of suspended crystals is further prolonged by using oleaginous bases rather than aqueous ones. In oleaginous suspensions, the tissue is first concerned with the oily vehicle and then with suspended particles. In order to increase viscosity, many oleaginous bases contain suspending agents with increasing viscosity, such as aluminum, calcium or magnesium stearate, or aluminum salts of alkylene or aralkyl phosphoric acids whose alkyl or aralkyl groups contain 6–18 carbon atoms. Most of the research on parenteral oleaginous suspensions has been done with penicillins. Oleaginous suspensions of procaine penicillin-G give longer duration of blood levels than aqueous suspensions.

Upon addition of aluminum stearate, the depot action can be further enhanced. For heparin, prolonged action has been obtained using emulsions for IM administration.

Precipitation of drug in tissue: Drug products from which the active ingredient precipitates upon IM administration are prepared using aqueous-organic solutions. The precipitation occurs either on change of pH from the environment of the tissue or by dilution of the aqueous-organic solvent. This principle has been employed for local anesthetics, but is not now in use because organic solvents may lead to irritation and inflammation of tissue.

Implants: Implants are a sterile solid drug product manufactured by compression of the drug alone or of the drug with a vehicle or by melting or sintering processes. Implants are administered by surgical methods using a large needle, through which the long solid-dosage form is instilled subcutaneously. Such solid-dosage forms may act for several months due to their low solubility and small surface area. In all cases of extravascular parenteral administration, the drug in the form of a drug product is administered into a relatively small, localized region, where it forms a type of depot from which the drug must leave by penetration and permeation to reach the blood or lymphatic system.

The absorption of solid drug particles from prolonged-action parenteral dosage forms depends primarily on the physical and chemical properties of the solid drug and the properties of the solution immediately surrounding it. As these solid particles are of very low solubility, absorption is therefore rate-limited by the rate of solution of the solid drug in the biological fluid in the tissue surrounding it. The site of implantation, as well as body movement, is probably of some influence on the rate of absorption, since different body regions differ in vascularity. From theoretical considerations, dissolution rate increases by increasing agitation or by body movement, which increases the blood supply to the area. Absorption rate is certainly influenced by the thickness of the diffusion layer surrounding the implanted drug. The diffusion layer itself can be influenced by body movement or differences in blood flow in different regions.

A fibrous tissue capsule is formed around the deposited solid in most cases following administration of solid particles IM or subcutaneous (SC), whether in the form of crystals, granules, pellets, or implants. Usually, this capsule formation starts somewhere between 72 hours and one week after application. Temperature has an influence on the diffusion coefficient, the solubility, and the diffusion-layer thickness of an implanted substance. Since the diffusion coefficient is inversely proportional to the viscosity of a fluid medium, viscosity increases when the temperature is reduced, which results in a decrease of diffusion coefficient. Solubility is reduced by lowering the temperature, resulting in a decrease of absorption rate. The diffusion layer around the implanted solid is influenced by temperature, since viscosity increases.[37]

SC drug delivery systems: SC tissue is one of the most favorable sites for the long-term administration of drugs via controlled-release drug delivery systems. This popularity in application is due to several reasons: better patient compliance without interruption of treatment for nonmedical reasons, easy access of blood circulation by bypassing the impermeable stratum corneum layers, and convenience and simplicity of the process involved in subcutaneous implantation. The potential biomedical application of SC drug delivery systems is exemplified by the development of the SyncroMate-B estrud synchronizer, a subdermal implant for herd-breeding management. Syncro-Mate-B (Searle, Chicago) is a veterinary estrus-synchronization treatment which consists of a norgestomet-releasing subdermal implant of hydrophilic polyethylene glycomethacrylate, implanted between the skin and the conchal cartilage on the dorsal surface of one ear. The implant is left in place for 9 full days and is supplemented by an intramuscular injection of 3 mg norgestomet and 5 or 6 mg estradiol valerate in 2 ml sesame oil at the time of implantation.

The concept of SC controlled drug administration, as illustrated by the Syncro-Mate-B treatment, can be extended to other biomedical applications. For example, an animal model for chronic hypertension can be created by the controlled release of desoxycorticosterone acetate from subdermal silicone implants; a once-a-year implantation of a contraceptive in women can be achieved by the controlled release of a progestin, such as megestrol acetate, from subdermal silicone capsules; and long-acting antinarcotic formulations for addiction treatment can be developed by the controlled release of narcotic antagonists, such as naltrexone, from biodegradable homopolymers or copolymers of lactic acid and glycolic acid.

A.   Intravenous delivery

Beginning in the early 1960s, concern over medication errors and the proliferation of drugs delivered intravenously led to the growth of parenteral or IV admixture systems. At that time, hospital pharmacists assumed responsibility for preparing IV doses, as well as dispensing unit doses of oral and IM medication. Since that time, burette-type systems have given way to glass partial-fill piggyback containers with medication added or admixed in the pharmacy. These systems, in turn, led to several versions of plastic partial-fill containers that served as reservoirs for medication.[38]

As time passed, features of more desirable drug delivery systems began to emerge. Pharmacists demanded less expensive systems, minimization of supplies and labor, and the ability to standardize on a single system. This led drug manufacturers to market their drugs in containers that allowed administration to patients after reconstitution — the so-called drug manufacturer's piggyback. Premixed medication systems, with the drug in solution and ready for administration, were designed to reduce preparation labor to practically nil. They fell short of the ideal, however, because a large number of drugs lose potency within 24 hours of mixing and therefore cannot be premixed. Recently, drugs have been put in solution and frozen by the manufacturer to circumvent the stability question. But this is a costly procedure, and again, not all drugs are stable in this form.

The medical staffs of most hospitals recognize the problems associated with IV drug administration and impose limitations on nursing personnel regarding the administration of drugs by IV push. This limitation has led to hospital-wide use of various types of intermittent infusion devices, such as volume-control units, minibags, and minibottles, for the administration of scheduled IV medications. This satisfies the requirement that medications be diluted for IV administration, thus allowing nurses to give IV medications. It also requires the nurse and the pharmacist to make decisions about which medications can be given effectively with these intermittent infusion devices.

Volume control units: With the advent of antibiotics, particularly cephalothin, volume-control units gained wide use in hospitals in the 1960s and 1970s as a method for intermittent drug administration. Duma et al.[39] and Henry and Harrison[40] noted problems associated with these devices. These include increased potential for microbial contamination and drug-compatibility problems. After the introduction of minibottle (piggyback) containers in the early 1970s, Turco[41] devised a combined volume-control set-piggyback system for intermittent IV therapy. This system is safe, effective, and less costly than the minicontainer systems alone. Minicontainer systems, including minibottle and minibag containers, introduced in the early 1970s, supply diluent of 5% dextrose in water and normal saline in 50- or 100-ml containers. These containers allow the drug to be diluted and prepared by pharmacists, which is just one of minicontainer diluents many advantages.

In the 1970s and early 1980s, methods other than volume-control units for intermittent IV drug administration were explored. Partial-fill diluent piggyback containers were accepted and became widely used. More than 100 million piggyback containers are used annually in the U.S. alone. The introduction of powered DMPB and bulk containers in the early 1970s expedited the use of IV piggyback administration. Premixed LVPs (large volume parenterals) are now used widely containing KCl, lidocaine, heparin, theophylline, and dopamine. Premixed drug solutions and containers offer significant advantages to hospitals: they are convenient, save time, and reduce the potential for error and contamination.

Ready-to-use plastic containers: Another innovation in prefilled IV piggyback containers is the ready-to-use plastic container that requires no manipulation or dilution and is ready for direct IV infusion. Searle markets metronidazole (Flagyl) in Travenol's ready-to-use Viafles plastic IV containers, as well as in 500-mg lyophilized vials, which require reconstitution and buffering in 100-ml, ready-to-use glass containers.

Frozen premixes: Travenol delivers frozen drug products packaged in polyvinylchloride containers to hospitals. These frozen products are stored in a hospital pharmacy freezer and are thawed and used as needed. The following drugs are available in premixed frozen form: Ancef, cephalothin, Mefoxin, Cefizox, Claforan, penicillin-G, nafcillin, pipracillin, Tagamet, Fortaz, Zinacef, gentamicin, and others.

Reconstitution systems: Lilly supplies a non-PVC plastic piggyback container — Faspak — which contains the dry powdered form of a drug

(Keflin, Kefzol, Mandol, or ampicillin). When reconstituted with the appropriate dilutent, the diluted drug can be administered directly. The Faspak serves as the final delivery container. This avoids the transferring step that usually takes place when a powdered drug is reconstituted. A specialized dilution pump, the ADDS-100 system, is supplied to help in the reconstitution step.

Electronic equipment: A few years ago, electronic equipment for automated administration of intermittent secondary piggyback medications was introduced. These systems allow infusion programming, so that when the secondary infusion is completed, the system reverts automatically to the desired primary fluid flow rate. They save time, offer convenience, and reduce the number of IV sites lost as a result of dry secondary bottles when no check valve set normally is used or, if a check valve set normally is used, they reduce the possibility of the primary solution infusing at the secondary rate. These systems can reduce the need for multiple electronic equipment infusions, increase the precision of drug administration, and allow more optimal interpretation of serum drug level concentrations. One system can also limit the volume infused from the secondary container, introducing the possibility of cost savings through placing more than one dose in the secondary container.[42, 43]

B.   Buccal-controlled delivery

In order to deliver macromolecules, such as peptides, through mucosal tissues for systemic activity, it may be necessary to improve tissue permeability, inhibit protease activity, or decrease immunogenic responses. Ideally, this should only be accomplished in a well-circumscribed area. The mouth, because of its accessibility, will permit localization of controlled drug delivery systems to achieve this task. Given anatomical and physiological differences between oral mucosal tissue, the location of the drug delivery system should be carefully chosen.

First, because of the functions of the mouth (mastication, swallowing) and of salivary secretion, some areas have to be avoided. Secondly, there are different patterns of cell differentiation in keratinized and non-keratinized oral epithelia, which effects permeability. The ranking of these epithelial locations, in terms of permeability, is drug-dependent. Therefore, a controlled drug delivery system should be located where the mucosal tissue is permeable enough to allow the drug delivery system to be rate-limiting. Therefore, *in vivo* and *in vitro* methodologies are needed to compare permeabilities of different sites for a given drug. The work by Veillard et al.[44] describes a new methodology to compare permeabilities of different oral mucosal sites of the dog's mouth for a drug.

The analgesic effect of buccal morphine has been compared with that of intramuscular morphine in a prospective, double-blind study of 40 patients who experienced pain after undergoing elective orthopedic surgery. Twenty patients were randomly assigned to receive the buccal preparation and a placebo IM injection, and 20 patients, the intramuscular preparation and a placebo buccal tablet. The IM preparation achieved slightly higher peak-plasma morphine levels than the buccal preparation. However, plasma morphine levels declined more slowly after buccal administration. The drug's bioavailability was 46% greater after buccal administration. This route of administration may be of particular value in chronic pain due to malignant disease, in which muscle wasting and cachexia may limit the use of parenteral analgesics.

Forest Laboratories, Inc. has been at work on buccal formulations of morphine, scopolamine, and insulin. Forest is also researching use of the same technology in oral tablets to achieve a long-acting form of ibuprofen and Mellaril, a tranquilizer.

Zetachron also has a buccal delivery system. It provides zero-order release by a mechanism of polymer-surface erosion. Marion Merrell-Dow's Susadrin tablets are buccal tablets that use Forest Laboratories' Synchron system to release nitroglycerine in a controlled manner over a period of 6 hours. Buccal tablets are not swallowed, but are put in the buccal pouch between the cheeks and the gum. Several advantages of buccal delivery include reliable absorption, lack of first-pass metabolism, and slow and predictable release.[45-48]

C.   *Magnetically modulated systems*

The feasibility of magnetic control of intravascular materials was experimentally demostrated in the early 1960s.[49-52] This was followed by preliminary clinical trials with therapeutic vascular occlusion of an intracerebral aneurysm using carbonyl iron suspended in albumin solution and of a renal cell carcinoma using carbonyl iron mixed with liquid silicone.[53] Intravascular carbonyl iron confined in the kidney and intraperitoneal zinc ferrite were shown to produce no systemic toxic reaction. On the other hand, the putative biological effects of high-intensity magnetic fields were reported to induce transformation of cultured cells. However, no significant toxicity was experienced in patients exposed to transient magnetic fields.

Despite the optimism for the magnetic control of drug carriers, there are significant practical problems with this system.[54,55] First, this approach requires an electromagnet that generates magnetic fields sufficient for extracorporeal control of the carriers in deep organs. Second, the magnet is expected to permit simultaneous fluoroscopic monitoring for arterial catheterization. However, frequent or continuous generation of strong magnetic fields may interfere with fine fluoroscopic monitoring and produce severe problems in the x-ray generator. Further studies of strong magnetic-field toxicity are needed.

The loading device reported by Langer et al.[56] for controlled release of macromolecules is rectangular-shaped and consists of two glass plates. When the plates are shifted with respect to each other such that the upper and lower holes are offset, the magnetic beads remain in the holes. The plates with the beads are positioned over the polymer slab in the mold. When the plates are shifted back, so that all the holes are aligned, the magnetic steel beads drop onto the polymer slab in a uniform array. The device used for "triggering" a release acts by creating an oscillating magnetic field. As the magnet-mounted plate turns, the stationary polymer matrices are exposed to an oscillating magnetic field. A motorized speed regulator allows for variation of the field frequency.

Several sets of experiments using variable frequencies have been conducted. It was found that frequency strongly affected release rates. For example, after 180 hours of release, exposure of the slabs to frequencies of 155, 200, 290, and 325 rotations per minute resulted in increases over baseline of 133%, 150%, 450%, and 733%, respectively, when the oscillating field was turned on. Tests were also conducted to examine the effect of magnetic-field strength on release rates. In studies where increases in modulation upon exposure to the magnetic field were tested as a function of the strength of that field, a steep curve was obtained. By using the appropriate frequency and field strengths, increases in release rates due to the magnetic field could be as much as 30-fold over baseline.

Microscopic studies have been carried out on the mechanism of release. In these studies, it was observed that the area immediately surrounding the bead in the matrix is the first to be depleted of a drug. This observation, coupled with earlier findings that these matrices are highly porous, and that drugs are released through these pores, suggests that the beads may have an effect on the pores during exposure to the oscillating field. A suggested mechanism is that pores leading to the surface of the system are alternately dilated and constricted, thereby "milking" out the drug. Alternatively, new portals of exit and communication could form within the matrix due to internal effects on the matrix during magnetic exposure.

In another study, Morris et al.[57] reported that magnetically responsive albumin microspheres bearing doxorubicin and magnetite could be selectively localized *in vivo*, resulting in release of significant concentrations of drug in a defined area. By using appropriate magnetic parameters, 50 to 80% of the injected carrier could be targeted, thus eliminating systemic distribution and subsequent toxicity of the entrapped agent. In addition, it has been reported that a remission rate of 75% (based upon histological examination) was achieved in Yoshida sarcoma-bearing rats when adriamycin-containing magnetic microspheres were targeted to the tumor.

Morris et al.[57] have also studied magnetic albumin microspheres containing vindesine sulphate. They showed that a single dose of vindesine, if administered encapsulated in magnetic microspheres and targeted to the tumor site, can achieve 85% remission of the tumor. No evidence of metastases was found in animals treated with targeted vindesine at necropsy. The dramatic response to targeted vindesine is in contrast to control animals receiving either the free drug or drug encapsulated into microspheres but without magnetic localization. It is interesting to note that all animals receiving free vindesine died from the drug, however, animals receiving the same dose administered intraarterially, but encapsulated in microspheres, suffered no acute toxicologic problems. Nontargeted treatment of the tumor, however, even with this dosage, was ineffective. By sequestering the drug to a tumor via magnetic localization, one may use a much lower concentration of drug than is needed if the drug is given systemically.

It is anticipated that this mode of therapy will prove clinically useful in the treatment of localized primary lesions with well-defined blood supplies. Since has been demonstrated that microspheres slowly release drug into the tumor environment over time, multiple agents may, in theory, be delivered concomitantly or sequentially to achieve maximum tumoricidal effects. In this way, maximum chemotherapeutic effects may be achieved before drug resistance occurs as microspheres are readily phagocytosed by tumor cells. Finally, sustained release of entrapped drugs within the tumor may enhance the cytotoxic effect of the drugs, as they will be able to affect tumor cells at critical times when the cells pass through various phases of the cell cycle.

In a study by Ito et al.,[58] ultrafine magnetic ferrite granules were used as drug carriers in treating esophageal cancer. The 5-mg granules contained a mixture of hydroxypropyl cellulose and Carbopol 934. When the granules were flushed into an agar-gel tube, 90% were held in the region of the applied magnetic field. When the granules were administered to rabbits through a catheter, all the granules remained in the region of the magnetic field for 2 h after magnetic guidance for the first 2 min.

Magnetic delivery has also been used with antibiotics in patients with bacterial and fungal abscesses and other sequestered infections, such as prostatitis and osteomyelitis. Another potential use is for the delivery of fibrinolytic agents in the treatment of deep-vein thrombosis (DVT) and pulmonary embolism and to deliver urokinase and neutrophil-attracting peptides, such as FMLP, for example.[59,60]

D.   Intravaginal delivery

Some systemically active drugs, such as steroid hormones, may be effectively absorbed through the vaginal mucosa. The effectiveness of vaginal absorption has been demonstrated by the intravaginal administration of progesterone via a drug-impregnated suppository formulation. Using the vagina as the route of administration for contraceptive drugs has several advantages. Among these, the most practical one is that a drug-releasing vaginal device, such as a medicated, resilient vaginal ring, could permit self-insertion and removal and provide continuous administration of an effective dose level, thus ensuring better patient compliance. Additionally, this continuous "infusion" of drug through the vaginal epithelium may contribute to reducing systemic toxicity or inefficient biological activity resulting from the varying plasma drug levels that occur with the intermittent use of oral contraceptive pills. Also, a rather steady plasma plateau can be obtained within two or three days after insertion of the vaginal ring and may be attained throughout treatment with minimal fluctuation until removal of the ring.[61,62]

Hepatic "first-pass effects" and GI incompatibility can be bypassed when drugs are administered intravaginally. The perineum venous plexus, which drains the vaginal tissue and rectum, flows into the pudentum vein and ultimately into the vena cava, thus initially bypassing the portal circulation. This is in marked contrast to GI blood, as mentioned previously, which drains into the portal vein and passes directly through the liver before reaching the general circulation and the target tissues. Thus, the vaginal route may be of great value with drugs like progesterone and estradiol, which have poor bioavailability when taken orally because they are extensively inactivated by hepatic metabolism. In addition, the intravaginal route of administration can also be beneficial for drugs such as prostaglandins, which cause adverse GI irritation.

Intravaginal absorption of a therapeutic agent from a controlled-release drug delivery system, such as a medicated vaginal ring, can be visualized as having several consecutive steps. For the drug-dispersing vaginal ring, the steps consist of the dissolution of the finely ground, well-dispersed drug particles into the surrounding polymer structure, diffusion through the polymer matrix to the device surface, partition into and then diffusion across the vaginal fluid (which is sandwiched between the vaginal ring and vaginal walls), uptake by and then penetration through the vaginal wall, and transport and distribution of the drug molecules by circulating blood or lymph to a target tissue. The important features of this theoretical model are: the receding interface of the drug-dispersion zone/drug-depletion zone in the polymer matrix as the drug is released with time; an aqueous hydrodynamic diffusion layer (the vaginal fluid) sandwiched between the vaginal drug delivery device and the vaginal wall; and the vaginal wall composed of a lipid continuum with interspersed "pores" or an aqueous shunt pathway. The rate-controlling step in this whole course of intravaginal absorption of drug is dependent on the duration of vaginal residence of the medicated ring.

It is assumed that the finely ground particles are homogeneously dispersed throughout the polymer matrix structure, such that dissolution of drug in the polymer phase is not a rate-limiting step, and that a sharp interface is maintained between the drug-dispersion zone and the drug-depletion zone; the interface recedes continuously into the core of the device with time. It is also assumed that the total drug content per unit volume, including the undissolved particles, is much greater than the drug solubility in the polymer. The drug molecules are visualized as reaching the device surface by diffusion through the polymer matrix structure, with a negligible end diffusion, for simplicity of mathematical treatment. Under these conditions, a drug-concentration gradient is established that extends from the receding interface of the drug-depletion zone/drug-dispersion zone to the outer reaches of the vaginal tissue.

In medical practice, vaginal administration of drugs is limited almost exclusively to the treatment of local disorders, such as fluor albus and other infections. Thus, amoebicides, sulfonamides, antibiotics, and disinfectants are frequently prescribed or sometimes combined with local anesthetics and astringents. Estrogens are also given to restore the vaginal mucosa. In contraception, spermicidal compounds have been applied. In 1980, prostaglandins as abortion-inducing compounds have also been administered by this or the rectal route. However, with the exception of steroids, it remains doubtful that there is much use for this route with respect to drugs that act systemically.[61]

An important aspect in the choice of a drug for vaginal aadministration is that it can remain there long enough to be effective. This will require sufficient solubility and dissolution rates, whereas no absorption should occur. The vaginal membrane transport obeys first-order kinetics for compounds such as aliphatic alcohols and alkanoic acids, and the membrane behaves as an aqueous diffusion layer in series with two parallel routes (i.e., lipoidal pathway and an aqueous pore pathway). Drugs that are to remain unabsorbed should perhaps be ones that remain ionized at vaginal pH, such as quaternary ammonium compounds. The pH at the surface of the absorbing membrane follows the luminal pH quite closely, and negligible amounts of the titratable species can be secreted. At times, the buffer species themselves influence the rate of membrane transport, either promoting (citrate and tromethamine) or decreasing it (borax). Other buffers are without effect (phosphate and phthalate). As these results refer to rabits, more data will be required on other species to permit extrapolation to the human situation.

The contraceptive vaginal ring provides a method of delivering steroids via the vagina. Because the ring may be left for 3 weeks or longer at a time, it provides a more convenient alternative to the pill for many users. The constant release, thus avoiding peaks and valleys of steroid concentration, and the mode of delivery means that, for equal doses, a lesser concentration reaches the liver than by oral delivery.

As with implants, the contraceptive rings that have been most explored have been made of Silastic. They are of toroid shape, with an overall diameter of 50 to 60 mm and a cross-sectional diameter of 7 to 9.5 mm. The dispersion of steroid within the ring depends upon the steroid and the desired dose. A homogeneous dispersion results in a decreasing release rate as the material near the surface is exhausted and the diffusion distance becomes greater. In the case of steroids of high solubility in Silastic, or in case only low doses are to be delivered, the steroid is confined to the center of the ring.

Further reduction in the amount delivered can be attained by making the core loading discontinuous. If the amount of steroid to be delivered is so large that the desired rate can be attained only if the diffusion distance is kept short, then constancy of rate of delivery can be approached by placing all of the steroid in a thin layer. This is the design that has been termed a "shell" ring.[62] By far, the most experience has been attained with rings delivering levonorgestrel (290 μg) and estradiol (180 μg) each day. The rings are designed for at least six cycles of use before replacement. These rings, like the usual combination pill, block ovulation in nearly all cycles.

The greater frequency of vaginal discharge among ring users contributes significantly to its discontinuation rate. Vaginitis leukorrhea, or vaginal discharge, was observed in 23% of ring users and 14% of pill users. Cervicitis, or cervical erosion, was not significantly elevated among ring users.[63–69]

Investigations of rings delivering other steroids have been discontinued for a variety of reasons. Norethindrone rings have not reliably inhibited ovulation even at high doses, and doses of 200 μg/day were associated with unsatisfactory bleeding patterns. Progesterone at 2.2 mg/day inhibited ovulation in only about half of the cycles. The addition of estradiol to the rings did not improve the pattern.[70,71]

Medroxyprogesterone acetate at dosages of 0.65 to 1.5 mg/day inhibits ovulation and gives good bleeding control. However, its evaluation was discontinued because of the difficulties in designing a ring that would deliver this dose of steroid over a several-month period and because of the questions regarding the safety of medroxyprogesterone acetate that followed the finding of mammary tumors in beagle bitches administered high chronic doses. The contraceptive vaginal ring appears to have assumed a place in fertility control. The magnitude of that role may depend on user perceptions of the convenience it offers as compared with alternative methods. Changes that enhance the convenience of use may also enhance its role[72–74] (see Figures 8.7 and 8.8).

Fildes and Hutchinson[75] have described a sustained-release delivery device containing a hydrophilic linear block, polyoxyalkylene-polyurethane copolymer, and, optionally, a buffer. A drug delivery device for releasing a drug at a continuous and controlled rate for a prolonged period of time has been reported by Higuchi and Hussain.[76] It is composed of polymeric material containing a drug and is permeable to passage by diffusion. The polymeric material is an ethylene-vinyl acetate copolymer having a vinyl acetate content of 4 to 80% by weight. In addition to ease of fabrication, this drug delivery device offers other important advantages. One of these is that diffusion of drugs, such as progesterone, through ethylene-vinyl acetate copolymers proceeds at a lower rate than through silicone rubber. This is important because it ensures that the rate of drug administration is controlled by diffusion through the polymer rather than by clearance from the surface of the device.[77,78]

Williams[79] has described an improved method of delivering drugs to the vagina wherein a water-soluble polymeric material, shaped in the form of a cartridge or sheath, is impregnated with a drug and inserted into the vagina. The drug is released as the polymer disintegrates in the vaginal fluid. In a modification of this invention, a tampon is inserted into the cartridge prior to insertion into the vagina. As the tampon expands to fill the vaginal cavity, it brings the polymer/drug system into close contact with the vaginal wall surface. The tampon serves to maintain the surface area and to absorb discharges that may result from certain infections.

Magoon et al.[80] have described a positive-pressure drug-releasing device. The positive-pressure mechanism includes a compression spring that exerts a constant force to reduce the size of a variable-volume chamber containing a drug solution capable of passing through a diffusion membrane and of being absorbed by the vaginal or uterine epithelium. One wall of the chamber includes a supported diffusion membrane; a second wall of the chamber, or a compartment of that chamber, takes the form of a plunger driven by the compression spring. Where the cavity constitutes the vagina, the device is additionally provided with flexible retaining elements that project radially outward from the end of the casing opposite from the end in which the diffusion membrane is supported. The result is a dependable and relatively simple drug delivery device that utilizes a positive-pressure mechanism and is not dependent upon osmotic pressure.

Roseman et al.[81] have described a vaginal contraceptive suppository having both a rapid release of active ingredient and prolonged duration of effectiveness. The suppository comprises a mixture of sodium starch glyco-late, a thickenning agent, and a vegetable oil base combined with a spermi-cide. The invention reported by Drobish and Gougeon[82] encompases devices used in the vagina to deliver spermicidal surfactants. By virtue of their unique construction and shape, the devices are foldable for easy insertion. Once in position at or near the cervical os, the devices open to cap or block the os and remain in position, so that access of the spermicidal surfactant to the cervical os is not interrupted.

Hughes[83] has described nonobstructive U-shaped devices for such pur-poses as supporting the uterus or for releasing spermicidal and other con-traceptive agents or deodorants. More specifically, this invention provides devices having U-shaped geometries which, when properly oriented, will not obstruct the portion of the vagina anterior to the cervix uteri so that the device does not produce interference or discomfort.

An intravaginal therapeutic system for the preprogrammed, unattended delivery of a drug is described by Wong.[84] The system is composed of a drug, a delivery module containing a reservoir for storing the drug, and a rate controller that maintains delivery throughout the life of the system. It also has an energy source for transferring drug from the reservoir to the vagina; a portal for releasing the drug from the module to the vagina; a platform that integrates the module into a unit size, shaped and adapted for insertion and retention in a vagina; and a therapeutic program that provides for the controlled release of drug to produce a beneficial effect over a prolonged period of time.

Laughlin[85] has reported that solutions of micelle-forming surfactant compounds can be enclosed in a container comprising a microporous mem-brane for release. Devices prepared in this manner are stable and do not suffer osmotic rupture when placed in body cavities in contact with body fluids. Rather, they provide controlled release of the surfactants. Proper selection of a surfactant provides a means for achieving various biological effects (e.g., antimicrobial or spermicidal activity).[86-90]

The efficacy and performance of a steroidal contraceptive preparation is influenced by the ratio of the progestogenic and estrogenic components. For oral contraceptives, the optimum ratio can easily be obtained by making tablets containing the required amounts of progestogen and estrogen. How-ever, for long-acting membrane-controlled delivery systems, this simple approach is less feasible, especially when the steroids have to be released in a ratio of 5–10 to 1. To achieve controlled release of 3-keto-desogestrel and ethinyl estradiol for at least 30 days from a vaginal delivery system in a 5–10 to 1 ratio, de Nijs et al.[91] developed a multicompartment intravaginal ring system. The system consists of two or more silicone rubber tubes — the shorter one containing both steroids, the longer one containing just the 3-keto-steroid — that are connected to form a ring by glass stoppers of a special shape. The shape and consistency of the glass stoppers prevent diffusion of ethinyl estradiol from the short compartment, thus preventing too large an effect. Administration of keto-desogestrel via the vaginal route showed a 1.5 times improved bioavailability than via the oral route.

E.   *Intrauterine delivery*

Development of intrauterine contraceptive devices (IUDs) began in the 1920s, with the first generation of IUDs constructed from silkworm gut and flexible metal wire. These early types of IUDs soon fell into disrepute because of the difficulty of insertion, the need for frequent removal as a result of pain and bleeding, and other serious complications. Subsequently, plastic IUDs of varying shapes and sizes were made available. Various inert, biocompatible, polymeric materials — such as polyethylene, ethylene/vinyl acetate copolymer, and silicone elastomer — were widely used to construct IUDs. The effectiveness of the nonmedicated plastic IUDs was found to be in proportion to the surface area of the device in direct contact with the endometrium; that is, large IUDs are more effective in preventing pregnancy than small ones. Unfortunately, the large devices also cause more endometrial compression and myometrial distension, leading to increased incidence of uterine cramps, bleeding, and expulsion of the IUDs.

Investigators have developed numerous IUDs in the last 20 years with the aim of eliminating these side effects. Unfortunately, variations in the shape or the size of IUDs have failed to minimize the side effects and, concurrently, to improve the contraceptive efficacy as much as was hoped. Therefore, efforts have been shifted to the improvement of intrauterine contraception via the inclusion of drugs in the IUDs. The controlled release of antifertility agents from IUDs was developed, and contraceptive metals, such as copper, were added to the IUD frame, and a progestin-releasing IUD was developed. The objectives were to add either antifertility agents to the more easily tolerated, smaller devices, such as the T-shaped device, to enhance their contraceptive effectiveness; or antifibrinolytic agents, such as ε-aminocaproic acid and tranexamic acid, to the larger, more effective IUDs to minimize the incidence of bleeding and pain.

IUDs have played a significant role in contraceptive practice since the mid-1960s. They do not necessarily depend upon drug delivery for their action, and devices consisting only of inert plastic, such as polyethylene, are still widely used. The mechanism of action of inert devices is not thoroughly understood, but a prominent theory is that they cause enough local inflammation to cause leukocytes to enter the uterus in large numbers, and the enzymes released interfere with implantation. There is also evidence that they interfere with sperm survival. The possibility of enhancing effectiveness while at the same time reducing the incidence of bleeding and pain has prompted the investigation of medicated IUDs. A reduction in bleeding and pain was expected because smaller devices could be used when effectiveness was attained with drug release. Two types of medicated devices have been introduced — those releasing copper and those releasing progestins.[92,93]

The copper devices consist of a plastic support wound with copper wire or fitted with copper collars. The metallic copper slowly undergoes oxidation and releases copper ions. It therefore constitutes a sustained-release dosage form. Devices in common use release about 20 µg of copper per day, although the amount released in the first few months of use may be as great as 100 µg/day, diminishing to 10 µg/day or less after periods of 1 or 2 years.[94] The amount of copper used is such that the copper will not be exhausted until 15 to 40 years of use, although with some wire-wound models, uneven corrosion may cause loss of discrete segments of the wire and thus greatly shorten the life of the device. Copper-bearing IUDs were introduced into distribution in the early 1970s and are widely used. The most effective copper-bearing devices have given annual pregnancy rates of one or less per 100 users.[95] This represents a significant improvement over the pregnancy rates experienced with inert devices.

IUDs delivering progestins may be expected to have progestational effects on the endometrium and to cause thickening of the cervical mucus, in addition to the effects on leukocyte infiltration characteristic of any foreign body placed in the uterus. The effects on cervical mucus may add significantly to antifertility effectiveness by inhibiting sperm access. A steroid-releasing IUD, Progestasert, was marketed by Alza Corporation in the mid-1970s.[96] Physically, the device consists of a T-shaped polyethylene support whose vertical arm is fitted with a sleeve containing the steroid. The sleeve consists of an inner reservoir of steroid, a silicone polymer, and an outer rate-regulating layer of polyethylene-vinyl acetate. Since the steroid is more soluble in the silicone polymer in the interior of the device than in its outer membrane of polyethylene vinyl acetate, the outer membrane is constantly exposed to a saturated solution of steroid in silicone.

The steroid thus has at all times a constant diffusion distance to the exterior of the device. *In vivo* results have shown a decline in release rate of about 25% in 1 year. A principal disadvantage of Progestasert in its present form is the required frequency of replacement (replacement is recommended after 1 year of use). An additional area of concern with the Progestasert device is the incidence of extrauterine pregnancies.[97]

A second steroid-releasing IUD uses levonorgestrel as the active agent. A particular advantage lies in the high potency of this steroid, coupled with its low solubility in Silastic, so that devices can readily be designed that will deliver contraceptive doses for many years. Both the devices used by Nilsson et al.[98] and El-Mahgoub[99] incorporate the steroid in a core in which it is mixed homogeneously with Silastic, with the release rate being modulated by a Silastic tube fitted over the core.

The levonorgestrel IUDs depress the endometrium, and the effectiveness of the devices undoubtedly depends on this effect and on the thickening of the cervical mucus. The doses used are not sufficient to block ovulation in most cycles. Although the plasma levels are low, as compared with those of pill, ring, and implant users, results in a comparative trial with copper IUDs indicated that levels were high enough to result in some systemic steroid effects. Increases in headaches, nervousness, depression, and acne were reported by about twice as many levonorgestrel IUD users as by users of the Nova T Copper IUD that was included in the same trials.[100]

A variant of the intrauterine IUD is an intracervical device. Intracervical devices have generally been received cautiously because they might serve to keep the cervix more open than IUDs and thus a better pathway for infection, and because of the high rates of expulsion experienced with intracervical devices in earlier trials. If these problems can be overcome, the devices are of interest because less skill is required for placement and because steroid-releasing intracervical devices might have differential effects, with more effect on cervical mucus and less on the endometrium than corresponding intrauterine devices (see Figures 8.7 and 8.8).

Cameron[101] has described a preparation for the purposes of a prolapsed uterus. The composition of this preparation (ointment) is alum, glycerol, and a soft solid carrier. It may also contain Epsom salts and a local anesthetic, such as procaine hydrochloride. The glycerol acts as a solvent for the alum and the Epsom salts. The ointment is preferably coated on a gauze pad and applied by placing it on the sore area of the uterus. The gauze pad may have a string attached to it for convenient removal.

An intrauterine device described by Lerner et al.[102] is composed of a plastic matrix having particulate material dispersed within it. This device has a contour that conforms to the midrange of the uterine cavity and has a number of lateral fins, which promote retention and permit accommodation to uterine contractions and variations in uterine shape extending outwardly from a central membrane portion.

Preferably, the intrauterine device is a composite formed of a plastic material, such as a copolymer of ethylene and vinyl acetate, polyethylene, polypropylene, polyvinyl chloride, nylon, or silicone rubber.[103,104] Most preferably, the plastic material is a copolymer of ethylene and vinyl acetate, such as UE 632 (U.S. Industrial Chemical Corp.), which contains 13 to 15% by weight vinyl acetate. In addition, the plastic matrix contains dispersed particulate material. The particulate material includes a metal and a metal salt, but may contain either alone. By way of example, metals that are satisfactory for contraception are copper, zinc, silver, platinum, or cadmium.[102]

A bioerodible intrauterine device that enables improved administration of pregnancy-interrupting drugs has been developed by Ramwell.[105] This drug delivery device, in its broadest aspects, comprises a body of polymer having drug dispersed through it, and is capable of bioeroding in the uterus over a prolonged period of time. The device is of a shape and size adapted for insertion and retention in the uterus or cervix uteri. As the body of polymer gradually erodes, it releases the dispersed drug at a controlled rate. Exemplary bioerodible materials include both natural and synthetic materials, such as structural proteins and hydrocolloids of animal origin, polysaccharides and other hydrocolloids of plant origin, and synthetic polymers. Such devices are useful for delivering all types of drugs to the uterus. However, these devices deliver with special efficiency progestational and estrogenic substances that have antifertility properties.

A polymeric device for the controlled release of progestational agents has been developed by Zaffaroni.[106] A local, contraceptively active steroid metabolite of progesterone is confined within the polymer. The polymeric material continuously meters the flow of an effective amount of the steroid to the uterus at a controlled rate. The material can be of suitable shape known to promote insertion and retention in the uterine cavity over short to prolonged periods of time. Alternatively, the polymeric release-rate-controlling material can be attached to an intrauterine device or intrauterine platform, which is effective for short- to long-term retention in the uterine cavity. In general, suitable devices can be obtained by distributing the steroid in a solid or gel matrix of the polymeric rate-controlling material, microencapsulating the agent, and then distributing the microcapsules in the polymeric rate-controlling material or confining the agent in a hollow container within the polymeric rate-controlling material.

Since this device is designed to control fertility for an extended period of time, such as 1 h to 3 or more years, there is no critical upper limit on the amount of steroid incorporated into the device, as it meters a regulated amount. Generally, the devices will contain from 250 mg to 5 g or more of agent.

A tubular device for suppression of fertility by the slow release of a progestin within the uterus has been described by Schommegna.[107] Test results have shown that ovulation and the menstrual cycle are not suppressed and that slow release of a progestin within the uterus produces superficial endometrial suppression. It is believed that this effect interferes with the reproductive process by making the endometrial surface unreceptive to the implantation of the fertilized ovum.

The progestin-containing capsule is maintained within the uterine cavity by an intrauterine device, to which it may be attached or of which it may be an integral part, the latter being preferred. This device comprises three capsules arranged in a triangular configuration and joined together by rounded juncture pieces. Each of the capsules comprises a short length (about 3 cm) of silicone elastomer tubing containing about 30 mg of a progestin, such as norgestrel. The juncture pieces are made of resilient polyethylene.

When fully assembled into the rounded triangular shape, the intrauterine device has sufficient rigidity to maintain its shape when not subjected to outside forces, but still is easily flexed as required for insertion into the uterine cavity. Once the device is in place within the uterine cavity, the capsules slowly release the progestin at a rate that varies with the length of the capsules, the thickness of the capsule walls, and the nature of the progestin. It has been found in clinical tests with progesterone-containing intrauterine T-shaped devices of this type that pregnancies are reduced to a substantially greater extent than would be expected from the mechanical action of the device. There were no pregnancies in patients in whom the device remained in position, and the capsule did not become depleted of progesterone.[108,109]

A method for treating hypermenorrhea by administering a progestational steroid to the uterine endometrium in low dosage over an extended duration of time has been described by Pharriss et al.[110] The system used administers 50 to 70 µg per day to the uterus over a prolonged period of one year. The system is made of ethylene-vinyl acetate copolymer, and the reservoir contains progesterone in silicone oil (see Figures 8.5 through 8.8).

F.   Rectal delivery

In the 18th century, a French pharmacist, Baumé, introduced cocoa butter as a vehicle for the preparation of suppositories, and this made further progress possible for the use of the rectal route for the administration of drugs. A great variety of fatty vehicles have been developed, both during and after World War II. Also, nonfatty vehicles have become available, and other dosage forms, such as ointments, microenemas, and soft-shell gelatin capsules, are in use for rectal administration.

The rectal route of administration can be utilized for both local and systemic effects. Suppositories and ointments for local effect are almost exclusively used for the relief of pain and itching due to hemorrhoids, with such common constituents as astringents, antiseptics, antipruritics, vasoconstrictors, and local anesthetics. However, suppositories can melt or soften in the ampulla-recti and spread through the rectum and will thus have at least partly passed the target (i.e., the anus).

For laxative purposes, retention enemas or suppositories of glycerine gelled by soap can be given, in addition to drugs. For the same purpose, suppositories releasing carbon dioxide after insertion, thereby stimulating defecation, have been usd. Retention enemas can also be used for local treatment, as in colitis; corticosteroids, either with or without antibiotics, are then dissolved or suspended in a moderately viscous aqueous medium. Two recent developments are microenemas and soft-shell gelatin capsules. Microenemas are supplied in a plastic container (Rectiole) with an application tube. After insertion of the tube, the container is emptied by compression. This permits the use of either aqueous or oily solutions for systemic application of drugs. Capsules used to achieve a systemic effect are filled with oil or paraffin. Of all the forms, fatty suppositories containing a suspended drug substance are the most widely used. Commonly used are suspensions of water-soluble substances in cocoa butter or in one of the many semisynthetic vehicles. These are prepared by hydrogenation of veg-

Classification of Drug Modification

Term	Type of Modification	Biologically Active Species	General Utility
I. Analog	Structural modification or substituent group synthesis	Active *per se*	Improve potency and specificity

Example

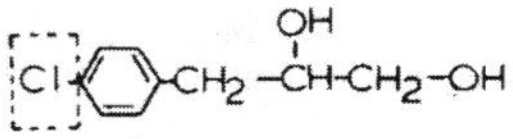

CI⟨ ⟩-CH₂-CH-CH₂-OH (with OH on middle carbon)

(Chlorophenesin)

| II. Prodrug | | | |
| a. Derivative Prodrug | Functional group derivative | Cleaved *in vivo* to active parent drug | Improve biopharmaceutical properties |

Example

$$NO_2-\langle\ \rangle-CH-CH-CH_2-O-C-C_{15}H_{31}$$

with HO, NH-C-CHCl₂ substituents

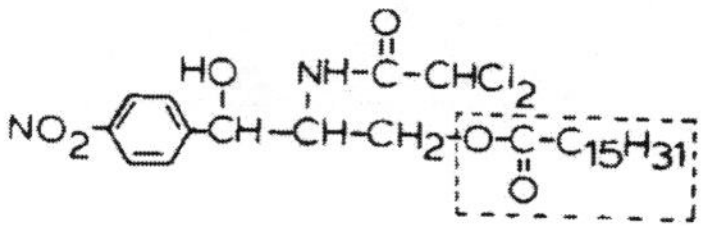

(Chloramphenicol Palmitate)

| b. Analog Prodrug | Structural modification or substituent synthesis | Metabolically transformed to active drug *in vivo* | Improve biopharmaceutical properties |

Example

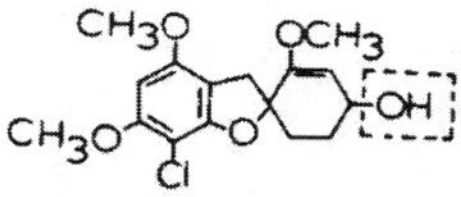

CH₃O, OCH₃, CH₃O, CI, OH

(Griseofulvin Alcohol)

| III. Derivative | Functional group derivative | Active *per se* | Improve potency and specificity and/or biopharmaceutical properties |

Example

$$CI-\langle\ \rangle-O-CH_2-CH-CH_2-O-C-NH_2$$

with OH substituent

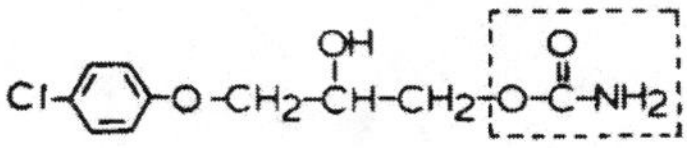

(Chlorphenesin Carbamate)

Figure 8.5 Classification of drug modification. (Copyright 1977 by the American Pharmaceutical Association, *Design of Biopharmaceutical Properties through Pro-Drugs and Analogs.* Reprinted with permission of the American Pharmaceutical Association.)

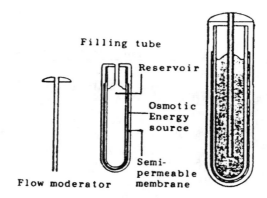

Figure 8.6 OSMET rectal system.

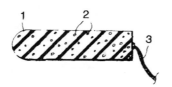

1. Section of Tampon
2. Microcapsules
3. String

Figure 8.7 Tampon impregnated with contraceptives. (From Johnson, J.C., Ed., *Sustained Release Medications*, Chemical Technology Review No. 177, 1980, 275. With permission.)

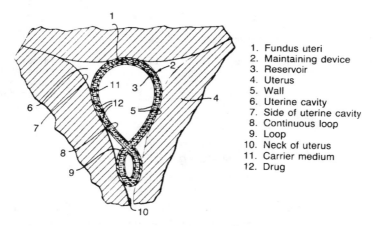

1. Fundus uteri
2. Maintaining device
3. Reservoir
4. Uterus
5. Wall
6. Uterine cavity
7. Side of uterine cavity
8. Continuous loop
9. Loop
10. Neck of uterus
11. Carrier medium
12. Drug

Figure 8.8 IUD with a replenishing drug reservoir. (From Johnson, J.C., Ed., *Sustained Release Medicatins*, Chemical Technology Review No. 177, 1980, 286. With permission.)

etable oils (e.g., coconut oil) or by esterification of glycerine with saturated fatty acids isolated from hydrolyzed vegetable fats.

Differences between vehicles thus occur (e.g., in hydroxyl number). The actual importance of this is not yet fully understood, but it seems essential that switching from one vehicle to another be avoided in order to prevent batch-to-batch variations. The same holds for bases containing extra emulsifying agents. The aqueous glycerinated gelatin vehicles are an exception and are only used for topical treatments. The macrogels are sometimes used for drugs that are fat-soluble or (e.g., for chloralhydrate).

Drug uptake from the rectum is not essentially different from that in other parts of the GI tract. Differences that do occur can be attributed to anatomy and physiology, rather than to specific membrane properties. Passive diffusion is still regarded as the main governing absorption mechanism. Therefore, solubility and partitioning parameters of the drug substance are of paramount importance. The lower rectum is surrounded by veins draining directly into the general circulation, whereas the upper and middle rectal veins lead to the vena porta. Because of many anastomoses between the two regions, a sharp separation cannot be assumed. The absorption step itself seems to follow the pH partition theory, at least in a quantitative sense. For drug design, the question is still open as to whether one has to adhere strictly, in this case, to molecules that are mainly un-ionized in the physiological pH range of 7.5 to 8.0. Currently, it still seems a good choice, although more evidence is becoming available that drugs that are completely ionized, like quaternary ammonium compounds, are also absorbed to a limited extent after rectal administration (i.e., <10%)

Depending on the nature of the vehicle and of the drug substance, different release mechanisms are involved. In water-soluble vehicles, mostly used for drugs like indomethacin that are poorly soluble in water and that have an appreciable solubility in fat, the drug will be present as a solution in PEG. In that case, the drug substance will be released as soon as contact has been made between vehicle and rectal fluid. Absorption will then be limited, either by membrane transport or by the diffusion rate in the aqueous contents of the rectum and the partitioning behavior between membranes and contents of the rectum. For drugs, such as indomethacin, it has been reported that *in vitro* release, and to a somewhat lesser extent *in vivo* absorption, is more rapid from a water-soluble than from a fatty vehicle. In cases where the drug substance is suspended in an aqueous vehicle, the particle size will be an additional parameter that may be rate-determining.

Many drug substances are liable to be bound by polyethylene glycols. The same considerations hold for microenemas, which contain the drug in PEG-containing solutions. But again, these types of delivery forms are only rarely used, and most emphasis has been placed on fatty vehicles, in particular, suspensions of relatively highly water-soluble drug substances. Principally, two different release mechanisms are possible: the suspended drug dissolves in the vehicle and is released through diffusion; and the suspended drug comes into contact with the aqueous rectal fluid and dissolves in it.

A model has been developed for suspension ointments, and in some instances, this model has been applied to suspension suppositories. Since suppositories melt fairly rapidly after insertion, a rather thin layer of a medium-viscosity suspension is formed. Assuming that the particles spread homogeneously with the vehicle, not all conditions under which the model operates are met. The particles will not remain distributed homogenously throughout the vehicle, but will reach an equilibrium position in the vehicle/ rectal fluid interface. This is because the viscosity of the melted suppository permits particles to settle. This is reflected in the observed rate of release from suppositories, which is far more rapid than predicted. Therefore, a release mechanism composed of three steps may be inferred. These steps are: approach of the suspended drug particles toward the interface between the melted vehicle and the aqueous rectal fluid, transport through that interface, and dissolution in the aqueous rectal fluid.

This transport process (the first step) may take place through two different driving forces. First, sedimentation is possible as soon as the viscosity is lowered during the melting process. This will be all the more important as the spreading area is smaller, and therefore the layer thickness of the melted mass remains larger. Second, the pressure waves occurring in the rectum may induce particle motion in the melted mass and thus collision with the interface, in which the particles will reach an equilibrium. Both processes would predict an influence of viscosity of the melted mass and also of the particle size of the drug. This latter observation is in contrast with the Higuchi ointment treatment, where no such influence is predicted. Also, particle concentration could be a factor, as it influences the viscosity of a melted mass. Particles will cross the interface (the second step), depending on their surface properties, in relation to the same properties of both liquid phases.

The dissolution process (the third step) is clearly an intrinsic property of the drug substance and can be derived by using the appropriate equations. There is one factor, however, that has to be considered (i.e., the surface exposed to the dissolving rectal fluid). The situation at the interface is not comparable to the one in which a particle dissolves in a stirred medium. The flow of liquid is negligible, and the particle continuously adjusts its position to maintain its equilibrium position as dictated by the surface forces. It is also relevant to know if one of the steps is rate-limiting and, if so, which one. Experiments have been performed in a model system consisting of different substances suspended in paraffin, as the fatty vehicle substitute, and water. For a highly soluble substance, the second and third steps are rapid and the release rate is limited by the first step, at least in the thickness layer used (1 cm).

The rectal route of administration has been reviewed by de Boer[111] and co-workers. The rectal route has received considerable attention as an alternative to oral administration, and is employed relatively frequently in pharmaceutical usage for either local or systemic effects. The successful enhancement of rectal absorption by the use of adjuvants has been extensively reported by Nishihata and co-workers,[112] who have discovered a number of potential adjuvants that facilitate transport across the rectal mucosa.

Modozeniec et al.[113] examined both rectal and oral delivery devices in rats, beagle dogs, and humans by noninvasive methods to determine *in vivo* release characteristics of experimental devices. The noninvasive procedures were minor modifications of the techniques performed by Beihn and Digenis.[114] The preliminary biopharmaceutical considerations for the rectal dosage forms described in this work showed that the data base exhibited considerable biovariability. Attempts to identify the formulation variables and the working mechanisms for rectal absorption required a more rigid explanation of the fate of the dosage form under *in vivo* release.

For these reasons, qualitative and quantitative information was obtained on the disposition of Witepsol H15 suppositories labeled with ^{99}Tc-HDP using external scintigraphic techniques in combination with lower GI radiographs. A variation in one of the subjects demonstrated that the insertion of the suppository blunt-end first or pointed-end first apparently made no difference in suppository movement or spreading behavior. The suppository generally stayed within 5 to 7 cm of the anal canal in the rectum. All subjects showed a negative biphasic slope of count activity from the original insertion site and a positive slope of activity from the area surrounding the original dosage form after an initial plateau. This plateau was interpreted as due to liquefaction and collapse of the suppository.

The major reasons for the biovariability experienced with the several rectal dosage forms studied appear to be the rate of liquefaction and the rate of spreading of the liquefied mass. As a major route of drug administration, rectal administration is relatively unaffected by food and diet and GI motility and is controlled only by defecation.

Hayakawa et al.[115] have determined the relative effectiveness of several penetration-enhancers on the rectal absorption of insulin across the isolated rectal membrane of the albino rabbit. These were DTA, polyoxyethylene 9-lauryl ether (POE), Na glycocholate (GC), Na taurocholate (TC), and Na deoxycholate (DC). Of the enhancers, 1% POE was as effective as 1% DC and 2.5 to 3% GC and much more effective than 0.01% EDTA. Increasing the EDTA concentration to 0.1% did not improve its effectiveness. However, it augmented the effectiveness of 1% GC approximately tenfold. To explain these results, it has been speculated that the main effect of GC was deaggregation of insulin, whereas that of EDTA was disruption of membrane integrity. Alternatively, it is possible that the membrane-disruptive effect of EDTA may occur only in an already damaged membrane.

Byrne and Aylott[116] have developed a slow-release suppository consisting of a linear polymer, water, and drug. The water is present in excess of more than 35 parts by weight. In general, the mechanical properties of suppositories containing between 35 and 40 parts by weight of water are not as good as the mechanical properties of suppositories containing approximately 50 parts by weight of water. A pharmaceutical vehicle for suppositories capable of releasing the effective ingredient over approximately 24 hours has been desired.

A pharmaceutical vehicle described by Aoda et al.[117] is characterized in that, in Ringer's solution, the vehicle is gradually swollen, cracks, disintegrates, and uniformly releases drug over a period of several to 24 hours. The vehicle is composed of a fatty acid glyceride having a melting point higher than 37°C; a water-soluble, low-viscous, and nonirritating organic substance having a particle size smaller than 28 mesh and a viscosity lower than 300 cps, as measured with respect to a 2% aqueous solution; an organic polymeric substance having a particle size smaller than 28 mesh that is capable of swelling upon contact with water; and a water-soluble, surface-active agent.

The industrial manufacture of suppositories normally involves a moulding process in which a molten mixture of suppository base and active agent is poured into molds. This procedure has certain disadvantages, in particular, the exposure of the active agent to elevated temperatures at which it may not be stable, the possibility of sedimentaion of active agent during the molding process, and the fact that high quantities of active agent may result in a mixture too viscous to pour. To overcome such problems, a simple compression process has been proposed, which may be effected on conventional tableting equipment, employing a mixture or granulate comprising the suppository base, active agent, and a binding agent, such as polyvinylpyrrolidone or sodium carboxymethylcellulose, in a solvent. This process may, however, result in suppositories of unsatisfactory biopharmaceutical or physical properties (e.g., low bioavailability of active agent, cracks, and other faults due to air entrapment, etc.).

de Buman et al.[118] have developed a compression process for the production of suppositories at a temperature of 10°C or below in the absence of an added binding agent. The suppositories made according to the de Buman procedure may contain any pharmacologically active agent that may be administered by the rectal, vaginal, or urethral routes. The amount of active agent pressed will naturally depend on its effective dose, the rate of absorption, and the suppository mass. In general, a suppository made according to the invention may contain up to 450 mg of active agent per gram suppository total weight.

Takagishi et al.[119] have developed a novel means for the administration of a drug in the form of a capsule that minimizes variation in absorbability. It has been observed that, when the drug is contained in the capsule in the form of a liquid, the osmotic pressure of the liquid plays an essential role in the absorption of the drug through the rectum, and the variation in absorbability of the drug among individuals can be minimized when the osmotic pressure of the liquid is substantially higher than the osmotic pressure of the rectal fluid. The hard-capsule shells used for rectal application are preferably composed of a mixed ester of cellulose.

Despite the advantages obtained with capsules for rectal applications, the developers have become aware of variable effectiveness of administration. That is, when a capsule containing either an aqueous or oleic prepration is rectally applied to a test animal, the disintegration of the capsule in the rectum and the absorbability of the drug through the rectum differ widely from animal to animal. As a result of the problem of nonuniformity of absorption, it has been concluded that the value of the osmotic pressure of the aqueous liquid contained in the capsule plays an important role in the disintegration of a rectally applied capsule.

Takagishi et al.[120] have also developed a novel and efficient means for the administration of a drug by rectal application. The drug capsule is formed of a hard-capsule shell made of a mixed ester of a cellulose ether (e.g., alkyl-hydroxyalkyl and hydroxyalkyl alkylcelluloses) esterified with aliphatic monoacyl groups and acidic succinyl groups. When the capsule is inserted into the rectum, the capsule shell disintegrates, and the drug is released into the rectum and absorbed as efficiently as with conventional suppositories.

The pharmaceutical composition for rectal administration in accordance with the invention by Kitao and Nishimura,[121] is generally used as a rectal suppository for a preparation prepared by dispersing a drug, an adjuvant, and other ingredients in a liquid oleaginous base to prepare a suspension or ointment and by filling the suspension or ointment in soft gelatin capsules or tubes. In preparing a pharmacological composition using the base for rectal preparation of this invention, the active substance is added to the base, followed by an antioxidant.

The development by Higuchi et al.[122] generally comprises the steps of preparing a drug form capable of being rectally administered, wherein the drug comprises an effective dosage amount absorbed into the bloodstream. A preferred form of suppository comprises a soft, elastic gelatin capsule having an outer shell that encloses the drug and the adjuvant in a suitable vehicle that will not attack the walls of the capsule. The shell encapsulates a preselected drug form and the adjuvant. The gelatin capsule shell may be formulated in accordance with conventional techniques for making filled, seamless, soft elastic gelatin capsules containing therapeutically effective unit dosage amounts of the drug. The present method and suppository permit the rapid clearance of the released drug into the bloodstream by way of the lower hemorrhoidal vein, instead of moving upward into the lower gut.

Roseman et al.[123] have described a medicated device adapted for a single, acute, and rate-controlled rectal or vaginal administration of a lipophilic prostaglandin. The device accomplishes drug administration at an essentially time-independent rate of dosage. Furthermore, the device results in depletion of the prostaglandin from the device at the conclusion of the single, acute use. The device comprises three elements: an inert, resilient support means contoured for easy vaginal or rectal insertion; an initial flexible, polymer film layer affixed to the support and containing the prostaglandin dispersed therein (this film is not rate-limiting); and a second polymer film, laminated onto the and providing a release rate, which is rate-limiting.

Michaels[124] has developed a dispenser for delivering a fluid or an agent to an environment of use. The dispenser comprises a wall formed of a laminate comprising a layer of a cross-linked hydrophilic polymer grafted to a layer of a non-cross-linked hydrophilic polymer. The wall-laminate surrounds an inner collapsible container made of an elastomeric material, which houses a fluid or a useful agent composition. In operation, the dispenser releases fluid or agent in response to the wall-laminate absorbing fluid from the environment and expanding, thereby exerting pressure on the container, which collapses and ejects fluid or agent from the dispenser. The dispenser can be sized, shaped, and adapted for dispensing drugs to the body cavities, body openings, for oral administration, for use as intramuscular implants, and for intrauterine, vaginal, cervical, nasal, ear, ocular, and dermal applications.

Recently, Alza developed OSMET, which is a rectal delivery system. Similar to the OROS system, this system consists of a semipermeable membrane, an osmotic energy source, and a drug reservoir. The unit is designed so that the collapsible reservoir that contains a solution of the drug for delivery is surrounded by an osmotic driving agent encapsulated in a semipermeable membrane. Alza's OSMET system has been used to provide controlled delivery of theophylline.

G.   Microspheres

Nonideal pharmaceutical, pharmacokinetic, and therapeutic properties often combine to reduce the effectiveness of cytotoxic compounds. For the vectoring of such compounds to target areas, liposomes, nanoparticles, and microspheres have been suggested. Since organ distribution of the latter is dependent upon their size and shape, it is reasonable to attempt second-order targeting of microspheres on this basis. At the time of clinical diagnosis, two general conditions apply to most tumor-bearing patients. The first concerns the various biological activities and surface properties of malignant cells, which interfere with their recognition and elimination — which, in turn, leads to a progressive biochemical imbalance between tumors and their hosts. Second, biochemical differences between tumor and host cells are almost always minimal and frequently quantitative rather than qualitative. The aim of targeted chemotherapy is to reduce the tumor/host imbalance by altering the distribution, uptake, or effects of drugs such that the tumor cells are damaged substantially more than normal cells.[125]

Albumin microspheres of various sizes and composition have been used extensively for lung scans and circulatory studies. The first-order distribution of microspheres is determined almost entirely by their size. For example, following the intravenous delivery of microspheres, more than 90% of those smaller than 1 to 1.4 microns in diameter are removed by the spleen and liver, whereas those larger than 10 microns are almost totally entrapped in the lungs by arteriolar and capillary blockade.

Following intra-arterial injection, small microspheres are again cleared by the reticuloendothelial system, but large microspheres are sequestered in the first capillary bed that the spheres encounter, with a negligible immediate spillover into secondary capillary systems. The use of albumin microspheres as carriers for antitumor compounds was first suggested by Kramer,[126] and they have been subsequently studied experimentally for doxorubicin HCl, daunorubicin HCl, 5-fluorouracil, and 6-mercaptopurine, among others.

Using models, it has been found that for polar organic molecules, their release from chemically cross-linked albumin microspheres is biphasic, with a large initial burst effect taking place — which can constitute between 60 and 90% of the initially incorporated drug. The burst effect has also been reported for heat-stabilized microspheres. To determine drug release from albumin microspheres, an online stream system has been developed. This enables release to be monitored under differing conditions.

The method uses a stainless-steel column filled with inert glass beads. Prior to study, some beads are removed from the column and replaced by the microsphere system under study. An eluent of fixed composition is then passed through the column using a high-performance, pulse-free pump. Eluate is then passed through the cell of a spectrophotometer. It is intended that the stream system should simulate the hydrodynamics of the microcirculation of tumors.

It has been clearly demonstrated that the release of alizarin, for example, can be manipulated simply by altering the contact of the microspheres with the cross-linker. Results to date indicate that judicious choice of cross-linking conditions can lead to reasonable release of polar and ionic drugs from albumin microspheres for periods ranging from minutes to days. Mass-balance studies have shown that the burst effect leaves between 10 and 40% of the incorporated drug still available for sustained release.[127–129]

Lipid microspheres are usually prepared from glycerides and lecithins, and are considered to be a convenient carrier for lipophilic drugs. Coating the surface of the lipid microspheres with a suitable polysaccharide shifts the negative surface charge slightly to a neutral value, effectively depressing Ca^{2+}-induced aggregation and fusion of the lipid microspheres and decreasing the fluidity of the surface.[130]

Prostaglandin E1 (PGE1) is a strong vasodilator and antiplatelet-aggregating agent and has been applied clinically to treat severe peripheral vascular disorders. Lipid microsphered (LM)PGE1 is a novel, improved, injectable preparation. It is seven times more potent in vasodilating activity than the conventional PGE1 preparation in diabetic rats.[131]

The incorporation of enzymes into bovine serum albumin microspheres and their subsequent release has been studied as a model system for the controlled release of labile protein drugs. Microspheres containing α-chymotrypsin, trypsin, or acetylated trypsin have been prepared by emulsifying an aqueous solution of albumin/enzyme in cottonseed oil or a 30% solution of Pluronic F88 in chloroform. Spheres were hardened with glutaraldehyde and resuspended in aqueous buffer solutions. The release of the enzymes into the suspending medium was assessed by measuring the hydrolytic activity of both suspension and supernatant towards synthetic substrates. Thus, these enzymes can be successfully loaded into microspheres while retaining their functional activity, both in the microsphere and after release.[132]

In one study, authors administered a gelling bioadhesive microsphere delivery system containing gentamicin using the nasal route. Lysolecithin was incorporated into the delivery system as an absorption enhancer, and the bioavailability of gentamicin was increased by a factor of 50%, compared with an increase of less than 1% for a simple nasal gentamicin solution.[133]

The solvent-evaporation process has been used to prepare a variety of drug-loaded microspheres. In this process, a drug and polymer are codissolved or codispersed in a volatile solvent, usually methylene chloride. The resulting mixture is emulsified in water, and the solvent is removed by evaporation to produce solid microspheres. When the drug and polymer are initially codissolved in a common solvent, a variety of physicochemical interactions can occur between them as solvent evaporation progresses. These interactions affect microsphere morphology, which, in turn, affects microsphere properties, such as release rate and stability. Some insight into the morphology of poly(d,l-lactide) microspheres and a series of ibuprofen-loaded ethylcellulose microspheres has been reported.[134]

Using a water-soluble substance with an unlimited solubility and a hydrophobic polymer (poly-caprolactone) with a molecular weight of approximately 30,000 dalton, microspheres (size 1 μm) were produced of the pure substance, which subsequently were coated with the poly-caprolactone using a spray-drying technique. Upon suspending the product, 50% of the entrapped substance was released after one hour. Radiolabeled bovine serum albumin has been entrapped in microderivatized starch (MW 28,000), which had been reacted with di-cyclohexyl-carbodiimide and coupled to the matrix, and *in vitro* release was determined radiometrically.[135]

Mathiowitz et al.[136] and Langer and Folkman[137] have described a method for the preparation of a bioerodible polyanhydride microspheres. The preparation occurs at room temperature in organic solvents, an important advantage for hydrolytically labile polymers, such as polyanhydrides. Previously, with polyanhydride microspheres, these authors employed a hot-melt technique to incorporate molecules into the polymers. While that approach has certain advantages, many drugs lose biological activity at high temperature. Therefore, the hot-melt technique can only be used with low-melting-point polymers. The new method permits the preparation of microspheres from polymers with high melting points and polyanhydride microspheres for several new polymers (e.g., copolymers of bis 1,3-(carboxy phenoxy propane)) copolymerized with sebacic acid or dodecanoic acid.

A sustained-release formulation of theophylline is desirable for maintaining plasma levels between 5 μg/ml and 20 μg/ml. Poly(methylmethacrylate) microspheres have been prepared using the solvent-evaporation method. Polyethylene glycol (PEG)400 was used to improve the rate of release of the drug from the microspheres. The ratio between theophylline and the polymer remained constant regardless of the size of the microspheres. The release of the drug from the microspheres was influenced by the drug-to-polymer ratio, the amount of PEG, and the diameter of the spheres. The release profile of the drug was altered by mixing differing ratios of microspheres of various formulations.[138]

A rapid decrease in plasma glucose has been observed after starch microspheres and insulin were administered intranasally as a dry powder. The degree of cross-linking affects the level of water uptake and swelling, and thus, release of insulin from spheres when tested *in vitro*. The ability to reduce plasma glucose levels was the same after the administration of either insoluble starch (MW 25,000) or starch microspheres. Water-soluble starch powder (MW 11,000) did not affect the plasma glucose level. The authors concluded that degradable epichlorohydrin cross-linked starch microspheres and starch powders promote the absorption of insulin in rats if the system is insoluble in water when administered intranasally.[139]

Bangs Laboratories (Carmel, IN) manufactures over 900 latex particles, microspheres made of polystyrene, and other polymers, copolymers, and terpolymers. Most popular and used commercially are their 1-μm superparamagnetic particles containing 12, 20, 40, or 60%, magnetite. They are truly superparamagnetic in that they respond to a magnet, but have no residual magnetism themselves They can be used for direct simple adsorption of proteins, and they have COOH or NH surface groups, which permit covalent attachment of ligands. Their surface activators can be used in ELISA tests, as these are designed for converting plates and tubes with hydrophobic surfaces (such as polystyrene, polyethylene, and polypropylene) to hydrophilic surfaces with carboxylic acid or amide functional groups for covalent attachment to proteins. These coatings permit thorough washing for "zero background" readings. The microspheres, beads, or particles have several applications, such as cell separation, cell tags, chemiluminescent assays, contrast agents, density calibrators, DNA probes, dyed markers for regional myocardial flow, flow cytometry standards, fluidized beds, magnetic resonance imaging, propping agents, and void sources for ceramics, to name a few. While companies like Bangs Laboratories and Rhone-Poulenc are involved in manufacturing these particles, Pharmacia is working on the use of microspheres in delivering anticancer drugs.

H.   Hydrogels

Hydrogels are usually considered to be cross-linked, water-swollen polymers having a water content ranging from 30 to 90%, depending on the polymer used. Because of their highly swollen nature, hydrogel membranes are usually quite permeable to hydrophilic or high-molecular-weight agents. This property, together with good biocompatibility, has led to the widespread use of hydrogels as rate-controlling membranes in devices for delivering proteins, such as insulin, aprotinin, tumor antigenesis factor, and leuteinizing hormone. Low-molecular-weight, water-soluble drugs often permeate hydrogels at too high a rate to be useful, but hydrogel membranes have found an application as rate-controlling barriers for water-insoluble drugs, such as steroids. Almost all hydrogel controlled-release devices have been monolithic systems, releasing the active agent following $t^{-1/2}$, or first-order, kinetics. Many hydrogels are made by free-radical polymerization of hydrophilic vinyl monomers. The initiation step is the formation of a free radical, usually by the addition of azo-type initiators, such as 2,2-azobis(2-methyl-propanenitrile), or peroxide initiators, such as benzoyl peroxide. Ultraviolet light or gamma radiation can also initiate the reaction. Propagation takes place by free-radical reaction with the vinyl monomer groups. Normally, a portion of the reaction mixture consists of difunctional vinyl compounds that provide a degree of cross-linking. The hydrophilicity of the gel is usually controlled by copolymerizing a hydrophilic and hydrophobic vinyl monomer into the gel. The permeability of a hydrogel is determined by the extent of cross-linking, the degree of hydration of the gel, the nature of the permeant, and the device design.

The quantity and type of solvent used in the polymerization mix can substantially affect the quality of the gel produced. For example, poly(hydro-xyethyl methacrylate), or poly(HEMA), only absorbs 35 to 40% of water, and therefore poly(HEMA) devices prepared from polymerization-reaction mixtures containing a greater amount of water contain water-filled voids and are translucent or opaque in appearance. Cross-linking usually reduces the water absorption of the polymer. Hydrogels may also be prepared in the absence of water and subsequently equilibrated with water or with a concentrated aqueous solution of the active agent. Other parameters to be controlled in the preparation of hydrogels are the temperature of polymerization and concentration of the initiator.

It has been proposed that water exists in two forms in gels: bound water closely associated with the polymer matrix (water of solvation) and bulk water lying between the polymer chains. Hydrophilic permeants of small molecular size have diffusion coefficients directly dependent on the water content of the hydrogel and independent of the chemistry of the polymer. There is a good correlation between the diffusion coefficient of sodium chloride and the reciprocal of the water content of the hydrogel over a variety of gels containing 10 to 70 wt% water. Diffusion coefficients in hydrogels decrease with increasing permeant size and with the degree of cross-linking, particularly as the size of the permeant approaches the size of the openings between the cross-links. Refojo and Leong[140] have determined the size of these openings by measuring the lowest molecular weight of the permeant that does not diffuse through the hydrogel. However, due to the nature of the system, hydrogels still have a relatively high permeability for all water-soluble agents, up to a fairly large molecular size.

The simplest form of controlled-release hydrogel is obtained by equilibriating the polymer, in either the dry or hydrated state, with a concentrated solution of the active material. This technique is useful for experimental studies, but commercial device preparation more often involves incorporation of the active compound into the polymerization mixture. Taking this approach for a biomedical device requires consideration of whether residual unremoved monomer would pose a problem. Hydrogels have been used to prepare reservoir devices, usually by coating a high-permeability monolithic core containing dispersed or dissolved active material with a less-permeable coating. For example, Lewis et al.[141] have used this technique to prepare a fluoride delivery system.

Hydrogels have been proposed as controlled-delivery systems for a variety of bioactive agents, such as contraceptives, ophthalmics, antibacteria agents, drug antagonists, antiarrhymics, anticancer drugs, anticoagulants, enzymes, and antibodies. They can be applied as inserts or implants or can be administered subcutaneously, intramuscularly, or perorally. In the development of controlled-release systems for opthalmological applications, hydrogels have been used as ocular insert devices, delivering the drugs directly to the eye. Soft contact lenses manufactured from poly(HEMA) have been found to prolong the action of pilocarpine and polymixin B when added in eyedrop form to human or animal eyes. Soft contact lenses presoaked with pilocarpine or phenylephrine give a more profound and prolonged ocular response than conventional eyedrop administration of the drugs.

Hydrogels prepared from polyethylene glycoldiacrylates, polyethylene dimethyl-acrylates, and copolymers with 2-acrylamidoglucose, 6-methacrylylgalactose, and methylene bisacrylamide have been studied as cervical dilator delivery systems for prostaglandins. Prostaglandins such as PGE^2 and PGF^2 have been shown to be effective for the induction of therapeutic abortion. However, systemic circulation of the prostaglandins causes concomitant side effects. Therefore, it would be desirable to apply the drugs in a controlled manner at the target organ. By utilizing the hydrogel devices, successful dilatation was achieved at low dosage rates with less chance for systemic side effects and clinical syndromes.[142]

Chien and Lau[143] prepared norgestomet-releasing hydrogels and studied *in vitro* and *in vivo* release behavior. *In vivo* studies were conducted by subcutaneous implanting of rods of hydrogels containing 5% norgestomet in the ears of cows.

The permeabilities of hydrogels for steroids has been extensively studied by Song et al.[144] Progesterones containing hydrogels were made from HEMA and mixtures of HEMA with methoxyethyl methacrylate (MEMA) and methoxyethoxyethyl methacrylate (MEEMA). Varying amounts of ethyleneglycol dimethacrylate (EGDMA) and tetraethyleneglycol dimethacrylate (TEGDMA) were used as cross-linking agents. Trilaminate hydrogel devices for continuous controlled release of fluoride to teeth have been fabricated by Coswar and Dunn[145] and sucessfully tested *in vivo*. The devices are composed of a core of a fluoride salt dispersed in a hydrogel. Copolymers of 2-hydroxyethyl methacrylate and methylmethacrylate were used as rate-controlling membranes. The zero-order-release dosage regimen could be varied by changing the composition of the polymer. Hydrogel devices have also been elaborated that provide zero-order release of narcotic antagonists and antibiotics.

Ionogenic hydrogels can be prepared by adding anionic or cationic monomers to the polymerization mixture. They also can be formed by modification of existing hydrogels (e.g., by partial hydrolysis of ester units). The effect of the incorporation of small quantities of ionogenic groups on bio-compatibility has been investigated, and the results have been briefly reviewed by Ratner and Hoffman.[146] The importance of charged groups on various aspects of biocompatibility is not clear. However, there are indications that charge density and the morphology of the device surface may be of greater importance than the total charge.

Gregonis et al.[147] have investigated the effect of small quantities of meth-acrylic acid (MAA) and dimethylaminoethyl methacrylate (DMAEMA) units on the swelling of hydrogels. It was reported that MAA units in their car-boxylate salt form gave a dramatic increase in the equilibrium water content of the gel, whereas the effect of the DMAEMA groups was less pronounced. According to Wichterle,[148] the presence of either acidic or basic groups in hydrogels causes a lower permeability for sodium chloride, whereas ampholyte structures increase its permeability. Abrahams and Rovel[149] have reported that the release of cyclazocine from tablets coated with a hydrogel membrane is more rapid, with increasing amounts of methacrylic acid units in the hydrogel. Consequently, the introduction of ionogenic groups may affect the rate of release of drugs from hydrogels.

Increasing the content of acidic or basic groups in the hydrogel matrix will lead to a material that can be described as an ion-exchange resin. Prin-cipally, ion-exchange resins, having the ability to swell in aqueous media, can be categorized as a special type of hydrogel material. Cationic and anionic ion exchangers have been used in the past to prolong the effect of drugs. Their use was based on the principle that acidic or basic pharmaceu-ticals, combined with appropriate resins, yield insoluble polysalt resinates. Biological evaluations of the coarse resinates performed on chickens, dogs, and sheep infected with various nematodes demonstrated the resinate to be more efficient than the pure drug. In most cases, the resinate exhibited 100% effectiveness. The practical and economical advantages of formulations that can kill all nematodes in one single treatment are obvious.[150,151]

The full-term, newborn infant has well-developed skin, which possesses excellent barrier properties. In contrast, the prematurely born infant has a poorly developed stratum corneum, resulting in higher skin permeability. This incomplete skin barrier may provide a convenient route of administra-tion for drugs intended for systemic therapy. Theophylline, which has been widely used in the treatment of apnea in premature infants, was chosen for the study. Theophylline hydrogel loading and difusivity and its *in vitro* trans-dermal permeation characteristics using a fetal pig skin model were initially investigated. Subsequent clinical studies demonstrated that theophylline loaded into a hydrogel system can permeate through the premature infant skin into the systemic circulation.[152]

Hydrogels normally consist of hydrophilic polymers that are covalently cross-linked to prevent their dissolution. Hydrogels prepared from "alloys"of hydrophobic and hydrophilic polymers have been investigated. These alloys are held together by ionic, dipole–dipole, and hydrophobic interactions, as well as hydrogen bonds. Water-absorption rate, water-sorption capacity, biocompatibility, biodegradation, and thermoplasticity can be controlled by selection of the proper composition and activation steps. The water-sorption capacities are pH-dependent, as are the swelling volumes. The fact that pH-induced changes are reversible indicates that these hydrogels can be useful for biological sensors and drug delivery systems. Pellets fabricated from these alloys and drugs, such as tetracycline, have demonstrated sustained release by an erosion mechanism *in vitro*. The alloys used in these studies were homogeneous mixtures of water-soluble poly(maleic anhydride) (PVA).[153]

Long-term oral drug delivery through the use of an enzyme-digestible "balloon" hydrogel can be achieved. Protein cross-linked hydrogels swell in the gastric environment to such an extent that gastric emptying is inhibited until they are enzymatically digested. The nonspecific enzymatic digestion ensures complete dissolution of the balloon hydrogels in the GI tract. The ability to control the extent of swelling and gel-disruption time of the balloon hydrogels presents an opportunity to achieve once-a-day or long-term oral controlled drug delivery.[154]

Water-soluble hydrogels of alkali metal alginate and glycerine have been found to be excellent wound dressings. The gels dry to an adherent, nontoxic, pliable protective film, which can be removed by water-washing when desired. The gels are also compatible with drugs, and hence can serve as vehicles or carriers for medication application to wounds, as well as a protective cover.

In general, the amount of medication in the composition ranges from approximately 0.01 to 10% by weight. The gel compositions are easily manipulated jelly materials and can be applied to a body surface. The applied gel coating has been found to dry on exposure to air at ambient temperature and form a nontoxic, transparent, flexible, and stretchable film that is tightly adherent to the body surface. Dried film-coatings of the compositions can be removed when desired by a simple water wash. In addition, reapplication of the composition over a previously applied area can be made without removing underlying layers of the composition. The transparency of this composition enables one to observe the wound underneath and closely follow the healing progress. Furthermore, its ability to stretch and bend without tearing or disturbing adherence to the wound enables it to be used over joints.[155]

Novel hydrogel compositions of diester cross-linked polyglucan and a process for their preparation has been described by Manning and Stark.[156] Amylose, dextran, and pullulan succinates and glutarates, when cross-linked, were found to have use as general fluid sorbants, have exceptional hemostatic activity, and have adherence to a wound and bioabsorption without causing undue irritation of the tissue or toxic effects. Reticulated hydrogel sponges made of the cross-linked diesters, which are particularly useful as general fluid sorbants, and those of amylose glutarate are good bioabsorbable hemostatic agents. The sponges are made by lyophilizing water-soluble salts of the mono- or half-esters, under process conditions of this invention in the presence of a reticulating agent. The resulting reticulated, porous, open-celled sponge is then cross-linked by heating the sponge under the dehydrating conditions to form diester cross-links. The sponge is highly porous, is moderately strong, and has the ability to retain up to 40 times its weight of isotonic saline. When neutralized with physiologically acceptable salts, the sponge has exceptional hemostatic activity, adherence to bleeding tissue, and bioabsorption without causing toxic effects.

Mueller and Good[157] have described an insoluble polymeric hydrogel that is suitable for oral, bucal, subcutaneous, or IM implant delivery. These implants can be used as artificial veins, devices for insertion into urethra, vagina, or anal cavity, or through the skin. Incorporation of the drug into the hydrogel may be accomplished either by dissolution or dispersion in the macromer or monomer solution prior to addition of the free-radical catalyst. Any of the drugs used to treat the body, both topical and systemic, can be incorporated as the active agent in the copolymeric carrier of this system.

I.   Microcapsules and microencapsulation

Microencapsulation is defined as a process whereby small solid particles or small liquid droplets are discretely surrounded or enclosed by an intact, thin shell of inert polymeric materials, such as ethylcellulose, cellulose acetate phthalate, ethylene vinyl acetate, poly(ethylene oxide), poly(vinyl alcohol), or gelatin.[158] The particle size may range from 5 to 500 μm in diameter, but microcapsules can be made less than 1 μm and up to 1000 μm in diameter. Microcapsules can be prepared by various methods and combinations of techniques. They are generally classified into the categories of coacervation or phase separation, interfacial polymerization, and mechanical methods, such as spray coating and polymer dispersion. The rationale for selecting ethylcellulose for the shell material is that this substance is commonly used as an additive in foods and drugs because of its high inertness and forms a stable, semipermeable, capsular membrane.

Ampicillin anhydrate microcapsules are fabricated by an organic phase-separation process. Microcapsules of the desired size (45 to 106 μm) are isolated from each batch by wet-sieving them with hexane using standard-mesh, stainless-steel sieves and a camel-hair brush. The microcapsules are then dried for at least 24 h in a vacuum chamber maintained at room temperature. All batches of microcapsules and ampicillin anhydrate evaluated in animals were sterilized with a 2.0- or 2.5-Mrad dose of gamma radiation at dry-ice temperature.[159]

Investigations have been conducted of proper dosage forms using microcapsules for anticancer drugs. Two types of core substances have been used: medicinal carbon with 5-fluorouracil adsorbed before and after capsulization. This was found to be a useful technique for slow release.[160]

With the goal of using short-acting sulfonamides with dihydrofolate reductase inhibitors in malaria, drug delivery systems have been fabricated for better pharmacokinetic and therapeutic profiles. Polymer and copolymer systems have been used to fabricate the multiunit dosage forms: microcapsules and micropellets. Comparative bioavailability studies were conducted for fasting and fed animals. With significant *in vitro* and *in vivo* correlation, drug release was prolonged compared to the uncapsulated drug.[161]

Microcapsules of pesticides have various advantages compared to conventional formulations, that is, longer residual efficacy, decrease in mammalian toxicity, decrease in phytotoxicity, decrease in fish toxicity, etc. However, in order to obtain these characteristics, particle design is important. In the case of the interfacial polymerization method, wall thickness, wall structure, capsule diameter, core materials, and additives cause change of capsule properties, that is, release mechanism, release rate, capsule strength, etc. The studies were conducted using fenitrothion, fenvalerate, and fenpropathrin microcapsules for agricultural use.[162]

Controlled-release bioadhesive microcapsules containing varying amounts of polyacrylic acid, hydroxypropylmethyl cellulose, and carboxymethyl cellulose have been developed. The microcapsules are loaded with radio-opaque barium sulfate. The microcapsules are mixed with bioadhesive agents, packed into standard capsules, and fed with water to fasting rabbits. The measurements for gastric emptying time and the time to reach the colon were conducted by repeated x-ray photography at regular intervals. Marked delay in gastric emptying time was observed compared to the control non-bioadhesive dosage form of barium sulfate. Intestinal transit time was consistant with the control, suggesting no interaction of the bioadhesive polymer with the intestinal mucosa.[163]

Studies have been carried out to elucidate some of the factors affecting release of a peptide, D-Trp-LHRH (luteinizing hormone releasing hormone) analog. Release rates of D-Trp-LHRH, which had been microencapsulated as the acetate salt, were measured in phosphate buffer. During these measurements, samples of microcapsules were taken for analysis by gel-permeation chromatography to obtain polymer molecular weight distributions, by nuclear magnetic resonance to determine ratios of acetate and terminal polymer carboxylate groups to D-Trp-LHRH and lactoyl to glycoyl ratios, and by scanning electron microscopy to monitor changes in the appearance of the microcapsules. This study suggests that release of D-Trp-LHRH from poly(glycolide-co-dl-lactide) microcapsules involves not only diffusion of the peptide through a porous structure created by degradation and dissolution of the polymer matrix, but also binding of the basic peptide to terminal polymer carboxylate groups. Thus, the polymer matrix appears to behave as a weak acid ion-exchange resin during the second phase of peptide release. Subsequent degradation of the polymer matrix in the third phase permits resumption of peptide release.[164]

Synthetic double-stranded RNA can be a potent inducer of interferon, which is a nonspecific inhibitor of viral replication. Poly(I.C), therefore, has potential for use in the prevention of viral infections. One of the major disadvantages, however, of using poly(I.C) therapeutically is its poor bioavailability due to rapid clearance from the body. In an attempt to enhance its bioavailability, an injectable, biodegradable microcapsule formulation has been developed which is designed to release poly(I.C) at a preprogrammed rate and duration. Several prototype batches of poly(I.C) microcapsules have been prepared using a phase-separation microencapsulation process.[165]

Microencapsulation technology has potential in the development of new mammalian cell-culture techniques, membrane bioreactors, and as new forms of treatment for a number of metabolic diseases of various organs. Goosen and McKnight[166] studied chemical modification of deacetylated chitin for the microencapsulation of mammalian cells. The molecular weight of the chitosan was a key factor in membrane formation with alginate. The type of terminating (reactive) group or distance of the group from the main polymerization did not appear to be a major factor in membrane synthesis.

Microencapsulation of living tissue in a biocompatible, semipermeable membrane has great clinical potential in the treatment of hormone-deficient diseases, such as diabetes. The success of such treatment is highly dependent on the physical properties of the microcapsules if the problems of immune rejection are to be overcome. Maleki et al.[167] studied the effects of the chemical composition and solution viscosity of alginate, and also of poly-l-lysine molecular weight on microcapsule shape and permeability. These authors report that highly spherical alg-lysine-alg microcapsules with an ultra smooth surface can be formed by the correct choice of the alginate sample, and that the permeability of the membranes may be controlled by the molecular weight of poly-lysine used in the encapsulation procedure.

Retinoids are experimental vitamin A-like compounds under investigation because of their potential to prevent chemical carcinogenesis without the toxicity of vitamin A. Inclusion of these unstable materials in the diets of test animals requires that the compounds be protected from oxidation, light, moisture, and decomposition induced by bacteria and by elevated temperatures. Swynnerton et al.[168] have prepared stabilized, encapsulated forms of certain synthetic retinoids.

Although a number of encapsulated formulations and enteric-coated tablets containing ethiofos gave excellent results in *in vitro* screening tests, oral administration in beagle dogs and rhesus monkeys provided only low plasma concentrations of unchanged drug and the unbound form of the metabolite. Subsequent experiments with radiolabeled ethiofos indicated that the drug was rapidly metabolized in the GI tract following its release. Thus, the objective of developing formulations of ethiofos that were stable under acidic conditions, yet would give release near neutral pH, was accomplished.[169]

Several methods are available for preparing reservoir microcapsules. Most can be classified under one of three categories: coacervation, coagulation, or fluidized bed coating. Reservoir microcapsules are characterized by a drug core surrounded by a polymer wall. Drug release from reservoir microcapsules is zero-order and follows Flick's first law, as long as the drug is present as an excess solid in equilibrium with a saturated solution. These microcapsules typically contain 80% drug. Solvent evaporation has recently become popular for preparing microspheres, especially in combination with biodegradable polyester polymers. This technique, however, produces monolithic microspheres in which the drug is dissolved or suspended in the polymer. Drug release from microspheres is first-order and decreases with time nonlinearly. Typically, drug loading is about 20%. The use of fluidized bed processes for the preparation of injectable microcapsules from biodegradable and other polymers was first described in 1976. This highly versatile technique has been used to prepare microcapsules from several drugs, such as progesterone, lidocaine, norethindrone, levonorgestrel, testosterone, methadone, and estradiol. The microcapsules prepared ranged from a few to 1000 microns in diameter. Most of the biodegradable polyesters have been used for preparing microcapsules by this process. These include polylactide, polyglycolide, and caprolactone-co-lactide. Other polymers used have been ethylcellulose, polyvinyl alcohol, and cellulose acetate phthalate.[170]

Chattaraj et al.[171] have investigated the development of a viable microencapsulated controlled-release drug delivery system. Microcapsules containing ranitidine hydrochloride, which was selected as the core material, were prepared by phase-separation coacervation of ethylcellulose in nonaqueous solvents. The effects of different concentrations of the coacervation-inducing agent polyisobutylene on drug release were studied.

While microencapsulation is used in the formulation of several drug products, two recent successful products include A.H. Robin's Micro-K and Parke Davis' ERYC. Micro-K extencap is a hard gelatin capsule containing small crystalline particles of potassium chloride. Each particle of potassium chloride is microencapsulated by a patended process of the Eurand Company with a polymeric coating, which allows for controlled release of potassium and chloride ions over an 8- to 10-h period. The microencapsulation process avoids the likelihood of highly localized concentrations of potassium chloride and potential mucosal ulceration in the GI tract.

Damon Biotech has developed a unique living-cell encapsulation technique called Encapcel, which can be utilized to deliver drugs. This technique is especially suitable for new pharmaceutical products emerging from the biotechnology industry that need to be administered on a repeated basis, but can be damaged by conventional drug delivery methods. In the Encapcel technique, a particular drug is encapsulated using very small pores in the surrounding capsule membrane. Through diffusion, the drug flows out of the pores until each capsule is emptied. After emptying, the capsule dissolves.

J.   *Microparticles — nannoparticles*

Cultivation of anchored cells *in vitro* requires adhesion to a substrate. Cells do not attach directly, but rather, attach and spread on an extracellular matrix that is deposited on the substrate. Collagen is a component of the extracellular matrix and has proven in the past to be an effective promoter of cell attachment and growth in monolayer cultures. SoloHill collagen microcarriers use denatured collagen (gelatin) coated on a copolymer plastic sphere. Most cell lines attach and grow rapidly on SoloHill collagen microcarriers. The microcarriers are solid spheres, so there are no requirements for hydration and no problems with absorption of toxic materials during long-term use or breakdown of the bead during freeze-thaw cell harvesting. This has practical advantages in large-scale applications in two ways. First, the amount of media spent in hydration of competitive microcarriers increases the effective cost, and second, the resulting increase in handling steps increases the chance of contamination.

The microcarriers are solid so that toxic materials are not absorbed and harvesting by way of freeze-thaw or ultrasonication is not difficult. Proteolytic enzyme harvesting is gentle and rapid, with viable cell recovery of better than 95%. Furthermore, harvested cells have been successfully replated on monolayer cultures, as well as plastic, glass, and collagen substrates. The ease with which anchorage-dependent cells can be harvested and replated suggests that glass microcarriers may be used in intermediate stages of scale-up applications. Whatever viable infected cells are required, the use of SoloHill glass microcarriers has met with success.

Under development at SoloHill are industrial processes in which particulate material, such as microcarriers, is held in liquid suspension, often requiring filters to separate the particles from the liquid (harvested cells and spent media). The commonly used woven-wire screen is actually three-dimensional in nature and in a short time clogs (known as "blinding"). SoloHill has developed a two-dimensional biofilter, which all but eliminates blinding. Using spirally wound triangular-shaped wire to form a cylinder, with the apex pointing inward, the media and harvested cells are drawn through the slots and carried up the center of the biofilter. The microcarriers remain in the bioreactor to be reused or discarded.

SoloHill macroporous and collagen-coated macroporous microcarriers may be used where anchorage-dependent cells will be damaged, even in gentle stirring. Made from a polystyrene-like material, the porosity is greater than 90% by volume. Pore diameter can be controlled from 20 to 150 microns, with high uniformity of pore size per bead. All pores are interconnected, with uniform channels ranging from 0.5 to 25 microns. The microcarriers appear to be highly permeable to fluids, therefore nutrients, as well as excreted products or biowaste, may be freely exchanged. Micrometer sizes are available in the 250-micron range, but these can be modified. Materials are nontoxic, and collagen coating is expected to aid in rapid attachment and spreading[172] (see Figures 8.9 through 8.13).

SoloHill has also developed an advanced technology that has been used to modify surface collagen microcarriers to greatly enhance cell attachment. The FACT (fast attachment collagen treated) microcarriers are available in the same sizes and specific gravities as their standard collagen-coated counterparts. Attachment is much quicker due to the propri-

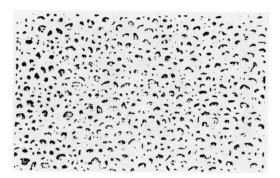

Figure 8.9 Macroporous microcarriers. (From SoloHill Engineering, Inc., Ann Arbor, MI, brochure. With permission.)

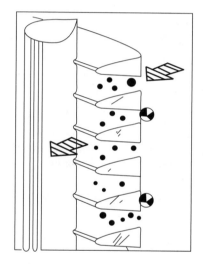

Figure 8.10 Biofilter. (From SoloHill Engineering, Inc., Ann Arbor, MI, brochure. With permission.)

etary surface modification. Spreading is rapid due to the presence of the collagen extracellular matrix.

Biodegradable microparticles of cross-linked starch (maltodextrin) have been designed by Artursson et al.[173] as carriers of proteins and low molecular weight drugs *in vivo.* Macromolecules are immobilized in the microparticles in high yields (i.e., up to 40% of the dry weight of the immobilized protein). The optimal conditions of immobilization were investigated by varying the concentration of starch and acryloyl groups and the amount of additional cross-linking agent. Exclusion of the cross-linking agent gave maximum immobilization of the micromolecules. Microparticles based on starch with small amounts of acryloyl groups were completely degraded after incubation with amyloglucosidase.

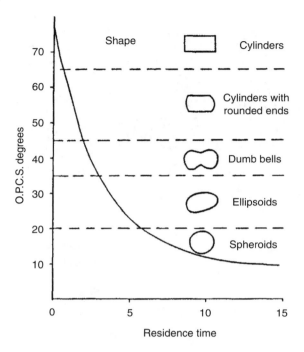

Figure 8.11 The change in shape represented by OPCS (one plane critical stability) values during successful spheronization. (From Capsugel, *Capsule Update*, division of Warner-Lambert, Greenwood, SC. With permission.)

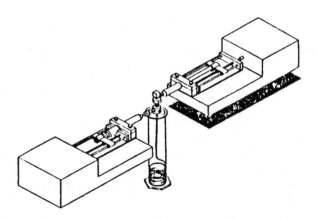

Figure 8.12 Device to spin the fibers. (From DiLuccio, R.C. et al., *Proc. 14th Symp. Controlled Release of Bioactive Materials*, Aug. 2–5, 1987, Controlled Release Society, Inc., Lincolnshire, IL. With permission.)

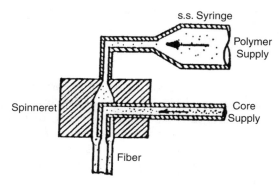

Figure 8.13 Spinnert diagram. (From DiLuccio, R.C. et al., *Proc. 14th Int. Symp. Controlled Release of Bioactive Materials,* Aug. 2–5, 1987, Controlled Release Society, Inc., Lincolnshire, IL. With permission.)

Natural macromolecules, such as proteins or celluloses, appeared to offer the most promise as degradable bases for nanoparticles. For example, the general production method has successfully yielded nanoparticles of human serum albumin, bovine serum albumin, ethylcellulose, casein, and gelatin from a group of suitable macromolecules. Gelatin was selected as a model macromolecule because of its ready availability, low antigenicity, and previous use in parenteral formulations.[174] Human serum albumin was selected because of its ability to bind drugs and its potential use in medicine. The process by which nanoparticles can be made was derived from the coacervation method of microencapsulation.

Colloidal preparations are widely used in nuclear medicine as carriers of radioisotopes for study of the morphology, blood flow, and functions of various organs in the body. One of the most common preparations for visualizing the liver is ^{99m}TC-sulfur colloid, which has an average particle size of 1 μm.[175] Human serum albumin (HSA) microspheres of similar size and labeled with technetium have been proposed for the assessment of reticuloendothelial function, since they have a more uniform particle size than the sulfur colloid.[176]

Gelatin, and to a lesser extent albumin, contain large amounts of lysine. Fluorescein isothiocyanate (FITC) is known to conjugate to amino groups, particularly in lysine. If FITC can be conjugated to the surface of gelatin or to albumin nanoparticles, it would show that such surface amino groups are not totally consumed in the glutaraldehyde cross-linking process. These amino acid surface sites may be utilized to bind drug molecules, and then the nanoparticle system may be used to deliver the drug to its desired site of action. The results of experimentation with FITC-labeled nanoparticles have two important ramifications. First, it seems that free amino groups are available on the surface of nanoparticles; these surface sites might be suitable for drug or pro-drug binding. Second, since some tumor lines appear to be able to take up nanoparticles, and since it seems possible to incorporate cytotoxic agents into nanoparticles, a new delivery system for cancer therapy may be devised.[177]

K.   Colloids

Colloidal dosage forms, such as emulsions, liposomes, suspensions, and microspheres, represent important ways of delivering drugs, both orally and parenterally. The recent interest in liposomes, as discussed previously, has stimulated the use of other colloids for the targeting of drugs and therapeutic agents to specific organs and sites in the body. Emulsion systems, both in simple and multiple varieties, have been of considerable use in cancer chemotherapy.[178]

Yamahira and colleagues[179] have studied the effect of lipid formulations on drug absorption and gastric emptying. They have found that the absorption of a highly lipid-soluble model drug depends upon the volume of lipid administered as well as the lipid's viscosity. They also reported on absorption and the digestibility of oily vehicles and compared a digestible medium-chain triglyceride to poorly digestible N-α-methylbenzyl-linoleamide. They concluded that the digestibility of the lipid vehicle was the major factor promoting the absorption of a model drug with high lipid solubility, no doubt through an effect on GI mobility and transit time.

Noguchi et al.[180] have studied the lymphatic transport of lipid-soluble compounds, such as Sudan Blue and vitamin A, concluding that both bile salts and phosphatidylcholine were needed for efficient lymphatic transport. Nakamoto and associates[181] investigated the enhancement of lymphatic transport of orally active agents by both oil-in-water (o/w) and water-in-oil (w/o) emulsions. Somewhat surprisingly, they found that the w/o emulsions gave the best effect. Ogata and associates[182] reported enhanced absorption of methyl orange from an o/w emulsion system when it was compared to an aqueous system; they proposed that the adsorption of methyl orange at the surface of the emulsion droplets accounted for the effect.

Parenterally administered emulsions can serve a number of different purposes. Parenterals can help administer a poorly water-soluble drug achieve a sustained-release effect or obtain site-specific delivery. Dardel and colleagues[183] described an emulsion system based upon a commercial soybean-oil emulsion for intravenous administration of diazepam. Diazepam has poor water solubility, and its intravenous administration in a formulated solution can produce side effects, such as pain and thrombophlebitis. The emulsion system considerably reduces these side effects, but does not alter the bioavailability of the drug. Jeppson and Ljunberg[184] have described the parenteral administration of a variety of drugs using modified vegetable-oil emulsions. In the case of intravenously administered barbiturates, they reported that the emulsion system offered a prolonged period of action.[185] Similar types of enhancement have been investigated for w/o emulsion systems used for the administration of medicinal agents by intramuscular or subcutaneous routes.

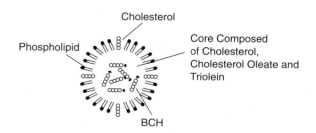

Cholesterol

Phospholipid

Core Composed
of Cholesterol,
Cholesterol Oleate and
Triolein

BCH

Figure 8.14 Schematic representation of VLDL-resembling phospholipids submicron emulsion-containing cholesterol-based drug, BCH. (With permission, Wiley, *J. Pharm. Sci.*, 91, 6, 1405, 2002.)

Useful information can be obtained from studies on other types of parenteral emulsions, for example, emulsions used as diagnostic agents (iodinated systems), as parenteral nutrition (fat emulsions), or as synthetic blood substitutes (fluorocarbon emulsions). Various oils of vegetable origin (soybean, cottonseed, and safflower) are regarded as nontoxic and biodegradable. In contrast, mineral oils (such as liquid paraffin and squalene) are not biodegradable. Such properties can affect the clearance of emulsion systems and, consequently, the fate of a drug contained therein.

A variety of fluorocarbon liquids have also been evaluated in animals and, more recently, in man as constituting a readily available substitute for red blood cells. The route of administration and the intended use for the emulsion will dictate particle size. With intravenous emulsions, for example, there are rigid requirements regarding globule size. Large globules can produce emboli in certain blood vessels. Toxicity, in general, is also related to particle size and particle-size distribution of colloidal systems, including emulsions.[186,187]

Other colloidal systems are also under active investigation for parenteral administration of drugs. The use of magnetic microspheres for site direction of drug substances has been described. These microspheres are based upon albumin and are biodegradable, but what differentiates them from other microspheres is their iron oxide content. Drugs can be incorporated into these microspheres, and it is possible to increase significantly the concentration of anticancer agents at certain targets by using a powerful magnetic field. Another approach involves development of small particles in the 50 to 500 μm range by the polymerization of micellar systems. These particles have been termed nanocapsules and can be made from biodegradable materials, such as polycyanacrylates (see Figure 8.14).[188,189]

L.   Microemulsions

An interesting characteristic of microemulsions is that when even a small amount of a mixture of surfactant and cosurfactant is added to a biphasic water–oil system, a theromodynamically stable, optically transparent, isotropic mixture is formed spontaneously.[190] The diameter of the droplets in a microemulsion is in the range of 100 to 1000 Å, whereas the diameter of droplets in a kinetically stable macroemulsion is 5000 Å. Because the droplets are small, a microemulsion offers advantages as a carrier for drugs that are poorly soluble in water.

Microemulsions can also make oil-soluble drugs easier to administer by making water an external phase. Microemulsions were first introduced by Hoar and Schulman in 1943.[191] They obtained a microemulsion by first preparing a normal emulsion of soap, water, and hydrocarbon and then adding a medium-chain alcohol, such as pentanol. A transparent "solution" resulted when a certain concentration of alcohol was added to the emulsion. The hydrophilic–lipophilic balance (HLB) system has been used for the selection of surfactants for microemulsions. Using this system, w/o microemulsions are formed using emulsifiers within the HLB range of 3 to 6, while o/w microemulsions are formed within the range of 8 to 18. The choice of emulsifiers is determined by the average HLB requirement of the proposed microemulsion.[192,193]

Several physiological applications of microemulsions have been reported in the literature.[194,195] Artificial blood composed of fluorocarbon oil in water is a unique example of a system in which microemulsions have an important role. Certain fluorocarbon oils are able to store oxygen and release it in the presence of carbon dioxide; however, to be practical, such an oil must be made miscible with blood. Microemulsions with a dispersed phase of less than 1000 Å are practical because they can pass through the capillaries. Microemulsions can also be used to prepare oral liquid dosage forms of hydrophobic drugs. These dosage forms are easy to administer to children and people who have difficulty swallowing solid dosage forms.

There are several other advantages of formulating drugs in microemulsions. For example, a drug administered in microemulsion will be immediately available for absorption and, in most cases, is more rapidly and more efficiently absorbed than the same amount of drug administered in a tablet or capsule. Microemulsions are excellent delivery forms for certain hormones, diuretics, and antibiotics. Furthermore, for the absorption of a hydrophobic drug, such as indomethacin, which has very low aqueous solubility, a microemulsion would be an ideal delivery system.

Halbert and co-workers,[196] have experimented with the incorporation of lipid-soluble antineoplastic agents into a microemulsion. They mixed lipid-soluble cytotoxic agents with low-density lipoproteins (LDLs) and incorporated them into a microemulsion. LDLs have aroused interest as novel drug carriers for cytotoxic agents. They have targeting potential because rapidly dividing cells require large quantities of cholesterol for cell-membrane synthesis. When cytotoxic agents are incorporated into a system with LDLs, it is thought that the system will preferentially deliver the drugs to cancer cells, providing a more specific drug delivery system.

Jayakrishan and colleagues[197] have demonstrated how commercial surfactants solubilize hydrocortisone. Their study provides a guideline for the

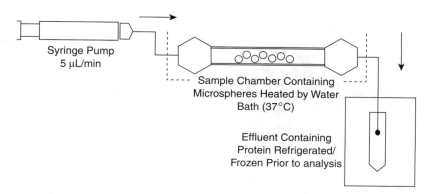

Figure 8.15 Illustration of the system used for the *in vitro* release of protein from microspheres. (With permission, Kluwer Publ., *Pharm. Res.* 19, 7, 1046, 2002.)

formulation of cosmetic and pharmaceutical emulsions. In other research, microemulsions have been used to study the clinical potency of analgesics, such as methyl salicylate,[198] and tetracycline hydrochloride formulations.[199]

Medical-grade silicone elastomers, commonly referred to as polydimethyl-siloxanes (PDMS), are biocompatible polymers useful as matrices for transdermal drug delivery systems (TDDS). Until recently, delivery of drugs from hydrophobic PDMS were limited to lipophilic and nonionic drugs, such as steroids. More recently, it has been demonstrated that enhanced release of hydrophilic and ionic drug species, such as morphine sulfate, sodium salicylate, sulfanilamide, and indomethacin, can be achieved from silicone matrices when coformulated with the appropriate hydrophilic excipients.

Aguadisch et al.[200] immobilized drugs in hydrophilic and hydrophobic microemulsions in silicone matrices and characterized the release kinetics of progesterone, propranolol, and indomethacien from these microemulsion reservoir-type elastomer matrices (see Figures 8.15 through 8.17).

M.   Hollow fibers

Certain characteristics of fibers make them attractive as possible candidates as drug delivery systems.[201] Their inherent high surface/volume ratio and high-loading capacity make them particularly useful devices to deliver drugs at specified rates. These systems can be formulated by proper selection of materials that would allow them to be hydrophilic, bioadhesive, pH-sensitive, and biodegradable. Fibers have been considered for drug delivery by a number of investigators. Dunn and Lewis[202] have proposed the use of "melt spinning" technology to develop delivery systems that are capable of prolonging delivery of contraceptive steroids. Eenink et al.[203] have found that poly-L-lactic acid can be spun by wet spinning to produce a biodegradable fiber delivery system that can be loaded after they are formed. These fibers have been reported to be potential candidates for subdermal delivery of medications.

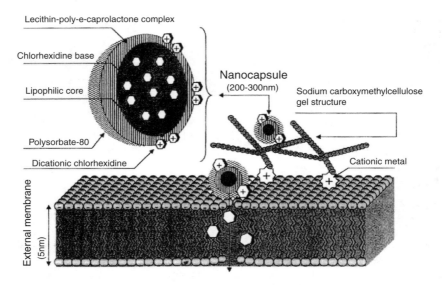

Figure 8.16 Schematic representation of a possible adsorption mechanism of chlorhexidine base-loaded PCL nanocapsules onto stratum corneum-associated bacteria membrane. (With permission, Elsevier, *J. Control Rel.*, 82, 319–334, 2002.)

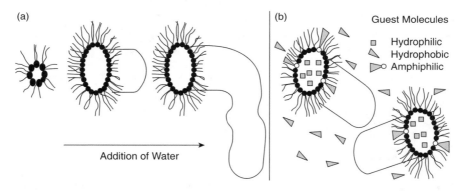

Figure 8.17 Microemulsion-based gels: (a) schematic representation of the formation of lecithin gels upon addition of water to small phosphatidyl choline reverse micelles in apolar solvents; (b) localization of solubilized guest molecules within lecithin gels (Reprinted courtesy of Elsevier Science. With permission, Advanstar, Elsevier, *Pharm. Tech.*, March 2002, 150.)

The work by DiLuccio et al.[204] describes the method of preparation of loaded hollow fibers by use of a phase-inversion spinning process. In this process, a solution of the sheath polymer and the drug suspended or dissolved in the lumen fluid are pumped simultaneously through a coaxial spinning die and quenched in a coagulant, causing formation of the fibers. After being formed, the fibers can be cut into uniform lengths and utilized for oral delivery of drugs (see Figures 8.12 and 8.13).

The release properties of salicylic acid and chlorpheniramine maleate from two hollow fiber fabrics have been investigated by Britton et al.[205] The two fabrics that were studied included a hollow nonwoven rayon fabric and a nonwoven polyester fabric. Scanning electron microscopy verified the presence of both drugs in the hollow fibers. The dissolution studies indicated that after a short burst effect, a slow release of drug over a 3- to 4-h time period could be achieved.

N. Ultrasonically controlled

Controlled-release systems using polymers as rate-controlling membranes were first introduced in the 1960s. However, one problem central to this field is that all the systems so far developed display release rates that are either constant or decay with time. However, there are a number of situations in which augmented delivery could be beneficial, such as insulin for diabetic patients, gastric acid inhibitors for ulcer control, antianginals, and others. Examples of various control techniques include pumps that can be activated by pH stimuli, nonerodible polymers containing enzymes that cause the polymer to swell and regulate delivery in response to external stimuli, pH-sensitive erodible polymers containing enzymes in hydrogels that degrade more rapidly in response to external stimuli, lectin drug systems that release additional drug due to affinity of an external molecule for the lectin, and temperature-sensitive polymers and polymer drug-magnetic systems that release additional drug in response to an oscillating external magnetic field.[206]

Kost et al.[207] have introduced the use of ultrasound to externally regulate the release of drug from polymeric matrices. The bioerodible polymers were composed of polyanhydrides and copolymers of poly(bis-carboxyphenoxy) propane with sebacic acid anhydride. The mechanism by which ultrasound enhances drug release from subcutaneously implanted bioerodible polymeric material is currently under investigation. One possible explanation is that ultrasound enhances the penetration of water into the polymer, exposing more linkages for hydrolysis and therefore higher degradation and release rates (see Figure 8.18).

O. Liquid-crystalline phases

Lyotropic liquid-crystalline phases have been investigated *in vitro* for use as sustained-release systems. It has been shown that the isotropic, cubic phase of a lipid/water mixture in water in these applications serves as a thermodynamically and kinetically stable matrix.[208] The formation of lyotropic liquid-crystalline (LC) phases in ternary and quaternary polar lipid/water/ peptide systems has also been investigated. Released peptide was determined by immunoreactivity of the peptide in plasma. It was found that the peptide was released from the LC phase and systematically absorbed in pseudo-zero-order during the observation period. The authors proposed that lyotropic LC phases may act as a parenteral depot for peptides and that the

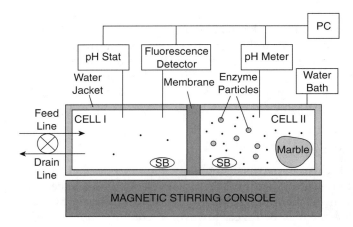

Figure 8.18 Diagram of test cell for rhythmic pulsatile delivery of GnRH. Both Cells I and II are 80 ml and are charged with 75-ml solutions, which are stirred vigorously using magnetic stir bars (SB) and maintained at 37°C by circulation from a waterbath through water jackets. Cell I is fed at 1.36 to 1.38 ml/min by 50 mM saline containing and 50 mM glucose and 0.01 wt.% bronopol (antibacterial), is drained at equal rate, and in pH stated at 7.0. Cell II initially contains glucose-free saline solution, a 12.5-g piece of marble, and small particles of polyacrylamide gel containing enzymes. Small dots refer to f-GnRH molecules, initially introduced at 1 µg/ml into Cell II. pH in Cell II is monitored by a pH meter, and appearance of f-GnRH in Cell I is recorded by a spectrofluorimter, with both instruments sending data to a personal computer. (With permission, Elsevier, *J. Control Rel.*, 81, 1–6, 2002.)

peptide can be protected against biological degradation when incorporated in the LC phase.[209]

P.   *Time-controlled "explosion systems"*

A new type of controlled-release system named time-controlled "explosion systems" (TES) is a mass of spheres containing metoprolol tartrate as a model drug and a swelling agent (low-substituted hydroxypropylcellulose, L-HPC). The spheres are coated with ethylcellulose (EC) for the purpose of releasing the drug after a certain period of time. The lag time produced was found to be proportional to the thickness of the membrane. The transit and behavior of the TES has been studied by recovering the particles from the GI tracts of beagle dogs following oral administration. These studies demonstrated that TES can act as a controlled-release system by combining the particles with different lag times.[210]

Q.   *Mammalian cells*

The use of mammalian cells as potential vehicles for the delivery of plant toxins to specific sites *in vivo* has been investigated. Ricin is a potent plant toxin isolated from the beans of the castor oil plant *Ricinus communis*. It is composed of two polypeptide chains (A and B) linked by a disulphide bond. The B chain of the toxin binds to cell-surface receptors containing terminal galactose residues. This toxin is internalized by the cell, and the A chain is liberated into the cytoplasm. The action of the A chain is enzymic. Once in the cytoplasm, it rapidly inhibits protein synthesis by inactivating 60S ribosomal subunits. The natural capacity of cells to internalize such a toxin by receptor-mediated endocytosis, and to later release some of their contained toxin to the extracellular space, has been described.[211] In 1978, Sandvig et al.,[212] reported the release of radiolabeled TCA-precipitable material from cells that had been treated with ^{125}I-ricin. This result suggested that some of the toxin internalized by cells could evade degradation by the lysosomal system and cycle back to the cell surface in an intact form.

R. Sutures

Antimicrobial sutures developed by Stephenson[213] are characterized by a multifilament structure impregnated with an antimicrobial agent and surface-coated with a covering of polyurethane polymer. The concentration of antimicrobial agent within the suture is preferably from 0.5 to 2%, although concentrations outside these ranges can be used with good results. The suture may be impregnated with antimicrobial solution by any convenient method, such as dipping, spraying, or soaking. The impregnated suture may be dried over hot rolls, in a warm-air oven, by a continous stream of warm air, or by any other convenient method. Drying temperatures and times are selected to avoid degradation of the suture or antimicrobial compositions. In general, temperatures of 80 to 100°C give rapid drying with no adverse effect on either the suture or the antimicrobial compound.

The report by Gilbert[214] has described iodine-polyvinylpyrrolidone products in which the iodine is bound within solid polyvinylpyrrolidone, with solidified cinnamic alcohol adherently distributed throughout. The novel solid iodine-containing emulsion applied with an applicator stick or swab enables iodine to be activated when the emulsion comes in contact with the moisture or temperature of the skin, blood, or blood serum, which liquifies the cinnamic alcohol at about 37 or 38°C.

According to Leveen and Joyce,[215] prolonged germicidal properties can be obtained with elemental iodine, a polymer of 2-pyrrolidone, and a polymeric poly-basic acid, which is isotonic to the skin and has a molecular configuration sufficient to slowly release carboxyl groups and stay free of absorption by the body. A polymeric acid (molecular weight 250,000) is preferred as the third component. The amount of acidic activity extender incorporated into the new "iodofor" composition may range from 5 to about 50 parts by weight of the total pyrrolidone-iodine composition, but is preferably within a range of about 10 to 20. It has been found that such a level is adequate to maintain the entire composition sufficiently acidic to maintain its bactericidal activity.

An alternative mode of this system is the formation of a new biocidal suture material. In this case, a polymer of 2-pyrrolidone is melt-spun into a continuous fiber. This fiber is then dipped into a hot solution of an aqueous alcoholic tincture of iodine at a temperature of 110°F, for 30 seconds to one minute. Approximately 15% of the total weight of elemental iodine is taken up. While the suture is still warm, it is dipped into a warm solution of polyacrylic acid (M.W. 250KD) until 10% by weight of the poly-pyrroli-done-iodine complex is impregnated. This product is then dried at room temperature to form a biocidal suture having long-term activity, as well as excellent tensile strength and knotting ability. Since the suture is biocidal, it may be woven into a polyfilament.

S.   Microsealed drug delivery

The microsealed drug delivery (MDD) system is so named on the basis of the fact that a drug reservoir (a suspension of solid drug in a water-miscible hydrophilic polymer) is dispersed homogeneously, as numerous microscopic spheres, in a cross-linked polymer matrix. The sizes of the microscopic, drug-containing, liquid-compartment spheres show a normal, bell-shaped distribution, which ranges from 5 to 50 microns. This microscopic dispersion of drug reservoir is achieved by high-energy shearing agitation during the cross-linking of the polymer matrix. Typical examples of the MDD system are testosterone-releasing transdermal therapeutic devices; contraceptive ste-roids, such as norethindrone-releasing vaginal ring-type delivery devices; cylinder-shaped drug delivery devices for he long-term intrauterine delivery of estradiol, and norgestomet released in a subdermal implant for the sub-cutaneous controlled administration to achieve estrus synchronization in livestock (see Figure 8.19).[216]

VI.   Recent advances

The buccal delivery system reported by 3M Company (Cydot) consists of a flexible mucoadhesive matrix composed of a blend of poly(acrylic acid) (Carbopol 934 P) and polyisobutylene (Vistanex). The patch device is unidi-rectional with a polyurethane backing layer. The patch is intended for appli-cation to the upper gum. A transmucosal therapeutic system was also reported for the buccal delivery of LHRH, with results indicating the feasi-bility of controlled-release transmucosal delivery of the peptide drug. The review by Shojael et al.[221] discusses and lists several novel buccal delivery systems containing a variety of therapeutic agents and lists components used as oral mucosal-permeation enhancers.

Baur[224] has reviewed material trends in colonic drug delivery. An exam-ple of a simple-matrix dosage form for colon targeting is gum tablets with embedded dexamethasone.

In this delivery system, methacrylic acid copolymers, cellulose acetate phthalate (CAP), or hydroxypropyl methylcellulose phthalate are used as

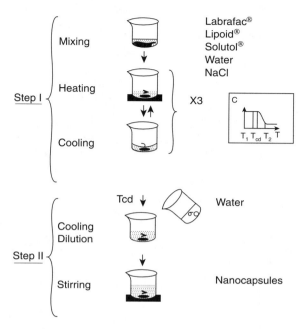

Figure 8.19 Formulation process of lipidic nanocapsules. Step I corresponds to the determination of the cooling-dilution temperature (T_{cd}) after applying three temperature cycles to the system. Step II leads to the formation of nanocapsules by the fast addition of cold water. (With permission, Kluwer Publ., *Pharm. Res.*, 19, 6, 875, 2002.)

conventional enteric-coating materials. A few pro-drugs, such as olsalazine, balsalazine, ipsalazine, and glycoside pro-drugs, such as beta-D glucosides of dexamethasone, prednisolone, naloxone, and nalmefene, could be better targeted for colon delivery.[263,264,269,270] Another pro-drug group is composed of drug-dextran-conjugates. Microbially controlled drug delivery systems to the colon are also reported and also studied when coating the matrix and hydrogel formulations with cross-linked chondroitin, pectins, oectates, and cross-linked guar with several drugs. Calciumpectinate has shown promising results in the colon targeting of insulin. A unique idea was the use of a pressure-controlled capsule in colonic targeting. The inner surface of this capsule is coated with an ethylcellulose. The capsule prepared in this way does not disintegrate in the stomach or in the small intestine, but it disintegrates in the colon due to the colonic peristalsis and releases its drug (see Figures 8.20 and 8.21).[224,225]

Nokhodchi and Farid[222] discuss microencapsulation of paracetamol by various emulsion techniques using cellulose acetate phthalate. These authors microencapsulated paracetamol using the emulsion solvent evaporation (ESE), modified emulsion solvent evaporation (MESE), and emulsion non-solvent addition (ENSA) methods. All three methods were reproducible in terms of the drug content, microcapsule size, and release rate of the drug

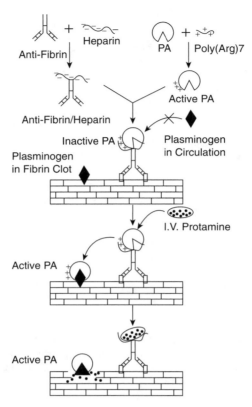

Figure 8.20 Schematic diagram of the ATTEMPS approach. (With permission, Elsevier, *J. Control. Rel.*, 78, 67–79, 2002.)

from the microcapsules. However, significant differences resulted among the three methods in terms of the time necessary for microcapsule formation, drug content, microcapsule size, and drug-release rate. These were not due to batch-to-batch variation.

Acetazolamide has been a highly effective drug for the treatment of glaucoma. However, its use has been limited because of its low solubility and poor permeability characteristics, which cause it to be unsuitable for topical administration. Its current use as an oral dosage form has been associated with a large number of side effects. Singla et al.[223] discuss novel approaches for the topical delivery of this agent. They discuss use of viscosity-imparting agents, gels, liposomes, and cyclodextrins.

Pro-drugs have been used to overcome poor solubility, insufficient stability, incomplete absorption across biological membranes, and premature metabolism to active species. Therefore, various novel attempts were made using pro-drugs as delivery systems, for example, topical delivery of 5-fluorouracil (5-FU) 1,3-bisalkylcarbonyl-5-FU pro-drugs, O-butyryl ester of tilisolol for ophthalmic insert, stabilized dipeptides D-Glu-Ala and D-Asp-Ala

Strategy

Visible-Light Irradiation

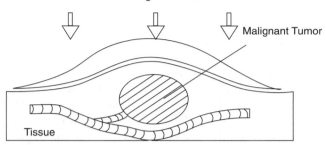

The Photoreactive Gelatin Solution Premixed with an Anticancer Drug
was Spread on a Tissue and Irradiated with Visible Light.

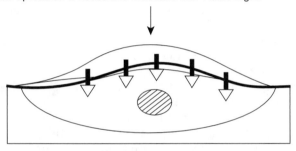

The Drug Release May Inhibit
Tumor Growth, Angiogenesis and Metastasis.

Figure 8.21 Strategy in device directed therapeutic drug delivery system. (With permission from *J. Control Rel.*, 78, 125–131, 2002.)

as pro-moieties for benzyl alcohol (oligopeptide transporter), 5′-O-ester pro-drugd of 3′-azido-2′,3′-dideoxythymidine (AZT) for HIV infection, polyethylene glycol conjugated drugs and pro-drugs, pro-drug of phyllohydroquinone, liposomes containing water-soluble pro-drugs of paclitaxel for the treatment of ovarian and breast cancer, diacyl glyceryl ester pro-drugs of naproxen for slow skin releaase in the skin,[272–275,277,278] Leuenkephalin analogue and ester pro-drugs thereof, cathepsin B-sensitive dipeptide pro-drugs of paclitaxel (Taxol), mitomycin C and doxorubicin, the use of esters of pro-drugs for oral delivery of beta-lactam antibiotics, pro-drugs of gestodene for matrix-type transdermal delivery, immunoliposomes containing 5-fluorouridine pro-drugs, beta-glucuronyl carbamate-based pro-drugs of paclitaxel, and thymidylate synthase inhibitors as potential candidates for ADEPT (antibody-directed enzyme pro-drug therapy). Pro-drugs of Ara-C, for their apoptotic activity, biphenyl acetic acid-beta-cyclodextrin conjugates as colon-targeting pro-drugs, vitamin K pro-drugs, and O-cyclopropane carboxylic acid ester pro-drugs of various beta-blocking agents were investigated.[282,284,286]

Microparticles have an important place in drug delivery. For example, recently, the following studies[297–300] were undertaken for their use: biodegradable poly(DL-lactide glycolide) as a vehicle for allergen-specific vaccines; cationic microparticles for immune stimulatory cpG DNA delivery; inhalable microparticles for the treatment of pulmonary tuberculosis; microparticles entrapping p-DNA-poly(amino acids) complexes for vaccine delivery; microparticles for intranasal immunization; lipid microparticles for parenteral controlled-release device for peptides; fabrication of porous poly(epsilon-caprolactone) microparticles for protein release; preparation of collagen-modified hyaluronan microparticles as antibiotics carriers; porous biodegradable microparticles for delivery of pentamidine;[302–310] microparticles for delivering therapeutic peptides and proteins to the lumen of the small intestine (e.g., elatin microparticles as a protein micronization adjuvant); microparticles for lectin-mediated mucosal delivery, controlled release of transforming growth factor-beta 1 (TGF-beta 1), containing biodegradable polymer microparticles to a bone defect; glucose oxidase-containing microparticles of poly(ethylene glycol)-grafted cationic hydrogels; preparation of magnetic iron–carbon composite microparticles for delivery of anticancer agents;[311–320] production of Eudragit microparticles; formulations of poly(D,L-lactic-co-glycolic acid) microparticles for rapid plasmid DNA delivery; microparticles in MF59; a potent adjuvant combination for a recombinant protein vaccine against HIV-1; PLG microparticles of oral vaccine delivery; antibiotic release from biodegradable PHBV microparticles; development of chitosan-cellulose multicore microparticles for controlled drug delivery; biodegradable microparticles as a delivery system for measles virus cytotoxic T-cell epitopes; and biodegradable microparticles containing colchicine or a colchicine analogue.[321–332]

Gel-microemulsions were used as vaginal spermicides and intravaginal drug delivery vehicles to improve bioavailability through the vaginal/rectal mucosa of microbiocidal drug substances against sexually transmitted diseases. Microemulsions were used also for peridontal anesthesia, indomethacin, phopholipid-based flurbiprofen, and testosterone. Aspirin-tableted microcapsules and preparations of microemulsions using polyglycol fatty acid esters as surfactants for the delivery of protein drugs were also evaluated (see Figures 8.22 and 8.23).[334–346]

Polyphasphazone-based microspheres for insulin delivery were prepared following different procedures: suspension-solvent evaporation, double emulsion-solvent evaporation, and suspension/double emulsion-solvent evaporation. All preparations stimulated anti-insulin antibody production that constantly increased over a period of 8 weeks. Chronic intraperitoneal insulin delivery was achieved using a mechanical pump.

Tozaki et al.[271] reported on the enhanced absorption of insulin and Asu(1,7)eel-calcitonin using novel azopolymer-coated pellets for colon-specific drug delivery, and lipid emulsions as vehicles for enhanced nasal delivery of insulin was investigated. Insulin was delivered using a trans-

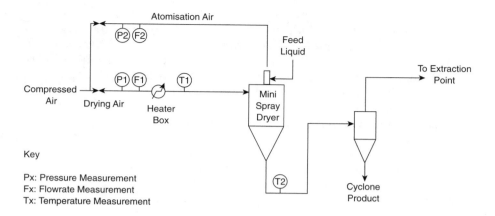

Figure 8.22 Schematic of spray-drying system. (With permission, Elsevier, *J. Control Rel.*, 82, 429–440, 2002.)

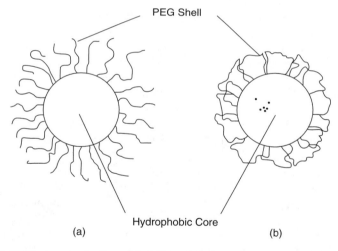

Figure 8.23 PEG-coated micelles with different PEG configurations: (a) PEG anchored to one end, (b) PEG anchored to both ends. (With permission, Wiley, *J. Pharm. Sci.*, 91, 6, 1463, 2002.)

dermal system containing flexible lecithin vesicles and continuous subcutaneous infusion.

Zinc insulin was successfully encapsulated in various polyester and polyanhydride nanosphere formulations using Phase Inversion Nanoencapsulation (PIN). A number of properties of this formulation, including size, release kinetics, bioadhesiveness, and ability to traverse the GI epithelium, are likely to contribute to its oralefficacy. Renard et al.[242] reported on insulin delivery with plasmid DNA. Simple-to-use tools, such as pen devices, were also introduced for insulin delivery. Kawashima[277] reported on the pulmonary delivery of insulin with nebulized DL-lactide/glycolide copolymer (PLGA) nanospheres to prolong hypoglycemic effect. Insulin has been delivered by transdermal iontophoretic and by surface-coated liposomes. Chetty and Chien[280] and Trehan and Ali[281] have described recent novel approaches for insulin delivery. Katre et al.[282] discuss multivesicular liposome (Depo-Foam) technology for the sustained delivery of insulin-like growth factor-I (IGF-I). Ando et al.[283] reported on nasal insulin delivery in rabbits using soybean-derived sterylglucoside and sterol mixtures as novel enhancers in suspension dosage forms. Takenaga et al.[284] reported on microparticle resins as a potential nasal drug delivery system for insulin. Insulin has also been delivered via an enhancer-free ocular device. Kagatani et al.[286] reported on electroresponsive pulsatile depot delivery of insulin from poly(dimethylaminopropylacrylamide) gel in rats. Saudek[287] discuss novel forms, alternate delivery systems, and formulations of insulin. Edelman et al.[288] reported on insulin release from an implantable, polymer-based system with simultaneous release of somatostatin. Kubota et al.[289] found that portal insulin delivery is superior to peripheral delivery in the handling of portally delivered glucose. Taylor et al.[290] reported on the delivery of insulin from aqueous and nonaqueous reservoirs that is governed by a glucose-sensitive gel membrane. Kim and Park[291] discuss modulated insulin delivery from glucose-sensitive, hydrogel dosage forms, and Bremseth and Pass[292] reported on their observations on the delivery of insulin by jet injection. Li et al.[293] discuss gellan film as an implant for insulin delivery. Gellan gum is an anionic polysaccharide produced by the aerobic fermentation of *Pseudomonas elodea* in batch culture. Lee and McAuliffe[294] discuss photomechanical transdermal delivery of insulin *in vivo*, and Mitra and Perzon[295] reported on the enhanced pulmonary insulin delivery by lung lavage fluid and phospholipids. Kisel et al.[296] reported on the liposomes, with phosphatidylethanol as a carrier for the oral delivery of insulin in rats, and Venugopalan et al.[297] discuss preparation and characterization of pelleted, bioadhesive, polymeric nanoparticles for the buccal delivery of insulin.

Charrueau et al.[253] have discussed poloxamer 407 as a thermogelling and adhesive polymer for rectal administration of short-chain fatty acids. Sznitowski et al.[254] investigated diazepam lipospheres based on Witepsol and lecithin intended for oral or rectal[267] delivery. Burstein et al.[255] reported on the absorption of phenytoin from rectal suppositories formulated with a polyethylene glycol base. It appeared that absorption of phenytoin from polyethylene glycol rectal suppositories in healthy subjects was highly variable and unpredictable; therefore, this formulation could not be recommended. Kim and Ku[256] reported on the enhanced absorption of indomethacin after oral or rectal administration of a self-emulsifying system containing this agent to rats. Dash et al.[257] reported on the development of a rectal nicotine-delivery system for the treatment of ulcerative colitis. Barichello et al.[258] found enhanced rectal absorption of insulin-loaded Pluronic F-127 gel containing unsaturated fatty acids. Miyazaki et al.[259] observed that thermally reversible xyloglucan gels can be used for rectal drug delivery; indomethacin was used in this study. According to Cook et al.,[260] cisapride was administered rectally in horses. However, they found that this method is not clinically useful. Sallai et al.[261] found that trimethoprim was suitable for further clinical pharmacological investigation. Watanabe et al.[262] reported on pharmacodynamics of recombinant human granulocyte colony-stimulating factor (rhG-CSF) after administration of a rectal dosage vehicle; it was found to be a promising drug delivery system. According to Van Os et al.,[263] azathioprine delivered to the colon by delayed-release oral and rectal foam formulations considerably reduced systemic 6-mercaptopurine bioavailability.

The therapeutic potential of these colonic delivery methods, which can potentially limit toxicity by local delivery of high doses of azothioprine, should be investigated in patients with inflammatory bowel disease. Pharmacokinetics of temazepam, apomorphine, and propylene glycol were studied.[268] The data presented by Kondo et al.[266] suggested that alpha-cyclodextrin in combination with xanthan gum is particularly effective in improving the rectal bioavailability of morphine from hollow-type suppositories. Miyazaki et al.[267] suggested that thermally gelling poloxamine Synperonic T908 solution can be used as a vehicle for rectal drug delivery. Antimalarials have also been used in rectal suppositories. The data presented by Noach et al.[269] indicate that although verapamil is able to enhance the absorption of hydrophilic compounds *in vivo*, practical application of this agent for this purpose did not seem feasible. Diwan and Park[252] found that pegylation enhances protein stability during encapsulation in PLGA microspheres.

Wildemeersch and Schacht[247] reported on a pilot study on the treatment of menorrhagia with a novel "frameless," intrauterine, levonorgestrel-releasing drug delivery system. The FibroPlant levonorgestrel IUSD is effective in significantly reducing the amount of menstrual blood loss in women with menorrhagia. Strong endometrial suppression is the principal mechanism explaining both the effect on menstrual blood loss and the contraceptive performance. The low daily release rate of levonorgestrel from the FibroPlant levonorgestrel results in a low incidence of hormonal side effects and reduces the likelihood of amenorrhagia.[249] According to Lahteenmaki et al.,[248] the use of the levonorgestrel intrauterine system (see Figure 8.24) is a good conservative alternative to hysterectomy in the treatment of menorrhagia and should be considered before hysterectomy or other invasive treatments.

According to Sohonen et al.,[249] local progestin delivery via a levonorgestrel-releasing intrauterine system was effective in suppressing the endometrium and in eliminating bleeding in women receiving estrogen replacement therapy. Varila et al.[250] reported that intrauterine levonorgestrel effectively protects against endometrial hyperplasia. In most women, it induces amenorrhagia, which is only temporarily affected by replacement of the LNG IUS. Maruo et al.[251] reported that LNG IUS resulted in a decrease in endometrial proliferation and an increase in apoptosis in endometrial glands and stroma. The increase in apoptosis associated with increased Fas antigen expression and decreased Bcl-2 protein expression in the endo-

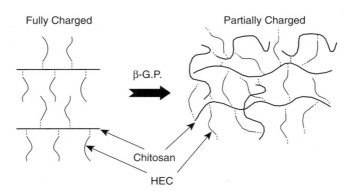

Figure 8.24 Role of β-G.P. in hydrogel formation with chitosan and HEC (left: fully charged and highly stretched chitosan repel each other to cause an intermolecular distance too large for HEC bridging; and right: partially neutralized with β-G.P. and highly flexible chitosan with a small intermolecular distance that allows bridging by HEC for hydrogel formation). Chain entanglement is also considered. (With permission, Wiley, *J. Pharm. Sci.*, 91, 7, 1669, 2002.)

metrium may be one of the underlying molecular mechanisms by which LNG IUS insertion causes the atrophic change of the endometrium. A multiload Cu25 intrauterine contraceptive device releasing 1.5 micrograms of 3-keto-desogestrel daily is able to reduce menstrual blood loss to a very low level and to replete body-iron stores in women with or without menorrhagia.[247] Higher doses had no superior effect.

D'Cruz and Uckun[244] reported on gel-emulsions as vaginal spermicides and intravaginal drug delivery vehicles. These emulsions have unprecedented potential as dual-function microbicidal contraceptives to improve vaginal bioavailability of poorly soluble antimicrobial agents without causing significant vaginal damage. Woolfson et al.,[245] in their review, discuss a range of drug delivery platforms suitable for intravaginal administration, including hydrogels, vaginal tablets, pessaries/suppositories, particulate systems, and intravaginal rings. Lamb et al.[246] reported on the inclusion of an intravaginal progesterone insert plus GnRH and prostaglandin F2alpha for ovulation control in postpartum-suckled beef cows. An improved intravaginal controlled-release prostaglandin E_2 insert for cervical ripening term has been reported.[248] In this study, 65% of PGE2-group patients had a successful outcome versus 44% of control patients (P = 0.001).

Janes et al.[238] described polysaccharide colloidal particles as delivery systems for macromolecules, such as DNA molecules. To date, the *in vivo* efficacy of the chitosan-based colloidal carriers has been reported for two different applications, while DNA-chitosan hybrid nanospheres were found to be acceptable transfection carriers; ionically cross-linked chitosan nanoparticles appeared to be efficient vehicles for the transport of peptides across the nasal mucosa, and according to Jones et al.,[239] polymer chemical structure is a key determinant of physicochemical and colloidal properties of polymer-DNA complexes for gene delivery. Lambert et al.[240] described polybutylcyanoacrylate nanocapsules containing an aqueous core as a novel colloidal carrier for the delivery of oligonucleotides (see Figures 8.25 and 8.26).

Orienti et al.[229] reported on hydrogels formed by cross-linked poly(vinyl alcohol) as colon-specific, sustained-release drug delivery systems. Vancomycin HCl was used in this study. The degree of cross-linking of ethylene glycol diglycidyl ether and the extent of substitution with oleoyl chloride were found to influence the drug release. Elvira et al.[227] reported on starch-based biodegradable hydrogels with potential biomedical applications as drug delivery systems. The design and preparation of novel biodegradable hydrogels developed by the free-radical polymerization of acrylamide and acrylic acid, and some formulations with bis-acrylamide, in the presence of a cornstarch/ethylene-co-vinyl alcohol copolymer blend (SEVA-C), is reported. The mechanical properties of the xerogels were characterized by tensile and compressive tests, as well as by dynamo-mechanical analysis (DMA).

A new family of nanoscale materials on the basis of dispersed networks of cross-linked ionic and nonionic hydrophilic polymers was reported by Vinogradov et al.[228] One example is the nanosized cationic network of cross-linked poly(ethylene oxide) and polyethyleneimine nanogel. Efficient cellular uptake and intracellular release of oligonucleotides immobilized in this nanogel have been demonstrated. Antisense activity of an oligonucleotide in a cell model was elevated as a result of the formulation of oligonucleotide with the nanogel. This delivery system has a potential of enhancing oral and brain bioavailability of oligonucleotides, as demonstrated using polarized epithelial and brain microvessel endothelial cell monolayers. Blanco et al.[230] reported on *in vivo* drug delivery of 5-fluorouracil using poly(2-hydroxyethyl methacrylate-co-acrylamide) hydrogels. Han et al.[231] described lactitol-based poly(ether polyol) hydrogels for controlled-release chemical and drug delivery systems, while Shantha and Harding[232] reported on the preparation and *in vitro* evaluation of poly(N-vinyl-2-pyrrolidone-polyethylene glycol diacrylate)-chitosan interpolymeric, pH-responsive hydrogels for oral drug delivery. Peppas et al.[233] described poly(ethylene glycol)-containing hydrogels for drug delivery, and Chiu et al.[234] reported on the synthesis and characterization of pH-sensitive dextran hydrogels as a potential colon-specific drug delivery system. Cytarabine trapping in poly(2-hydroxyethyl methacrylate) hydrogels in drug delivery systems was reported by Teijon et al.,[235] and according to Zhang et al.,[236] hydrogels can also be used in transdermal drug delivery. Azo polymeric hydrogels containing 5-fluorouracil for colon-targeted drug delivery was reported by Shantha and Harding.[237]

Finally, insulin can be effectively delivered using external and implantable pumps. Selam,[241] in a review, described management of diabetes with glucose sensors and implantable insulin pumps from 1960s to the period of the 1990s. Tenjarla[334] reported on the evolution toward the development of totally implantable rotary blood pumps and Bakshi and North[243] described implantable pumps for drug delivery to the brain.

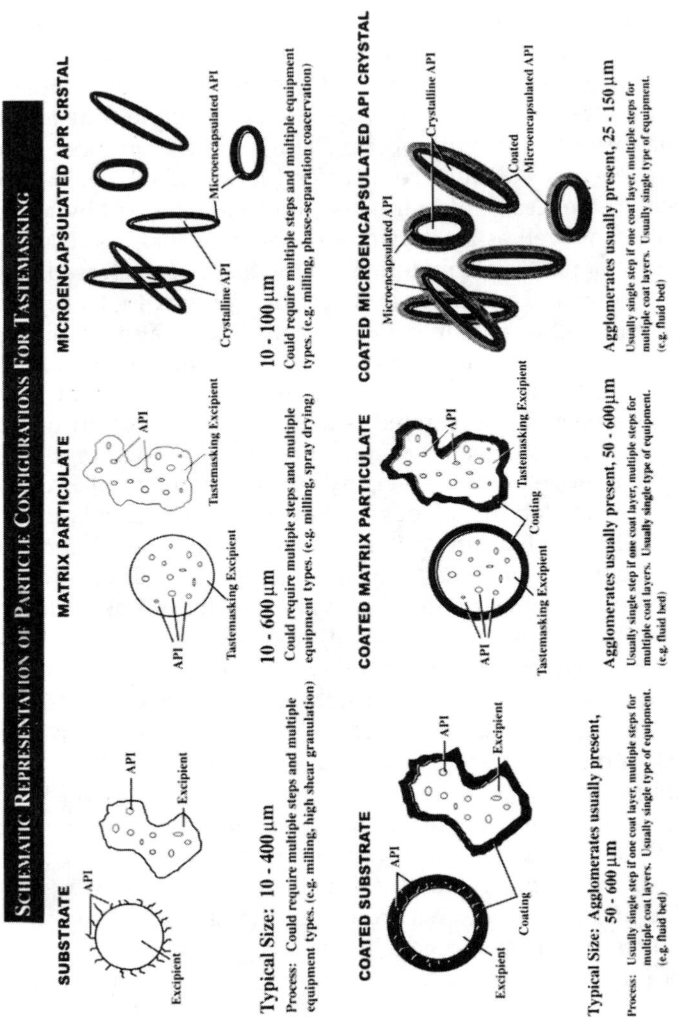

Figure 8.25 Schematic representation of particle configurations for tastemasking. (With permission, Russell Publ., *Am. Pharm. Rev.*, 3, 3, 8, 2002.)

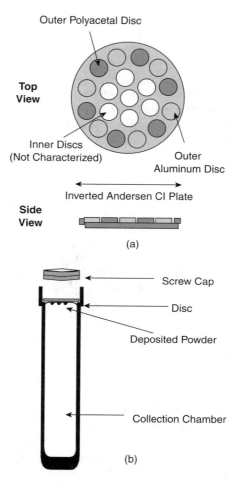

Figure 8.26 Schematic diagram of (a) polyacetal and aluminum disks positioned on the collection plate of the Andersen cascade impactor, and (b) centrifugal cell assembly. (With permission, Kluwer Publ., *Pharm. Res.*, 3, 322, 2002.)

VII. Summary

Demand for sustained-release and accurate delivery of pharmaceuticals has created a vast market for alternative drug delivery systems. The industry now includes transdermal patches and matrices, nasal delivery systems, ambulatory infusion pumps, oral osmotics, and liposomes. These technologies administer lower dosages at specific sites and reduce the adverse side effects commonly caused by conventional therapies for cancer, diabetes, and other chronic conditions.[217,218]

Despite impressive growth rates in recent times, the market for programmable drug delivery systems is still in its infancy. In 1989, therapeutic agents with various programmed drug delivery systems approached $1.6 billion in sales. Uncorrected for inflation, that market exceeded to $4.5 billion by 1995. Some of the significant factors contributing to this dynamic growth include bioerodible materials finding increased utilization for a number of therapeutic areas, monoclonal antibodies and liposome delivery systems becoming more commonplace, microspheres seeing a marked increase in utilization; and the use of narcotic analgesics and drug-behavior modification systems dramatically expanding the market associated with central nervous system agents.

References

1. Yalkowsky, S.H. and Morozowich, W., *Drug Design*, Vol. 9, Ariens Academic Press, Inc., 1980.
2. Stella, V.J., Mikkelton, T.J., and Pipkin, J.D., Pro-drugs: The control of delivery via bioreversible chemical modification. In *Drug Delivery Systems*, Juliano, R.L., Ed., Oxford Univ. Press, Oxford, 1980.
3. Roche, E.B., Ed., *Design of biopharmaceutical properties through pro-drugs and analogs*, APhA Academy of Pharmaceutical Sciences, Washington, D.C., 1977.
4. Notari, R.E., *Alteration of pharmacokinetics through structural modification*, APhA Academy of Pharmaceutical Sciences, Washington, D.C., 1977, 68.
5. Amidon, G.L., Pearlman, R.S., and Leesman, G.D., *Design of pro-drugs through consideration of enzyme-substrate specificities*, APhA Academy of Pharmaceutical Sciences, Washington, D.C., 1977, 281.
6. Nelson, S.D., *Alteration of drug metabolism through structural modification*, APhA Academy of Pharmaceutical Sciences, Washington, D.C., 1977, 316.
7. Morozowich, W., Cho. M.J., and Kezdy, F.J., *Application of physical organic principles to pro-drug design*, APhA Academy of Pharmaceutical Sciences, Washington, D.C., 1977, 344.
8. Sinkula, A.A., *Design of improved taste properties through structural modification*, APhA Academy of Pharmaceutical Sciences, Washington, D.C., 1977, 422.
9. Bodor, N. and Kaminski, J.J., Pro-drugs and site-specific chemical delivery systems, *Ann. Reports Med. Chem.*, 22, 303, 1987.
10. Handley, A.J., Portable heparin injector, *The Lancet*, 2, 313, 1970.
11. Mobile Infusion Pumps for Ambulatory Patients, Products Bulletin, Cormed., Middleport, NY, 1978.
12. Tucker, E.M., The latest developments in drug delivery systems, *Conf. Proc., Pharm. Tech.*, 13, 1980.
13. Nielsen R.L., The insulin pump: an advance in diabetic control, *Drug Therapy*, June 1985, 133.
14. Campbell, R.K., Insulin infusion pumps for home care patients, *U.S. Pharmacist*, November 1987, 97.
15. Blackshear, P.J. and Rohde, T.D., Artificial devices for insulin infusion in the treatment of patients with diabetes mellitus. In *Controlled Drug Delivery*, Vol. 2, Clinical Applications, Bruck, S.D., Ed., CRC Press, Boca Raton, FL, 1983.
16. Clark, L.C. Jr. and Lyons, S.C., Electrode systems for continuous monitoring in cardiovascular surgery, *Ann. N.Y. Acad. Sci.*, 102, 29, 1964.
17. Updike, S.J. and Hicks, G.P., The enzyme electrode, *Nature* (London), 214, 986, 1967.

18. Bessman, S.P. and Schultz, R.D., Prototype glucose-oxydase sensor for the artificial pancreas, *Trans. Acad. Soc. Artif. Intern. Org.*, 19, 361, 1973.
19. March, W., Engerman, R., and Rabinovitch, B., Optical monitor of glucose, *Trans. Acad. Soc. Artif. Intern. Org.*, 25, 28, 1979.
20. Kadish, A.H., Automation control of blood sugar, I. A servomechanism for glucose monitoring and control, *Am. J. Med. Electron.*, 3, 82, 1964.
21. Pfiffer, E.F., Thum, C., and Clemens, A.H., The artificial beta cell: a contunuous control of blood sugar by external regulation of infusion system (Glucose-Controlled Insulin Infusion System [GCIFS]), *Horm. Metab. Res.*, 6, 339, 1974.
22. Albisser, A.M., Libel, B.S., Ewart, T.G., Davidovac, Z., et al., Clinical control of diabetes by artificial pancreas, *Diabetes*, 23, 397–404, 1974.
23. Clemens, A.H., Chang, P.H., and Myers, R.W., The development of Biostator, a glucose-controlled insulin infusion system (GCIFS), *Horm. Metab. Res. Suppl.*, 8, 23, 1977.
24. Bechard, S., Yamaguchi, N., and McMullen, J.N., *In vitro* and *in vivo* release of insulin from porous polymeric implants, *Proc. Int. Symp. Control Rel. Bioact. Mater.*, 14, 57, 1987.
25. Heller, J., Pangburn, S.H., and Penhale, D.W., Use of bioeridible polymers in self-regulative drug delivery system, *Proc. Int. Symp. Control Rel. Bioact. Mater.*, 107, 1987.
26. Siddiqui, O., Shi, W., and Chien, Y.W., Transdermal iontophoretic delivery of insulin for blood glucose control in diabetes, *Proc. Int. Symp. Control Rel. Bioact. Mater.*, 174, 1987.
27. Watler, P.K. and Sefton, M.V., A piezoelectric micropump for insulin delivery, *Proc. Int. Symp. Control Rel. Bioact. Mater.*, 231, 1987.
28. Sefton, M.V., Sugamori, M.E., and Broughton, R.L., Microencapsulation of mammalian cells in hydrophilic polyacrylates by interfacial precipitation, *Proc. Int. Symp. Control Rel. Bioact. Mater.*, 279, 1987.
29. Choay, A. and Choay, H., *Ann. Pharm. Fr.*, 5, 420, 1947.
30. Langer, R., Brown, L., and Edelman, E., Controlled release and magnetically modulated systems for macromolecules. In *Recent Advances in Drug Delivery Systems*, Anderson, J.M. and Kim, S.W., Eds., Plenum Press, New York and London, 249, 1984.
31. Siegel, R.A. et al., Sintered polymers for sustained macromolecular drug release, In *Recent Advances in Drug Delivery Systems*, Anderson, J.M. and Kim, S.W., Eds., Plenum Press, New York and London , 315, 1984.
32. Kim, S.W. et al., Self-regulating insulin delivery system, In *Recent Advances in Drug Delivery Systems*, Anderson, J.M. and Kim, S.W., Eds., Plenum Press, New York and London , 123, 1984.
33. Horbett, T.A. et al., A bioresponsive membrane for insulin delivery, In *Recent Advances in Drug Delivery Systems*, Anderson, J.M. and Kim, S.W., Eds., Plenum Press, New York and London, 209, 1984.
34. Goriya, Y., Bahoric, A., Marliss, E.B., Zinman, B., and Albisser, A.M., Glycemic regulation using a programmed insulin delivery device, III. *Diabetes*, 28, 558–564, 1979.
35. Schade, D.S., Eaton, R.P., Friedman, N.M., and Spencer, W.J., Normalization of plasma insulin profiles with intraperitoneal insulin infusion in diabetic man, *Diabetologia*, 19, 35–39, 1980.

36. Ritschel, W.A., Parenteral dosage forms with prolonged action. In *Drug Design*, Ariens, E.J., Ed., 75, 1973.
37. Ballard, B.E. and Nelson, E., in *Remington's Pharmaceutical Sciences*, 14th ed., Mack Publ., Easton, PA, 1970, 1699.
38. Kringel, J., The new intravenous systems: the latest developments in drug delivery systems, *Pharm. Tech.*, 17, 1987.
39. Duma, R.I., Warner, J.F., and Dalton, H.P., Septicemia from intravenous infusions, *N. Eng. J. Med.*, 284, 257–260, 1971.
40. Henry, R.H. and Harrison, W.L., Problems in the use of volume control sets for intravenous fluids, *Am. J. Hosp. Pharm.*, 29, 485–490, 1972.
41. Turco, S.J., New intravenous drug delivery systems, *Am. J. Hosp. Pharm.*, 17, 1987.
42. Current Status of Health Care Industry Under DRGs (Report A1578), Frost and Sullivan, Inc., New York, December 1986.
43. Rapp, R.P., Wermeling, D.P., and Piecoro, J.J. Jr., Guidelines for the administration of commonly used intravenous drugs, *Drug Intel. Clin. Pharm.*, 18, 217–232, 1984.
44. Veillard, M.U., et al., *Proc. Int. Symp. Control. Rel. Bioact. Mater.*, 14, 22, 1987.
45. Tyle, P., Ed., *Drug Delivery Devices: Fundamentals and Applications*, Vol. 32, Marcel Dekker, New York, 607, 1988.
46. Tyle, P., Ed., *Specialized Drug Delivery Systems: Manufacturing and Production Technology*, Vol. 41, Marcel Dekker, New York, 1990, 475.
47. Osborne, D.W. and Amann, A.H., Eds., *Topical Drug Delivery Formulations*, Marcel Dekker, New York, 1989, 448.
48. Juliano, R.L., Ed., *Biological Approaches to the Controlled Delivery of Drugs*, Annals N.Y. Acad. Sciences, Vol. 507, N.Y. Acad. Sci., 1987, 364.
49. Kato, T., Encapsulated drugs in targeted cancer therapy. In *Controlled Drug Delivery, Clinical Applications*, Vol. 2, Bruck, S.D., Ed., CRC Press, Boca Raton, FL, 1983, 189.
50. Widder, K.J., Senyei, A.E., and Flouret, G., Magnetic microspheres synthesis of a novel parenteral drug carrier, *J. Pharm. Sci.*, 68, 79, 1979.
51. Widder, K.J., Morris, A.M., Poore, G., Howard, D.P. Jr., and Senyei, A.E., Tumor remission in Yoshida sarcoma-bearing rats by selective targeting of magnetic albumin microspheres containing doxorubicin, *Proc. Natl. Acad. Sci.* (U.S.), 78, 579–581, 1981.
52. Meyers, R.H., Cronic, F., and Nice, C.M., Experimental approach in the use and magnetic control of metallic iron particles in the lymphatic and vascular system of dogs as a contrast and isotropic agent, *Am. J. Roentgenol. Radium Ther. Nucl. Med.* (N.S.), 90, 1068, 1963.
53. Turner, R.D., Rand, R.W., Bentson, J.R., and Mosso, J.A., Ferromagnetic silicone necrosis of hypernephromas by selective vascular occlusion to the tumor, *J. Urology*, 113, 455–459, 1975.
54. Barnothy, M.F., Biological effects of magnetic fields, *Prog. Biomatereol.*, 1, 392, 1974.
56. Langer, R., Brown, L., and Edelman, E., Controlled release and magnetically modulated systems for macromolecules: recent advances. In *Recent Advances in Drug Delivery Systems*, Anderson, J.M. and Kim, S.W., Eds., Plenum Press, New York and London, 249, 1983.
57. Morris, R.M. et al., Magnetic microspheres in drug delivery, In *Recent Advances in Drug Delivery Systems*, Anderson, J.M. and Kim, S.W., Eds., Plenum Press, New York and London, 221–227, 1983.

58. Ito, R., Machida, Y., Sannan, T., and Nagai, T., Magnetic granules: A novel system for specific drug delivery to esophageal mucosa in oral administration, *Int. J. Pharm.*, 61, 109–117, 1990.
59. Hsieh, D.T. and Langer, R., Zero-order drug delivery systems with magnetic control. In *Controlled Release Delivery Systems*, Roseman, T.D. and Mansdorf, S.Z., Eds., Marcel Dekker, New York, 1983.
60. Widder, K.J., Magnetic targeting of drugs. In *The Latest Develpoments in Drug Delivery System Conf. Proc.*, 21, 1983.
61. deBlaey, C.J. and Polderman, J., Rationals in the design of rectal and vaginal delivery forms of drugs. In *Drug Design*, Vol. 9, Academic Press, Inc., New York, 237, 1980.
62. Nash, H.A., Controlled-release systems for contraception. In *Medical Applications of Controlled Release*, Vol. 2, Langer, R.S. and Wise, D.L., Eds., CRC Press, Boca Raton, FL, 35, 1984.
63. Folkman, J. and Long, D.M., The use of silicone rubber as a carrier for prolonged drug therapy, *J. Surg. Res.*, 4, 139, 1964.
64. Segal, S.J. and Croxatto, H.B., Single administration of hormones for long-term control of reproductive function, *23rd Meet. Am. Fert. Assoc.*, Washington, D.C., April 14–16.
65. Croxatto, H., Diaz, S., Vera, R., Etchart, M., and Atria, P., Fertility control in women with progestogen released in microquantities from subcutaneous capsules, *Am. J. Obst. Gynec.*, 105, 1135–1138, 1969.
66. Nilsson, C.G., Lachteenmaki, P., and Lunkkainen, T., Levonorgestrel plasma concentrations and hormone profiles after insersion and after one year of treatment with a levonorgestrel IUD, *Contraception*, 21, 225, 1980.
67. Fanndes, A., Sivin, I., and Stern, J., Long-acting contraceptive implants: an analysis of menstrual bleeding patterns, *Contraception*, 18, 355, 1978.
68. Nash, H.A., Robertson, D.N., Moo Young, A.J., and Atkinson, L.E., Steroid release from silastic capsules and rods, *Contraception*, 367–394, 1078.
69. Snowden, R., The Progestasert and ectopic pregnancy, *Br. Med. J.*, 2, 1600, 1977.
70. Nash, H.A. and Jacjanicz, T., Contraceptive vaginal ring. In *Advances in Fertility Research*, Mishell, D.R. Jr., Ed., Raven Press, New York, 129, 1981.
71. Mishell, D.R. Jr., Moore, D.E., Roy, S., Brenner, P.F., and Page, M.A., Clinical performance and endocrine profiles with contraceptive vaginal rings containing a combination of estradiol and d-norgestrel, *Am. J. Obst. Gynec.*, 130, 55–62, 1978.
72. Victor, A., Jackanicz, T.M., and Johansson, E.D.B., Vaginal progesterone for contraception, *Fertil. Steril.*, 30, 631, 1978.
73. Mishell, D.R. Jr. and Lumkin, M.E., Contraceptive effect of varying doses of progestogen in Silastic vaginal rings, *Fertil. Steril.*, 99, 1970.
74. Thiery, M., Vandekerckhove, D., Dhont, M., Vermeulen, A., and Decoster, J.M., The medroxyprogesterone acetate intravaginal silastic ring as a contraceptive device, *Contraception*, 13, 605–617, 1976.
75. Fildes, F.J.T. and Hutchinson, F.G., U.S. Patent 4,235,988, 1980.
76. Higuchi, T. and Hussain, A., U.S. Patent 4,016,251, 1977.
77. Schopflin, G., U.S. Patent 4,012,497, 1977.
78. Heller, J. and Baker, R.W., U.S. Patent 4,014,987, 1977.
79. Williams, B.C., U.S. Patent 4,317,447, 1982.
80. Magoon, K.E., Evans, L.E., and Hembrough, F.B., U.S. Patent 4,312,347, 1982.
81. Roseman, T.J., Derr, G.R., and Schwartz, G., U.S. Patent 4,402,693, 1983.

82. Drobish, J.L. and Gougeon, T.W., U.S. Patent 4,304,226, 1981.
83. Hughes, A.G., U.S. Patent 4,066,075, 1978.
84. Wong, P.S., U.S. Patent 4,402,695, 1983.
85. Laughlin, R.G., U.S. Patent 4,067,961, 1978 and 4,145,408, 1979.
86. Chvapil, M., U.S. Patent 4,274,410, 1981.
87. Vorys, N., U.S. Patent 4,372,951, 1983.
88. Homm, R. and Katz, G., U.S. Patent 3,875,300, 1975.
89. Cornfeld, E., U.S. Patent 3,918,452, 1975.
90. Gordon, M., U.S. Patent 3,814,809, 1974.
91. de Nijs, H. et al., The multicompartment intravaginal ring: Preliminary pharmacokinetics in female volunteers, *Proc. Int. Symp. Control. Rel. Bioact. Mater.*, 14, 297, 1987.
92. Brazean, G.A., Modern drug delivery systems for contraception, *Pharm. Int.*, 6, 69, 1985.
93. Nash, H.A., Controlled-release systems for contraception. In *Medical Applications of Controlled Release*, Vol. 2, Langer, R.S. and Wise, D.L., Eds., CRC Press, Boca Raton, FL, 35, 1984.
94. Moo-Young, A.J. et al., Copper levels in certain tissues of rhesus monkeys and of women bearing copper IUDs. In *Analysis of Intrauterine Contraception*, Hefnawi, F. and Segal, S.J., Eds., American Elsevier, New York, 439, 1975.
95. Sivian, I. and Tatum, H.J., Four years of experience with the TCu 380 Ag intrauterine contraceptive device, *Fertil. Steril.*, 36, 159, 1981.
96. Pharriss, B.B., Clinical experience with intrauterine progesterone contraceptive system, *J. Reprod. Med.*, 20, 155, 1978.
97. Martinez-Manantan, J. et al., Clinical experience with the intrauterine progesterone-releasing system. In *Analysis of Intrauterine Contraception*, Hefnawi, F. and Segal, S.J., Eds., Elsevier, New York, 173, 1975.
98. Nilsson, C.G., Lachteenmaki, P., and Luukkainen, T., Patterns of ovulation and bleeding with a low levonorgesterol-releasing device, *Contraception*, 21, 155, 1980.
99. El-Mahgoub, S., The norgestrel T IUD, *Contraception*, 22, 27, 1980.
100. Higuchi, T. and Hussain, A.A., U.S. Patent 4,188,951, 1980.
101. Cameron, M.R., U.S. Patent 4,265,883, 1981.
102. Lerner, I..S., Davis, H.J., and Earl, T.J., U.S. Patent 3,834,378, 1974.
103. Shaw, S.T., U.S. Patent 4,381,001, 1983.
104. Heller, J. and Baker, R.W., U.S. Patent 4,180,064, 1979.
105. Ramwell, P.W., U.S. Patent 3,888,975, 1975.
106. Zaffaroni, A., U.S. Patent 3,895,103, 1975.
107. Schommegna, A., U.S. Patent 3,911,911, 1975.
108. Zaffaroni, A., U.S. Patent 3,896,819, 1975; 3,948,262, April 6, 1976; and 3,993,073, November 23, 1976.
109. Zaffaroni, A., U.S. Patent 3,845,761, 1974.
110. Pharriss, B.B., Erickson, R.R., and Tillson, S.A., U.S. Patent 4,014,988, 1977.
111. de Boer, A.G., Moolenaar, F., de Leede, L.G., and Breimer, D.D., Rectal drug administration: clinical pharmacokinetic considerations, *Clin. Pharmacokinet.*, 7, 285–311, 1982.
112. Nishihata, T. et al., Adjuvant effects on rectal absorption, The Alfred Benzon Symposium 17, *Optimization of Drug Delivery*, Bundgaard, H., Hansen, A.H., and Kefod, H., Eds., Munksgaard, Copenhagen, 17, 1982.

113. Modozeniec, A.R. et al., Noninvesive monitoring of the *in vivo* release characteristics of rectal drug delivery devices. In *Recent Advances in Drug Delivery Systems*, Anderson, J.M. and Kim, S.W., Eds., Plenum Press, New York, 321, 1984.

114. Beihn, R.M. and Digenis, G.A., Noninvasive dissolution measurement using perturbed angular correlation, *J. Pharm. Sci.*, 70, 1325, 1981.

115. Hayakawa, E., Yamamoto, A., and Lee, V.H.L., Synergistic effects of penetration enhancers on insulin absorption across the isolated rectal membrane, *Program and Abstracts of 15th Int. Symp. Control. Rel. Bioact. Mater.*, Switzerland, 1988, 128.

116. Byrne, G.A. and Aylott, R.I., U.S. Patent 4,265,875, 1981 and 4,292,300, 1982.

117. Aoda, Y. et al., U.S. Patent 4,344,968, 1982.

118. deBuman, A., Riva, A., and Sucker, H., U.S. Patent 4,369,784, 1983.

119. Takagishi, Y. et al., U.S. Patent 4,405,597, 1983.

120. Takagishi, Y. et al., U.S. Patent 4,402,692, 1983.

121. Kitao, K. and Nishimura, K., U.S. Patent 4,338,306, 1982.

122. Higuchi, T., Nishihata, T., and Rytting, H.J., U.S. Patent 4,406,896, 1983.

123. Roseman, T.J. et al., U.S. Patent 4,237,888, 1980 and 4,308,867, 1982.

124. Michaels, A.S., U.S. Patent 4,367,741, 1983.

125. Tomlinson, E. et al., Albumin microspheres for intra-arterial drug targeting. In *Recent Advances in Drug Delivery Systems*, Anderson, J.M. and Kim, S.W., Eds., Plenum Press, New York and London, 199, 1984.

126. Kramer, P.A., Albumin microspheres as vehicles achieving specificity in drug delivery, *J. Pharm. Sci.*, 63, 1646, 1974.

127. Yapel, A.F., U.S. Patent 4,147,767, 1979.

128. Longo, W.E., Iwata, H., Lindheimer, T.A., and Goldberg, E.P., Preparation of hydrophilic albumin microspheres using polymeric dispersing agents, *J. Pharm. Sci.*, 71, 1323–1328, 1982.

129. Morris, R.M. et al., Magnetic microspheres in drug delivery. In *Recent Advances in Drug Delivery Systems*, Anderson, J.M. and Kim, S.W., Eds., Plenum Press, New York and London, 221, 1984.

130. Sumamoto, J. et al., Stable cell-recognizable lipid microspheres for delivery of lipophilic drugs, *Program and Abstracts of 15th Int. Symp. Control. Rel. Bioact. Mater.*, August 15–19, 1988, Paper No. 78.

131. Okamoto, H. et al., Possible mechanisms for the enhanced efficacy of lipid microspheres of prostaglandin E preparation, *Program and Abstracts of 15th Int. Symp. Control. Rel. Bioact. Mater.*, August 15–19, 1988, Paper No. 186.

132. Shankland, K. and Whateley, T.C., Release of enzymes from microspheres and nanoparticles, *Program and Abstracts of 15th Int. Symp. Control. Rel. Bioact. Mater.*, August 15–19, 1988, Paper No. 259.

133. Illum, L. et al., Nasal administration of gentamicin using a novel microsphere delivery system, *Int. J. Pharm.*, 46, 3, 261, 1988.

134. Dubernet, C. et al., A physicochemical study of the morphology of ibuprofen-loaded microspheres, *Proc. Int. Symp. Control. Rel. Bioact. Mater.*, 14, 236, 1987.

135. Schroder, U., Lager, C., and Norrlow, O., Carbo-lactic microspheres, graft polymerization of PLA to starch microspheres, *Proc. Int. Symp. Control. Rel. Bioact. Mater.*, 14, 238, 1987.

136. Mathiowitz, E. et al., Developments in polyanhydrides microspheres, *Proc. Int. Symp. Control. Rel. Bioact. Mater.*, 14, 242, 1987.

137. Langer, R. and Folkman, J., Polymers for the sustained release of proteins and other macromolecules, *Nature*, 263, 797, 1976.

138. Pongpaibul, Y., Maruyama, K., and Iwatsuru, M., Formation and *in vitro* evaluation of theophylline-loaded poly(methylmethacrylate) microspheres, *J. Pharm. Pharmacol.*, 40, 530–533, 1988.

139. Bjork, E. and Edelman, P., Characterization of degradable starch microspheres as a novel delivery system for drugs, *Int. J. Pharm.*, 62, 2–3, 187, 1990.

140. Refojo, M.F. and Leong, F.L., Microscopic determination of the penetration of proteins and polysaccharides into poly(hydroxyethyl methacrylate) and similar hydrogels, *J. Polym. Sci.: Polym. Symp.*, 66, 227, 1979.

141. Lewis, D.H., Cowsar, D.R., and Hamilton, M.D., Hydrophobic polymers as excipients for biologically active agents. In *Proc. 5th Int. Symp. Cont. Rel. Bioact. Mater.*, Univ. of Akron, Akron, OH, 2, 1978.

142. Kliment, K. et al., U.S. Patent 3,689,634, 1972.

143. Chien, Y.W. and Lau, E.P.K., Controlled drug release from polymeric delivery devices, IV. *In vitro-in vivo* correlation of subcutaneous release of norgestomet from hydrophilic implants, *J. Pharm. Sci.*, 65(4), 488, 1976.

144. Song, S.Z., Cardinal, J.R., Kim, S.H., and Kim, S.W., Progestin permeation through polymer membrane, V. Progesterone release from monolithic hydrogel devices, *J. Pharm. Sci.*, 70, 216–219, 1981.

145. Coswar, D.R. and Dunn, R.L., *Biodegradable and nonbiodegradable fibrous delivery systems in long-acting contraceptive delivery systems*, Zatuchini, G.L., et al., Eds., Harper & Row Publishers, Philadelphia, 1984, 145.

146. Ratner, B.D. and Hoffman, A.S., Synthetic hydrogels for biomedical and related applications, Andrade, J.D., et al., ACS Symp. Ser. 31, Washington, D.C., chap. 1.

147. Gregonis, D.E. et al., *The Chemistry of Some Selected Hydrogels*, Andrade, J.D., Ed., ACS Symp. Ser. 31, Washington, D.C., chap. 7.

148. Wichterle, O., U.S. Patent 3,397,376, 1976 and 3,896,806, 1975.

149. Abrahams, R.A. and Rovel, S.H., Biocompatible implants for the sustained zero-order release of narcotic antagonists, *J. Biomed. Mater. Res.*, 9, 355, 1975.

150. Schacht, E.H., Hydrogel drug delivery systems: physical and ionogenic drug carriers. In *Recent Advances in Drug Delivery Systems*, Anderson, J.M. and Kim, S.W., Eds., Plenum Press, New York and London, 1984.

151. Ishikawa, S., Kobayashi, M., and Sawejima, M., Evaluation of the rheological properties of various kinds of carboxyvinyl polymer gels, *Pharm. Bull.*, 36(6), 2118, 1988.

152. Kurihara, T. et al., Hydrogel systems in the transdermal administration of therapeutic agents to the premature neonate, *15th Int. Symp. Control. Rel. Bioact. Mater.*, Basel, Switzerland, 1988, paper No. 128.

153. Laughlin, T.J. et al., Hydrogel delivery systems based on polymer alloys, *Proc. Intl. Symp. Control. Rel. Bioact. Mater.*, 14, 39, 1987.

154. Park, K. and Park, H., Enzyme-digestible balloon hydrogels for long-term oral drug delivery: synthesis and characterization, *Proc. Int. Symp. Control. Rel. Bioact. Mater.*, 41, 1987.

155. Mason, A.D. Jr. et al., U.S. Patent 4,393,048, 1983.

156. Manning, J.H. and Stark, J.H., U.S. Patent 4,002,173, 1977.

157. Mueller, K.F. and Good, W.R., U.S. Patent 4,304,591, 1981.

158. Luzzi, L.A., Microencapsulation: review article, *J. Pharm. Sci.*, 59, 1367, 1970.

159. Setterstrom, J.A., Tice, T.R., and Myers, W.E., Development of encapsulated antibiotics for topical administration to wounds. In *Recent Advances in Drug Delivery Systems*, Anderson, J.M. and Kim, S.W., Eds., Plenum Press, New York, 185, 1984.

160. Ishibashi, K. et al., Preparation of microcapsules containing 5-fluorouracil adsorbed on medicinal carbons, *Program and Abstracts 15th Int. Symp. Control. Rel. Bioact. Mater.*, Basel, Switzerland, 1988, 68.

161. Das, S.K., Chattaraj, S.C., and Gupta, B.K., Controlled release of antimalarials from microcapsules and microparticles, *Program and Abstracts 15th Int. Symp. Control. Rel. Bioact. Mater.*, Basel, Switzerland, 1988, 170.

162. Tsuji, K., Microencapsulation of pesticide-particles: Design and biological characteristics, *Program and Abstracts 15th Int. Symp. Control. Rel. Bioact. Mater.*, Basel, Switzerland, 1988, 170.

163. Chattraj, S.C., Das, S.K., and Gupta, B.K., The development of bioadhesive microcapsules and assessment for delaying the gastrointestinal transit in rabbits, *Program and Abstracts 15th Int. Symp. Control. Rel. Bioact. Mater.*, Basel, Switzerland, 1988, 251.

164. Lawter, J.R. et al., Drug release from poly(glycolide-CO-DL-lactide) microcapsules, *Proc. Int. Symp. Control. Rel. Bioact. Mater.*, 14, 99, 1987.

165. Tice, T.R. et al., Development of injectable controlled-release poly(I.C) microcapsules for the inhibition of viral replication, *Proc. Int. Symp. Control. Rel. Bioact. Mater.*, 14, 275, 1987.

166. Goosen, M.F.A. and McKnight, C.A., Chemical modification of deacetylated chitin for the microencapsulation of mammalian cells, *Proc. Int. Symp. Control. Rel. Bioact. Mater.*, 14, 277, 1987.

167. Maleki, M. et al., Effect of alginate composition and poly-L-lysine molecular weight on alginate-poly-L-lysine-alginate microcapsule properties, *Proc. Int. Symp. Control. Rel. Bioact. Mater.*, 14, 281, 1987.

168. Swynnerton, N.F. et al., Encapsulation of retinoids for administration in laboratory diets, *Proc. Int. Symp. Control. Rel. Bioact. Mater.*, 14, 301, 1987.

169. Lew, C.W. et al., Stabilization of antiradiation compounds by microencapsulation, *Proc. Int. Symp. Control. Rel. Bioact. Mater.*, 14, 303.

170. Nuwayser, E.S. and DeRoo, D.J., Microencapsulation with microfluidized beds, *Proc. Int. Symp. Control. Rel. Bioact. Mater.*, 14, 304, 1987.

171. Chattaraj, S.C., Das, S.K., and Gupta, B.K., *In vitro-in vivo* correlation of drug release from ethyl cellulose microcapsules, *Proc. Int. Symp. Control. Rel. Bioact. Mater.*, 14, 308, 1987.

172. SoloHill Engineering, Inc., private communication.

173. Artursson, P. et al., Characterization of polyacryl starch microparticles as carriers for proteins and drugs, *Pharm. Intern.*, March 1985, Abst. No. 31.

174. Hassig, A. and Stampfli, K., Plasma substitutes: past and present, *Bibl. Haematol.*, 33, 1, 1969.

175. McAfee. J.G., and Subramanian, G., In *Clinical Scintillation Imaging*, 2nd ed., Freeman, L.M. and Johnson, P.M., Eds., Grune and Stratton, NY, 13, 1975.

176. Scheffel, U., Rhodes, B.A., Natarajan, T.K., and Wagner, H.N. Jr., Albumin microspheres for study of the reticuloendothelial system., *J. Nucl. Med.*, 13, 498–503, 1972.

177. Ward, H.A. and Fothergill, J.E., In *Fluorescent Protein Tracing*, 4th ed., Nairn, R.C., Ed., Churchill Livingstone, London, 22, 1976.

178. Davis, S.S., Colloids as drug delivery systems, *Pharm. Tech.*, June 1987, 110.

179. Yamahira, Y. et al., Biopharmaceutical studies on lipid-containing oral dosage forms: Relationship between drug absorption and gastric emptying of lipid formulations, *J. Pharm. Dyn.*, 1, 160, 1978.

180. Noguchi, T., Jinguji, Y., Kimura, T., Muranishi, S., and Sezaki, H., Mechanism of the intestinal absorption of drugs from oil-in-water emulsions, VII. Role of bile in the lymphatic transport of lipid-soluble compounds from triolein emulsions, *Chem. Pharm. Bull.*, 23, 782–786, 1975.

181. Nakamoto, Y., et al., Enhancement of lymphatic transport of 1-(2-tetrahy-dro-furoyl)-5-flurouracil by water-in-oil emulsion, *J. Pharm. Dyn.*, 2, 45, 1979.

182. Ogata, H., Kakemi, K., Furuya, A., Fujii, M., and Muranishi, S., Mechanism of the intestinal absorption of drugs from oil-in-water emulsions, V. Enhanced absorption of methyl orange adsorbed at oil/water interface in emulsions, *J. Pharm. Dyn.*, 23, 716–724, 1975.

183. Dardel, O., Mebuis, C., and Mossburg, T., Diazepam in emulsion form for intravenous use, *Anesth. Scand.*, 20, 221, 1976.

184. Jeppson, R. and Ljunberg, S., Intraarterial administration of emulsion formulations containing cyclandelate and nitroglycerine, *Acta. Pharm. Suec.*, 10, 129, 1973.

185. Jeppson, R., Effects of barbituric acids using an emulsion from intravenously administration, *Acta. Pharm. Suec.*, 9, 81, 1972.

186. Davis, M.A. and Taube, R.A., Pulmonary perfusion imaging: acute toxicity and safety factors as a function of particle size, *J. Nucl. Med.*, 19, 1209, 1978.

187. Fujita, T., Sumaya, T., and Yokoyama, K., Fluorocarbon emulsions as a candidate for artificial blood: correlation between particle size of the emulsion and acute toxicity, *Eur. Surg. Res.*, 3, 436, 1971.

188. Herbert, W.J., Multiple emulsions: a new form of mineral-oil antigen adjuvant, *Lancet*, Part ii, 771, 1965.

189. Birrenbach, G. and Speiser, D.P., Polymerized micelles their use as adjuvants in immunology, *J. Pharm. Sci.*, 65, 1763, 1976.

190. Bhargava, H.N., Narurkar, A., and Lieb, L.M., Using microemulsions for drug delivery, *Pharm. Tech.*, March 1987, 46.

191. Hoar, T.P. and Schulman, J.H., Transport water-in-oil dispersions: the oleo-pathic hydromicelle, *Nature*, 152(3847), 102, 1943.

192. Hamlin, R.M. and Shah, D.O., Structure of water in microemulsions: electrical, birefringence and nuclear magnetic resonance studies, *Science*, 171, 483, 1971.

193. Shinoda, K. and Freiberg, S., Microemulsions: colloidal aspects, *Adv. Colloid Interface Sci.*, 4, 281, 1975.

194. Leland, C.C., U.S. Patent 3,911,138, 1975.

195. Prince, L.M., *Emulsions in Biological Horizons in Surface Science*, Prince, L.M. and Sears, D.F., Eds., Academic Press, New York, 353, 1973.

196. Halbert, G.W, Stuart, J.B., and Florence, A.T., The incorporation of lipid-soluble antineoplastic agents into microemulsions: protein-free analogs of low-density lipoproteins, *Int. J. Pharm.*, 21, 219, 1984.

197. Jayakrishan, A., Kakaiarasi, K., and Shah, D.O., Microemulsions evolving technology for cosmetic applications, *J. Soc. Cosmet. Chem.*, 34, 335, 1983.

198. Shah. D.O., High-resolution NMR (220 MC) studies on the structure of water in microemulsions and liquid crystals, *Ann. N.Y. Acad. Sci.*, 204, 125, 1973.

199. Ziegenmeyer, J. and Fuehrer, C., Microemulsionen als topische Arzneiform, *Acta Pharm Technol.*, 26(4), 273, 1980.

200. Aguadisch, L.M., et al., Controlled release of progesterone, propranolol and indomethacin from a solid-state microemulsions reservoir-type silicone transdermal delivery system, *Proc. 14th Int. Symp. Control. Rel. Bioact. Mater.,* 263, 1987.

201. DiLuccio, R.C. et al., Hollow-fiber delivery systems, I. Preparation, *Proc. 14th Int. Symp. Control. Rel. Bioact. Mater.,* 188, 1987.

202. Dunn, R.L. and Lewis, D.H., In *Controlled Release of Pesticides and Pharmaceuticals,* Lewis, D.H., Ed, 1981, 125.

203. Eenink, M.J.D. et al., Biodegradable hollow fibers for the controlled release of drugs, *Proc. Int. Symp. Control. Rel. Bioact. Mater.,* 12, 49, 1985.

204. DiLuccio, R.C. et al., Hollow-fiber delivery systems, II. Oral drug releases *in vitro* and *in vivo* (dogs) evaluation, *Proc. Int. Symp. Control. Rel. Bioact. Mater.,* 190, 1987.

205. Britton, P. et al., Controlled drug delivery from hollow fibers, *Rel. Bioact. Mater.,* Paper No. 69, 1988.

206. Kost, J., Leong, K., and Langer, R., Ultrasonically controlled drug delivery, *Rel. Bioact. Mater.,* 14, 186, 1987.

207. Kost, J. et al., Glucose-sensitive membranes containing glucose oxidase activity: Swelling and permeability studies, *J. Biomed. Res.,* 19, 1133, 1985.

208. Rehmberg, G., Andreasson, A., and Lofroth, J., Liquid-crystalline phases as delivery systems, *Int. Symp. Control. Rel. Bioact. Mater.,* 15, 118, 1988.

209. Eriksson, B., Leander, S., and Ohlin, M., Liquid-crystalline phases as delivery systems, *Int. Symp. Control. Rel. Bioact. Mater.,* 15, 118, 1988.

210. Ueda, S. et al., Design and development of time-controlled explosion system (TES) as a controlled drug delivery system, *Int. Symp. Control. Rel. Bioact. Mater.,* 15, 127, 1988.

211. McIntosh, D. and Davies, A.J.S., *Proc. Int. Symp. Control. Rel. Bioact. Mater.,* 14, 217, 1987.

212. Sandvig, K., Olsnes, S., and Pihl, A., Binding uptake and degradation of the toxic proteins abrin and ricin by toxin-resistant cell variants, *Eur. J. Biochem.,* 82, 13, 1978.

213. Stephenson, M., U.S. Patent 4,024,871, 1977.

214. Gilbert, J.G., U.S. Patent 4,094,967, 1978.

215. Leveen, H.H. and Joyce, P.J., U.S. Patent 4,113,852, 1978.

216. Chien, Y.W., Microsealed drug delivery system: theoretical aspects and biomedical assessments. In *Recent Advances in Drug Delivery Systems,* Anderson, J.M. and Kim, S.W., Eds., Plenum Press, New York, 367, 1984.

217. Davis, B.K., Control of diabetes with polyacrylamide implants containing insulin, *Experientia,* 28, 349, 1972.

218. Tuttle, M.E., Baker, R.W., and Laufe, L.E., Slow-release aprotinin delivery of intrauterine device-induced hemorrhage, *J. Memb. Sci.,* 1, 351, 1980.

219. Bos, G.W. et al., Hydrogels for the controlled release of pharmaceutical proteins, *Pharm. Tech.,* 25, 110–120, 2001.

220. Garg, S. et al., Compendium of pharmaceutical excipients for vaginal formulations, *Pharm. Tech. Suppl.,* 14–24, 2001.

221. Shojael, A.H. et al., Systemic drug delivery via the buccal mucosal route, *Pharm. Tech.,* 25, 70–81, 2001.

222. Nokhodchi, A. and Farid, D., Microencapsulation of paracetamol by various emulsion techniques using cellulose acetate phthalate, *Pharm. Tech.,* 26, 54–60, 2002.

223. Singla, A.K. et al., Novel approaches for topical delivery of acetazolamide, *Pharm. Tech.*, 26, 24–34, 2002.

224. Baur, K.H., Colonic drug delivery: review of material trends, *Am. Pharm. Rev.*, 4, 8–16, 2001.

225. Bansal, A.K., Product development issues of powders for injection, *Pharm. Tech.*, 26, 2002.

226. Orienti, I. et al., Hydrogels formed by cross-linked poly(vinyl alcohol) as sustained drug delivery systems, *Arch. Pharm.* (Weinheim), 335, 89–93, 2002.

227. Elvira, C. et al., Starch-based biodegradable hydrogels with potential biomedical applications as drug delivery systems, *Biomaterials*, 23, 1955–1966, 2002.

228. Vinogradov, S.V. et al., Nanosized cationic hydrogels for drug delivery: Preparation, properties and interactions with cells, *Adv. Drug Deliv. Rev.*, 54, 135–1147, 2002.

229. Orienti, T.R. et al., Hydrogels formed by cross-linked polyvinylalcohol as colon-specific drug delivery systems, *Drug Dev. Ind. Pharm.*, 27, 877–884, 2001.

230. Blanco, M.D. et al., *In vivo* drug delivery of 5-fluorouracil using poly(2-hydroxyethyl methacrylate-co-acrylamide) hydrogels, *J. Pharm. Pharmacol.*, 52, 1319–1325, 2000.

231. Han, J.H. et al., Lactitol-based poly(ether polyol) hydrogels for controlled-release chemical and drug delivery systems, *J. Agri. Food Chem.*, 48, 5278–5282, 2000.

232. Shantha, K.L. and Harding, D.R., Preparation and *in vitro* evaluation of poly(N-vinyl-2-pyrrolidone-polyethylene glycol diacrylate)-chitosan interpolymeric pH-responsive hydrogels for oral drug delivery, *Int. J. Pharm.*, 207, 65–70, 2000.

233. Peppas, N.A. et al., Poly(ethylene glycol)-containing hydrogels in drug delivery, *J. Control. Release*, 62, 81–87, 1999.

234. Chiu, H.C. et al., Synthesis and characterization of pH-sensitive dextran hydrogels as a potential colon-specific drug delivery system, *J. Biomater. Sci. Polym. Ed.*, 10, 591–608, 1999.

235. Teijon, J.M. et al., Cytarabine trapping in poly(2-hydroxyethylm methacrylate) hydrogels: drug delivery studies, *Biomaterials*, 18, 383–388, 1997.

236. Zhang, I. et al., Hydrogels with enhanced mass transfer for transdermal drug delivery, *J. Pharm. Sci.*, 85, 1312–1316, 1996.

237. Shantha, K.L. et al., Azo polymeric hydrogels for colon-targeted drug delivery, *Biomaterials*, 16, 1313–1318, 1995.

238. Janes, K.A. et al., Polysaccharide colloidal particles as delivery systems for macromolecules, *Adv. Drug Deliv. Rev.*, 47, 83–97, 2001.

239. Jones, N.A. et al., Polymer chemical structure is a key determinant of physicochemical and colloidal properties of polymer-DNA complexes for gene delivery, *Biochem. Biophys. Acta.*, 1517, 1–18, 2000.

240. Lambert, G. et al., Polyisobytylcyanoacrylate nanocapsules containing an aqueous core as a novel colloidal carrier for the delivery of oligonucleotides, *Pharm. Res.*, 17, 707–714, 2000.

241. Selam, J.L., External and implantable insulin pumps: Current place in the treatment of diabetes, *Exp. Clin. Endocrinol. Diabetes*, 109(Suppl. 2), s333-s340, 2001.

242. Renard, E. et al., Implantable insulin pumps: Infections most likely due to seeding from skin-flora determine severe outcomes of pump-pocket seromas, *Diabetes Metab.*, 27, 62–65, 2001.

243. Bakshi, S. and North, R.B., Implantable pumps for drug delivery to brain, *J. Neurooncol.*, 26, 133–139, 1995.

244. D'Cruz, O.J. and Uckun, F.M., Gel-microemulsion as vaginal spermicides and intravaginal drug delivery vehicles, *Contraception*, 64, 113–123, 2001.

245. Woolfson, A.D. et al., Drug delivery by the intravaginal route, *Crit. Rev. Ther. Drug Carrier Syst.*, 17, 509–555, 2000.

246. Lamb, G.C. et al., Inclusion of an intravaginal progesterone insert plus GnRH and prostaglandin F2alpha for ovulation control in postpartum-suckled beef cows, *J. Anim. Sci.*, 79, 2253–2259, 2001.

247. Wildemeersch, D. and Schacht, E., Treatment of menorrhagia with a novel "frameless" intrauterine levonorgestrel-releasing drug delivery system: a pilot study, *Eur. J. Contracept. Reprod. Health Care*, 6, 93–101, 2001.

248. Lahteenmaki, P. et al., Open randomized study of use of levonorgestrel-releasing intrauterine system as alternative to hysterectomy, *Brit. Med. J.*, 316(7138), 1122–1126, 1998.

249. Sohonen, S. et al., Three-year follow-up of the use of a levonorgestrel-releasing intrauterine system in hormone replacement therapy, *Acta. Obstet. Gynecol. Scand.*, 76, 145–150, 1997.

250. Varila, E. et al., A five-year follow-up study on the use of a levonorgestrel intrauterine system in women receiving hormone replacement therapy, *Fertil. Steril.*, 76, 969–973, 2001.

251. Maruo, T. et al., Effects of the levonprgestrel-releasing intrauterine system on proliferation and apoptosis in the endometrium, *Hum. Reprod.*, 16, 2103–2108, 2001.

252. Diwan, M. and Park, T.G., Pegylation enhances protein stability during encapsulation in PLGA microspheres, *J. Control. Release*, 73, 233–244, 2001.

253. Charrueau, C. et al., Poloxamer 407 as a thermogelling and adhesive polymer for rectal administration of short-chain fatty acids, *Drug Devel. Ind. Pharm.*, 27, 351–357, 2001.

254. Sznitowski, M. et al., Investigation of diazepam lipospheres based on Witepsol and lecithin intended for oral or rectal delivery, *Acta. Pol. Pharm.*, 57, 61–64, 2000.

255. Burstein, A.H. et al., Absorption of phenytoin from rectal suppositories formulated with a polyethylene glycol base, *Pharmacotherapy*, 20, 562–567, 2000.

256. Kim, J.Y. and Ku, Y.S., Enhanced absorption of indomethacin after oral or rectal administration of a self-emulsifying system containing indomethacin to rats, *Int. J. Pharm.*, 194, 81–89, 2000.

257. Dash, A.K. et al., Development of a rectal nicotine delivery system for the treatment of ulcerative colitis, *Int. J. Pharm.*, 190, 21–34, 1999.

258. Barichello, L.M. et al., Enhanced rectal absorption of insulin-loaded Pluronic F-127 gel containing unsaturated fatty acids, *Int. J. Pharm.*, 183, 125–132, 1999.

259. Miyazaki, S. et al., Thermally reversible xyloglucan gels as vehicles for rectal drug delivery, *J. Control. Release*, 56, 75–83, 1998.

260. Cook, G. et al., Pharmacokinetics of cisapride in horses after intravenous and rectal administration, *Am. J. Vet. Res.*, 58, 1427–1430, 1997.

261. Sallai, J. et al., Experiences with the rectal use of trimethoprim, *J. Pharm. Pharmacol.*, 49, 496–499, 1997.
262. Watanabe, Y. et al., Pharmacodynamics and pharmacokinetics of recombinant human granulocyte colony-stimulating factor (rhG-CSF) after administration of a rectal dosage vehicle, *Biol. Pharm. Bull.*, 19, 1059–1063, 1996.
263. Van Os, E.C. et al., Azathioprine pharmacokinetics after intravenous, oral, delayed-release oral and rectal foam administration, *Gut*, 39, 63–68, 1996.
264. Hanff, L.M. and Rutten, W.J., Pharmacokinetic aspects of rectal formulations of temazepam, *Pharm. World Sci.*, 18, 114–119, 1996.
265. Kolloffel, W.J. et al., Pharmacokinetics of propylene glycol after rectal administration, *Pharm. World Sci.*, 18, 109–113, 1996.
266. Kondo, T. et al., Combination effects of alpha-cyclodextrin and xanthan gum on rectal absorption and metabolism of morphine from hollow-type suppositories in rabbits, *Biol. Pharm. Bull.*, 19, 280–286, 1996.
267. Miyazaki, S. et al., Thermally gelling poloxamine Synperonic T908 solution as a vehicle for rectal drug delivery, *Biol. Pharm. Bull.*, 18, 1151–1153, 1995.
268. Van Laar, T. et al., Pharmacokinetics and clinical efficacy of rectal apomorphine in patients with Parkinson's disease: a study of five different suppositories, *Mod. Discov.*, 10, 433–439, 1995.
269. Noach, A.B. et al., Absorption enhancement of a hydrophilic model compound by verapamil after rectal administration to rats, *J. Pharm. Pharmacol.*, 47, 466–468, 1995.
270. Caliceti, P. et al., Polyphosphazene microspheres for insulin delivery, *Int. J. Pharm.*, 211, 57–65, 2000.
271. Udelsman, R. et al., Intraperitoneal delivery of insulin via mechanical pump: surgical implications, *Langenbecks Arch. Surg.*, 385, 367–372, 2000.
272. Tozaki, H. et al., Enhanced absorption of insulin and (Asu[1,7])eel-calcitonin using novel azopolymer-coated pellets for colon-specific drug delivery, *J. Pharm. Sci.*, 90, 89–97, 2001.
273. Mitra, R. et al., Lipid emulsions as vehicles for enhanced nasal delivery of insulin, *Int. J. Pharm.*, 205, 127–134, 2000.
274. Guo, J. et al., Transdermal delivery of insulin in mice by using lecithin vehicles as a carrier, *Drug Deliv.*, 7, 113–116, 2000.
275. Carino, G.P. et al., Nanosphere-based oral insulin delivery, *J. Control. Release*, 65, 261–269, 2000.
276. Bohannon, N.J., Insulin delivery using pen devices: Simple-to-use tools may help ypung and old alike, *Postgrad. Med.*, 106, 57–58, 61–64, 1999.
277. Kawashima, Y. et al., Pulmonary delivery of insulin with nebulized DL-lactide/glycolide copolymer (PLGA) nanospheres to prolong hypoglycemic effect, *J. Control. Release*, 62, 279–287, 1999.
278. Kanikkannan, N. et al., Transdermal iontophoretic delivery of bovine insulin and monomeric human insulin analogue, *J. Control. Release*, 59, 99–105, 1999.
279. Iwanaga, K. et al., Application of surface-coated liposomes for oral delivery of peptide: effects of coating the liposome's surface on the GI transit of insulin, *J. Pharm. Sci.*, 88, 248–252, 1999.
280. Chetty, D.J. and Chien, Y.W., Novel methods of insulin delivery: an update, *Crit. Rev. Ther. Drug Carrier Syst.*, 15, 629–670, 1998.
281. Trehan, A. and Ali, A., Recent approaches in insulin delivery, *Drug Dev. Ind. Pharm.*, 24, 589–597, 1998.

282. Katre, N.V. et al., Multivesicular liposome (DepoFoam) technology for the sustained delivery of insulin-like growth factor-I(IGF-I), *J. Pharm. Sci.*, 87, 1341–1346, 1998.

283. Ando, T. et al., Nasal insulin delivery in rabbits using soybean-derived steryl-glucoside and sterol mixtures as novel enhancers in suspension dosage forms, *Biol. Pharm. Bull.*, 21, 862–865, 1998.

284. Takenaga, M. et al., Microparticle resins as a potential nasal drug delivery system for insulin, *J. Control. Release*, 52, 81–87, 1998.

285. Lee, Y.C. et al., Systemic delivery of insulin via an enhancer-free ocular device, *J. Pharm. Sci.*, 86, 1361–1364, 1997.

286. Kagatani, S. et al., Electroresponsive pulsatile depot delivery of insulin from poly(dimethylaminopropylacrylamide) gel in rats, *J. Pharm. Sci.*, 86, 1273–1277, 1997.

287. Saudeck, C.D., Novel forms of insulin delivery, *Endocrinol. Metab. Clin. North Am.*, 26, 599–610, 1997.

288. Edelman, E.R. et al., Quantification of insulin release from omplantable polymer-based delivery systems and augmentation of therapeutic effect with simultaneous release of somatostatin, *J. Pharm. Sci.*, 85, 1271–1275, 1996.

289. Kubota, M. et al., Portal insulin delivery is superior to peripheral delivery in handling of portally delivered glucose, *Metabolism*, 45, 150–154, 1996.

290. Taylor, M.J. et al., The delivery of insulin from aqueous and nonaqueous reservoir governed by a glucose-sensitive gel membrane, *J. Drug Target.*, 3, 209–216, 1995.

291. Kim, J.J. and Park, K., Modulated insulin delivery from glucose-sensitive hydrogel dosage forms, *J. Control. Release*, 77, 39–47, 2001.

292. Bremseth, D.L. and Pass, F., Delivery of insulin by jet injection: recent observations, *Diabetes Technol. Ther.*, 3, 225–232, 2001.

293. Li, J. et al., Gellan film as an implant for insulin delivery, *J. Biomater. Appl.*, 15, 321–343, 2001.

294. Lee, S. and McAuliffe, D.J., Photomechanical transdermal delivery of insulin *in vivo*, *Lasers Surg. Med.*, 28, 282–285, 2001.

295. Mitra, R. and Perzon, I., Enhanced pulmonary delivery of insulin by lung lavage fluid and phospholipids, *Int. J. Pharm.*, 217, 25–31, 2001.

296. Kisel, M.A. et al., Liposomes with phosphatidylethanol as a carrier for oral delivery of insulin: studies in the rat, *Int. J. Pharm.*, 216, 105–114, 2001.

297. Venugopalan, P. et al., Pelleted bioadhesive polymeric nanoparticles for buccal delivery of insulin: preparation and characterization, *Pharmazie*, 56, 217–219, 2001.

298. Tirucherai, G.S. et al., Pro-drugs in nasal drug delivery, *Expert Opin. Biol. Ther.*, 1, 49–66, 2001.

299. Beall, H.D. and Sloan, K.B., Topical delivery of 5-fluorouracil(5-FU) by 1,3-bis-alkylcarbonyl-5-FU pro-drugs, *Int. J. Pharm.*, 231, 43–49, 2002.

300. Kawakami, S. et al., Controlled-release and ocular absorption of tilidolol utilizing ophthalmic insert-incorporated lipophilic pro-drugs, *J. Control. Release*, 76, 255–263, 2001.

301. Parang, K. and Wiebe, L.I., Novel approaches for designing 5′-O-ester pro-drugs of 3′-azido-2′,3′-dideoxythymidine (AZT), *Curr. Med. Chem.*, 7, 995–1039, 2000.

302. Greenwald, R.B. and Conover, C.D., Poly(ethylene glycol)-conjugated drugs and pro-drugs: A comprehensive review, *Crit. Rev. Ther. Drug Carrier Syst.*, 17, 101–161, 2000.
303. Takata, J. et al., Pro-drugs for systemic bioreductive activation-independent delivery of phyllohydroquinone: An active form of phylloquinone (vitamin K1): preparation and *in vitro* evaluation, *Biol. Pharm. Bull.*, 22, 1347–1354, 1999.
304. Greenwald, R.B. et al., Drug delivery systems based on trimethyl lock lactonization: Poly(ethylene glycol) pro-drugs of amino-containing compounds, *J. Med. Chem.*, 43, 475–487, 2000.
305. Ceruti, M. and Crosasso, P., Preparation, characterization, cytotoxicity and pharmacokinetics of liposomes containing water-soluble pro-drugs of paclitaxel, *J. Control. Release*, 63, 141–153, 2000.
306. Fredholt, K. et al., Chemical and enzymatic stability as well as transport properties of a Leu-enkephalin analogue and ester pro-drugs thereof, *J. Control. Release*, 63, 261–273, 2000.
307. Dubowchik, G.M. et al., Cathepsin B-sensitive dipeptide pro-drugs, 2. Models of anticancer drugs paclitaxel (Taxol), Mitomycin C and doxorubicin, *Bioorg. Med. Chem. Lett.*, 8, 3347–3352, 1998.
308. Mizen, L. and Burton, G., The use of esters as pro-drugs for oral delivery of beta-lactam antibiotics, *Pharm. Biotechnol.*, 11, 345–365, 1998.
309. Lipp, R. et al., Pro-drugs of gestodene for matrix-type transdermal drug delivery systems, *Pharm. Res.*, 15, 1419–1424, 1998.
310. Crosasso, P. et al., Antitumoral activity of liposomes and immunoliposomes containing 5-fluorouridine pro-drugs, *J. Pharm. Sci.*, 86, 832–839, 1997.
311. Springer, C.J. et al., Pro-drugs of thymidylate synthase inhibitors: potential for antibody-directed enzyme pro-drug therapy (ADEPT), *Anticancer Drug Res.*, 11, 625–636, 1996.
312. Wipf, P. et al., Synthesis of chemoreversible pro-drugs of ara-C with variable time-release profiles: biological evalyuation of their apoptotic activity, *Bioorg. Med. Chem.*, 4, 1585–1596, 1996.
313. Takata, J. et al., Vitamin K pro-drugs, 2. Water-soluble pro-drugs of menahydroquinone-4 for systemic site-specific activity, *Pharm. Res.*, 12, 1973–1979, 1995.
314. Hovgaard, L. et al., Drug delivery studies in Caco-2 monolayers: synthesis, hydrolysis and transport of O-cyclopropane carboxylic qcid ester pro-drugs of various beta-blocking agents, *Pharm. Res.*, 12, 387–392, 1995.
315. Oku, N. et al., Therapeutic efficacy of 5-fluorouracil pro-drugs using endogeneous serum proteins as drug carriers: a new strategy in drug delivery system, *Biol. Pharm. Bull.*, 18, 181–184, 1995.
316. Batanero, E. et al., Biodegradable poly(DL-lactide glycolide) microparticles as a vehicle for allergen-specific vaccines: a study performed with Ole e 1, the main allergen of olive pollen, *J. Immunol. Methods*, 259, 87–94, 2002.
317. Sharma, R. et al., Inhalable microparticles containing drug combinations to target alveolar macrophages for treatment of pulmonary tuberculosis, *Pharm. Res.*, 18, 1405–1410, 2001.
318. Benoit, M.A. and Ribet, C., Studies on the potential of microparticles entrapping pDNA-poly(aminoacids) complexes as vaccine delivery systems, *J. Drug Target.*, 9, 253–266, 2001.
319. Vajdy, M. and O'Hagan, D.T., Microparticles for intranasal immunization, *Adv. Drug Deliv. Rev.*, 51, 127–141, 2001.

320. Reithmeier, H. et al., Lipid microparticles as a parenteral controlled device for peptides, *J. Control. Release*, 73, 339–350, 2001.

321. Lin, W.J. and Huang, L.I., Fabrication of porous poly(epsilon-caprolactone) microparticles for protein release, *J. Microencapsul.*, 18, 577–584, 2001.

322. Lee, J.E. and Park, J.C., Preparation of collagen-modified hyaluronan microparticles as antibiotics carriers, *Yonsei Med. J.*, 42, 291–298, 2001.

323. Mandal, T.K. and Bostanian, L.A., Porous biodegradable microparticles for delivery of pentamidine, *Eur. J. Pharm. Biopharm.*, 52, 91–96, 2001.

324. Amorim, M.J. and Ferreira, J.P., Microparticles for delivering therapeutic peptides and proteins to the lumen of the small intestine, *Eur. J. Pharm. Biopharm.*, 52, 39–44, 2001.

325. Morita, T. et al., Preparation of gelatin microparticles by co-lyophilization with poly(ethylene glycol): characterization and application to entrapment into biodegradable microspheres, *Int. J. Pharm.*, 219, 127–137, 2001.

326. Bagwe, R.P. and Kanicky, J.R., Improved drug delivery using microemulsions: rationale, recent progress, and new horizons, *Crit. Rev. Ther. Drug Carrier Syst.*, 18, 77–140, 2001.

327. Lu, L. et al., TGF-beta1 release from biodegradable polymer microparticles: its effects on marrow stromal osteoblast function, *J. Bone Joint Surg. Am.*, 83-A, Suppl. 1 (pt. 2), S82–891, 2001.

328. Clark, M.A. and Hirst, B.H., Lectin-mediated mucosal delivery of drugs and microparticles, *Adv. Drug Deliv. Rev.*, 43, 207–223, 2000.

329. Podual, K. et al., Dynamic behavior of glucose oxidase-containing microparticles of poly(ethylene glycol)-grafted catioic hydrogels in an environment of changing pH, *Biomaterials*, 21, 1439–1450, 2000.

330. Rudge, S.R. et al., Preparation, characterization and performance of magnetic iron-carbon composite microparticles for chemotherapy, *Biomaterials*, 21, 1411–1420, 2000.

331. Esposito, E. et al., Production of Eudragit microparticles by spray-drying technique: influence of experimental parameters on morphological and dimensional characteristics, *Pharm. Dev. Technol.*, 5, 267–278, 2000.

332. Tinsley-Brown, A.M. et al., Formulation of poly(D,L-lactic-co-glycolic acid) microparticles for rapid plasmid DNA delivery, *J. Control. Release*, 66, 229–241, 2000.

333. O'Hagan, D.T. et al., Microparticles in MF59: a potent adjuvant combination for a recombinant protein vaccine against HIV-1, *Vaccines.*, 18, 1793–1801, 2000.

334. Tenjarla, S., Microemulsions: an overview and pharmaceutical applications, *Crit. Rev. Ther. Drug Carrier Syst.*, 16, 461–521, 1999.

335. Scherlund, M. and Malmsten, M., Thermosetting microemulsions and mixed micellar solutions as drug delivery systems for periodental anesthesia, *Int. J. Pharm.*, 194, 103–116, 2000.

336. Delgado, A. and Lavelle, E.C., PLG microparticles stabilized using enteric coating polymers as oral vaccine delivery systems, *Vaccine*, 17, 2927–2938, 1999.

337. Park, K.M. and Lee, M.K., Phospholipid-based microemulsions of flurbiprofen by the sponraneous emulsification process, *Int. J. Pharm.*, 183, 145–154, 1999.

338. Nokhodchi, A. et al., Effects of hydrophilic excipients and compression pressure on physical properties and release behavior of aspirin-tableted microparticles, *Drug Dev. Ind. Pharm.*, 25, 711–716, 1999.

339. Sendil, D. et al., Antibiotic release from biodegradable PHBV microparticles, *J. Control. Release*, 59, 207–217, 1999.
340. Muramatsu, N. and Nakauchi, K., A novel method to prepare monodisperse microparticles, *J. Microencapsul.*, 15, 715–723, 1998.
341. Remunan-Lopez, C. and Lorenzo-Lamosa, M.L., Development of new chitosan-cellulose multicore microparticles for controlled drug delivery, *Eur. J. Pharm. Biopharm.*, 45, 49–56, 1998.
342. O'Hagan, D.T. et al., Recent advances in vaccine adjuvants: the development of MF59 emulsion and polymeric microparticles, *Mol. Med. Today*, 3, 69–75, 1997.
343. Kreuter, J., Nanoparticles and microparticles for drug and vaccine delivery, *J. Anat.*, 189(pt3), 503–505, 1996.
344. Partidos, C.D. et al., Biodegradable microparticles as a delivery system for measles virus cytotoxic T cell epitopes, *Mol. Immunol.*, 33, 485–491, 1996.
345. Ho, H.O. et al., Preparation of microemulsions using polyglycerol fatty acid esters as surfactant for the delivery of protein drugs, *J. Pharm. Sci.*, 85, 138–143, 1996.
346. Gradus-Pizlo, I. et al., Local delivery of biodegradable microparticles containing colchicine or a colchicine analogue: effects on restenosis and implications for catheter-based drug delivery, *J. Am. Coll. Cardiol.*, 26, 1549–1557, 1995.
347. Boisdron-Celle, M. et al., Preparation and characterization of 5-fluorouracil-loaded microparticles as biodegradable anticancer drug carriers, *J. Pharm. Pharmacol.*, 47, 108–114, 1995.

section five

Regulatory considerations and global outlook

chapter nine

Regulatory considerations for drug delivery systems

I.   Introduction

Before 1938 in the U.S., there were practically no Food and Drug Administration (FDA) regulations dealing specifically with drugs. A law in 1906 banned adulteration and misbranding, and it was enforced by court actions based on inspections and the laboratory analysis of drug samples. The U.S. Congress designated the U.S. Pharmacopoeia and the National Formulary as official standards for the strength, quality, and purity of drug products.

A drug that did not meet these standards simply had to be labeled to show the differences.

The toxicity law approved on June 25, 1938, required that regulations be drafted to carry out its provisions. One of these contained the first version of the prescription legend. Another regulation defined what constituted "newness" in a drug and required the filing of a new drug application (NDA) to show the drug's safety. Also included in these first regulations were those for the control of cosmetics. Medical devices, however, were covered in the general regulations for human and veterinary drugs. Far from inhibiting drug innovation, the required additional research seems to have increased innovation; at least 90% of the drugs marketed since 1938 are considered to be new in a medical and legal sense. Drug regulation based on NDAs consequently became the principal system of drug control in the U.S.

World War II greatly stimulated the development of drugs. The most important of these drugs was penicillin, which was critically needed to treat battlefield casualties. Because penicillin was subject to unpredictable variations in purity and potency, which could make the difference between a lifesaving drug and a dangerous one, arrangements were made by the War Production Board to have every batch tested by the FDA. In 1945, when output of the drug justified civilian distribution, Congress enacted amendments to continue the controls originally set up for military procurement. Antibiotic drug regulations are still in effect as of today.

The greatest change in U.S. drug regulation occurred in 1962, when Congress passed a series of amendments dealing with the prescription-legend drugs. These amendments usually are referred to as the drug effectiveness amendments because they added effectiveness to safety as a requirement for FDA approval. Equally important, if not more so, was the requirement that drug manufacturers operate in conformity with current good manufacturing practices (cGMPs). Wide differences in quality control had existed among drug firms. Congressional hearings showed that this variability was a dangerous situation. Public safety required an improved way to ensure that all drug producers met standards already shown to be attainable.

As stated in the FDA's 1962 annual report, "These drug amendments, designed to ensure greater safety, effectiveness, and reliability in prescription drugs, are a milestone in the protection of public health. Drug manufacturers will be required to conduct their establishments in conformity with good manufacturing practices, using controls that will rule out inadequate facilities and poorly trained operators, to ensure that drugs have the identity and strength and meet the quality and purity characteristics they are represented to possess."[1]

Industry expertise was the major component of the cGMP regulations, combined with the FDA's experience gained in thousands of inspections and hundreds of court cases. Put simply, cGMPs spell out proper ways to run a drug-manufacturing business. The regulators work to protect consumers by preventing errors and violations of the law instead of merely punishing violators after harm has been done. In 1973, the U.S. Supreme Court strongly endorsed this type of regulation. In deciding cases that involved drug effectiveness, the court held that FDA regulations could spell out the specifics of what the law requires and how to comply with it.

In recent years, the science of biopharmaceutics has shown convincingly that products containing the same active ingredients can exhibit marked differences in therapeutic effect. In other words, the medical usefulness of a pharmacologically active substance may depend greatly, or even entirely, on its administration in a properly devised dosage form. From this knowledge, delivery systems have been developed that administer drugs to patients at rates that take proper account of the pharmacokinetic properties of the drug. Rate-controlled systems have shown potentially significant applications in pharmaceutical development and marketing under the Drug Price Competition and Patent Restoration Act, which was enacted in 1984. This act has fundamentally reordered the methods by which drugs are developed and marketed, and has lead to the discovery and exploration of exciting new therapies for new and existing pharmaceutical agents. It has also created vast new markets for generic drugs. At the same time, it has rewarded research-based manufacturers that can distinguish their products from the competition by features such as longer dosage schedules, better safety profiles, new indications, or new combinations.

Incorporating distinguishing features in a product is possible with currently available rate-controlled delivery systems. It is made easier, moreover, by provisions of the act, such as those governing the release of safety and effectiveness data and ANDA (abbreviated new drug application)-variance provisions — or combinations of these. For a pioneer firm, using rate-controlled technology to refine drug selectivity and thereby reduce adverse reactions and unwanted side effects entitles a manufacturer to ANDA-exclusivity for an approved product. In the process, the technology provides the manufacturer with an opportunity to establish specifications and seek labeling tailor-made to the pharmacokinetics of the product — including its specific action and the onset, intensity, and duration of that action. This serves to make the product difficult or costly for generic manufacturers and marketers to replicate, even after the product becomes ANDA-eligible. For innovators who are not the originator of the drug, rate-controlled technology provides an opportunity to enter a market by way of applying some therapeutic advance to an established pharmaceutical agent and developing the market for that product during the period of ANDA-exclusivity.

ANDA-exclusivity is a recent, if not entirely new, concept in drug law, originating in the 1983 Orphan Drug Act. ANDA-exclusivity may be defined as a time-limited statutory exemption from generic competition for a drug product that possesses some distinctive feature or innovation that makes it, in effect, a new or better therapy. There are similarities between ANDA-exclusivity and patent protection, but in most respects, the two are quite different. Patent-term restoration extends only to a patent covering an NCE (new chemical entity) and will not be in effect until the end of the 17-year patent life of the new entity. ANDA-exclusivity, on the other hand, protects the finished dosage form of a drug product, whether patented or not, provided that the product in its finished form is sufficiently distinguishable from current therapy.[2]

The ANDA-exclusivity provisions take effect immediately upon the approval of the drug. ANDA-exclusivity provisions can even protect products that are composed of off-patent drugs or naturally occurring or other nonpatentable substances. They can also protect new combinations of existing drugs. Finally, they can protect drugs that have been marketed overseas, but the remaining patent life of which is so short that they have never been thought to be worth the expense involved in seeking U.S. approval. More than 25% of the 200 largest-selling drugs, totaling sales of some $2.5 billion, became ANDA-eligible the day the act took place, and 50 of these are pre-1962 drugs and account for some $1.4 billion in sales. Existing drugs utilizing new and novel delivery systems can conceivably fall in this category.

The regulatory requirements relating to controlled-release dosage forms first appeared in a regulation published approximately 25 years ago by the FDA. It defined the conditions under which the drugs delivered in a controlled-release formulation would be regarded as new drugs within the meaning of the federal Food, Drug, and Cosmetic Act, Section 201. Since then, there has been a proliferation of controlled-release dosage forms that have little rationale and provide no advantage over the same drugs in conventional dosage forms. There has also been an increase in the use of controlled-release labeling claims. Controlled-release dosage forms have been described in various ways, such as delayed-action, extended-action, gradual-release, prolonged-release, protracted-release, repeated-action, slow-release, sustained-release, depot, retard, and timed-release dosage forms. Any of these terms, or similar terms which impart the same idea, are permitted by the FDA in labeling to designate a controlled-release product.

A milestone in the evolution of controlled-release dosage forms was made with the development of several new innovations. For example, the inventions of polymer-medicated controlled-release drug delivery systems for long-term medication. The development of the progesterone-releasing Progestasert intrauterine device (IUD) for 1-year intrauterine contraception, the pilocarpine-releasing Ocusert system for weekly management of glaucoma, and the scopolamine-releasing Transderm-Scop system for 72-h prevention and treatment of motion sickness exemplify it. Regulatory approval of these controlled-release drug delivery systems has been granted by the FDA, and, in the future, the FDA plans to expedite NDAs or ANDAs, provided the industry improves on submission of data for approval.

II.   Current status of drug delivery technology

A.   Regulatory requirements

As the world of pharmaceutical research and development matures, so do FDA regulations. Issues that faced early drug developers are now accepted as a matter of course by the FDA. Regulatory reverberations are painful and costly for those who do not comply. Commonly, the development for marketing of drugs and biological therapeutics occurs in three stages: preclinical investigation (for IND submission), clinical investigation (for NDA submission), and marketing approval. Traditionally, the period of clinical investigation is divided into three phases, namely, Phase I, Phase II, and Phase III. Phase IV can be invoked for post-marketing surveillance.

The Center for the Study of Drug Development estimates the cost of developing a new drug at $230 million. The Pharmaceutical Manufacturers Association estimates the average time for drug development at over 10 years — at least 1 year in preclinical development and an average of 6.4 years in human clinical trials. A prudent approach for quality regulatory planning throughout these phases, and ultimately product introduction into the market, is to know the system well, seek FDA advice, and develop data and submissions that will expedite the regulatory process. The FDA now cites manufacturers for deficiencies that the agency previously found acceptable. The FDA can, and does, seize products, request recalls, enjoin manufacturing, and, if it finds a manufacturer chronically not in compliance, it can take legal action to close the facility.[3–8]

The FDA recognizes that expediting the drug review process is important to maintaining the pharmaceutical industry's vitality and independence. Regulatory affairs leading to product development and registration after the IND is filed are important. Once the matter of determining the appropriate FDA-center jurisdiction is determined, the IND receives a nontechnical administrative review. Assuming the submission is complete, it is then sent for technical review, and a team of reviewers convenes to evaluate it. Each team member reviews the application and submits a report to the group leader. The group leader makes a recommendation to the division director. The director may approve the application or request additional studies.

It is important to recognize that the product's medical, legal, and marketing future can depend on its package insert. Typically, this may include the following: proprietary name of the drug; the established U.S. adopted name (USAN); the dosage form; a statement of sterility (if applicable); the pharmacologic or therapeutic class; the chemical name and structure of the drug; and any other important physical or chemical information, such as radiation data, clinical pharmacology, indications and usage, contraindications, warnings, precautions, adverse reactions, drug abuse and dependence, overdosage, and information about how it is supplied. In addition, the package insert may contain specific labeling requirements.

The following is a brief summary of some of the categories of pre-approval drug applications evaluated by the FDA. IND is the short name for a "Notice of Claimed Investigational Exemption for a New Drug." The filing of an IND with the FDA exempts a new drug shipped in interstate commerce for clinical testing from the requirement that an approved new drug application be on file with the FDA. An IND submission consists of essential chemical, manufacturing, and quality-control information; preclinical (animal) information; a plan of clinical study (including information about the investigator and facilities for the study); and certain legal commitments relating to the new drug.

As mentioned previously, NDA is the abbreviation for "New Drug Application." An approved NDA is required before a new drug may be legally marketed in interstate commerce. An NDA includes full reports of investigations to show that the drug is safe and effective; a full list of components; a full statement of the composition of the drug; a full description of the methods, facilities, and controls used for manufacture, processing, and packaging the drug; samples of the drug, components, and standards that may be required; and specimens of the labeling.

Drugs approved for safety only (approved before the passage of the 1962 amendments) were reviewed under a contract with the National Academy of Sciences-National Research Council (NAS-NRC) for effectiveness. The FDA published its findings based on its review of the NAS-NRC reports. Additional data from industry were accepted and also reviewed. On the basis of this review, if the FDA concluded a drug was ineffective for an indication, it required the indication be deleted from the labeling. Approval for marketing was withdrawn for drugs for which there were no effective indications.

This overall process is known as the Drug Efficacy Study Implementation (DESI) Project. When the FDA concluded that a drug approved between 1938 and 1962 on the basis of safety only was also effective, the indications for which the drug could be labeled and promoted were published in the Federal Register. Subsequent manufacturers of the same drug products are not required to provide animal and clinical evidence of the drug's safety and effectiveness. They are required, however, to obtain approval of an ANDA before the drug product can be marketed. These applications contain information on the formulation, composition, manufacture, and labeling of the product and on its bioequivalence to a standard product.

Prior to passage of the Drug Price Competition and Patent Term Restoration Act of 1984, ANDAs were accepted only for products that were identical to the specific drugs and dosage forms cited in the Federal Register notices; such notices were, in turn, limited to drugs that were originally approved prior to 1962. With passage of new legislation, similar ANDA requirements are now in effect for drugs approved after 1962. In practical terms, drugs approved between January 1, 1982 and September 24, 1984 will not be eligible for ANDAs for 10 years after their approval. New chemical entities (NCEs) approved after September 24, 1984 must have at least five years of exclusive marketing before an ANDA can be submitted.

The first step in the ANDA process is submission of the application to the Division of Generic Drugs. The application is dated, and this date of receipt, in most instances, signals the start of the 180-day statutory review period. The application is then routed to the Consumer Safety Officer or Consumer Safety Technician for the administrative review. At this point, an application is reviewed for acceptability and completeness. The criteria for acceptability are inclusion in the list entitled "Approved Prescription Drug

Products List with Therapeutic Equivalence Evaluations (the Orange Book)"[6] and approval of an NDA prior to January 1, 1982. The latter requirement assures that the drug is not subject to any exclusivity provision of the Waxman–Hatch legislation. If a firm is interested in submitting an ANDA for a drug product not on this list, the firm may seek a determination as to whether or not the drug product is an acceptable candidate for submission as an ANDA. In order to get this determination, the firm is required to file a citizen's petition, as indicated in the Federal Register. If the application is acceptable and complete, it is assigned an ANDA number and a request is prepared for inspection of the applicant's facility, the actual manufacturers of the active ingredient(s), and any outside facilities involved in the manufacturing, testing, or packaging of the drug product. The applicant may not market the drug until notified that the ANDA has been approved.

"Paper NDA" was a term applied to NDAs submitted in response to the FDA's policy to accept for evaluation NDAs for drugs first marketed after 1962 that relied totally upon the published scientific literature for evidence of safety and effectiveness. This policy was implemented in a memorandum dated July 31, 1978, by the Associate Director for New Drug Evaluation (the Finkle Memo). With the passage of the ANDA/patent restoration legislation in 1984, there is little or no value in using the paper NDA route.

A supplemental NDA is a proposal by the applicant to make a particular change in an already approved NDA. This change may be a new indication for use or a change in manufacturing methods or controls, labeling, container, etc. An NDA may also be subject to a supplement proposing a change after approval.

Antibiotic Form 5 is a "Request to Provide for Certification of a New Antibiotic Product." This application is similar to the NDA (i.e., a Form 5 must be approved for safety, effectiveness, labeling and manufacture, just like an NDA, before the new antibiotic product can be legally marketed). In addition, a monograph must be developed describing the tests and specifications for the antibiotic product. Whether exempt from certification by the FDA or not, the applicant still must assure that each batch meets the monograph's specifications.

Antibiotic Form 6 is "Data to Accompany or Precede Every Initial Request for Certification of a Batch of an Antibiotic Drug." After a Form 5 is approved and a monograph is published in the Federal Register, a new manufacturer may propose to duplicate an approved antibiotic drug by filing a Form 6. The Form 6 is analogous to an NDA. After obtaining an approved Form 6, unless exempted from certification, each batch of the antibiotic is tested by the FDA. Each batch must pass the tests and specifications in the published monograph for certification before marketing. The approval process for antibiotics was not affected by the ANDA/patent restoration legislation approved in 1984.

DMF is the abbreviation for "Drug Master File." In order to protect trade secrets, and at the same time disclose sufficient information to the FDA to get marketing approval, it is important to prepare regulatory submissions carefully. This is an important role of the regulatory affairs professional, who often finds submitting a master file an attractive solution. A master file is unusual in the sense that the FDA neither approves nor disapproves it; the agency reviews it only in association with other submissions. The primary submission may be declared approved, approvable, or not approved. If the information in the master file is unacceptable, the FDA may recommend modifications to the master file. Although the agency may refuse to approve the primary submission, it will not disapprove the master file. Unlike many other regulatory submissions, a master file is required by neither the law nor FDA regulations.

A sponsor can use master files in different ways. One is to incorporate information into a regulatory submission by reference to the master file. This strategy can be useful when a sponsor produces several products that contain a common active ingredient or uses a common procedure to manufacture several products. The sponsor can describe the manufacture of the drug substance in a single-drug master file and can then incorporate this information into each NDA by cross-reference to the DMF.

Five types of master files are currently recognized by the FDA:

1. Type I — Manufacturing site, facilities, operating procedures and personnel
2. Type II — For drugs: drug substance, drug intermediate, drug products, or material used in preparation of drug substance or intermediate. For devices: materials or subassembly
3. Type III — Packaging materials
4. Type IV — For drugs: components used in drug products (excipients, colors, flavors, essences). For devices: contract packaging or other contract manufacturing
5. Type V — FDA accepted reference information.[9]

Because one of the primary uses of master files is to allow a second party to cross-reference the information therein, the master file holder is responsible for identifying to the FDA who is authorized to do so. All or any part of the master file may be incorporated into an IND, NDA, ANDA, another DMF, an export application, or an amendment or supplement to any of these. A master file holder may make additions, changes, or deletions to the master file, but must inform all persons authorized to reference the master file of these changes.

The master file holder is responsible for filing an annual update report. The report must contain an updated list of persons authorized to reference the DMF. A master file holder may appoint an agent or representative for the master file. Domestic master file holders need not appoint an agent; foreign master file holders, however, are encouraged to engage a U.S. agent.

Biotechnology companies rarely use Type I master files for biological products because the establishment license application (ELA) usually contains the information included in Type I master files. The Center for Devices and Radiological Health (CDRH) accepts device master files only if the information will be cross-referenced in a second party's device-related sub-mission. Submission of a device master file for cross-reference to the holder's own device submission is unacceptable. An organization that does contract manufacturing, sterilization, or packaging for an investigational device exemption (IDE), pre-market approval application (PMA), or 510(k) holder may submit a master file describing facilities, manufacturing procedures, or quality-control procedures. When the operation is subject to cGMP regula-tions, the master files must address all appropriate cGMP issues.

As with all new drugs in conventional dosage forms, the regulatory approval of a controlled-release drug product (new drug delivery system) requires submission of scientific documents from the pharmaceutical firm to substantiate the clinical safety and efficacy of the controlled-release prod-uct and to demonstrate its controlled-release characteristics. The require-ments for regulatory approval can be outlined as follows:

1. For drugs that have been published in the Federal Register as safe and effective in conventional dosage forms:
   a. Controlled clinical studies may be required to demonstrate the safety and efficacy of the drugs in a controlled-release formulation.
   b. Bioavailability data of drugs delivered in controlled-release for-mulations are also required and may be acceptable in lieu of clinical trials.
2. For drugs that have been published in the Federal Register as safe and effective in controlled-release dosage forms:
   a. Bioavailability data are required and acceptable when comparable to data from an approved controlled-release drug product.
   b. The labeling must be identical to the reference standard with regard to effectiveness and side effects. Without appropriate clin-ical studies, the labeling cannot be modified to make any different claims of clinical effectiveness and side effects.
   c. Bioavailability studies that have been performed under steady-state conditions to demonstrate comparability to an ap-proved immediate-release drug product are acceptable for sup-porting a labeling for dosage administration.

B.   Bioavailability data

Bioavailability data are required in the submission of a new drug application for a controlled-release drug product in accordance with the "Bioavailability Requirements for Controlled-Release Formulations," as specified in the Fed-eral Register. The FDA bioavailability regulations call for firms to provide the following information for their controlled-release drug products:

1. The drug product meets the controlled-release claims made for it.
2. The bioavailability profile established for the drug product rules out the possibility of any dose dumping.

3. The drug product's steady-state performance is equivalent to a currently marketed noncontrolled-release or controlled-release drug product with the same active drug ingredient or therapeutic moiety which has been subjected to an approval for full new drug application.
4. The drug product's formulation provides consistent pharmacokinetic performance between administrations.

C.   *The reference standard*

The reference standard for comparative studies should include one of the following:

1. A solution or suspension of the same active drug ingredient or therapeutic moiety
2. A currently marketed, approved, noncontrolled-release drug product containing the same active drug ingredient or therapeutic moiety
3. A currently marketed controlled-release drug product subject to an approved full new drug application containing the same active drug ingredient or therapeutic moiety.

The bioavailability data, consisting of blood level or urinary excretion rate profiles performed under steady-state conditions, may be acceptable in lieu of clinical trials if it can be demonstrated that the blood levels or urinary excretion rates are comparable to those achieved by multiple doses of the same drug in appropriate conventional dosage forms (for drugs under classification A-1), or to an equivalent dose of the same drug in appropriate controlled-release dosage forms (for drugs under classification A-2). In this case, the labeling must clearly state the recommended dosing regimen, and the claims of effectiveness and side effects must be identical with the reference dosage forms. At times, a multiple-dose steady-state study design in normal subjects or patients may be required for drugs under classification A-1 to establish comparability of dosage forms or to support drug labeling.

Any labeling claims of clinical advantage, such as greater effectiveness or reduced incidence of side effects, must be substantiated by appropriate, well-controlled clinical studies.

Clinical testing would also be required if there is substantial evidence that the drug effectiveness is related to a rate of change in drug level, i.e., pseudo-steady-state, rather than to the absolute blood level achieved at steady-state.

D.   *Requirements to demonstrate drug controlled-release*

To demonstrate the performance of a controlled-release formulation or drug delivery system, two kinds of data are required.

1. In vitro *drug release data*

The drug release-rate profiles are generated from a well-designed, reproducible *in vitro* testing method, such as the dissolution test for solid dosage forms. The test should be sensitive enough to detect any changes in formulation parameters and lot-to-lot variations. A meaningful *in vitro/in vivo* correlation should have been established. The key elements are reproducibility of the method, proper choice of medium, maintenance of perfect sink conditions, and control of solution hydrodynamics.

2. In vivo *bioavailability data*

The key elements in *in vivo* data are pharmacokinetic profiles; bioavailability data, either comparable to the reference dosage form with the same labeling for indications and side effects or nonequivalent to the reference dosage form with demonstration of safety and efficacy to support a different labeling; and reproducibility of *in vivo* performance. It should be feasible to demonstrate the controlled-release nature of a drug from a controlled-release formulation through both *in vitro* and *in vivo* methods. The manufacturers of controlled-release drug products are urged to develop reproducible and sensitive *in vitro* methods to characterize the release mechanisms of the controlled-release drug products they have developed and intend to market. The *in vitro* tests developed can be utilized to predict the bioavailability of the controlled-release dosage forms and can also be relied upon to assure lot-to-lot performance.

Any new controlled-release formulation should offer two advantages. It should allow the maximum percentage of the dose in the formulation to be absorbed and, second, it should be capable of minimizing patient-to-patient variability. One commonly used approach in the development of controlled-release formulations is to modify the rate of release of a drug from the formulation by pharmaceutical manipulation. This may result in alteration of the drug-absorption rate and its plasma levels. Therefore, one must assure that the absorption efficiency of the drug is not appreciably impaired and that variability is not increased.

The selection of drug candidates for controlled-release formulation is of vital importance. Drugs which are known or suspected of undergoing hepatic, first-pass metabolism should not be formulated in a controlled-release dosage form that slows down their rate of absorption, unless this is justified by the fact that an active metabolite is generated in the process. On the other hand, there is little medical rationale for drugs with a long biological half-life (i.e., greater than 12 h) to be formulated in a controlled-release formulation, since the drugs are long-acting themselves, unless the development of a controlled-release formulation will offer some convenience to the patient and result in better patient compliance.

In recent years, novel drug delivery systems have been designed to deliver drugs at predetermined rates over prolonged periods of time. Among them can be included such therapeutic systems as the Ocusert, Progestasert, and Transderm systems. All such new drug delivery systems are considered new drugs requiring full new drug applications as a basis of approval.

In addition to safety and efficacy considerations for these drug products, biopharmaceutic and pharmacokinetic issues need to be addressed by the manufacturer. The key elements that need to be established are reproducibility of the new delivery systems, a defined bioavailability profile that rules out the possibility of dose dumping, demonstration of reasonably good absorption relative to an appropriate standard, and a well-defined pharmacokinetic profile that supports the drug labeling. The basis for the approval of such a controlled-release drug delivery system, from a biopharmaceutic standpoint, consists of the following data: reproducibility of plasma drug levels, defining of pharmacokinetic parameters to support drug labeling; and demonstration that the plasma concentrations are within reasonable therapeutic limits of those achieved with the oral dosage form.

In general, clinical trials might be needed to support certain dosage claims (i.e., every 12 or 24 h). Such trials may not only support maintenance dosage recommendations, but may also document more reliable drug delivery. Regulatory approval of a controlled-release drug product in terms of bioavailability requirements requires demonstration of bioavailability, controlled-release characteristics, reproducibility of *in vivo* performance, and evidence to support clinical safety, efficacy, and the rationale, as reflected in the labeling.

For the clinical development of new products, compliance with cGMP regulations is required when producing clinical trial materials. The product must be produced in a qualified facility, using qualified equipment and validation processes. At early clinical stages, when a single batch of drug product may be produced, and when significant formulation and processing changes may make batch replication difficult or inexact, only limited validation may be possible. The FDA, nonetheless, believes that it is vital to make investigational products in conformance with cGMPs. Product contamination and wide variations in potency can potentially produce substantial toxicity and wide variability in pharmacological activity of the drug. Product safety, quality, and uniformity may affect the outcome of a clinical investigation that will, in large measure, determine whether or not the product will be approved for marketing.

Both nonclinical and clinical research are required to conform to quality-control principles. cGMP regulations govern nonclinical laboratories engaging in studies intended to support applications for research or marketing permits for regulated products. Facilities are inspected routinely, approximately every two years, and any time the FDA has reason to carry out a "for cause" inspection. Establishment inspection reports are issued, and, when necessary, the FDA may issue a warning letter or disqualify a facility or an investigator. Criminal investigations can lead to charges of fraud, untrue statements of material facts, bribery, illegal gratuities, or criminal negligence. Studies carried out at disqualified facilities or by disqualified investigators can be rejected; that is, they cannot be used to support claims of safety and efficacy — an important factor to consider when identifying contract vendors of toxicology and clinical research services.[10]

Protocols are narrative documents that describe the general conduct of operations or activities in GMP facilities. Protocols contain company policies or commitments and cite more specific documents — such as standard operating procedures (SOPs) — that unify individual activities within or between departments. In effect, protocols describe systems of cGMP for the routine rituals of conduct in a facility that ensure consistent, reliable operations. Protocol commitments usually include company or departmental policy, standards, and acceptance criteria. Neither the Code of Federal Regulations nor guideline documents specifically mention protocols, except in association with validation. Although they are not required documents, the information and commitments they contain are required. Using protocols may minimize FDA prior-approval requirements. The article by DeSain[11] discusses protocols as documents that unify, direct, and control activities in a GMP manufacturing environment. Throughout inspections and audits by clients and regulators, protocol documents provide a clear, organized map of the often overwhelming sea of SOPs, specifications, and product-processing events.

The FDA has increased its attention to preapproval activities and is now giving more scrutiny to GMP and NDA integrity issues. The FDA policies for system validation during new drug development have undergone significant changes. The FDA expects firms to provide adequate assurances that drugs have the identity, strength, quality, and purity characteristics that they are purported or represented to possess. Even before the 1978 GMP revisions introduced the requirement for validations, the agency expected firms to use sound scientific methods during the development of new drugs and during their manufacture for clinical trials.

In the wake of the generic drug scandal, the FDA has increased the number of preapproval inspections. As the FDA increased its scrutiny of integrity and GMP compliance for new drugs, many firms were found to have problems. When preapproval inspections detect problems with either integrity or inadequate validation of equipment or processes, there are problems for all concerned. The FDA must decide if the problems are significant enough to withhold approvals of NDAs. Firms have to be in a position to justify at all times the validity of their processes.[12]

Since 1987, the FDA has published a large number of guidelines that describe the format and content of applications and documents submitted to the agency. Examples include guidelines on such topics as general principles of validation, aseptic processing, stability, pharmacokinetics, documentation, drug master files, microbiology, etc. In 1991, the agency published two guidelines that are particularly significant for manufacturing and systems validation for new drug products. In March 1991, the agency published a revised edition of *the Guideline on the Preparation of Investigational New Drug Products* (human and animal).[11] This document provides information about some of the unique aspects of GMPs for research and development activities and highlights some of the GMP sections about which questions are often asked. These guidelines address many of the unusual aspects of scaling up from research to commercial production, and provide guidance about record-retention requirements.

In September 1991, the FDA published a revision to the *Guide to Inspection of Bulk Pharmaceutical Chemicals*. This document is relevant to the raw-material active ingredients that may be used in formulating new drug products. The guide identifies some of the important systems that may have an influence on bulk drug quality. GMPs (Part 211) apply only to finished pharmaceuticals, but the guide emphasizes the requirement that drugs must be made in accordance with good manufacturing practices. The guide cites a dozen specific manufacturing and control systems that parallel the sections contained in the GMP regulations, including raw materials, buildings, equipment, production and process control, etc. Guidance is provided about acceptable practices. The agency considers it important that firms have adequate data to demonstrate the suitability of ingredients used to make finished pharmaceuticals. This document helps clarify some of the issues that have been controversial in the past.

Tetzlaff[12] presents information about the FDA preapproval inspection program that has been in effect since October 1990. During the past few years, the policies and procedures used by the agency were designed to ensure that information submitted to the FDA is factual and complete. The FDA is giving greater priorities to NDA integrity and process validation for new drugs. Manufacturers should realize that the FDA will be giving greater scrutiny to the data submitted, and they must be prepared to support the validation of their equipment, facilities, and processes. The FDA and the industry must work closely together to ensure that the needs of each are satisfied.[13,14]

In another article, Tetzlaff[15] describes current issues in documenting computer-system validation and operation from the standpoint of an FDA investigator. The GMP regulations require that automated systems be routinely calibrated or checked according to a written program designed to ensure proper performance. Written records of the checks and inspections must be maintained to demonstrate adequate performance monitoring. Each firm must develop its own record-keeping system to define completely and clearly what the systems are supposed to do and to provide documented evidence that processes perform in the manner expected, and that automated system documentation will conform to the intent of the GMP guidelines.

Early in the drug-development phase, a drug is first prepared in small quantities for initial clinical studies. Larger amounts of the drug are prepared, usually varying in formulation, as the number and size of the studies increase. Although the formulation used in the definitive clinical studies requires a bioavailability determination, it is not unusual for bioavailability studies to have been conducted early on a number of formulations.

Shah et al.[16] discuss the FDA's views regarding the scale-up of controlled-release dosage forms. In the development of a new version of an already approved and marketed drug product (i.e., for an ANDA), the usual

custom is first to determine the marketed product's *in vitro* release characteristics. A small batch formulation is prepared matching the *in vitro* release
characteristics of the patented marketed product. It is then studied to determine *in vivo* performance. The product is approved for marketing if it meets
stability requirements, the usual ANDA criteria, and appropriate *in vitro* and
in vivo requirements. In this instance, the issue of scale-up becomes quite
important (unlike the approval process for NCEs), since the investigator not
only lacks formulation development experience with the critical manufacturing variables, but also lacks knowledge of the *in vivo-in vitro* formulation
normally obtained through the IND phase.

Dissolution is commonly considered the most significant *in vitro* measurement of product performance for solid dosage forms. Although dissolution is only one of the processes involved in drug absorption, it is an
essential step. Consequently, until more refined models for predicting oral
bioavailability are developed, this one measure of performance must be
relied upon. Because performing biostudies on every manufactured batch is
impractical, formulators must be able to rely on *in vitro* testing to ensure
batch-to-batch uniformity and consistency in bioavailability. For the *in vitro*
test to be predictive, and therefore, useful and meaningful, it should correlate
well with the product's *in vivo* performance. Also, for the *in vitro* test to be
reliable, its specifications must be relevant to critical manufacturing and
bioavailability variables. The manufacturing variables critical for batch
scale-up depend on the nature of the product, especially for oral controlled-release formulations, which vary, from extended-release suspensions
to soluble, insoluble, and erosion matrices to microencapsulated products.

The FDA's Office of Generic Drugs has recently established an interim
guideline regarding the minimum batch size and scale-up considerations for
nonantibiotic, immediate-release, solid oral dosage forms. The pilot-batch
size should be ≥10% of the proposed commercial scale-up production batch,
contain ≥100,000 solid oral dosage units, and have 3 months of accelerated
stability and comparative dissolution data (for ANDAs). The drug product
is required to be manufactured in a production facility that is in compliance
with GMPs and using equipment appropriate for production of that marketed product. The Office of Generic Drugs' interim guideline permits a
tenfold batch scale-up, provided that the company submits appropriate process controls, validation data, finished-product test data, dissolution data,
and stability data from the scale-up batch.

The objective of batch scale-up is to develop an economically feasible
procedure that ensures bio- and therapeutic equivalence. Production is generally a more efficient process than the experimental process. The successful
scale-up of any process involving pilot or production-size equipment
depends greatly on the existence of an effective laboratory development
program. Scale-up of a batch from laboratory to pilot to production usually
requires a number of scale-up stages or phases. Each stage or phase of the
scale-up should be carefully evaluated. All aspects of the development program should be understood and validated. All process and product data

should be collected and analyzed to define the process equipment requirements and to determine product quality achieved. Raw material variability,
process control latitude, product quality variations, and process equipment
limitations should be considered and, when appropriate, characterized by
sensitive *in vitro* dissolution studies or other appropriate objective measures.

During the scale-up phase, it is essential to critically analyze process
parameter sensitivity (flexibility) in order to optimize the in-process variables. The most common variables, especially in the manufacture of tableted
dosage forms, include the raw materials, processes, and equipment involved
in mixing, drying, milling, and coating. Some of the variables are also common to other finished dosage forms, such as capsules. As mentioned previously, the *in vitro* dissolution test is recognized as the single most important
quality-control test to assess lot-to-lot product uniformity and bioequivalence. Consequently, this test has been used to measure the influence of
different manufacturing variables on the finished product. Other important
factors for consideration are raw material processing, coating process,
in vitro-in vivo correlation, and relationships between critical manufacturing
variables and *in vitro* dissolution.

The production batch formula often provides for the use of a range of
inactive ingredients. It is important to know what happens to *in vitro* dissolution rates when the batch is prepared with either extreme of the ingredients. All ranges identified in the batch formula should ensure the quality of
the final product. The effect of variation in process modification sometimes
may not be apparent or detectable by *in vitro* testing when the freshly manufactured product is evaluated. However, effects on product stability and
shelf life may be different and should be investigated carefully. Following
approval of the generic drug biobatch or of the NDA pivotal clinical trial
batch, complete records should be maintained concerning any changes in
formulation or manufacturing process. Such changes — including scale-up
— should be reported.

Every production batch must have the same performance characteristics
as those of the FDA-approved batch. This will ensure that the product meets
the standards of the lot submitted in support of the application, and thus
can be assumed safe and efficacious. With present state-of-the-art knowledge, it may be impossible to develop an appropriate, sensitive, *in vitro*
procedure that can be used to characterize certain controlled-release preparations. In these cases, the test is not useful for detecting process changes,
and scale-up will require biostudies. Finally, it should be emphasized that
these scale-up considerations have been developed based on accumulated
experience and knowledge in the field of biopharmaceutics and have not
been challenged in the manufacturing arena. These considerations should
be revised as the current state of knowledge progresses and with increasing
expertise of pharmaceutical technology.[17–21]

The FDA considers transdermal drug delivery (TDD) systems to be new
drugs intended for the treatment or prevention of a systemic disease or condition, as opposed to topical drugs intended for a local effect. All such drugs

are considered to be controlled-release dosage forms and, therefore, require a demonstration of controlled-release characteristics to support drug labeling. ANDA submissions of a transdermal dosage form are approvable, provided that the release mechanism, adhesives, etc. are similar and the blood level or urinary data are equivalent to the approved product. TDD systems require demonstration of safety, both in terms of local irritation and systemic toxicity.

In the event that systemic toxicity of an active therapeutic moiety is defined in the scientific literature, e.g., nitroglycerine, scopolamine, etc., the agency may waive the demonstration of animal systemic toxicity, but may require additional clinical testing for safety or efficacy in human subjects. Where blood level comparisons of the transdermal medication to an already established systemic route of administration of the same drug (e.g., IV, IM, or PO) are available, and comparable, systemic safety issues may be ruled out.

Clinical testing for efficacy is required for TDD systems involving new drug entities and may be required to support new efficacy claims on already marketed drugs. Biopharmaceutic considerations can play an immense role in the latter determinations, since the FDA may be able to rely on blood level comparisons in cases where the pharmacodynamic effects of a drug are well defined, employing a systemic or oral route of drug administration. Clinical efficacy data should be supplied to support a new indication or any claim of superior efficacy. Any claim as to enhanced or superior reproducibility or prolonged therapy will require appropriate bioavailability/pharmacokinetic studies to support drug labeling. In certain instances, additional metabolic studies in man may be required to define the metabolism of the drug where it is suspected that significant alteration in metabolic pathways may be encountered due to differences in hepatic-portal or GI metabolism.

The types of studies required as a basis for approval of an NDA need to be customized and are largely dictated by the following considerations: nature of the active drug; availability of marketed systemic dosage form of the same drug; medical and biopharmaceutic rationale; literature data on safety, efficacy, and pharmacodynamics of the drug entity; and agency experience with the drug or drug delivery system.

It should be stressed that these drug delivery systems require careful scientific evaluation based on the pharmacologic and pharmacokinetic properties of the drug and drug delivery systems. Drugs with a narrow therapeutic index or drugs that require patient titration may need additional specialized studies to define safety, efficacy, and labeling requirements. Such studies need to be customized. In most instances, where systemic toxicity of the drug entity is well known, further animal toxicity testing is obviated. Where toxicity data are required, such requirements should parallel other systemic drugs of the same pharmacological class.

E.   Bioequivalence

Biopharmaceutic considerations are pivotal for TDD systems since they determine which specific kinds of clinical or toxicological studies need to be performed. There is an absolute need to define the dosage for the delivery system in terms of the rate and extent of drug delivery; the pharmacokinetics and metabolism of the active therapeutic moiety itself, where such information is lacking; and *in vivo* reproducibility of the drug delivery system. It should be stressed that the pharmacokinetics and metabolism of a drug delivered from a TDD system may differ significantly from that administered orally due to bypassing of liver or GI metabolism. In such instances, the pharmacokinetic profile of the drug should be similar to intravenous infusion, which delivers the drug by a zero-order mechanism. In evaluating TDD systems, there is a need to evaluate the site of drug administration in order to optimize drug delivery (since skin permeability varies, only tested sites are approved and indicated in labeling); consider parameters such as optimal skin area for drug administration and blood flow at that site, etc.; and assess the role of the skin in controlling (and in some instances, sustaining) drug delivery to the systemic circulation.[22]

For most drugs, the bioavailability and pharmacokinetic parameters are defined using oral or intravenous dosage administration. TDD systems in general deliver the drug at a rate comparable to an intravenous infusion rate. Therefore, ideally, the bioavailability and pharmacokinetics of a TDD system should be defined in comparison to an intravenous dose. In cases where an IV dose is not available, an oral or IM dose may be employed. Transdermal scopolamine, for example, has been compared to oral and intramuscular drug administration, as well as intravenous infusion. In that study, scopolamine was comparable to a zero-order infusion over a three-day period. The rate of drug delivery was designed to maintain plasma levels necessary for its antiemetic effect (for motion sickness) while at the same time avoiding side effects (e.g., drowsiness and tachycardia) associated with oral dosing.

In considering systemically effective drug delivery systems using absorptive surfaces other than the GI tract, one cannot ignore the likelihood that such dosage forms will generate significantly different metabolites and pharmacokinetic profiles than those obtained from oral dosage forms. For example, where a first-pass effect is associated with oral drug delivery, it would be necessary to demonstrate that a systemically effective TDD system avoids first-pass liver metabolism associated with the oral dosage form. In addition, the transdermal dosage form is likely to deliver a drug over a longer period of time. These pharmacokinetic differences have been demonstrated in two systemically effective nitroglycerine products (sublingual tablets and transdermal patches). The data showed that cutaneous absorption of nitroglycerine from a TDD system results in detectable plasma levels for 24 h, in contrast to plasma levels for only 15 min following a sublingual administration.

In the case of clonidine, steady-state blood levels and urinary recovery have been compared following transdermal and oral administration. The transdermal patch, applied on the upper outer arm, was worn for 7 days. Oral drug was administered twice daily for 4 consecutive days. The steady-state blood levels, Cmax, Cmin, and urinary excretion data from the patch were comparable to that obtained with the oral dosage regimen.[22]

In addition to defining the pharmacokinetic profile of a new drug delivery system, it is necessary to demonstrate the brand-to-brand and batch-to-batch (within a brand) drug-release reproducibility. This can be achieved by comparison of different batches of the drug delivery system in the same patients or by development of a suitable *in vitro* procedure.

The stratum corneum, especially the deeper, horny layers, can sometimes act as a drug reservoir and modify transdermal permeation characteristics of some drugs. Therefore, at the time of evaluating TDD systems, the protocol should be designed to allow for a determination as to whether the tissue serves as a drug reservoir or not. In the case of scopolamine, the skin does serve as a tissue reservoir, whereas in the case of transdermal nitroglycerine, it does not. This can be accomplished by following blood or urinary drug levels after the patch is removed.

The basis of approval of TDD systems from a biopharmaceutics standpoint consists of a demonstration that the plasma concentrations of the active moiety are comparable to those of an approved dosage form (if the profile of active metabolites generated is different from the administration of the approved dosage form, some clinical studies may be required), demonstration of batch-to-batch reproducibility, and, defined pharmacokinetic parameters to support drug labeling. It may not always be feasible or desirable to define the bioavailability profile of a TDD system relative to an IV dose (bolus or zero-order infusion). The use of other routes of drug administration providing additional pharmacokinetic data may be desirable in order to permit appropriate labeling.

Bioavailability data are required as part of the submission of an NDA, as noted earlier. Because of the lack of acceptable correlative *in vivo/in vitro* data for controlled-release products at this time, *in vitro* data is not acceptable for approval of additional dosage strengths. In the case of multiple-strength controlled-release products, the Division of Biopharmaceutics (FDA) requires multiple-dose, steady-state and single-dose studies on the highest strength of all controlled-release products. In addition, a single-dose crossover study will be required for each additional lesser-dosage strength for NDA/ANDA approval, provided the system is linear and dose proportionality can be established. The single-dose crossover study will include the dosage strengths on which multiple studies were done. In the case of controlled-release capsule dosage forms involving identical beaded material, where the various dosage strengths differ from each other only in the amount of material each capsule contains, then a single- and multiple-dose study will only be required for the highest dosage strength. Other strengths could be approved solely on the basis of comparative dissolution, depending upon the ancillary information provided.

Typically, the FDA evaluation of controlled-release drug products contains the following aspects. In conventional (i.e., immediate-release) preparations, drug absorption is usually quite rapid and most often dependent upon the concentration of the drug in the GI fluids. Elimination is usually slower in that the elimination rate constant, K_e, is considerably smaller than the absorption-rate constant, K_a. An important fact about controlled-release preparations is that they often involve the opposite, i.e., K_a is considerably smaller than K_e. The purpose of a controlled-release preparation is to deliver sustained drug levels. In this particular case, absorption is considerably less rapid, and, in fact, is designed into the drug-dosage system to be slower than the rate of elimination. Because in these (controlled-release products), K_a is smaller than K_e, pharmacokineticists have termed it a "flip-flop model." Consideration must also be given to the "therapeutic window." In this case, one is concerned with what percentage of time steady-state systemic drug concentration is within the clinically effective range.

The selection of a particular drug candidate for controlled-release formulation is obviously of vital importance. Depot preparations of penicillin provide an outstanding example of a useful controlled-release formulation. Insulin is another example of a drug that has been prepared in controlled-release forms, with the result that the management of diabetes has been simplified.

It is usually not possible for a controlled-release drug product to be properly evaluated by single-dose administration. There usually is a need to determine whether controlled-release dosage can achieve well-defined therapeutic plasma levels or equivalent plasma levels obtained by an immediate-release dosage form administered to healthy volunteers or patients. It should be emphasized that bioequivalence employing the superimposition principle need not be demonstrated for purposes of product approval.

By definition, the rate of absorption for a controlled-release dosage form will differ appreciably relative to the immediate-release dosage forms or other systems and provide greater convenience or better patient compliance. What needs to be established is satisfactory bioavailability and pharmacokinetics to support drug labeling. The following criteria should be met: satisfactory steady-state plasma levels should be obtained with the test drug and reference drug in sufficient patients or volunteers to warrant comparison; determination of adequate steady-state should be established by comparison of Cmin values (trough values) on three or more consecutive days; failure to achieve satisfactory steady-state in a large percentage of subjects indicates either lack of patient compliance or dosage failure; comparison of pharmacokinetic parameters (e.g., Cmin, "AUC" values, etc.) should be limited only to subjects who achieve steady-state conditions; comparison of "AUC" during a dosing interval is only proper if both the test drug and reference drug are at steady-state.

Other relevant information regarding these aspects can be found in the Code of Federal Regulations, the U.S. Pharmacopoeia, and symposia presented through several Controlled Release Society workshops.[23]

III. Submission of documents for manufacture and quality

A. Control of drug products

The following section considers the documentation of the manufacturing process used to produce dosage forms and the accompanying quality-control systems intended for raw materials, in-process materials, and the finished dosage form suitable for administration. The information contained herein does not necessarily involve mandatory requirements; however, it offers guidance on acceptable approaches to meeting regulatory requirements. Different approaches may be followed, but the applicant is encouraged to discuss significant variations in advance with the FDA reviewers to preclude expending time and effort in preparing a submission that the FDA may later determine to be unacceptable. The information and data discussed here relate to the identity, strength, quality, and purity of the dosage form and the procedures for assuring that all batches manufactured conform to the appropriate specifications. Information relating to the container, closure, stability, and labeling is not included here, since it can found be in the FDA's guidelines.

Information included in a DMF to satisfy the documentation needed to evaluate any particular part of the manufacture and quality control for a drug product is acceptable, provided the reference is specific, current, and applicable to the drug product described in the application. However, the agency will consider the information in a DMF only if written authorization is granted with specific reference to pertinent sections, including dates of submission of the DMF.

1. Drug product (NDAs and ANDAs)

The following information should be included in the application:

Components: Provide a list of components, including all substances and process materials used in producing a defined finished drug or a placebo product. List all substances used in the finished product, whether or not they remain in the finished product, and state the quality designation or grade for each material. Identify each component by its established name, if any, or by complete chemical name, using structural formulas when necessary, for specific identification. If any proprietary preparations or other mixtures are used as components, their identity should include a complete statement of composition and other information that will properly describe and identify these materials. Justify proposed alternatives for any listed substances by demonstrating that the use of these alternatives does not significantly alter the stability and bioavailability of the drug product and the suitability of manufacturing controls.

Composition, statement of composition: A statement of the quantitative composition should specify, by unit dose, a definite weight or measure for each active drug substance and a definite weight, measure, or appropriate range for all other ingredients contained in the drug product.

Batch formula: Provide a complete list of the ingredients and the amounts to be used for the manufacture of a representative batch of the drug product. Submit a separate batch formula for each formulation of the drug product. All ingredients should be included in the batch formula whether or not they remain in the finished product

Specifications and analytical methods for inactive components: Provide acceptance specifications and the corresponding analytical methods for all inactive components of the formulation, regardless of whether they remain in the finished product. Limits and methods (applicable to the finished dosage form) for components that are removed in the manufacturing process should be included. Limits and methods must be included for potentially toxic components.

Manufacturer: State the name, location, and, where applicable, building number of each facility having a part in the manufacturing or controls of the drug product. This should include manufacturers of the bulk drug substances and the bulk drug product; contract packagers or labelers; contract laboratories performing quality-control tests on raw materials, drug substance, or the finished drug product; and suppliers of components used in the manufacture of the drug product.

Methods of manufacturing and packaging; production operations: To facilitate the evaluation of the production and control of the drug product, submit a copy of the proposed or actual master batch production and control records, or a comparably detailed description of the production process for a representative batch. Describe the manufacturing and packaging process for a representative batch, including a description of each production step, actual operating conditions, equipment to be utilized, and points of sampling for in-process controls. A schematic diagram of the production process is often helpful. Such a diagram should include a superimposed materials flow plan, indicating the equipment used and the points of sampling.

Processing operations: Before reprocessing a drug product, the applicant should consider the effects of reprocessing on stability and bioavailability. To permit approval of the reprocessing of batches of bulk, in-process, and finished drug products that do not conform to established specifications, the original submission of an NDA may include proposals for reprocessing procedures that cover possible foreseeable deviations from specifications. Such reprocessing may require additional amounts of one or more of the components. However, the amounts added should not result in a component being present beyond the reasonable variations provided for the formulation. Reprocessing due to deviations not anticipated in the original NDA should be covered by a supplemental application.

Approval of reprocessing procedures must be obtained before release of the reprocessed drug or drug product. These supplements may be directed to the reprocessing of a specific lot/batch, or may be admitted as a new procedure. Supplemental applications for reprocessing should include a specific and complete description of the rejected material, including a statement of the deviations from the specifications; a detailed description of the proposed reprocessing procedure, including controls beyond those established for routine production; and a statement of the maximum time elapsed between the initial manufacture and the time of reprocessing and the storage conditions during this interval.

Specifications and analytical methods for the drug product: The goal of drug product manufacture is reproducibility within all specified limits. The significant chemical and physical parameters important to clinical response of the drug product should be defined at an early stage in the investigational studies, so that the transition to routine production lot manufacture may be conducted rationally. A well-organized drug application should demonstrate that the manufacturing, sampling, and control processes have been designed to provide a consistent product that, within any lot and on a lot-to-lot basis, does not vary beyond the established specifications.

Sampling methods: Describe the sampling plan that will be used to assure that the sample of the drug product obtained is representative of the batch. The plan should include both the sampling of production batches and the selection of subsamples for analytical testing. This plan will, of course, be applicable only to batches of that particular size, so procedures for scale-up or scale-down of this sampling plan to other batch sizes must also be provided. If samples are pooled, a justification must be given for pooling them.

In-process controls: The analytical controls used during the various stages of manufacturing and processing of the dosage form should be fully described. Where feasible, the in-process specifications should be supported by appropriate data that may include, but does not have to be limited to, representative master/batch production and control records. In particular, when these records are submitted in support of a supplemental application that proposes the deletion or broadening of specifications, the records should cover a consecutive series of batches. Information on in-process controls in manufacturing is essential to a thorough review of the manufacturing and processing of the drug.[24]

2.   Regulatory specifications and methods for drug products

Regulatory specifications are the defined limits within which test results for a drug substance or drug product should fall when determined by the regulatory methodology. The regulatory methodology is the procedure or set of procedures used by the FDA to ascertain whether or not the drug substance or drug product is in conformance with the approved regulatory specifications in the NDA. The regulatory tests and specifications should be designed to ensure that the dosage form will meet acceptable therapeutic and physicochemical standards throughout the shelf life of the marketed product. As such, regulatory specifications normally include all criteria that apply to the bulk dosage form, those related to the packaged product, and those that indicate the presence or absence of degradation.

Regulatory specifications may differ from in-house product-release specifications. All drug products require assay and identity tests and specifications.

For compendial products, the specifications and tests in the United States Pharmacopoeia/National Formulary (USP/NF) monographs may satisfy relevant requirements. Additional specifications or alternate analytical methods may be required as necessary. Broader limits than those in the USP/NF monograph will not ordinarily be approved as regulatory specifications unless the labeling indicates that the product differs from the official monograph. When alternate analytical methods that are equivalent to, or that are an improvement over, the compendial methods are submitted to the agency, the applicant is encouraged to simultaneously ask the U.S. Pharmacopoeia Convention (USPC) to change or modify the methodology in the monograph. Assay and identity specifications using a well-characterized reference standard and description of physical characteristics are required. A description of other attributes should also be considered for inclusion, depending on the type of dosage form. The following list is advisory, and is not exhaustive, and the omission of a parameter from the list should not lead to the conclusion that it cannot be the subject of a regulatory test under appropriate circumstances.

Tablets, capsules, and other solid dosage forms: Uniformity of dosage units, rate of release of the active ingredient from the dosage form by methodology as appropriate for the dosage form, moisture content, where applicable. Special consideration should be given to dosage forms in which a major component is known to be hygroscopic and softening or melting points for suppositories.

Solutions (including sterile solids for injection): Clarity, limit of particulate matter, assay of preservative, isotonicity (for injectable and ophthalmic products), and pH determination; sterility of injectable and ophthalmic products; apyrogenicity of injectable products; leakage test for ampoules; aerosols; pouch packets; stripes; tubes; etc., metering tests; specifications; container pressure for aerosols; completeness and clarity of constituted solutions.

Suspensions: Assay of preservative and pH determination, sterility of injectable and ophthalmic products, apyrogenicity of injectable products, particle size specifications, resuspendibility, viscosity, sedimentation rates, caking and syringability of suspensions, and metering tests, specifications, and container pressure for aerosols.

Creams, emulsions, and ointments: Assay of preservative and pH determination, sterility where required, homogenicity, and uniformity of dosage units as appropriate.

Transdermal delivery systems: *In vitro* release rates and uniformity of dosage units.

Diluent solutions: Full-acceptance specifications and analytical methods, including assays for preservatives, should be included for diluents with dry solids or for liquid concentrates; sterile plastic devices containing active drugs; *in vitro* release rates; sterility; and limits for residual ethylene oxide and its decomposition products, as applicable; in addition to the identity of all plastic components and additional physical tests, such as frame memory, resiliency, tensile strength, and seal integrity of the immediate package.

Placebos: A suitable test demonstrating the absence of the drug substance in the placebo.

Investigational formulations (INDs): The following information should be included in the application. Provide a list of all components, including all substances and in-process materials used in producing a defined investigational drug product or placebo product. List all substances used in the manufacture of a drug product, whether or not they appear in the dosage form, and state the quality designation or grade for each material. Each component should be properly identified by its established name, if any, or by complete chemical name, using structural formulas when necessary for specific identification. If any proprietary preparations or other mixtures are used as components, their identity should include a complete statement of composition and other information that will properly describe and identify them. Justify proposed alternatives for any listed substances. An amendment should be filed for any significant changes in formulation not proposed in the initial IND. Submit a quantitative statement of composition. It should specify an appropriate range or a definite weight or measure for each ingredient contained in the investigational drug product and contain a batch formula representative of that to be used for the manufacture of the investigational drug product. Each formulation of defined dosage forms, potencies/strengths, or significant changes of inactive ingredients should be identified with a formulation number or other appropriate designation.

Include all ingredients in the batch formula regardless of whether they remain in the investigational drug product. The content of new drug indicated in the statements of composition and the representative batch formula should be on the basis of 100% potency/strengths, as stated on the label. Any calculated excess of an ingredient over the label declaration should be designated as such, and percent excess should be shown. Explain any overage in the batch formula, other than that added to compensate for losses in manufacturing.

3. Methods of manufacturing and packaging

A document describing proposed production and packaging operations should be submitted for IND phases. Although it would lack certain features of the final record, it should be as complete as possible under the circumstances.

Specifications and analytical methods for investigational drug products: The product tests and specifications appropriate to investigational drug products are not as well developed as when an NDA is submitted. However, the safety of investigational products can be assured only if appropriate analytical information is provided. It is necessary to realize that the developmental studies of such methods are not so clearly separated into Phases I, II, and III as the clinical studies. The following is presented as a general IND development sequence intended to provide guidance for the development of product information during the investigational phases. The ultimate goal of this sequence is the development of product tests and specifications in the form that will eventually be submitted with an NDA. The level of detail for specifications and analytical methods set forth here should be considered as an ultimate goal. However, the fact that an item may not be included here in the discussion should not be viewed as justification for its omission at a later development stage of an IND.

Phases I and II: An assay method including adequate acceptance specifications for content of the new drug substance in the dosage form should be submitted. The initial limits need not be overly narrow, but should be appropriately tightened as experience with the drug accumulates. Because the assay alone might not serve as a satisfactory identity test, using a different method may be necessary during these phases. Chemical and physical tests characterizing the dosage form should be included for solid oral dosage forms, such as uniformity and dissolution profile in an appropriate medium. Sterility tests, a measure of particulate content, and apyrogenicity testing should be included for injectables. The assay or other procedure should make use of a reference standard or interim standard, and analytical data to support its integrity should be submitted. Information should also be submitted to support the specificity, linearity, precision, and accuracy, as discussed before, which is applicable to specific quantitative methods used to test the dosage form.

Phase III: Provide a full description of the identity tests, assay methods, and acceptance specifications, as well as any other appropriate chemical and physical characteristics of the dosage form. These should approach NDA requirements in the level of detail provided, including the suitability of specifications, and data to confirm the adequacy of the analytical methodology. *In vitro* dissolution rate tests and specifications should be submitted for solid dosage forms. Information in support of any reference standard should be comparable to that expected in an NDA submission.

Placebos: For matching placebos used in clinical studies, a full description should be provided of the precautions that will be taken to ensure the absence of the new drug substance from the placebo preparation. The placebo and active dosage form should be as similar as possible in physical characteristics and identical in packaging.

4.   Current FDA draft guidelines and regulations

The following pages include the latest developments and changes in the FDA guidelines for drug delivery systems involving nasal aerosols and nasal sprays, vaccines, peptide formulation, solid oral dosage forms, implants, liposomes, monoclonal antibodies, transdermal drug delivery, access to managing computer records and the relevant security requirements.

   a.   Nasal aerosols and nasal sprays.   The draft guideline is intended to provide recommendations to the manufacturers who are planning product-quality studies to establish bioequivalence in support of abbreviated new drug applications for locally acting drugs in nasal aerosols and nasal sprays. For solution formulations, *in vitro* methods can be relied upon for bioequivalence and for suspension formulations. *In vivo* studies would have to be conducted to determine the delivery of the drug to local nasal sites of action and the systemic exposure of the administered dose. It is appropriate that the ingredients of the proposed product be within 5% of the innovator product, and the same standards for impurity profiles and degradants be applied to both products. The guideline is specific about the need to match the container and closure system of the innovator "as close as possible in all critical dimensions." Harrison[26] has outlined the draft guideline for the proposed *in vitro* testing program. Details regarding batch requirements for *in vitro* bioequivalence testing, appropriate design of local nasal delivery study, and appropriate design of systemic exposure/absorption study are given. There are significant differences of opinion in what constitutes appropriate bioequivalance guidelines for nasal products, which have broad implications for the industry in particular. The FDA has formed the oral inhalation and nasal drug products expert panel in an attempt to resolve the several issues. Uppoor discusses bioavailability and bioequivalence studies for new oral inhalation aerosols and nasal spray products.[28] According to this author, bioavailability and bioequivalence characterization for locally acting, orally inhaled, and nasal products generally necessitates *in vitro*/pharmacokinetic/ pharmacodynamic/clinical studies For systemically acting drug products, however, pharmacokinetic data alone may be sufficient to demonstrate bioequivalence. Pharmacokinetic studies are the first choice to characterize systemic exposure of nasal and oral inhalation products. Hansen et al.[29] discuss developing consensus-based guidelines or orally inhaled and nasal drug products.

Between October 1998 and June 1999, the FDA issued three draft guidelines for the industry for metered-dose inhaler, dry-powder inhaler, drug products chemistry, manufacturing and controls documentation, nasal spray and inhalation solution, suspension and spray drug products, including dose-content uniformity. While a few issues have remained unsolved, the industry and the FDA have taken significant steps to address the need for science-based regulations for orally inhaled and nasal products. Finally, Woodhouse[25] has listed important tests for inhalation products: dose/medication delivery, dose-content uniformity, dose through life, shot weight, number of actuations, particle/droplet sizing, cascade impaction, laser diffraction, microscopic testing, particle size, particulate matter, spray patterns, plume geometry, assay, total drug content, impurities and degradation products, net content fill weight, identification, appearance, moisture, pressure testing, exciepient testing, microbial limits, and extractables and leachables testing. Some of these listed are common for other forms of drug delivery.

Delivery of drugs via the inhalation route poses some unique safety and efficacy considerations. These issues are both product- and indication-specific. Drug products developed for pulmonary indications must consider the sensitivity of the population to irritants and allergens. In addition, it cannot be assumed that different populations (COPD versus asthma versus CF; adult versus pediatric) will respond identically to device/formulation changes. Conversely, drug products developed for systemic delivery must always take into account that chronic disease or acute lung processes may change absorption and delivery characteristics. The International Pharmaceutical Aerosol Consortium on Regulation and Science (IPAC-RS) is an industry association formed with the explicit purpose of advancing science-based, data-driven regulations for orally inhaled and nasal drug products (OINDP). Pulmonary route is preferred for the treatment of many pulmonary diseases, but each patient population presents unique safety/efficacy challenges. Pulmonary route used for systemic delivery must consider airway function, acute and chronic lung processes, special sensitivities, and other issues for safety, efficacy, and consistency of effect. The Nasal Spray and Inhalation Solution, Suspension and Spray Products-Chemistry, Manufacturing and Controls Documentation was published in the July 5, 2002, Federal Register. The guideline notes that the closure system's ability to properly deliver the drug is crucial to the formulation's effectiveness. The selection of a suitable pump for a given set of formulation characteristics (e.g., viscosity, density, surface tension, rheological properties) is of paramount importance for the correct performance of the pump, and ultimately, the drug product, according to the guideline.[27,28]

   b.   Vaccines. The Center for Biologics evaluation and research (CBER) regulates biological products, including vaccines. The regulations provided in Title 21 of CFR describe the following areas relevant to vaccine development: standards to be used in biologics production, adequate and well-controlled clinical trials, good manufacturing practices, institutional review boards, environmental impact assessment requirements and the protection of human subjects. Passive surveillance systems, such as the vaccine adverse event reporting system, coadministered by the Centers for Disease Control and Prevention and the FDA, have been post-licensure to gather additional data on vaccine safety. Pregnancy registries have been established for varicella and lyme vaccines. Pregnancy registries should be considered for new vaccines administered to women of childbearing age, particularly those with novel components not previously licensed or with live, attenuated products. As part of an efficacy study, attempts should be made to identify immune correlates of protection. Immunogenicity data are critical for evaluating manufacturing consistency and for bridging across different populations and different vaccine regimens. For U.S. licensure of combination vaccines, the FDA follows the specific provisions in the CFR. In 1997, the FDA issued a "Guidance for industry for the evaluation of combination vaccines for preventable diseases: Product testing and clinical studies," which discusses the general considerations for the production and testing of combination vaccines. This document provides general guideline on how the regulations might be implemented in the preclinical and clinical testing of combination products. During the preclinical development of combination vaccines, the issue of compatibility of the combined components is a major issue. It is important to evaluate the compatibility of all components of the combination vaccine. Regulatory challenges in demonstrating the clinical safety of combination vaccines include the choice of the appropriate control arm, i.e., separate injections of the components or, alternatively, a "standard of care" vaccine, such as a U.S. licensed vaccine. Demonstrating the effectiveness of combination vaccine has certain regulatory challenges. Large-scale field trials demonstrating field efficacy may be needed if a combination vaccine consists of novel components or if the product is the first application of a particular combination to a new target population. Such efficacy studies should be conducted in the intended or closely similar target population.

The use of live, attenuated viral and bacterial organisms for delivering foreign antigens is an active area of product development. Vectored vaccines often pose challenges for the development of appropriate informed consent. As with any live organism, careful consideration should be given to the ease with which a vector can be eliminated from the host if such a situation becomes necessary. Finally, the impact of the vector on the environment should be evaluated. In evaluating the efficacy or immunogenicity of vectored vaccines, appropriate immunological assays should be developed and standardized prior to initiating pivotal studies. If the vectored vaccine is intended to protect against multiple diseases, demonstration of efficacy or immunogenicity is necessary for all components for which an indication is sought. Currently, the only adjuvant used in U.S.-licensed products is aluminum compounds. In the case of novel adjuvants, it is recommended that additional preclinical toxicity studies be performed. Clinical studies should be aimed at demonstrating the clinical advantage of the new adjuvant, as well as the compatibility of the adjuvant with other vaccine components in terms of efficacy or immunogenicity.

As new methods for antigen delivery are developed, CBER faces new regulatory challenges. According to Falk and Ball,[30] for novel vaccine delivery systems, the demonstration of safety should consider possible long-term effects, such as prolonged stimulation of the immune system and the potential for inducing immunological tolerance. Clinical studies evaluating the safety of DNA vaccines should consider potential for incorporation into the host genome. In determining the effectiveness of novel vaccine delivery systems, such as transgenic edible, intranasal, and transcutaneous vaccines, one challenge has been determining the optimal dose of the study agent. As these products enter clinical development, discussions between the sponsor and CBER to address these areas of concern should be initiated as early in the clinical development as possible.[31,32,34,46]

    c.   *Peptide formulation.*   Recently, demands for effective delivery systems for peptide drugs and vaccines has led to research and development in the area of new drug delivery technology. In addition to parenteral administration, other peptide delivery systems have been developed to administer peptides through the gut, sinus, mouth, and lungs. Niu and Chiu[33] have discussed peptide formulation and stability issues with regards to parenteral, oral, and nasal delivery systems. In the parenteral delivery systems, aspects such as solution formulation, lyophilized powder formulation, and depot formulation are important. In the latter system, poly(lactic-co-glycolic) (PLGA) copolymer is commonly used. During manufacture of the PLGA depot formulation, the following common assurances should be considered: copolymer, organic solvents, copolymer-peptide complexes, sterilization, *in vitro* and *in vivo* correlation of peptide release, peptide size, and the diluent or the suspending vehicles. In the case of oral delivery systems, there are two issues involved with respect to the manufacture of the peptide tablets. They are heat granulation and the dissolution test. In the case of nasal delivery systems, particle size, preservatives, and adsorption are the important issues. According to these authors, many peptide delivery systems have been approved for marketing. Formulations for each route of administration are unique and have special characteristics, but in careful examination of these delivery systems, common features appear to surface. For example, in both liquid and lyophilized powder formulations, the sterilization process and loss of peptide concentration (potency) due to adsorption are critical issues during formulation. During manufacture of PLGA-depot formulations, issues of purity and average molecular weight of the PLGA copolymer, residual organic solvents, duration, temperature used to remove solvents, and water, particle size, and sterilization process need to be carefully considered.

  d. Solid oral dosage forms. Dissolution testing remains a potentially powerful and nearly always useful method for obtaining data related to quality and potentially clinical performance of dosage forms, especially solid oral dosage forms. However, dissolution is not always a surrogate for bioequivalence, which necessitates human testing for determination of bioequivalence in many instances. The key confidence in dissolution testing is the strength of the relationship between dissolution and bioequivalence, or the ability of dissolution testing to predict *in vivo* performance. Therefore, the availability of an IVIVC, as well as the type of dissolution testing conducted, are important considerations. Please refer to FIP guidelines for dissolution testing of solid oral products, Final Draft and the FDA draft guidance extended-release solid oral dosage forms-development, evaluation and application of *in vitro/in vivo* correlations.

  Malinowski[35] has discussed regulatory concerns regarding these aspects for Europe, Japan, and North America. In the U.S., the draft guidance was released in 1996. This guidance provides recommendations to pharmaceutical scientists related to various aspects of IVIVC for oral extended-release drug products, particularly as utilized in the NDA/ANDA review process. It presents a comprehensive perspective on methods of developing IVIVC, appropriate means of evaluating the predictability of IVIVC, and relevant applications for IVIVC in the areas of changes (e.g., formulation, equipment, process, and manufacturing site) and setting dissolution specifications. *In vitro* testing is important for: providing necessary process control and quality assurance, determining stability of the relevant release characteristics of the product, and facilitating certain regulatory determinations and judgments concerning, for example, minor formulations changes or changes in the site of manufacture. The author, in this review, has discussed important aspects such as biowaivers and setting dissolution specifications. Malinowski,[35] in another review, discussed different levels used in the correlation of IVIVC data. Experimental data considerations should be given to dosage form properties, internal versus external predictability, and therapeutic index of the drugs.

5. Implants

The FDA has proposed rules regarding pre-market approval for dental, silicone breast, intraocular implants in existing bone, and endosseous implants, among other things. The Office of Device Evaluation within the Center for Devices and Radiological Health of the FDA is the primary component responsible for pre-market review of medical devices. Dental devices are reviewed by the Dental Device Branch within ODE. Pre-market submissions to the FDA for dental endosseous implants should include complete characterization of the device and often may necessitate the inclusion of mechanical and other bench-testing and clinical data.

FDA documents are available that outline the information that should be included in the submissions. The guideline document also provides guidelines on clinical trials for dental implants. This guideline document addresses such issues as the number of patients and study sites, length of follow-up, post-implant assessment, and pooling of data. The central issue facing federal regulation of breast implants is that while such devices are not functionally necessary or needed for survival, the side effects may be harmful and have not been proven otherwise. The Medical Device Amendments of 1976 appear to require such evidence prior to the FDA permitting the unrestricted marketing of these devices. However, only recently have such requirements been imposed by the FDA. Recently, the FDA has approved the NuvaRing contraceptive implant, and Chiron Vision has filed an application to market intraocular implants for CMV retinitis. These implants release drugs into the systemic circulation, and the manufacturer would be require to follow the FDA guidelines and regulations that are similar to those described earlier.[36-39]

6. Monoclonal antibodies

In reviewing proposals that include several methods, the animal research committee is required by federal regulations to determine that the use of the methods for producing monoclonal antibodies (Mabs) is scientifically justified; that methods that avoid or minimize discomfort, distress, and pain (including *in vitro* methods) have been considered, and that such alternatives have been found unsuitable. The National Research Council Committee, on methods of producing monoclonal antibodies, states: "It is incumbent on the scientist to consider first the use *in vitro* methods for the production of mAb. When hybridomas fail to grow or fail to achieve a product consistent with scientific goals, the investigator is obliged to show that a good-faith effort was made to adapt the hybridoma in *in vitro* growth conditions before using the particular (ascites) method and that *in vitro* methods for producing mAb are appropriate in numerous situations, and it is the responsibility of the researcher to produce scientific justification for using the mouse ascites method."

The guidelines for the Ascites method include, e.g., priming, inoculation, harvesting Ascites fluid, and euthanasia. For immunomodulatory molecules, particular attention is paid to defining potential for increased risks of lymphoproliferative disorders, opportunistic infections, and immune impairment. To address the issues, a wide variety of preclinical studies, mainly in nonhuman primates, have been performed for the purpose of assessing the potential risk of drug-induced human toxicity. In some cases, homologous forms of the biologic agent and "humanized" transgenic models have been used to assess potential clinical risks. The sponsor's and regulatory authority's experienced judgment should determine whether or not purported benefits of the novel therapeutic agents are balanced by the potential short- and long-term risks.

In this field of development, preclinical models often need to reflect recent technology innovations; therefore, these models are not always "validated" in a conventional sense. Key components of protocol design for preclinical studies addressing the risks of the agents derived from the use of biotechnology include a safe starting dose in humans, identification of potential target organs and clinical parameters that should be monitored in humans, and identification of at-risk populations. One of the distinct aspects of the safety evaluation of biotechnology-derived pharmaceuticals is the use of relevant and often nontraditional species and the use of animal models of disease in preclinical safety evaluation. Subsequent to product approval, the incremental database of test results serves as a natural continuum for further evolving/refining specifications. While there is considerable latitude in the kinds of testing modalities finally adopted to establish product quality on a routine basis, for both drug products and drugs, it is important that the selection takes into consideration relevant significant product characteristics that appropriately reflect on identity, purity, and potency. Recently, the FDA has approved rituximab and indium-111 satumomab pendetide.[40–42]

For transdermal, liposomal, and monoclonal antibody delivery systems, Guidelines for Industry S7A Safety Pharmacology studies for human pharmaceuticals should also be followed. This guideline was developed within the Expert Working Group (Safety) of the International Conference of Harmonization of Technical Requirements for Registration of Pharmaceuticals for Human Use (ICH) and has been subjected to consultation by the regulatory parties, in accordance with the ICH process. This guideline generally applies to new chemical entities and biotechnology-derived products for human use. This guideline can be applied to marketed pharmaceuticals when appropriate (e.g., when adverse clinical events, a new patient population, or a new route of administration raises concerns not previously addressed). The size of the groups should be sufficient to allow meaningful scientific interpretation of the data generated. The sample size should take into consideration the size of the biological effect that is of concern for humans.

Safety pharmacology studies may not be needed for locally applied agents (dermal or ocular) where the pharmacology of the test substance is well characterized and where systemic exposure or distribution to other organs or tissues is demonstrated to be low. For biotechnology-derived products that achieve highly specific receptor targeting, it is often sufficient to evaluate pharmacology endpoints as a part of toxicology or pharmacodynamic studies; therefore, safety pharmacology studies can be reduced or eliminated for these products. For these products that represent a novel therapeutic class, or those products that did not achieve highly specific receptor targeting, a more extensive evaluation by safety pharmacology studies should be considered. For the timing of safety pharmacology studies in relation to clinical development, studies prior to first administration to humans, studies during clinical development, and studies before approval are important and, therefore, should be considered. Available information from toxicology studies adequately designed and conducted to address safety pharmacology endpoints, or information from clinical studies, can support this assessment and may replace safety pharmacology studies. The FDA is considering evaluating alternatives to dermatopharmacokinetics for determining bioequivalence of topical dermatological products. The FDA's draft guideline on determining bioequivalaence of topical dermatological drug products issued in June 1998 recommended the DPK skin-stripping technique. The human cadaver skin and transepidermal water-loss assays to assess the bioequivalence was considered. Both techniques predicted bioequivalence between the generic and brand products.

According to the FDA draft guideline, dosing for liposome drug products could be determined through comparative pharmacokinetic studies of liposomal and nonliposomal products containing the same active moiety. The draft guideline recommends a single-dose pharmacokinetic study, which would compare the absorption, distribution, metabolism, and excretion of the liposome and nonliposome formulations of the drug. The guideline notes that the pharmacokinetics of a drug in liposomal form are expected to be different from those of the same drug in nonliposomal form. Also recommended was the multiple-dose study and a dose-proportionality study over the expected therapeutic dose range after administration of the liposome drug product. The draft guideline also proposed the inclusion of a warning that a liposome product "is not equivalent to or cannot be substituted for other drug products containing the same drug substance." The Draft Guideline for Industry on Liposome Drug Products: CMC, Human Pharmacokinetics and Bioavailability and Labeling Documentation was published in the *Federal Register* on August 21, 2002.[43,44]

7. Computer access and security requirements

In a recent article, Lopez[45] has reviewed regulatory requirements that apply to computer resources and current technologies that can be used to mitigate threats to and vulnerabilities in computer resources. Computer security is used to regulate and record access to computer resources, as well as manage records residing in a computer. It is one of the main factors to consider when implementing environments that will manage electronic records set forth in FDA regulations or electronic records submitted in compliance with the Federal Food Drug and Cosmetic Act and the Public Health Service Act. The FDA defines electronic records as any combination of text, graphics, data, audio, pictorial, or other information represented in digital form that is created, modified, maintained, archived, retrieved, or distributed by a computer system. One example is the submission to the FDA of records and reports supporting the safety and efficacy of new human and animal drugs, biologics, medical devices, and certain food and color additives.

The advantage of using computer technologies supporting electronic submissions and inspections is that the FDA can review and analyze this information with automated tools, thereby reducing the review time. Trustworthiness is the key characteristic expected of all records by existing FDA regulations. According to the National Archives and Records Administration, reliability, authenticity, integrity, and usability are the characteristics used to describe trustworthy records from a record-management perspective. The FDA addresses the subject of the security of computer records in its CGMP regulations and associated policy guidelines. Specifically, 211.68(b) and a recent guideline require appropriate controls of computer resources to ensure that only authorized personnel make changes in master production, control, or other records. The compliance policy guideline 7132a.07 (inputs/outputs checking) includes specific requirements to establish the necessary controls of records. The main FDA regulation affecting computer resources performing functions covered by the FDA is 21 CFR Part 11, Electronic Records, Electronic Signatures, Final Rule. This rule allows the use of electronic records and electronic signatures for any documents that are required to be kept and maintained by FDA regulations. The good automated manufacturing practices (GAMPs) requirements concerning computer resources include protection of records, access controls authentication, audit-trail controls, computer systems time controls, authority checks, device checks, technical controls of open systems, signature/record linking, uniqueness of electronic signatures, and electronic signatures security. These requirements are key elements. The controls implemented as a result of security-related requirements are intended to build trusted records. Finally, the National Security Agency (NSA) has developed security configuration guidelines for Microsoft Windows® 2000 with the purpose of providing direction about the services that are available in the Windows 2000 environment and explaining how to integrate these services into network architecture.

References

1. Janssen, W.F., Since 1938 — a regulatory revolution, *Pharm. Tech.*, 12, 160–172, 1988.
2. Chew, N.J., Product development and registration, *Bio. Pharm.*, 4, 16–20, 1991.
3. Chew, N.J., Inspections, recalls, seizures: who's in control? *Bio. Pharm.*, 1, 14–19, 1988.
4. Wechsler, J., The lion roars, *Pharm. Tech.*, 15, 16–22, 1991.
5. Wechsler, J., Reassessing risk: the key to faster drug approvals, *Pharm. Tech.*, 11, 16–19, 1991.
6. Chew, N.J., Product development and registration: after the IND is filed, *Bio. Pharm.*, 5, 14–19, 1992.
7. Chew, N.J., Product development and registration: the final verdict, *Bio. Pharm.*, 5, 24–31, 1992.
8. Cook, J. and Meyer, G.F., Structure for success: speeding NDA reviews, *Pharm. Tech.*, 12, 62–70, 1992.
9. Hinman, D.J. and Chew, N.J., Master files: streamlining your submissions, protecting your secrets, *Bio. Pharm.*, 3, 12–18, 1990.
10. Chew, N.J., Clinical (and other concurrent) developments, *Bio. Pharm.*, 5, 12–16, 1992.
11. DeSain, C., Designing GMP and facility qualification master protocols, *Bio. Pharm.*, 5, 18–21, 1992.
12. Tetzlaff, R.F., Validation issues for new drug development, Part I. Review of current FDA policies, *Pharm. Tech.*, 16, 44–56, 1992.
13. Moore, R.E., The FDA's guidelines for bulk pharmaceutical chemicals: a consultant's interpretation, *Pharm. Tech.*, 16, 88–100, 1992.
14. Gorsky, I. and Nielsen, R.K., Scale-up methods used in liquid pharmaceutical manufacturing, *Pharm. Tech.*, 16, 112–120, 1992.
15. Tetzlaff, R.E., GMP documentation requirements for automated systems, Part I., *Pharm. Tech.*, 16, 112–123, 1992.
16. Shah, V.P., Skelly, J.P., Barr, W.H., Malinowski, H., and Amidon, G., Scale-up of controlled-release products, preliminary considerations, *Pharm. Tech.*, 16, 35–40, 1992.
17. *Regulatory Compliance Manual: The FDA Inspections before, during and after*, InterPharm Press, Buffalo Grove, IL.
18. DeSain, C., *Drug Devices and Diagnostic Manufacturing: the Ultimate Resource Handbook*, InterPharm Press, Buffalo Grove, IL, 1991.
19. Guarino, R., Ed., *New Drug Approval Process: Clinical and Regulatory Management*, InterPharm Press, Buffalo Grove, IL.
20. Mathieu, M., *New Drug Development*: *Regulatory Overview*, InterPharm Press, Buffalo Grove, IL.
21. Spilker, B., Ed., *Guide to Clinical Studies and Developing Protocols*, InterPharm Press, Buffalo Grove, IL.
22. *Bioequivalence Guidelines* (USA), InterPharm Press, Buffalo Grove, IL.
23. Gregory, G. and Chew, N.J., EEC directives in transition, *Bio. Pharm.*, 4, 20–23, 1991.
24. Stephenson, J., European strategy: myth, mystery or mistake, *Pharm. Tech.*, 15, 24–26, 1991.

25. Woodhouse, R.N. and Cummings, R.H., The pharmaceutical development of inhalation medicines and the value of outsourcing, *Pharm. Tech.*, 26, 90–95, 2002.

26. Harrison, L.I., Commentary on the FDA draft guidance for bioequivalence studies for nasal aerosols and nasal sprays for local action: an industry view, *J. Clin. Pharmacol.*, 40, 701–707, 2000.

27. Fink, J.B., Matching the right nebulizer with your patient for effective aerosol delivery, *AARC Times*, April 2001, 27–32.

28. Uppoor, V.R., Bioavailability and bioequivalence studies for new oral inhalation aerosols and nasal spray products, *Am. Pharm. Rev.*, 3, 8–11, 2000.

29. Hansen, G.F. and Evans, C., Developing consensus-based guidances for orally inhaled and nasal drug products, *Am. Pharm. Rev.*, 5, 20–25, 2002.

30. Falk, L.A. and Ball, L.K., Current status and future trends in vaccine regulation — USA, *Vaccine*, 19, 1567–1572, 2001.

31. Eccleston, D.S. et al., Rationale for local drug delivery, *Semin. Interv. Cardiol.*, 1, 8–16, 1996.

32. Piscitelli, D.A. and Young, D., Setting dissolution specifications for modified-release dosage forms, *Adv. Exp. Med. Biol.*, 423, 159–166, 1997.

33. Niu, C. and Chiu, Y., FDA perspective on peptide formulation and stability issues, *J. Pharm. Sci.*, 87, 1331–1334, 1998.

34. Davis, S.S., Meeting the challenges of viable delivery systems for peptide and protein pharmaceuticals, *Am. Pharm. Rev.*, 5, 29–36, 2002.

35. Malinowski, H. et al., Draft guidance for industry extended-release solid oral dosage forms: Development, evaluation and application of *in vitro–in vivo* correlations, *Adv. Exp. Med. Biol.*, 423, 269–288, 1997.

36. Weber, H.P. et al., Clinical trials on placement of implants in existing bone, *Ann. Periodontal.* 2, 315–328, 1997.

37. Scott, P.D. and Runner, S., The Food and Drug Administration and the regulation of clinical trials for endosseous implants, *Ann. Periodontal.*, 2, 284–290, 1997.

38. Palley, H.A., The evolution of FDA policy on silicone breast implants: a case study of politics, bureaucracy, and business in the process of decision making, *Int. J. Health Serv.*, 25, 573–591, 1995.

39. Eckert, S.E., Food and Drug Administration requirements for dental implants, *J. Prosthet. Dent.*, 74, 162–168, 1995.

40. Baertschi, S.W. and Kinney, H., Issues in evaluating the in-use photostability of transdermal patches, *Pharm. Tech.*, 24, 70–80, 2000.

41. Green, J.D. and Black, L.E., Overview status of preclinical safety assessment for immunomodulatory biopharmaceuticals, *Hum. Exp. Toxicol.*, 19, 208–212, 2000.

42. Serabian, M.A. and Pilaro, A.M., Safety assessment of biotechnology-derived pharmaceuticals: ICH and beyond, *Toxicol. Pathol.*, 27, 27–31, 1999.

43. Murano, G., FDA perspective on specifications for biotechnology products: from IND to PLA, *Dev. Biol. Stand.*, 91, 3–13, 1997.

44. Miele, L., Plants as bioreactors for biopharmaceuticals: regulatory considerations, *Trends Biotechnol.*, 15, 45–50, 1997.

45. Lopez, O., Technologies supporting security requirements in 21CFR Part 11, Part I, *Pharm. Tech.*, 26, 36–46, 2002.

46. Wiethoff, C.M. and Middaugh, C.R., Barriers to nonviral gene delivery, *J. Pharm. Sci.*, 92, 2, 203–217, 2003.

chapter ten

Drug delivery industry and the global outlook

According to Find/SVP market reports, U.S. sales in drug delivery systems surpassed $9 billion in 1999. The development of alternative drug therapies has been a major thrust over the past three decades. Alternative drug delivery devices, which cater to the increasing emphasis on cost-containment through outpatient care, include ambulatory infusion pumps, implanted infusion pumps, inhalers, other nasal delivery systems, injector pen systems, needleless systems, and transdermal systems. Emerging alternative drug delivery systems throughout the world include aerosol macromolecule and protein delivery systems, biologic and molecular systems, electrotransport and iontophoretic transdermal systems, and gene therapy.[1-8]

Despite the significant advances in the industry, it is estimated that fewer than 30% of the drugs currently on the market involve alternative drug delivery systems. Development has been slowed by the high costs of research and development of new technologies and by the lengthy procedures needed to secure approval from the regulatory agencies. Nonetheless, increasing concern over the high level of health care expenditures is expected to support the growth of cost-effective novel drug delivery systems.

While a few companies have addressed the demand for more convenience through the miniaturization of infusion pumps, other manufacturers continue to investigate ways of improving the administration of drugs. Companies such as Dura Pharmaceuticals have marketed completely novel systems for dry compounds, while others are advancing dissolution, electrotransport, liposome, and soft gelatin encapsulation technologies. However, most have focused on the lucrative area of sustained-release and transdermal patches, technologies with demonstrated capacities to extend product life and improve the therapeutic effectiveness of the active ingredient.[9-15]

Reasons for intense interest in developing new drug delivery systems have been improving conventional dosage forms, exclusivity for existing drugs, high cost for developing new drugs with new molecular entities, delivery of bioengineered compounds, and enhanced efficacy and safety. Market share for conventional dosage forms, controlled-release, and novel delivery systems has been 90%, 10%, and less than 1%, respectively. However, in the future, for cost-containment and fast approval for marketing, controlled-release formulations with both rate-modulation and targeting capabilities will prove to be an essential component of effective therapeutic regimens.

According to Freedonia Group, Inc. reports, during the past decade, in a 5-year time period, drug delivery systems demands increased by 5% annually and drug delivery system end uses increased by 12%. This prospectus clearly demonstrates the judicial use of drug delivery systems as a valuable decision-making tool for the pharmaceutical industry.[16–19] Business strategies and market drivers from an industry perspective include a list of items, such as negotiating licensing agreements for new drug delivery technologies; forming strategic partnerships; watching market and consolidation trends in the drug delivery industry; leveraging a technology platform into a commercial strategy; targeting a pharmaceutical product pipeline, capitalizing on new drug delivery technologies, novel technologies, partnering in research and development, portfolio management, pricing, reimbursement and regulatory implications of novel systems within managed care, and government programs; and scrutinizing drug delivery companies from a Wall Street perspective.[20–24]

The global outlook for the development of drug delivery systems appears to be encouraging. This observation is supported by the numerous drug delivery systems listed in the following table. The developers and manufacturers of these delivery systems (see Table 10.1) are located throughout the world,[23,24] although concentrated in the U.S., Europe, and Japan. The data presented here is partial, but representative of the current status of drug delivery systems.[25–28]

In addition to these drug delivery systems, there are several other novel delivery systems that have been simultaneously developed. The categories of these systems are the following:

1. Controlled drug delivery systems, such as Snaplets, Eucaps Multipor, AdMMS, Angie, BioSert, submicronized fat emulsion delivery system, SES formula, Detach, Flo-tab, Flui-Dose, IPDAS, MICROCAP, microCRYSTAL, MicroDROPLET, Micro-Release, MOSTS, NANO-ZOME, OLipHEX, Oncholab, pHEMS, POLiM, ProLease, Pulsincap, fat-dissolving dosage form (FDDF), site-specific targeted delivery in the colon (STDC), Emisphere, Pegnology, HALO, and HIPN (heterogeneous interpenetrating polymer networks).
2. Transdermal drug delivery systems, such as Pediapatch, Plantar-Patch, Trans-Plantar, Trans-Ver-Sal, Dermaflex, Powerpatch, and cation-activated topical delivery systems.
3. Dental drug delivery systems, such as transoral mucosal anesthetic delivery system (TMADS) and PT-system (an acryl film).
4. Miscellaneous drug delivery systems, such as chemical delivery system for taste masking, immunoliposomes, osmicated liposomes,

Table 10.1 Developers/manufacturers of drug delivery systems

Drug	Drug delivery system	Developer/manufacturer
Ibuprofen	EUCAPS	Euderma, Ciba-Geigy Sankyo
Ibuprofen	Synchron technique	Forest Labs.
Ibuprofen	Liquitard sustained	Eurand Release Technique
Ibuprofen	MICROCAP multiparticulate dosing system	Eurand
Ibuprofen	Softgel (Scherersol) formulation	R.P. Scherer
Indomethacin	IV	Dumex
Indomethacin	Transdermal	KOWA
Indomethacin	Repro-Dose	Hafslund Nycomed
Ketoprofen	Transdermal	Hisamatsu
Ketoprofen	INDAS	Elan
Piroxicam	Topical gel	KRKA, Hyal Pharm
Lithium	Synchron technology	Forest Labs, Johnson & Johnson
Glucagon	Intranasal	Akzo, Novo-Nordisk
Testosterone	Sublingual transdermal	Gynex, TheraTech, CEPA
Contraceptive	Transdermal	Warner Lambert
Estradiol	Transdermal	TheraTech, Solvay
γ-Interferon	Erythrocyte delivery	Novacell
Immunomodulators	Erythrocyte delivery	Novacell
Glucosamyl Muramyl analogs	Liposomes	Immunotherapeutic
Hexamethylmelamine	Microemulsion	Biotech Develop Corp.
Lomustine	Redox drug delivery	PharmTec
Methotrexate	Biodegradable gel-like matrix	Matrix Pharma
Carbamazepine	Molecusol cyclodextrin delivery	PharmTec
Dexmedetomidine	Transdermal	Cygnus
Dihydroepi-androsterone	Transdermal	Pharmedic
Inositol hexaphosphate	Erythrocyte delivery	Novacell
Alprenoxine-HCl	Site-specific delivery	Xenon Vision
Ketoprofen	INDAS	Elan
Diclofenac	Ophthalmic	Wakamoto Pharm.
Diclofenac	Topical	Hyal Pharma
Flurbiprofen	Ophthalmic	Boots, Allergen
Hyaluronic acid	Ophthalmic	Seikagaku Kogyo
Lovobunolol	Ophthalmic	Warner Lambert, Allergen
Ofloxacin	Ophthalmic	Daiichi, Allergen, Bausch & Lomb
Pilocarpine	Soluble ophthalmic delivery	Diversified Tech.
Suprofen	Ophthalmic	CuSi
Metoclopramide	Nasal	Nastech, Rugby

Table 10.1 Developers/manufacturers of drug delivery systems (Continued)

Drug	Drug delivery system	Developer/manufacturer
Ribavarin	Brain-specific carrier system	Pharmos
Gentamicin	Liposomes	The Liposome Co., 3M
Zidovudine	Redox delivery	Pharmos
Asparaginase	Erythrocyte delivery	Novacell
Daunorubicin	Liposome	Vestar
Butorphenol	Nasal	Nastech, Bristol-Myers Squibb
Diazepam	Rectal solution	Dumex
Tetrahydroacridine	Redox brain delivery	Pharmos
Tetrahydrocannabinol	Molecusol cyclodextrins	Pharmos
Valproate sodium	Brain-specific delivery	Pharmos
Amphotericin	Liposome	Vestar, Fujisawa
Histamine H2-receptor antagonists	Nasal	Nastech
Antiemetics	Nasal	Nastech
Doxorubicin (Evacet)	Liposome	The Liposome Co.
CDP870	Pegylation technology	Inhale Therapeutics
Insulin (Exubera)	Inhalation	Aventis/Pfizer
Neulasta	Inhalation	Amgen
Pegasys	Inhalation	Roche
Somavert	Inhalation	Pharmacia
Risperidol (antipsychotic)	Oros	J & J (Alza)
Topamax (antiepileptic)	Oros	J & J (Alza)
Ortho Evra	Contraceptive patch	Ortho-McNeill
Lotemax (loteprednol)	Ophthalmic	Bausch & Lomb
Alrex	Ophthalmic	Bausch & Lomb
Singulair (montekulast)	Inhalation	Merck
Nasonex (mometasone)	Inhalation	Schering-Plough
Beconase (corticosteroid)	Inhalation	GSK
Vancenase (corticosteroid)	Inhalation	Schering-Plough
Pulmicort respules	Inhalation (Budesonide)	AstraZeneca
Flonase (fluticasone)	Inhalation	GSK
Azmacort triamcinolone)	Inhalation	Rhone Poulenc Rorer
Climara (estradiol)	Transdermal	3M-Berlex
Zomig (Zolmitriptan)	Nasal spray	AstraZeneca
Interferon beta-1a	Inhalation	Inhale Therap
Spiros	Aerosol	Dura
Pulmosol (proteins)	Inhalation	Inhale Therap
Larger particles	Inhalation	Alkermes
Therap. agents	Inhalation	Aradigm
Powder formulations	Transdermal	Powder Tech
E-Trans	Iontophoresis	Alza
Macroflux	Transdermal	Alza
Sono-Prep Syst	Ultrasound-transdermal	Sontra Medical
Therap. agents	Microchip drug delivery	MicroCHIPS
Depofoam	Extended release	Skye-Pharma

Table 10.1 Developers/manufacturers of drug delivery systems (Continued)

Drug	Drug delivery system	Developer/manufacturer
Concerta	OROS-Tech	Alza
Duros/Alzamer	Implant	Alza
Proteins	ReGel/Oligosphere	MacroMed
Medisorb/Prolease	Microspheres	Alkermes
Macromolecules	Carrier Tech	Emisphere
Vaccines, insulin, proteins	Orasomes	Endorex
Macromolecules	Oral/Promdas/Locdas	Elan
Rapamune (immunosuppressant)	Nanocrystal Tech	Elan

stealth liposomes, pyran oil as diluents, caragennan complexes, collagen-based liposomes and the use of HYAFF membranes, and TOGA gene delivery.

Drug delivery is playing a significant role in the pharmaceutical industry such that new drug delivery systems and a diverse range of technology options have emerged. The drug delivery market is currently estimated to be worth approximately $50 billion, and worldwide sales could reach as much as $100 billion by 2005. Big pharmaceutical companies, unfortunately, are experiencing "dry" product pipelines. Consequently, they are looking to acquire drug delivery companies as a means of filling their gaps.

A recent industry survey estimated that there are more than 300 companies engaged in the development and licensing of drug delivery technology. By merging with a drug delivery company, the big pharmaceuticals add to their core business by extending the exclusivity and life cycle of a marketed product, enhancing patient compliance, improving the biopharmaceutical properties of a new chemical entity, or enabling delivery via a new route.

Sometimes, a higher risk is worth taking in areas of high unfulfilled medical need, where the new delivery technology can potentially enable the innovative NCE to significantly advance the current standard of care and become a commercial blockbuster medicine.

The final goal has been winning in the marketplace, which is where we ultimately want to get to first and quickly. These products have to be developed and launched before loss of exclusivity. For a product (either old or new) in a drug delivery system, the same "Go/No-Go" rules apply for its development for the market. The attraction of increased revenues through product sales is likely to lead to numerous mid-sized drug delivery companies becoming fully integrated pharmaceutical companies. A recent survey has estimated that, on average, big pharmaceuticals have about five drug delivery deals per year and smaller pharmaceuticals have about two delivery deals per year.

More than half of the current drug delivery market is based on technologies for the oral delivery of drugs. Oral dosage forms will remain as the primary dosage form; however, in the future, alternative routes of administration are likely to increase in prominence. Development and adoption of delivery technologies will be influenced by trends in pharmaceutical discovery portfolios, therapeutic area focus, and patient demographics. Increased prominence of biotechnology-derived products in the marketplace will play a major role in shaping drug delivery technologies. Current estimates are that biotechnology products will contribute $120 billion by 2010, and needleless delivery systems are predicted to increase to about $1 billion by 2005. However, just as any conventional drug could be recalled or removed from the market, either NCE or an established drug in a drug delivery system could experience a similar fate. For example, Wyeth recently discontinued production of Norplant, a levonorgestrel implant for contraception, as women and health care professionals continued to report adverse effects with this product.

It is likely that during the next several years, extensive work on these delivery systems or those that are similar to these will be continued. Additional drug delivery systems and methods may include, for example, refinements in timed-capsule delivery, contact lenses soaked with antibiotics, plastic wafers that can convey medications into the bloodstream quickly, and a powder consisting of microsponges that transmit antibiotic transdermally where they are sprinkled.[29,30]

New drugs will continue to be developed, but at a slower pace due to higher costs and government regulations. However, the advent of drug delivery systems — that is, more patches and specific chemical compounds (e.g., liposomes, cyclodextrins, etc.) designed to extend the life of drugs — may well enhance the future of the research-based pharmaceutical companies. Through these systems, products can have extended patent life and be produced at lower cost, and products that have not been commercially available due to high production costs will now be commercially viable.[31-35]

References

1. Madley, S.W., Oral delivery of macromolecules and continued movement shape the drug delivery industry, *Contract. Pharma.*, April/May 2002, 36–44, 2002.
2. Roth, G.Y., Delivering profits, *Contract. Pharma.*, April/May 2000, 50–54, 2000.
3. Henry, C.M., *Special Delivery C&E News*, Sept. 18, 2000, 49–65.
4. Henry, C.M., *Drug Delivery, C&E News*, August 26, 2002, 39–45.
5. Horspool, K.R., Future strategies for the drug delivery industry, *Am. Pharm. Rev.*, 5, 20–24, 2002.
6. Charlish, P., *Scrip Magazine*, May 2000, 27–32.
7. Drews, J., *Drug Discovery Today*, 2000, 5, 2–4.
8. Jain, K.K. in *Drug Delivery Technologies and Markets*, Informa Publishing Group, Ltd., 2000, 144.
9. Kermani, F. and Findley, G., in *The Application of Drug Delivery Systems: Current Practices and Future Strategies*, CMR International, Epsom, U.K., 2000.
10. Langer, R., Drug delivery and targeting, *Nature*, (Suppl. 6679) 1998, 392, 5–10.
11. Pulazzinnini, A. and Segantini, L., *Scrip Magazine*, May 2001, 7.
12. Putney, S.D., *Pharmaceutical News*, 1999, 6, 7–10.

13. Shi, M. et al., *Modern Drug Discovery*, July 2001, 27–32.

14. Tinebo, K. and Siebert J.M., Presentation at the Sixth Annual Drug Delivery Partnerships Meeting, Los Angeles, January 28–30, 2002.

15. Park, K. and Mresny, R.J. Eds., Controlled drug delivery: designing technologies for the future, *ACS Symposium Series 752*, American Chemical Society, Oxford University Press, New York, 2000.

16. Shao, J. et al., A cell-based drug delivery system for lung targeting, I. Preparation and pharmacokinetics, *Drug Deliv.*, 8, 61–69, 2001.

17. Pignatello, R. and Amico, D., Preparation and analgesic activity of Eudragit RS100 microparticles containing diflunisal, *Drug Deliv.*, 8, 35–45, 2001.

18. Singh, M. and Kosoon, N., Receptor-mediated gene delivery to HepG2 cells by ternary assemblies containing cationic liposomes and cationized asialoorosomucoid, *Drug Deliv.*, 8, 29–34, 2001.

19. Quadir, M. et al., Development and evaluation of nasal formulations of ketorolac, *Drug Deliv.*, 7, 223–229, 2000.

20. Sinha, J. et al., Targeting of liposomal andrographolide to *L. donovani*-infected macrophages *in vivo*, *Drug Deliv.*, 7, 209–213, 2000.

21. Risbud, M.V. and Bhonde, R.R., Polyacrylamide-chitosan hydrogels: *in vitro* biocompatibility and sustained antibiotic release studies, *Drug Deliv.*, 7, 69–75, 2000.

22. Dass, C.R. and Walker, T.L., A microsphere-liposome (microplex) vector for targeted gene therapy of cancer, II. *In vivo* biodistribution study in a solid tumor model, *Drug Deliv.*, 7, 15, 2000.

23. Petrikovics, I., McGuinn, W.D., et al., *In vitro* studies on sterically stabilized liposomes (SL) as enzyme carriers in organophosphorous (OP) antagonism, *Drug Deliv.*, 7, 83–89, 2000.

24. (a) Dass, C.R. and Jessup, W., Apolipoprotein A-I, phospholipid vesicles and cyclodextrins as potential anti-atherosclerotic drugs: delivery, pharmacokinetics and efficacy, *Drug Deliv.*, 7, 161–182, 2000; (b) Mishra, P.R. and Jain, N.K., Reverse biomembrane vesicles for effective controlled delivery of doxorubicin HCl, *Drug Deliv.*, 7, 155–159, 2000; (c) Allen, C. et al., PCL-b-PEO micelles as a delivery vehicle for FK506: Assessment of a functional recovery of crushed peripheral nerve, *Drug Deliv.*, 7, 139–145, 2000.

25. Wechsler, J., Harmonizing clinical trials, *Applied Clinical Trials*, 1, 14–22, 1992.

26. Reinhart, S.P. and Trotter, J.P., Incorporating economic analysis into clinical trials, *Applied Clinical Trials*, 1, 46–50, 1992.

27. (a) The businessman's guide to EC legal developments, InterPharm Press; (b) Future system for the free movement of medicinal products in the European community, InterPharm Press; (c) Product liability in Europe, InterPharm Press; (d) EC drug registration, notes for guidance, InterPharm Press; (e) Guide to working in a Europe without frontiers, InterPharm Press; (f) EC Pharmaceuticals after 1992, InterPharm Press; (g) 1992 and the European pharmaceutical industry, The EC directives, InterPharm Press; (h) EUCOMED harmonization of medical device regulation in Europe, InterPharm Press; (i)Therapeutics in Australia, InterPharm Press; (j) Guide to medical device registration in Japan, InterPharm Press; (k) The Japanese pharmaceutical challenge, InterPharm Press; (l) Pharmaceutical innovations: recent trends, future prospects, InterPharm Press; (m) Multinational drug companies: issues in drug discovery and development, InterPharm Press.

28. Stephenson, J., Who gains, who loses from a European formulary?, *Pharm. Tech.*, 15, 26–29, 1991.

29. Rolf, D., Chemical and physical methods of enhancing transdermal drug delivery, *Pharm. Tech.*, 12, 130–141, 1988.
30. Schlom, J., Monoclonal antibodies in cancer therapy: the present and the future, *Pharm. Tech.*, 12, 56–60, 1988.
31. (a) Pharmaceutical dosage forms: Disperse systems, InterPharm Press; (b) Chien, Y., Novel drug delivery systems: Fundamentals, development concepts, biomedical assessments, InterPharm Press; (c) Drug development: From laboratory to clinic, InterPharm Press; (d) Groves, M.J., *Parenteral Technology Manual*, InterPharm Press, 1989.
32. Hamrell, M.R. and Chew, N.J., New development strategies for life-threatening illnesses., *Bio. Pharm.*, 5, 18–21, 1992.
33. (a) Kydonieus, A., Ed., *Treatise on Controlled Drug Delivery: Fundamentals, Optimization and Application*, Marcel Dekker, New York, 1992; (b) Pardridge, W.M., *Peptide Drug Delivery to the Brain*, Raven Press, 1991; (c) Tomlinson, E. and Davis, S.S., Eds., *Site-Specific Drug Delivery*, John Wiley & Sons, New York, 1986; (d) Juliano, R.L., Ed., Biological approaches to the controlled delivery of drugs, *Annals. of N.Y. Acad. Sci.*, 1987; (e) Shaw, J.M., Ed., *Lipoproteins as Carriers of Pharmacological Agents*, Marcel Dekker, New York, 1991; (f) Chien, Y.W., Su, K.S.E., Chang, S., *Nasal Systemic Drug Delivery*, Marcel Dekker, New York, 1989; (g) Davis, S.S., Illum. L. McVie, J.G., and Tomlinson, E.. *Microspheres and Drug Therapy: Pharmaceutical, Immunological and Medical Agents* Elsevier, 1984; (h) Kydonieus, A.E. and Berner, B., *Transdermal Delivery of Drugs*, Vols. 1–3, CRC Press, Inc., Boca Raton, FL, 1987; (i) Guiot, P. and Couvreur, P., *Polymeric Nanoparticles and Microspheres.*, CRC Press, Inc., Boca Raton, FL, 1986; (j) Tyle, P. and Ram, B.P., *Targeted Therapeutic Systems*, Marcel Dekker, New York, 1990; (k) Wise, D.L., *Biopolymeric Controlled Release Systems*, Vols. 1–2, CRC Press, Inc., Boca Raton, FL, 1984; (l) SaeHore, M.E., Bucci, M., and Speiser, P., Eds., *Ophthalmic Drug Delivery: Biopharmaceutical, Technological and Clinical Aspects*, Liviana Press, Springer-Verlag, Padova, Italy, 1987; (m) Roerdink, F.H. and Kroon, A.M., Eds., *Drug Carrier Systems*, John Wiley & Sons, New York, 1989; (n) Rodwell, J.D., Ed., *Antibody-Mediated Delivery Systems*, Marcel Dekker, New York, 1988; (o) Ansel, H.C. and Popovich, N.G., *Pharmaceutical Dosage Forms and Drug Delivery Systems*, Lea & Febiger, Philadelphia, 1990; (p) Gregoriadis, G., Senior, J., and Poste, G., *Targeting of Drugs with Synthetic Systems*, Plenum Press, New York, 1986; (q) Krowczynski, L., *Extended-Release Dosage Forms*, CRC Press, Inc., Boca Raton, FL, 1987 (r) Hsieh, D.S.T., *Controlled-Release Systems: Fabrication Technology*, Vols. 1 and 2, CRC Press, Inc., Boca Raton, FL, 1988; (s) Tirrell, D.A., Donaruma, L.G., and Turek A.B., Eds., Macromolecules as drugs and as carriers for biologically active materials, *N.Y. Acad. Sci.*, New York, 1985; (t) Thompson, K. and Burrill, G.S., Pharmacoeconomics and health care reform, *Bio. Pharm.*, January-February, 7, 50–52, 1994; (u) Wechsler, J., Healthcare takes center stage in Washington, *Pharm. Tech.*, 17(1), 16, 1993; (v) Knowles, M.R., Surviving health care system reforms, *Pharm. Executive*, 14(4), 38, 1994; (w) Wagner, J.R., Angst, health care reform and the German market, *Pharm. Executive*, 14(7), 38, 1994.
34. Varma, R.K. and Garg, S., Current status of drug delivery technologies and future directions, *Pharm. Technol. On-line*, 25 (2), 1–14, 2001.
35. Kannan, V., Kandarapu, R., and Garg, S., Optimization techniques for the design and development of novel drug delivery systems, Part 1, *Pharm. Tech.*, February 2003, 74–90.

Index

A

Abbreviated New Drug Application (ANDA), 4, 391, 392, 394, 395, 402, 403, 405, 409
Abortion inducer, 339
Abrin, 86
Absorption, gastrointestinal, 211
Acetylation, 85
Acne treatment, 224
Acrylic acid polymers, 82
Acrylic resins, 171
Actibase, 231
Actiderm, 232
Actifed, 179
Acutrim, 160, 182
ADD-Vantage System, 302
Adhesives, 79–83, 101, 154, 174–175
    intranasal applications, 263
    microcapsules, 343
    microspheres, 336
    ophthalmic applications, 276
    pressure-sensitive, 215, 216, 224
    transdermal system applications, 215–216, 224
Adjuvants, 13, 53, 212, 330
Adriamycin, 8, 22, 37, 50, 86, 298, 316
Aerosol systems, 254
Agar, 169, 278, 317
Alarms, 121, 122, 301
Albumin microspheres, 316, 334, 335
Albuterol, 15, 221, 237, 298
Alginates, 94, 95, 138, 174, 187, 237
Alginic acid, 95, 272
Alizarin, 335
Alkaloid-tannic acid complexes, 174
Allergy relief, 219
Alphafetoprotein, 50
Alphatocopherol nicotinate, 17, 20

Alprenoxine HCl, 427
Alzamer, 99
Alzheimer's disease, 46, 220
Amantadine, 101
Amine, volatile, 185
Amine drug complexes, 174
Aminocaproic acid esters, 233
Aminoglycosides, 262
Amitryptyline, 224
Amphetamine, 168, 174
Amphipathic drugs, 18
Amphotericin, 8, 428
Ampicillin, 188, 314
Analgesics, see Pain relief; specific drugs
Analogs, 290
Anaquest, 222
Ancef, 313
ANDA, 4, 391, 392, 394, 395, 403, 405, 409
Angiotensin II receptor, 49
Anthracenone derivatives, 224
Anthracyclines, 22, 46
Anthralin, 222
Anti-arrhythmia control, 305
Antibiotic drugs, see specific drugs
Antibodies, see Monoclonal antibodies
Antibody-directed enzyme prodrug therapy (ADEPT), 49, 361
Antibody imaging, 49
Anticancer drugs, see Cancer chemotherapy; specific drugs
Anticoagulants, heparin-releasing polymers, 89–90
Antiemetics, 428
Antiepileptic drugs, 125
Antigenic heterogeneity, 45
Antigen-presenting cells, 50
Antihistamines, 193, 220
Anti-inflammatory agents, 85
Antimicrobial sutures, 357–358

H

I